Intestinal inflammation: Implications for Therapeutic Interventions in IBD

Intestinal inflammation: Implications for Therapeutic Interventions in IBD

Editor: Daisy Ross

FOSTER ACADEMICS

www.fosteracademics.com

www.fosteracademics.com

FOSTER ACADEMICS

Cataloging-in-Publication Data

Intestinal inflammation : implications for therapeutic interventions in IBD / edited by Daisy Ross.
p. cm.
Includes bibliographical references and index.
ISBN 978-1-63242-959-9
1. Inflammatory bowel diseases. 2. Intestines--Abnormalities. 3. Intestines--Diseases.
4. Intestines--Diseases--Treatment. 5. Gastroenteritis. I. Ross, Daisy.
RC862.I53 I58 2020
616.344--dc23

Foster Academics,
118-35 Queens Blvd., Suite 400,
Forest Hills, NY 11375, USA

ISBN 978-1-63242-959-9 (Hardback)

Contents

Preface

Inflammatory bowel disease refers to diseases which involve the chronic inflammation of the digestive tract. There are primarily two types of inflammatory bowel diseases, namely, ulcerative colitis and Crohn's disease. Ulcerative colitis involves long-lasting inflammation in the innermost lining of the large intestine. Crohn's disease is characterized by the inflammation of the lining of the digestive tract. Some of the symptoms which accompany these diseases are severe diarrhea, weight loss, fatigue and abdominal pain. It is caused by immune malfunction. An abnormal immune response can lead to the immune system attacking the cells in the digestive tract. This book contains some path-breaking studies in the field of inflammatory bowel disease. It elucidates the concepts and innovative models around therapeutic interventions with respect to this disease. This book is appropriate for students seeking detailed information in this area as well as for experts.

Significant researches are present in this book. Intensive efforts have been employed by authors to make this book an outstanding discourse. This book contains the enlightening chapters which have been written on the basis of significant researches done by the experts.

Finally, I would also like to thank all the members involved in this book for being a team and meeting all the deadlines for the submission of their respective works. I would also like to thank my friends and family for being supportive in my efforts.

Editor

1

Initiation of an Inflammatory Response in Resident Intestinal Lamina Propria Cells-Use of a Human Organ Culture Model

Jutta Schröder-Braunstein[1]*, Judith Gras[1], Benedikt Brors[2], Sonja Schwarz[1], Timea Szikszai[1,5], Felix Lasitschka[3], Guido Wabnitz[1], Antje Heidtmann[1], Young-Seon Lee[1,8], Serin Schiessling[1,4], Christine Leowardi[4], Mohammed Al-Saeedi[4], Alexis Ulrich[4], Antonia Engelke[6], Johannes Winter[7], Yvonne Samstag[1], Thomas Giese[1], Stefan Meuer[1]

1 Institute of Immunology, University Hospital Heidelberg, Heidelberg, Germany, **2** Division of Theoretical Bioinformatics, German Cancer Research Center (DKFZ), Heidelberg, Germany, **3** Institute of Pathology, University Hospital Heidelberg, Heidelberg, Germany, **4** Department of Surgery, University Hospital Heidelberg, Heidelberg, Germany, **5** Department of Anesthesiology, University Hospital Heidelberg, Heidelberg, Germany, **6** Department of Surgery, Salem Hospital, Heidelberg, Germany, **7** Department of Surgery, St. Vincentius Hospital, Speyer, Germany, **8** Department of Gastroenterology, Hepatology, and Endocrinology, Hannover Medical School, Hannover, Germany

Abstract

Resident human lamina propria immune cells serve as powerful effectors in host defense. Molecular events associated with the initiation of an intestinal inflammatory response in these cells are largely unknown. Here, we aimed to characterize phenotypic and functional changes induced in these cells at the onset of intestinal inflammation using a human intestinal organ culture model. In this model, healthy human colonic mucosa was depleted of epithelial cells by EDTA treatment. Following loss of the epithelial layer, expression of the inflammatory mediators *IL1B, IL6, IL8, IL23A, TNFA, CXCL2*, and the surface receptors CD14, TLR2, CD86, CD54 was rapidly induced in resident lamina propria cells *in situ* as determined by qRT-PCR and immunohistology. Gene microarray analysis of lamina propria cells obtained by laser-capture microdissection provided an overview of global changes in gene expression occurring during the initiation of an intestinal inflammatory response in these cells. Bioinformatic analysis gave insight into signalling pathways mediating this inflammatory response. Furthermore, comparison with published microarray datasets of inflamed mucosa *in vivo* (ulcerative colitis) revealed a significant overlap of differentially regulated genes underlining the *in vivo* relevance of the organ culture model. Furthermore, genes never been previously associated with intestinal inflammation were identified using this model. The organ culture model characterized may be useful to study molecular mechanisms underlying the initiation of an intestinal inflammatory response in normal mucosa as well as potential alterations of this response in inflammatory bowel disease.

Editor: Jörn Karhausen, Duke University Medical Center, United States of America

Funding: This work was funded by the Deutsche Forschungsgemeinschaft (SFB 938, project O, M, and Z2) (www.dkfz.de). The funders had no role in study design, data collection and analysis, decision to publish, or preparation of the manuscript.

Competing Interests: The authors have declared that no competing interests exist.

* E-mail: jutta.schroeder-braunstein@urz.uni-heidelberg.de

Introduction

Investigations aimed at understanding molecular events underlying intestinal inflammation are largely focused on chronic processes, summarized as inflammatory bowel diseases (IBD). Moreover, such studies are mostly performed in symptomatic, i.e. ongoing pathological situations: in the murine system following treatment with artificial agents such as dextran sulfate (DSS) [1]; in humans, tissues derived from inflamed intestine in Crohn's disease, ulcerative colitis etc. Needless to say, experiments with human material are rather scarce when compared to investigations in experimental animal models. Given, therefore, that so far only symptomatic disease situations have been studied, it seems not surprising that all established therapies to treat IBD are of symptomatic nature [2,3].

As yet, virtually nothing is known concerning the conditions driving intestinal inflammation at its very onset. The central and obvious question, namely, how resident immune effector cells of the intestine differentiate from their physiologic quiescent stages into activated, inflammation producing cell types remains unanswered.

In this regard, previous data published by others and ourselves employing human mucosal tissues virtually exclude the possibility that intestinal T lymphocytes, one major effector population in inflammation, are, under physiological conditions, able to mount adaptive immune responses since their T cell receptor (TCR) reactivities are strongly inhibited by a number of local mechanisms [4–9]. Furthermore, innate recognition of commensal microbes is restricted by low or absent expression of pattern recognition receptors (PRR), like CD14, TLR4, and PRR-associated signalling molecules in lamina propria myeloid cells (LPMO) [10–13].

Here, we make an attempt to address the onset of intestinal inflammation in a standardized organ culture model employing healthy human colonic tissues. Once exposed to ethylenediaminetetraacetic acid (EDTA), which leads to the detachment of the luminal epithelial layer [14], resident lamina propria cells undergo a vigorous activation process. The present study describes their phenotypical and functional changes at a molecular level. We propose that this model has the potential to collect important information on those molecular mechanisms that drive the initiation of intestinal inflammation.

Materials and Methods

Tissue Samples

Gut specimens were derived from individuals undergoing resection for localized colon cancer or benign colonic diseases (e.g. diverticular disease). Microscopically normal colonic mucosa was dissected from the surgical specimen near the resection margin and immediately subjected to the experimental procedures.

For analysis of *DUSP2* gene expression in normal and inflamed intestinal tissue, transmural gut specimens (snap frozen in liquid nitrogen immediately after surgical resection) were provided by the Institute of Pathology, University Hospital Heidelberg. Inflamed gut specimens were derived from patients suffering from ulcerative colitis (UC) or Crohn's disease (CD). The diagnosis was confirmed by histopathological and clinical criteria prior to qRT-PCR analysis. Specifically, samples considered to be inflamed were characterized by dense mononuclear cell infiltrations, crypt abscesses/cryptitis, erosions or ulcerations. Normal control tissue was obtained from individuals suffering from localised colon cancer or benign colonic disease.

Antibodies

For immunoflourescent staining of tissue sections the following primary antibodies were employed: CD68, 1 µg/ml (clone: PGM-1, Dako Cytomation, Hamburg, Germany); CD14, 1 µg/ml (clone: TÜK4, Dako); CD86, 10 µg/ml (clone: FUN-1, BD Pharmingen, Heidelberg, Germany). Isotype- and concentration-matched control antibodies (Dako) served as negative controls.

For flow cytometric analysis the following mAb were purchased from BD Bioscience (Heidelberg, Germany): CD3 V450, CD14 FITC, CD33 PE-Cy7, CD86 AF700, HLA-DR V500, CD117 APC.

"Loss of Epithelial Layer" (LEL) Organ Culture

Mucosal specimens were washed extensively in RPMI 1640 (Life Technologies, Paisley, UK) containing antibiotics prior to removing the mucus layer by dithiothreitol (DTT) treatment (1 mM, 10 min; Sigma, St. Louis, MO, Germany). Subsequently, punches of defined surface area were prepared and denuded of epithelial cells by exposure to 0.7 mM EDTA (Sigma) in HBSS (without Ca^{2+} and Mg^{2+}; Life Technologies) at 37°C in a shaking water bath for 30 min (50 ml EDTA/HBSS per punch) [14]. This incubation was repeated three times with two washing steps (10 min in HBSS/antibiotics) after each incubation period.

Where indicated, total mucosa specimens of the same surface area were cultured under identical conditions.

Isolation of Lamina Propria and Peripheral Blood Leukocytes

Lamina propria leukocytes (LPL) were isolated by enzymatic tissue digestion according to a modified method of Bull and Bookman [14]. Briefly, after depletion of the epithelial layer (see above) mucosal tissue was cut into 2–4 mm pieces and digested in a shaking waterbath at 37°C for 1.5 h using collagenase IV (70 µg/ml; Sigma) and deoxyribonuclease I (100 µg/ml; Sigma) in RPMI 1640 containing 2% fetal calf serum (Sigma), 2% L-glutamine (Life Technologies), and antibiotics. The resulting cell suspension was separated from undigested tissue by filtration through a 70 µm nylon mesh (BD Bioscience, Heidelberg, Germany). For further purification, the cell suspension was subjected to Percoll (GE Healthcare, Munich, Germany) and Ficoll-Hypaque (GE Healthcare) density gradient centrifugation.

Peripheral blood was taken during the operation. Peripheral blood mononuclear cells (PBL) were obtained by Ficoll-Hypaque (GE Healthcare) density gradient centrifugation.

Gene Expression Analysis by qRT-PCR

Tissue samples were disrupted with the aid of a RiboLyser device (ThermoHYBAID, Heidelberg, Germany) in lysing matrix "D" tubes (Q-BIOgen, Heidelberg, Germany) containing 400 µl lysis buffer from the MagnaPure mRNA Isolation Kit II (ROCHE Diagnostics, Mannheim, Germany). 300 µl of the lysate was collected and mixed with 600 µl capture buffer containing oligo-dT. After centrifugation at 13000 rpm for 5 min, 880 µl of this mix was transferred into a MagnaPure sample cartridge and mRNA was isolated with the MagnaPure-LC device using the mRNA-II standard protocol. MRNA was reverse transcribed using AMV-RT and oligo- (dT) as primer (First Strand cDNA synthesis kit, Roche) according to the manufactures protocol. Primer sets optimized for the LightCycler (RAS, Mannheim, Germany) were developed and provided by SEARCH-LC GmbH (Heidelberg, Germany). The qRT-PCR was performed with the LightCycler FastStart DNA Syber Green I kit (RAS) according to the protocol provided in the parameter specific kits. To correct for differences in the content of mRNA, the calculated transcript numbers were normalized according to the expression of the housekeeping gene peptidylprolyl isomerase B (*PPIB*). Values were thus given as transcripts per 1000 transcripts of *PPIB*.

Double Immunofluorescence Staining of Tissue Sections

Staining was performed on 2 µm sections of formalin fixed, paraffin embedded human colon tissue. After deparaffinization in graded alcohols, heat induced antigen-retrieval was achieved by incubating the slides in a pressure cooker for 5 min in citrate buffer, pH 6.0. Double immunofluorescence staining was performed using a combination of CD68 (mouse mAb, IgG3) and either CD14 (mouse mAb, IgG2a) or CD86 (mouse mAb, IgG1κ). Incubations were performed overnight at 4°C in antibody diluent (DCS, Hamburg, Germany). Biotinylated rabbit anti-mouse IgG1, (2 µg/ml; Zymed, San Francisco, CA, USA), biotinylated rabbit anti-mouse IgG2a (4 µg/ml; Zymed) and sheep anti-mouse IgG3 (1:100, lot number AAM05; AbDserotec, Oxford, UK) served as secondary antibodies (30 min at room temperature). DyLight488-conjugated donkey anti-sheep antibody (green fluorescence; 8 µg/ml; Dianova), and Cy3-conjugated streptavidin (red fluorescence; 2 µg/ml; Dianova) were used as secondary reagents (30 min at room temperature). Slides were mounted and viewed with a TCS SL confocal microscope (Leica Microsystems, Wetzlar, Germany).

For quantification, $CD14^+$ and $CD86^+$ cells were counted in an area (lamina propria) defined by 100 $CD68^+$ cells. Three different areas were evaluated per experiment. In order to allow for consistent and comparable results within/between the different experimental conditions areas densely populated by $CD68^+$ subepithelial macrophages were excluded from the analysis.

Flow Cytometry

1×10^5 to 1×10^6 cells were incubated with a cocktail of up to six antibodies labelled with different fluorochromes. Peripheral blood monocytes (PBMO) were identified as $CD33^+$ $CD3^-$ cells. $CD33^+$ $CD3^-$ lamina propria myeloid cells (LPMO) [15] were further distinguished from mast cells by lack of or low CD117 expression. Flow cytometric analysis was performed using an LSR II (BD Biosciences) and FACSDiva v6 software (BD Bioscience). Doublets were identified by plotting FSC-A versus FSC-H and excluded from the analysis. As negative controls the (auto)fluorescence of the myeloid cell populations (stained with CD33PE-Cy7/CD3 V450, and CD117 APC (LPMO), respectively) was determined.

Laser-Capture Microdissection (LMD)

12 μm thick cryosections were prepared from flash frozen colonic tissue samples collected prior to culturing as well as after loss of the epithelial layer (LEL-M 5 h). After transfer to NF 1.0 PEN membrane coated slides (Carl Zeiss MicroImaging, Munich, Germany) sections were treated with DTT (1 mg/ml) for 5 min and stored in 100% EtOH at −20°C. Immediately before laser-capture microdissection, sections were stained with Cresyl Violet (0.1% in 100% EtOH; Sigma) and subsequently dehydrated by immersion in 100% EtOH and Xylene (Roth, Karlsruhe, Germany). LMD was performed for 1 h each using the PALM MicroBeam (Carl Zeiss MicroImaging). Microdissected tissue was collected using opaque AdhesiveCaps (Carl Zeiss MicroImaging).

Microarray Analysis

RNA was isolated with the RNeasy Micro Kit (Qiagen, Hilden, Germany) according to the manufacturer's instructions for microdissected samples, using glycogen (Sigma) as a carrier. RNA quantity and integrity was determined using the Agilent 2100 Bioanalyzer (Agilent Technologies, Waldbronn, Germany). All samples had a RNA integrity number (RIN) between 3.1 and 6.6. The mean RIN of RNA samples directly sampled by LMD ($t=0$ h) was 5.1±1.67 compared to 3.9±0.75 after 5 h ($t=5$ h) incubation. Samples were stored at −80°C until microarray analysis.

Microarray analysis was performed using the whole genome cDNA-mediated Annealing, Selection, extension and Ligation (WG-DASL) Assay (Illumina, San Diego, CA, USA) employing a minimum of 200 ng of total RNA per sample (≥40 ng/μl; input 5 μl). Four replicates were measured for each time point. The analysis was conducted at the Genomics and Proteomics Core facility of the German Cancer Research Center (DKFZ), Heidelberg, Germany. Complete microarray data have been submitted to the GEO repository and are available under the accession number GSE56448.

Analysis of Microarray Data

Microarray data were normalized by variance stabilizing normalization (vsn) [16]. Differential expression has been calculated by the test implemented in the limma package [17], and P values adjusted for multiple testing by the method of Benjamini and Hochberg [18]. Over-representation analysis of GeneOntology (GO) terms ('biological process' branch only) was calculated by GOstats [19] using the hypergeometric test conditional on the GO structure. Heatmaps were calculated on gene-wise z-transformed data by hierarchical clustering (complete linkage method, Euclidean distance) on rows. All calculations were performed in R v.3.0.0 [20] with the following extension packages: lumi v.2.12.0 [21], limma v.3.16.8 [17], GOstats v.2.26.0 [19], and GO.db v.2.9.0. For comparison with published data [22], we took the list of limma results for all probes from the microarray and selected those genes that had a corrected P value of less than 0.01 and absolute log2-fold change of at least one. This resulted in 439 up-regulated and 297 down-regulated genes, respectively. To calculate significance of overlap, 1000 random lists of length 439 were drawn from all microarray probes in [22] and overlap calculated with genes found to be differentially expressed in the LEL model. The distribution of sizes of intersection sets was used to calculate empirical P values (given as "<0.001" if the observed size was never exceeded by data from any random list).

TUNEL Assay

Apoptosis was analysed using the TACS 2 TdT-DAB *In Situ* Apoptosis Detection Kit (Trevigen, Gaithersburg, MD, USA). The assay was performed according to the manufacturer's instructions.

Ethics Statement

All human studies were approved by the ethics committee of the University of Heidelberg and performed in accordance with the principles laid down in the Declaration of Helsinki. Written informed consent was obtained from the patients.

Results

Induction of Inflammatory Gene Expression in Resident Lamina Propria Cells following EDTA-mediated Loss of the Epithelial Layer

Healthy colonic mucosa of defined size was prepared from freshly obtained human surgical specimens and depleted of epithelial cells by exposure to EDTA under standardized conditions. Mucosal tissue was harvested prior to culturing (total mucosa (TM) $t=0$ h), during or immediately after loss of the epithelial layer ("loss of the epithelial layer" mucosa (LEL-M) $t=3/4/5$ h); Fig. 1A). As a control, total mucosa (including the epithelial layer) was cultured for 5 h prior to harvesting (TM $t=5$ h).

We chose to employ qRT-PCR in order to evaluate the tissue expression of a selected number of "conventional" inflammatory genes. As shown in Fig. 1B, expression of the cytokine genes *IL6, IL8, IL1B, IL23A, TNFA, IFNG* as well as the chemokine gene *CCL2* was markedly upregulated in LEL-M ($t=3/4/5$ h) when compared to mucosa prior to culturing, which contained only low numbers of these transcripts. Transcript levels of all inflammatory mediators analysed were also higher in LEL-M at $t=5$ h when compared to total mucosa cultured for the same period of time (TM $t=5$ h). *IL12B* mRNA was not consistently detected in EDTA treated mucosa (data not shown). Note that treatment of peripheral blood (PBMC) and lamina propria (LPMC) mononuclear cells (isolated by enzymatic digestion), respectively, with EDTA using similar conditions as employed for epithelial cell detachment from mucosal tissue did not cause upregulation of *IL6, IL8, IL1B* and *IL23A* transcript numbers (*CCL2, IFNG, TNFA* not tested) (Fig. 1C).

Induction of Co-stimulatory Molecules and Pattern Recognition Receptors in Resident Lamina Propria Cells Following EDTA-mediated Loss of the Epithelial Layer

Pattern recognition receptors and co-stimulatory molecules are critically involved in innate and adaptive immune responses [23,24]. Under homeostatic conditions, their expression has been described to be detectable only at low levels in the intestinal lamina propria [10–12]. We therefore examined the effect of EDTA-mediated loss of the epithelial layer on the expression of the genes encoding the PRR *CD14, TLR2*, as well as the co-stimulatory molecules *CD86* and *CD54* in mucosa cells. As shown in Fig. 2A, transcript levels of these genes were upregulated in mucosal tissue within 3 h after starting to inflict LEL (5 h LEL-M versus 0 h TM) while being not or marginally altered in total

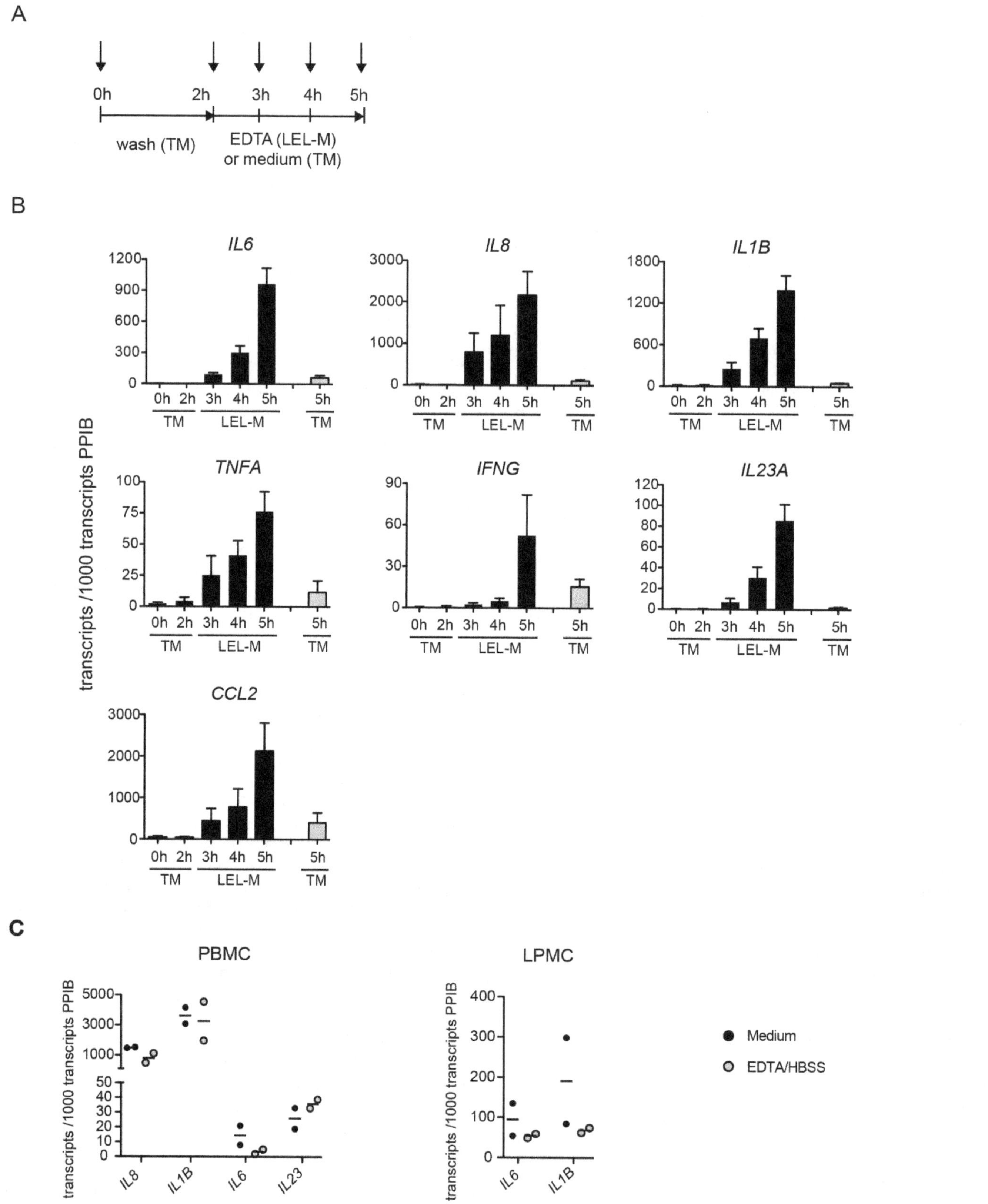

Figure 1. Induction of inflammatory gene expression in resident lamina propria cells following loss of the epithelial layer. (**A**) Time scheme of the LEL model. Arrows indicate time points of tissue collection. Tissue samples were collected prior to culturing (TM t = 0 h), after washing (TM t = 2 h), as well during and after completion of epithelial cell release by EDTA treatment (LEL-M t = 3/4/5 h). As a control, tissue samples were collected from TM cultured for 5 h (TM t = 5 h). (**B**) LEL induces gene expression of *IL1B, IL6, IL8, IL23A, TNFA, IFNG*, and *CCL2* in resident lamina propria cells. Transcript levels of cytokines/chemokines were determined by qRT-PCR in tissue samples collected as described in (A). Shown are the mean normalized transcript numbers ± SEM of at least 4 independent experiments. Gray bars represent transcript levels of TM (t = 0/2/5 h), black bars

represent transcript levels of LEL-M (t = 3/4/5h). (**C**) EDTA treatment does not induce inflammatory cytokines in PBMC or LPMC. PBMC and LPMC, respectively, were exposed to 0.7 mM EDTA/HBSS or medium (RPMI/2% FCS) for 3 h. Subsequently, transcript levels of *IL6, IL8, IL1B*, and *IL23A* were determined by qRT-PCR (*IL8* and *IL23A* not tested for LPMC). The results of two independent experiments are shown.

mucosa cultured for the same period of time (5 h TM versus 0 h TM).

In parallel, protein expression of CD14 and CD86, respectively, was determined in formalin-fixed tissue samples collected prior to culturing and immediately after epithelial cell depletion by immunohistological analysis. As shown in Fig. 2B, expression of both surface receptors was not detectable in lamina propria cells in the presence of an intact epithelial layer (TM t = 0 h) - in accordance with a previous study [25]. After 5 h of culture of total mucosa (TM t = 5 h) some CD14$^+$ and CD86$^+$ cells, respectively, which were negative for the macrophage marker CD68 (green fluorescence) appeared in the lamina propria. Note that at this time point signs of epithelial layer disintegration were already detectable by Hematoxylin-Eosin staining (see Figure S1). Importantly, following detachment of epithelial cells (LEL-M t = 5 h) higher numbers of CD14$^+$ as well as CD86$^+$ CD68$^-$ cells than in the medium control (TM t = 5 h) could be observed in the lamina propria (Fig. 2B and 2C). Notably, the expression pattern of CD86 and CD14 in mucosal cells as observed in the organ culture model resembles that in intestinal inflammation *in vivo* (ulcerative colitis) (see Figure S2).

In line with the *in situ* results, expression of CD14 and CD86 was detectable on lamina propria myeloid cells (LPMO; CD33$^+$ CD3$^-$ CD117$^-$) rapidly isolated after epithelial cell detachment (by enzymatic digestion of the lamina propria) as determined by flow cytometry. Expression levels on LPMO were comparable to those on autologous peripheral blood monocytes (PBMO; CD33$^+$ CD3$^-$) (see Figure S3A). Both myeloid cell populations expressed HLA-DR with significantly higher levels being detectable on LPMO than on PBMO. Note that neither EDTA nor enzymatic treatment (as employed for the isolation of LPL) of PBL resulted in an upregulation of CD14 and CD86 surface expression on PBMO (see Figure S3B, C).

Early Inflammatory Gene Expression Profile of Resident Lamina Propria Cells

Given that our investigation so far contained the bias of arbitrary selection of inflammatory "markers", we in addition decided to perform a global gene expression analysis. In order to focus on the features of immunocompetent cells in the intestine with regard to their phenotypic and functional changes over time, frozen tissue samples collected prior to culturing (TM t = 0 h) as well as immediately after EDTA treatment (LEL-M t = 5 h) were subjected to laser-capture microdissection (LMD) of the lamina propria (LP). Subsequently, mRNA was extracted for global gene expression analysis followed by bioinformatic evaluation. As shown in Fig. 3, microarray analysis of four individual experiments (replicates R1–R4 for each of the two experimental conditions (TM-LP t = 0 h and LEL-LP t = 5 h)) yielded reproducible results. Compared to microdissected lamina propria prior to culturing (t = 0 h), 1119 genes were differentially regulated in the lamina propria following EDTA treatment (t = 5 h) with 488 genes being significantly up-, and 631 genes significantly downregulated (cut-off: adjusted p value <0.01). Table 1 lists the top 40 upregulated genes, respectively, ranked by fold change (for a complete list of all differentially regulated genes see Table S1). Importantly, among these significantly upregulated genes were also some of those observed to be upregulated using qRT-PCR (see Fig. 1), namely *IL6, IL8, IL1B, IL23A* and *CCL2*. An increase in gene expression of *IFNG* as well as *TNFA* was also observed though not at a statistically significant level (data not shown). Given that a number of epithelial cell specific genes were included within the dataset of downregulated genes (likely due to some epithelial cell contamination of the microdissected lamina propria preparation), the subsequent functional analysis was at this point restricted to the dataset of significantly upregulated genes only.

In order to gain insight into biological processes occurring during the initiation of an inflammatory response in the organ culture model, an analysis of overrepresentation of gene ontology (GO) categories in our dataset of upregulated genes was performed (Table 2: top 30 significantly over-represented GO terms; for a complete list of all significantly over-represented GO terms see Table S2). Among the GO categories identified were many representing basic features of an inflammatory response, namely "regulation of response to stress" [26], "positive regulation of defense response" [27], "regulation of an inflammatory response", "blood vessel development" [28], "(chemo)taxis" [26] and "interleukin-1 production" [29]. Furthermore, according to this analysis, NF-κB activation, cAMP and cytokine induced responses as well as the unfolded protein response seem to be important signaling events determining initial activation processes in lamina propria cells. In addition, several GO terms identified cover aspects of the innate response to bacteria suggesting that such microorganisms (or molecules derived from the latter) may contribute to the induction of the inflammatory response in the organ culture model. Alternatively, non-bacterial stimuli eliciting expression of similar gene sets may participate in this response. Of note, significant induction of apoptotic processes in lamina propria cells following LEL as proposed by the GO term analysis could not be substantiated experimentally by TUNEL assay (see Figure S4).

Inflammatory Events in the LEL Model Partially Reflect those Occurring in Intestinal Inflammation *in vivo*

To address (1) the *in vivo* relevance of the organ culture model and (2) the central point whether early activation processes occurring in the *in vitro* system differ from events that exist in symptomatic human colonic diseases, our data collected from the *in vitro* systems were subjected to a comparative analysis with published data from microarray analyses from inflamed colonic tissue (ulcerative colitis (UC)). In the absence of any published gene expression profiling studies using microdissected lamina propria cells, UC data sets generated based on the examination of total biopsy tissue were employed for this comparative analysis [22].

As illustrated in the Venn diagram (Fig. 4A), 57 of 488 significantly upregulated and 134 of 631 downregulated genes in our *in vitro* model were also found to be upregulated and downregulated, respectively, in active UC samples when compared to normal (non-inflamed) gut samples [22]. This corresponds to a significant enrichment of genes differentially expressed in UC (as identified by Granlund *et al.* [22]) in our dataset ($p < 0.001$ for up- and downregulated genes, respectively, as determined by a permutation test with 1000 lists of random genes). Among the shared upregulated genes (see Table S3) were also biomarkers for clinical and/or endoscopic disease activity in UC, such as *IL8, CXCL2, LCN2*, and *MMP9* [30–32]. In addition to *IL8* (see Fig. 1), increased *CXCL2* gene expression in LEL-M (t = 5 h) vs. TM (t = 0 h and t = 5 h) was confirmed by qRT-PCR (Fig. 4B; other markers not tested). As expected, *S100A8* and *S100A9* genes,

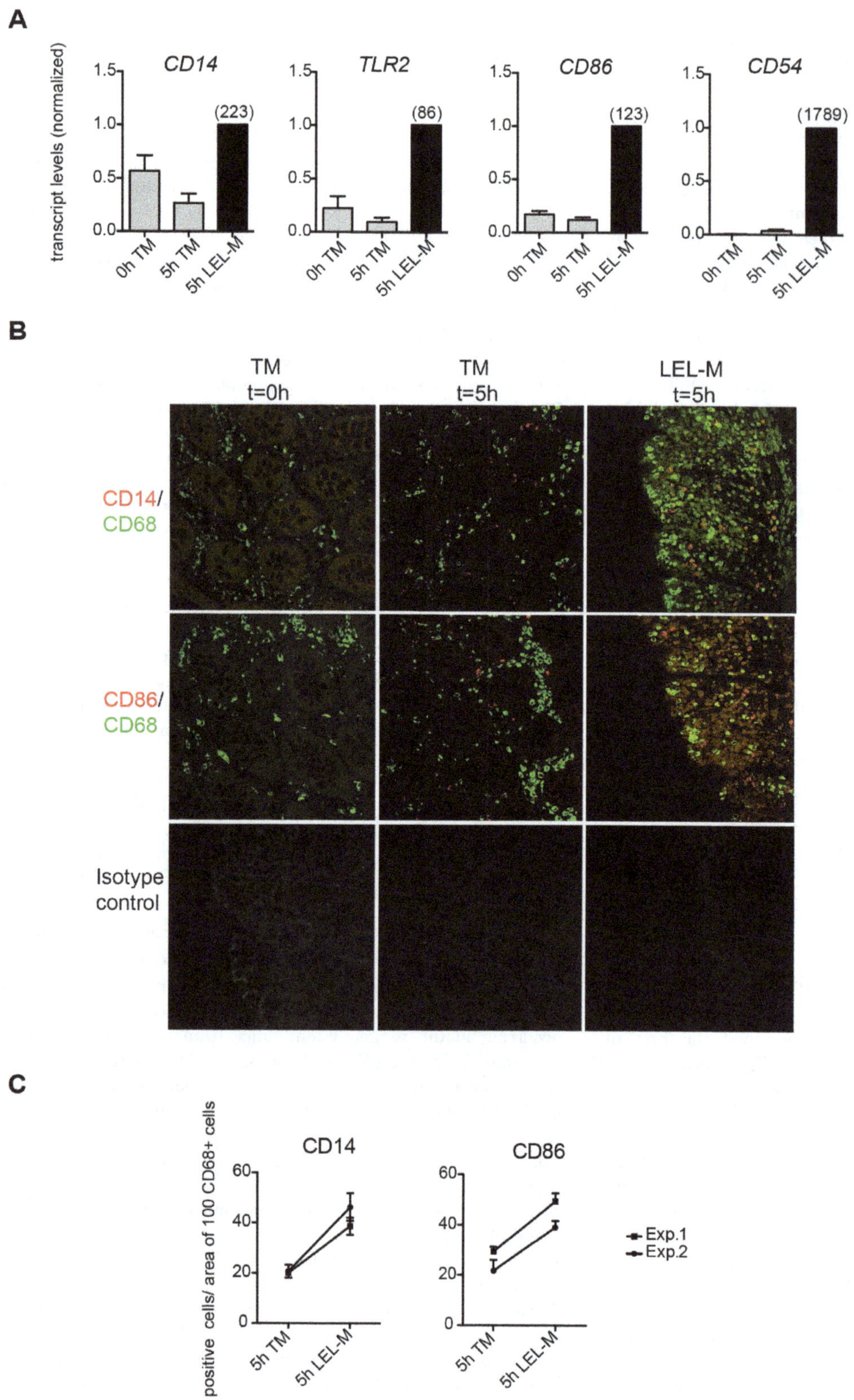

Figure 2. Expression of surface receptors in resident lamina propria cells following loss of the epithelial layer. (**A**) LEL induces gene expression of *CD14*, *CD86*, *TLR2*, and *CD54* in resident lamina propria cells *in situ*. Tissue samples of total mucosa (TM) were collected prior to culturing (0 h TM) and simultaneously from both TM and LEL mucosa after completion of epithelial cell release by EDTA treatment (5 h TM, 5 h LEL-M) (see Fig. 1a). Subsequently, transcript levels of *CD14*, *TLR2*, *CD54*, and *CD86* were determined by qRT-PCR. Transcript numbers (normalized to 1000 transcripts *PPIB*) of "5 h LEL-M" were set to 1, and those of all other conditions were calculated as a fraction/multiple of 1. Shown are the mean normalized transcript numbers ± SEM of three or four independent experiments. Numbers in brackets indicate the absolute transcript numbers normalized to 1000 transcripts *PPIB*. Gray bars represent transcript levels of TM (0 h, 5 h), black bars represent transcript levels of LEL-M (5 h). (**B**) LEL induces

protein expression of CD14 and CD86 in resident lamina propria cells *in situ*. Double immunofluorescence staining of CD68 (green) and CD14 or CD86 (red) in healthy total mucosa prior to culturing (TM t = 0 h) and after 5 h of culture (TM t = 5 h) as well as in mucosa immediately after LEL (LEL-M t = 5 h). Colocalization of both antigens is shown by yellow signals in the overlay. Magnification: x40. LEL enhances the expression of CD14 and CD86 on some $CD68^{+}$ and a large pool of $CD68^{-}$ cells. The results represent one of three independent experiments. **(C)** Quantification of $CD14^{+}$ and $CD86^{+}$ cells in TM 5 h and LEL-M 5 h, respectively. The mean numbers (± SEM) of $CD14^{+}$ and $CD86^{+}$ cells, respectively, per area of 100 $CD68^{+}$ cells were determined with three areas/experimental condition being evaluated. Shown are the results of two independent experiments.

IBD biomarkers preferentially expressed in peripheral blood myeloid cells (granulocytes, monocytes) [33] migrating into the tissue in response to inflammatory stimuli, were not observed to be upregulated in the LEL model. Notably, a comparison of our dataset with publicly available results (Top 200 differentially regulated genes) of a meta-analysis of IBD gene expression profiles [34] gave similar results (data not shown). These observations clearly demonstrate that key inflammatory events as observed in intestinal inflammation *in vivo* are at least partially reproduced by the organ culture model *in vitro*.

Not surprisingly, the majority of differentially regulated genes in the organ culture model differ from those differentially regulated in active UC (Fig. 4A) [22]. Their potential clinical relevance – in particular with respect to the initial phase of an intestinal inflammatory response- needs to be further evaluated. In this regard it is interesting to note that several of the genes detected to be solely upregulated in our organ culture model have been prioritized as key genes linked to gene loci identified to be associated with UC (or inflammatory bowel disease (IBD) in general) in genome wide association studies [35] (GWAS; see Table S4).

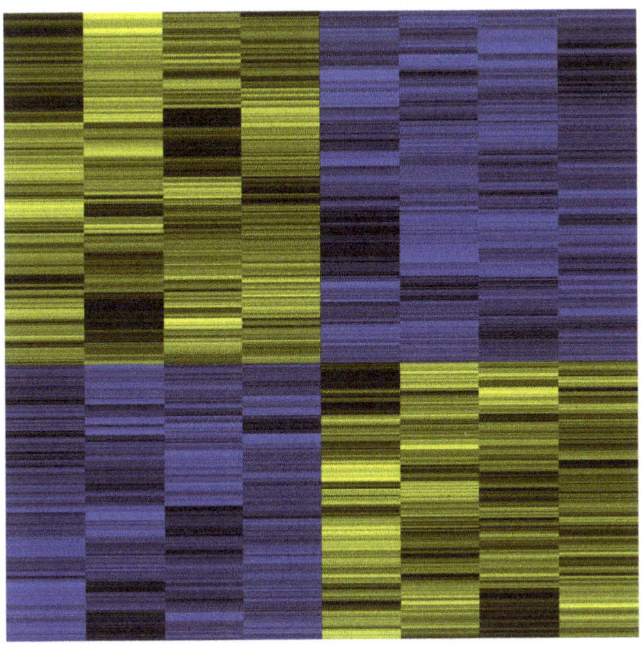

Figure 3. Early inflammatory gene expression profile of resident lamina propria cells. Frozen tissue samples collected prior to culturing (TM 0 h) and immediately after release of the epithelial layer (LEL-M 5 h) were subjected to laser-capture microdissection of the lamina propria. Following RNA extraction, global gene expression profiles of lamina propria cells were obtained by microarray analysis. Shown is a heatmap of significantly regulated genes in LEL-LP 5 h vs. TM-LP 0 h (four matched replicates (R1–R4) for each time point replicates representing four independent experiments). Colors show expression relative to the average (black), higher (yellow), or lower (blue) relative expression, respectively. Data have been transformed to gene-wise zero mean and unit variance (z transform). Rows have been re-ordered by hierarchical clustering (complete linkage, Euclidean distance metrics).

Furthermore, for one of the genes observed to be significantly upregulated in the LEL model, dual specific phosphatase 2 (*DUSP2*), we tried to confirm its differential expression in intestinal inflammation *in vivo*. DUSP2, a regulator of MAP kinases, is induced in human leucocytes following stimulation. It may potentially represent an important signaling module involved in the initiation of intestinal inflammation as it has been demonstrated to promote inflammatory responses in rheumatoid arthritis in mice [36,37]. As shown in Fig. 4C, induction of *DUSP2* expression in the LEL model as observed by global gene expression profiling was confirmed by qRT-PCR (left panel). Importantly, in agreement with this result in the LEL model *in vitro*, significantly higher expression levels of this gene were observed in inflamed tissue of UC vs. normal control tissue (NC) *in vivo* ($p<0.05$). Increased *DUSP2* transcript numbers were also detected in inflamed CD tissue, however at a lower level. Note that the low induction of transcript levels of *DUSP2* in UC and CD vs. NC tissue when compared to the LEL model may be due to the fact that different types of tissue were used for these analyses (UC/CD/NC: transmural tissue; LEL model: mucosa).

Discussion

Inflammation represents a fundamental defense response of the body to infection and tissue damage, which aims at the restoration of homeostasis [26]. In the human intestinal mucosa, molecular processes determining the onset of an inflammatory response in resident lamina propria cells are as yet largely unknown. However, knowledge of these processes would not only help to understand basic principles of the initiation of an intestinal immune response but also potentially promote the identification of novel drug targets for remission maintaining therapy and/or the discovery of biomarkers predicting relapse in IBD [38]. Importantly, it could also provide the basis for unraveling etiologically relevant alterations of early inflammation in IBD.

Here, we characterized the initiation of an inflammatory response in resident lamina propria cells in a human intestinal organ culture model. In this model, an inflammatory response was initiated in lamina propria cells following EDTA mediated loss of the epithelial layer. Damage of the epithelial layer due to disruption of tight junctions, epithelial cell death, erosions, and ulcers represents an early pathogenic event in intestinal inflammation *in vivo*, e.g. in acute enteric infections caused by invasive or toxin- producing pathogens [39–42]. It is associated with inflammatory cellular infiltrates of the mucosal tissue, which are largely missing in infections caused by non-invasive pathogens that do not induce significant epithelial cell damage [43,44]. Furthermore, aphthoid lesions represent one of the earliest pathological mucosal manifestations in Crohn's disease [45].

The inflammatory response elicited in resident lamina propria cells following loss of the epithelial layer (LEL) was characterized

Table 1. Top 40 upregulated genes in the LEL model.

Gene symbol	logFC[1]	adj. P.Val[2]
IL6	5,1	7,50E-05
CSF3	5,0	1,84E-05
C2CD4B	4,7	5,43E-05
SERPINA3	4,5	9,16E-05
RND1	4,4	4,81E-06
FAM71A	4,3	1,53E-04
CSF3	4,2	1,39E-03
EGR3	4,2	2,41E-06
IL8	4,1	2,69E-04
C2CD4B	4,1	1,02E-04
CXCL2	4,0	6,15E-06
ICAM4	4,0	1,99E-05
MAFF	4,0	1,95E-04
MAFA	4,0	2,89E-04
ADAMTS4	3,9	4,76E-04
ATF3	3,9	3,03E-04
ICAM4	3,8	2,39E-05
FOSL1	3,8	4,85E-06
ABL2	3,8	2,14E-04
ARC	3,7	6,61E-04
GEM	3,7	3,79E-04
TNFSF9	3,7	1,64E-05
AMPD3	3,7	2,16E-03
GFPT2	3,7	5,27E-06
NR4A1	3,7	6,55E-03
MOB4	3,7	2,09E-03
CCL21	3,6	1,39E-03
UBC	3,6	1,64E-03
C2CD4B	3,6	4,81E-06
EGR3	3,6	2,39E-04
SOCS3	3,6	8,86E-07
HAS1	3,6	2,37E-03
NA	3,5	4,99E-04
RGS16	3,4	6,37E-05
NR4A1	3,4	7,89E-05
DES	3,4	4,77E-04
CALCA	3,3	3,75E-03
ATF3	3,3	4,84E-04
RRAD	3,3	2,87E-06
NFKBIZ	3,3	2,59E-03

[1]log base 2 of fold change.
[2]P value from moderated t test, adjusted by the Benjamini & Hochberg method [18].

by a rapid upregulation of canonical inflammatory mediators, e.g. *IL1B*, *IL8*, as well as co-stimulatory and pattern recognition receptors. With regard to the latter our results provide at least partial mechanistic insight into the previous observation that lamina propria myeloid cells migrated out of the intestinal mucosa during a 12 h culture period following epithelial cells depletion express these receptors [46]. Information on the global transcriptional response induced in the LEL model was obtained by microarray analysis of laser-capture microdissected lamina propria.

Insight into molecular processes including signaling pathways involved in the initiation of an intestinal inflammatory response in resident lamina propria cells was provided by bioinformatic GO term analysis of the set of differentially regulated genes in this

Table 2. Over-representation of GO terms in dataset of upregulated genes in the LEL model.

GO Term	P value[1]	Count[2]	Size[3]
positive regulation of cell death	1,08E-09	38	442
positive regulation of NF-kappaB transcription factor activity	5,08E-09	17	104
cellular response to biotic stimulus	1,06E-08	17	109
positive regulation of phosphate metabolic process	4,66E-08	45	662
response to bacterium	1,09E-07	29	337
response to nitrogen compound	2,11E-07	42	628
blood vessel development	4,37E-07	34	469
positive regulation of apoptotic process	4,92E-07	29	367
cellular response to hypoxia	8,40E-07	13	86
regulation of sequence-specific DNA binding transcription factor activity	1,10E-06	21	224
response to decreased oxygen levels	1,88E-06	21	226
response to cytokine stimulus	1,96E-06	34	497
cellular response to oxygen levels	2,09E-06	13	93
Hemopoiesis	3,61E-06	34	511
response to unfolded protein	4,21E-06	9	46
Aging	5,81E-06	18	186
regulation of transferase activity	5,99E-06	32	486
Ossification	6,77E-06	23	285
immune system development	7,93E-06	35	557
regulation of phosphorylation	1,14E-05	38	655
negative regulation of multicellular organismal process	1,15E-05	26	358
regulation of response to stress	1,19E-05	30	457
positive regulation of kinase activity	1,69E-05	29	433
negative regulation of apoptotic process	1,72E-05	36	598
Taxis	1,85E-05	36	600
cellular response to lipopolysaccharide	2,60E-05	9	57
interleukin-1 production	3,35E-05	8	45
regulation of inflammatory response	3,36E-05	17	192
toll-like receptor 3 signaling pathway	3,79E-05	10	73
negative regulation of phosphorylation	3,94E-05	18	214

[1]P value of hypergeometric test for over-representation (conditional on GO structure).
[2]Count: number of GO term associated genes in the dataset of upregulated genes.
[3]Size: total number of GO term associated genes.

model. While -according to this analysis- bacterial stimuli (likely present in the mucosal culture despite extensive washing steps) may contribute to the induction of this inflammatory response they are most likely not sufficient for triggering the latter given the low/lack of homeostatic expression of pattern recognition receptors and associated signaling molecules in lamina propria cells [10–13]. Furthermore, inflammatory gene expression was higher in LEL mucosa when compared to total mucosa, which was exposed to at least the same amount of potentially contaminating bacterial stimuli being present during culture for the same period of time (see Fig. 1B). Further studies using the LEL model may provide insight into upstream stimuli, e.g. danger molecules like ATP, mediating the initiation of an inflammatory response in lamina propria cells. In particular, it will be tested whether loss of epithelial cell derived factors, e.g. IL-10, TGF-β, which have been shown to contribute to the control of intestinal inflammation [47–49], is sufficient for activation of the latter cell population.

Many of the signaling events (e.g. NF-κB activation, response to cytokines) identified to contribute to early intestinal inflammatory responses in the LEL model are also known to be involved in later, chronic stages of intestinal inflammation suggesting that their activity could potentially be maintained for a prolonged period of time. This observation is in agreement with findings of a recent study showing that changes in (inflammatory) gene expression in peripheral blood leucocytes following severe injury in humans occur within hours and are maintained for up to one to three months until recovery of the patients [50]. Importantly, gene sets associated with the unfolded protein response (UPR) were found to be overrepresented in the dataset of upregulated genes in the LEL model. This is the first indication that the UPR is not only induced in epithelial cells during human chronic intestinal inflammation - as previously described [51,52] - but also in LP cells at the onset of an intestinal inflammatory response. Hence, genetic susceptibility for IBD linked to hypomorphic variants of the UPR-associated gene *XBP1* [51] may be associated with dysregulation of the UPR

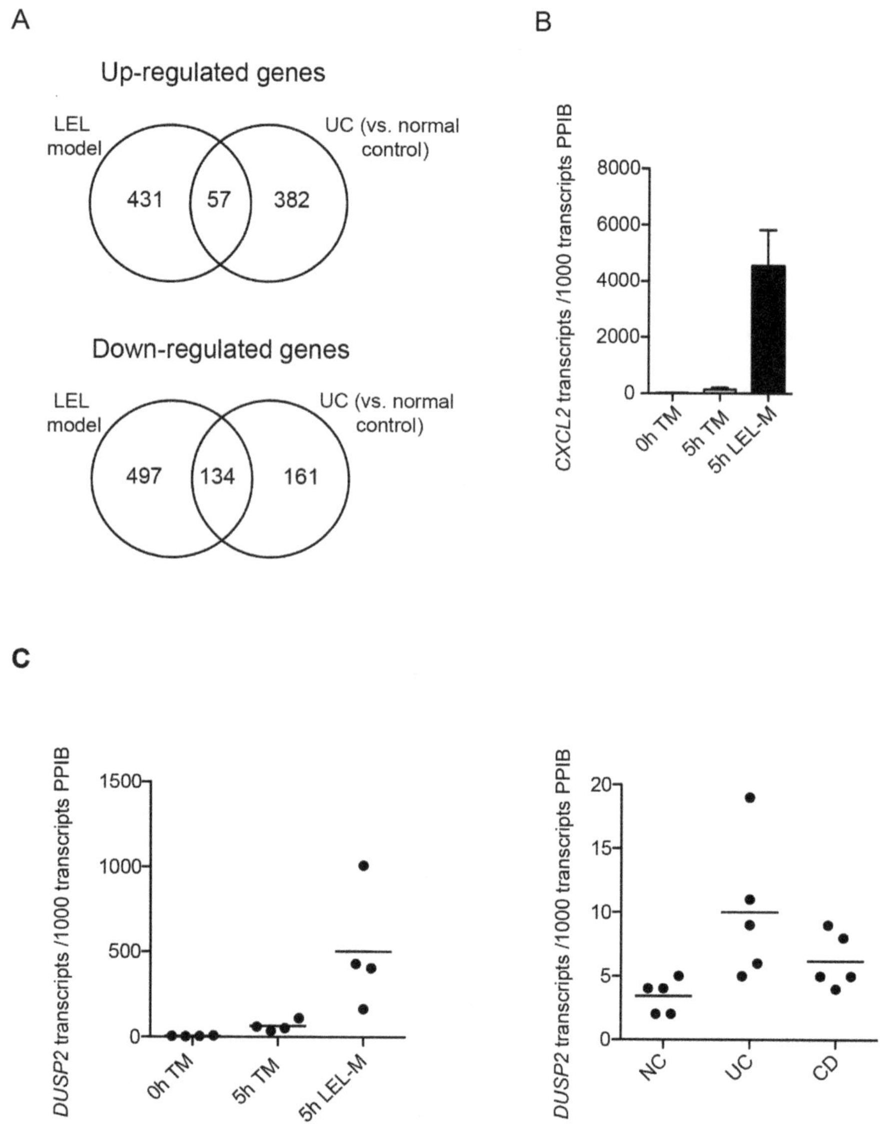

Figure 4. Inflammatory events in the LEL model partially reflect those occurring in intestinal inflammation *in vivo.* (**A**) The overlap of differentially expressed genes in the LEL model *in vitro* and in inflamed tissue obtained from ulcerative colitis patients (vs. normal control tissue) as published in Granlund *et al.* [22] is depicted by a Venn diagram. (**B**) Upregulation of the IBD biomarker gene *CXCL2* in the LEL model. Tissue samples of total mucosa (TM) were collected prior to culturing (0 h TM). Furthermore, tissue samples were collected simultaneously from both TM and LEL mucosa after completion of epithelial cell release by EDTA treatment (5 h TM, 5 h LEL-M) (see Fig. 1a). Subsequently, transcript levels of *CXCL2* were determined by qRT-PCR. Shown are the mean normalized transcript numbers ± SEM of three to four independent experiments. Gray bars represent transcript levels of TM (0 h, 5 h), the black bar represents transcript levels of LEL-M (5 h). (**C**) Identification of *DUSP2* as a novel gene upregulated in intestinal inflammation. *Left panel:* Tissue samples of total mucosa (TM) were collected prior to culturing (0 h TM). Furthermore, tissue samples were collected simultaneously from both TM and LEL mucosa after completion of epithelial cell release by EDTA treatment (5 h TM, 5 h LEL-M) (see Fig.1a). Subsequently, transcript levels of *DUSP2* were determined by qRT-PCR. Shown are normalised transcript numbers (including mean) as determined in four independent experiments. *Right panel:* Transcript levels of *DUSP2* were determined in transmural tissue samples of normal (NC) as well as of inflamed (UC, CD) gut by qRT-PCR. Shown are normalized transcript numbers (including mean) as determined in five different tissue samples of NC, UC, and CD, respectively.

not only in epithelial but also lamina propria cells. Importantly, we have collected evidence that the transcription factor C/EBPβ, a target of the UPR [53], is rapidly upregulated in lamina propria myeloid cells in intestinal inflammation (manuscript in preparation).

The relevance of the LEL model with regard to key inflammatory events occurring in inflammation *in vivo* is underlined by the observation that the set of differentially expressed genes in this model partially overlaps with that in inflamed tissue from UC patients (vs. normal colonic mucosa) as determined by Granlund *et al.* [22]. Importantly, among the genes upregulated in the organ culture model were also biomarkers for clinical or endoscopic disease activity in ulcerative colitis [30–32].

Clearly, the majority of genes observed to be differentially expressed in in the organ culture model differed from those differentially expressed in active ulcerative colitis and *vice versa.* This is not unexpected given that (1) the LEL model reflects the initial phase of inflammation whereas UC samples subject to gene expression profiling were taken during symptomatic stages of the disease (2) immigration of blood monocytes and granulocytes into inflamed tissue as taking place *in vivo* [26,54] cannot occur in the LEL model; (3) UC tissue samples are often obtained from patients receiving anti-inflammatory drug treatment, which may modulate inflammatory gene expression; (4) gene expression profiling of the LEL model was performed employing microdissected lamina propria in order to focus the analysis on immunocompetent cells located in this compartment, while microarray analysis of human intestinal tissue collected from UC patients was conducted with total mucosa; (5) IBD-linked genetic polymorphisms may be associated with a dysregulated inflammatory response in UC patients.

The clinical relevance of the genes differentially regulated solely in the LEL model is supported by the fact that several of these genes have been linked to UC/IBD susceptibility loci as identified by GWAS [35] (see Table S4). While differential expression of most of these genes - though not detected by global gene expression profiling- has been demonstrated in IBD in previous studies, differential expression of one of these IBD loci associated genes, *FOSL1*, in human intestinal inflammatory responses is reported here for the first time. FOSL1 belongs to the AP1 family of transcription factors [55]; its overexpression in mice has been demonstrated to ameliorate DSS-induced colitis [56]. Application of the LEL model to non-inflamed mucosa in UC vs. non-IBD may allow to determine a potentially altered regulation of *FOSL1* expression and other IBD loci associated genes in these patients thereby promoting the establishment of genotype-phenotype correlations.

Notably, *DUSP2*, a gene upregulated in the LEL model but not in IBD gene expression profiling datasets of Granlund *et al.* and the meta-analysis by Clark *et al.* (as far as data are available), was confirmed to be upregulated in intestinal inflammation *in vivo*. This result further supports the *in vivo* relevance of novel inflammation related genes as detected in the LEL model. Given its pro-inflammatory role in a murine model of rheumatoid arthritis, DUSP2 may positively regulate inflammatory responses also in intestinal immune cells [37].

Another implication of our findings relates to the interpretation of results gained in experiments using enzymatically isolated "resting" lamina propria leucocytes. Most protocols employed for the isolation of these cells include EDTA treatment of mucosal specimens for release of epithelial cells [14,57–59] as it has been applied in this study. According to our results cells subjected to this treatment during the isolation procedure may not exist in a resting state as observed under homeostatic conditions *in vivo* but rather exhibit features of activated cells.

In summary, molecular events associated with the initiation of an inflammatory response in human lamina propria cells are characterized for the first time using an intestinal organ culture model. The organ culture model may represent a valuable tool to elucidate molecular mechanisms underlying this initial activation of lamina propria cells in man. Furthermore, when applied to non-inflamed mucosa of IBD patients, it may help to determine potential alterations of the early mucosal inflammatory response in these patients and thereby support the discovery of disease-specific drug targets. Finally, it may be useful for identifying general (non-specific) drug targets for remission-maintaining therapy for these diseases.

Supporting Information

Figure S1 Hematoxylin-Eosin staining of total mucosa (TM) and mucosa depleted of epithelial cells (LEL-M). Signs of epithelial layer disintegration are detectable in TM cultured for 5 h (TM 5 h) in comparison to TM prior to culturing (TM 0 h).

Figure S2 Double immunofluorescence staining of CD68 (green) and CD14 or CD86 (red) in inflamed tissue in ulcerative colitis. Co-localization of both antigens is shown by yellow signals in the overlay. Magnification: ×40.

Figure S3 CD14 and CD86 are expressed on lamina propria myeloid cells (LPMO) rapidly isolated after LEL. (A) LPMO were rapidly isolated by enzymatic tissue digestion after detachment of the epithelial cell layer (LEL). Subsequently, surface expression of CD14 and CD86 was analyzed on PBMO (upper panel) and LPMO (lower panel) by flow cytometry. *Dot blots:* A gate was set on $CD33^+$ $CD3^-$ $CD117^-$ myeloid cells (blue). *Histograms:* Shown are the expression levels of HLA-DR, CD14 and CD86 on $CD33^+CD3^-CD117^-$ PBMO and LPMO, respectively. Results are representative of two independent experiments. **(B)** Treatment with EDTA does not affect CD14 and CD86 surface expression on PBMO. PBL were cultured in RPMI/10% FCS/antibiotics, HBSS/antibiotics, or HBSS/EDTA 0.7 mM/antibiotics for 1.5 h. Surface expression of CD14 and CD86 on $CD33^+CD3^-$ PBMO was determined by flow cytometry. Shown is the mean fluorescence intensity (MFI) of one of two independent experiments showing similar results. **(C)** Treatment with Collagenase/DNAse does not affect CD14 and CD86 surface expression on PBMO. PBMC were cultured in RPMI/2% FCS/antibiotics in the absence or presence of collagenase IV (45 U/ml)/DNAse I (27 U/ml) for 1.5 h. Surface expression of CD14 and CD86 on $CD33^+$ $CD3^-$ PBMO was determined by flow cytometry. Shown are % MFI of the untreated controls (100%) of two independent experiments.

Figure S4 Apoptosis is not significantly induced in lamina propria cells following LEL. The occurrence of apoptosis during the LEL organ culture was determined using an *in situ* terminal deoxynucleotidyl transferase dUTP nick end labeling (TUNEL) assay. Images show colonic cryosections at t = 0 h (TM) and t = 5 h (LEL-M). Apoptotic cells containing fragmented DNA (thereby indicating apoptosis) are stained brown with 3,3'-diaminobenzidine. Sections are counterstained with Methyl Green. The positive control was achieved with TACS-Nuclease^{TM}. Results are representative of two independent experiments.

Table S1 Complete list of all differentially regulated genes.

Table S2 Complete list of all significantly over-represented GO terms.

Table S3 List of overlapping genes upregulated in the LEL model (LEL-M 5 h vs. TM 0 h) and in UC vs. normal control according to Granlund *et al.* [22].

Table S4 Key genes of IBD associated gene loci as described by Jostins *et al.* [35] **included in the set of upregulated genes in the LEL model but not in UC vs. normal control according to Granlund *et al.*** [22].

Acknowledgments

We are grateful to Dieter Stefan, Jutta Scheuerer, Simone Fomuki, Daniela Merklinger, and Sabine Wentrup for excellent technical assistance. Furthermore, we thank Frank Autschbach for providing tissue specimens of patients suffering from ulcerative colitis/Crohn's disease as well as Bettina Jocher for logistic support regarding the acquisition of blood and colon specimens. This work was performed with support from the Genomics and Proteomics Core Facility of the DKFZ.

Author Contributions

Conceived and designed the experiments: JSB JG S. Schwarz SM TG. Performed the experiments: JG AH TS S. Schiessling YSL S. Schwarz FL. Analyzed the data: JSB JG BB FL TG GW TS. Contributed reagents/materials/analysis tools: CL MAS AU AE JW. Wrote the paper: JSB JG SM. Review: GW YS SM BB FL TG.

References

1. Okayasu I, Hatakeyama S, Yamada M, Ohkusa T, Inagaki Y, et al. (1990) A novel method in the induction of reliable experimental acute and chronic ulcerative colitis in mice. Gastroenterology 98: 694–702.
2. Danese S (2012) New therapies for inflammatory bowel disease: from the bench to the bedside. Gut 61: 918–932.
3. Ordas I, Eckmann L, Talamini M, Baumgart DC, Sandborn WJ (2012) Ulcerative colitis. Lancet 380: 1606–1619.
4. Pirzer UC, Schurmann G, Post S, Betzler M, Meuer SC (1990) Differential responsiveness to CD3-Ti vs. CD2-dependent activation of human intestinal T lymphocytes. Eur J Immunol 20: 2339–2342.
5. Qiao L, Schurmann G, Autschbach F, Wallich R, Meuer SC (1993) Human intestinal mucosa alters T-cell reactivities. Gastroenterology 105: 814–819.
6. Qiao L, Schurmann G, Betzler M, Meuer SC (1991) Activation and signaling status of human lamina propria T lymphocytes. Gastroenterology 101: 1529–1536.
7. De Maria R, Fais S, Silvestri M, Frati L, Pallone F, et al. (1993) Continuous in vivo activation and transient hyporesponsiveness to TcR/CD3 triggering of human gut lamina propria lymphocytes. Eur J Immunol 23: 3104–3108.
8. Sido B, Braunstein J, Breitkreutz R, Herfarth C, Meuer SC (2000) Thiol-mediated redox regulation of intestinal lamina propria T lymphocytes. J Exp Med 192: 907–912.
9. Sido B, Lasitschka F, Giese T, Gassler N, Funke B, et al. (2008) A prominent role for mucosal cystine/cysteine metabolism in intestinal immunoregulation. Gastroenterology 134: 179–191.
10. Qiao L, Braunstein J, Golling M, Schurmann G, Autschbach F, et al. (1996) Differential regulation of human T cell responsiveness by mucosal versus blood monocytes. Eur J Immunol 26: 922–927.
11. Hausmann M, Kiessling S, Mestermann S, Webb G, Spottl T, et al. (2002) Toll-like receptors 2 and 4 are up-regulated during intestinal inflammation. Gastroenterology 122: 1987–2000.
12. Smythies LE, Sellers M, Clements RH, Mosteller-Barnum M, Meng G, et al. (2005) Human intestinal macrophages display profound inflammatory anergy despite avid phagocytic and bacteriocidal activity. J Clin Invest 115: 66–75.
13. Smythies LE, Shen R, Bimczok D, Novak L, Clements RH, et al. (2010) Inflammation anergy in human intestinal macrophages is due to Smad-induced IkappaBalpha expression and NF-kappaB inactivation. J Biol Chem 285: 19593–19604.
14. Bull DM, Bookman MA (1977) Isolation and functional characterization of human intestinal mucosal lymphoid cells. J Clin Invest 59: 966–974.
15. Rogler G, Hausmann M, Vogl D, Aschenbrenner E, Andus T, et al. (1998) Isolation and phenotypic characterization of colonic macrophages. Clin Exp Immunol 112: 205–215.
16. Huber W, von Heydebreck A, Sultmann H, Poustka A, Vingron M (2002) Variance stabilization applied to microarray data calibration and to the quantification of differential expression. Bioinformatics 18 Suppl 1: S96–104.
17. Smyth GK (2005) Limma: linear models for microarray data. In: Gentlemen R, Carey V, S D, R I, W H, editors. Bioinformatics and Computational Biology Solutions unsing R and Bioconductor. New York: Springer. 397–420.
18. Benjamini Y, Hochberg Y (1995) Controlling the false discovery rate: a practical and powerful approach to multiple testing. J R Statist Soc B 57: 289–300.
19. Falcon S, Gentleman R (2007) Using GOstats to test gene lists for GO term association. Bioinformatics 23: 257–258.
20. Team RC (2013) R: A language and environment for statistical computing. Vienna, Austria: R foundation for Statistical computing.
21. Du P, Kibbe WA, Lin SM (2008) lumi: a pipeline for processing Illumina microarray. Bioinformatics 24: 1547–1548.
22. Granlund A, Flatberg A, Ostvik AE, Drozdov I, Gustafsson BI, et al. (2013) Whole genome gene expression meta-analysis of inflammatory bowel disease colon mucosa demonstrates lack of major differences between Crohn's disease and ulcerative colitis. PLoS One 8: e56818.
23. Chen L, Flies DB (2013) Molecular mechanisms of T cell co-stimulation and co-inhibition. Nat Rev Immunol 13: 227–242.
24. Moresco EM, LaVine D, Beutler B (2011) Toll-like receptors. Curr Biol 21: R488–493.
25. Rugtveit J, Bakka A, Brandtzaeg P (1997) Differential distribution of B7.1 (CD80) and B7.2 (CD86) costimulatory molecules on mucosal macrophage subsets in human inflammatory bowel disease (IBD). Clin Exp Immunol 110: 104–113.
26. Medzhitov R (2008) Origin and physiological roles of inflammation. Nature 454: 428–435.
27. Takeuchi O, Akira S (2010) Pattern recognition receptors and inflammation. Cell 140: 805–820.
28. Halin C, Detmar M (2008) Chapter 1. Inflammation, angiogenesis, and lymphangiogenesis. Methods Enzymol 445: 1–25.
29. Schroder K, Tschopp J (2010) The inflammasomes. Cell 140: 821–832.
30. Faubion WA Jr, Fletcher JG, O'Byrne S, Feagan BG, de Villiers WJ, et al. (2013) EMerging BiomARKers in Inflammatory Bowel Disease (EMBARK) Study Identifies Fecal Calprotectin, Serum MMP9, and Serum IL-22 as a Novel Combination of Biomarkers for Crohn's Disease Activity: Role of Cross-Sectional Imaging. Am J Gastroenterol 108: 1891–1900.
31. Stallmach A, Giese T, Schmidt C, Ludwig B, Mueller-Molaian I, et al. (2004) Cytokine/chemokine transcript profiles reflect mucosal inflammation in Crohn's disease. Int J Colorectal Dis 19: 308–315.
32. Zahn A, Giese T, Karner M, Braun A, Hinz U, et al. (2009) Transcript levels of different cytokines and chemokines correlate with clinical and endoscopic activity in ulcerative colitis. BMC Gastroenterol 9: 13.
33. Hessian PA, Edgeworth J, Hogg N (1993) MRP-8 and MRP-14, two abundant Ca(2+)-binding proteins of neutrophils and monocytes. J Leukoc Biol 53: 197–204.
34. Clark PM, Dawany N, Dampier W, Byers SW, Pestell RG, et al. (2012) Bioinformatics analysis reveals transcriptome and microRNA signatures and drug repositioning targets for IBD and other autoimmune diseases. Inflamm Bowel Dis 18: 2315–2333.
35. Jostins L, Ripke S, Weersma RK, Duerr RH, McGovern DP, et al. (2012) Host-microbe interactions have shaped the genetic architecture of inflammatory bowel disease. Nature 491: 119–124.
36. Rohan PJ, Davis P, Moskaluk CA, Kearns M, Krutzsch H, et al. (1993) PAC-1: a mitogen-induced nuclear protein tyrosine phosphatase. Science 259: 1763–1766.
37. Jeffrey KL, Brummer T, Rolph MS, Liu SM, Callejas NA, et al. (2006) Positive regulation of immune cell function and inflammatory responses by phosphatase PAC-1. Nat Immunol 7: 274–283.
38. Fiocchi C (2011) Early and late inflammatory bowel disease: why and how are they different? Curr Opin Gastroenterol 27: 317–320.
39. Coron E, Flamant M, Aubert P, Wedel T, Pedron T, et al. (2009) Characterisation of early mucosal and neuronal lesions following Shigella flexneri infection in human colon. PLoS One 4: e4713.
40. Phalipon A, Sansonetti PJ (2003) Shigellosis: innate mechanisms of inflammatory destruction of the intestinal epithelium, adaptive immune response, and vaccine development. Crit Rev Immunol 23: 371–401.
41. Riegler M, Sedivy R, Pothoulakis C, Hamilton G, Zacherl J, et al. (1995) Clostridium difficile toxin B is more potent than toxin A in damaging human colonic epithelium in vitro. J Clin Invest 95: 2004–2011.
42. van Spreeuwel JP, Duursma GC, Meijer CJ, Bax R, Rosekrans PC, et al. (1985) Campylobacter colitis: histological immunohistochemical and ultrastructural findings. Gut 26: 945–951.
43. Lorrot M, Vasseur M (2007) [Physiopathology of Rotavirus diarrhea]. Arch Pediatr 14 Suppl 3: S145–151.
44. Oberhuber G, Kastner N, Stolte M (1997) Giardiasis: a histologic analysis of 567 cases. Scand J Gastroenterol 32: 48–51.
45. Morise K, Yamaguchi T, Kuroiwa A, Kanayama K, Matsuura T, et al. (1994) Expression of adhesion molecules and HLA-DR by macrophages and dendritic cells in aphthoid lesions of Crohn's disease: an immunocytochemical study. J Gastroenterol 29: 257–264.
46. Mahida YR, Galvin AM, Gray T, Makh S, McAlindon ME, et al. (1997) Migration of human intestinal lamina propria lymphocytes, macrophages and eosinophils following the loss of surface epithelial cells. Clin Exp Immunol 109: 377–386.
47. Autschbach F, Braunstein J, Helmke B, Zuna I, Schurmann G, et al. (1998) In situ expression of interleukin-10 in noninflamed human gut and in inflammatory bowel disease. Am J Pathol 153: 121–130.
48. Glocker EO, Kotlarz D, Boztug K, Gertz EM, Schaffer AA, et al. (2009) Inflammatory bowel disease and mutations affecting the interleukin-10 receptor. N Engl J Med 361: 2033–2045.
49. Iliev ID, Mileti E, Matteoli G, Chieppa M, Rescigno M (2009) Intestinal epithelial cells promote colitis-protective regulatory T-cell differentiation through dendritic cell conditioning. Mucosal Immunol 2: 340–350.
50. Xiao W, Mindrinos MN, Seok J, Cuschieri J, Cuenca AG, et al. (2011) A genomic storm in critically injured humans. J Exp Med 208: 2581–2590.

51. Kaser A, Lee AH, Franke A, Glickman JN, Zeissig S, et al. (2008) XBP1 links ER stress to intestinal inflammation and confers genetic risk for human inflammatory bowel disease. Cell 134: 743–756.
52. Shkoda A, Ruiz PA, Daniel H, Kim SC, Rogler G, et al. (2007) Interleukin-10 blocked endoplasmic reticulum stress in intestinal epithelial cells: impact on chronic inflammation. Gastroenterology 132: 190–207.
53. Chen C, Dudenhausen EE, Pan YX, Zhong C, Kilberg MS (2004) Human CCAAT/enhancer-binding protein beta gene expression is activated by endoplasmic reticulum stress through an unfolded protein response element downstream of the protein coding sequence. J Biol Chem 279: 27948–27956.
54. Ryan GB, Majno G (1977) Acute inflammation. A review. Am J Pathol 86: 183–276.
55. Karin M, Liu Z, Zandi E (1997) AP-1 function and regulation. Curr Opin Cell Biol 9: 240–246.
56. Takada Y, Ray N, Ikeda E, Kawaguchi T, Kuwahara M, et al. (2010) Fos proteins suppress dextran sulfate sodium-induced colitis through inhibition of NF-kappaB. J Immunol 184: 1014–1021.
57. Carrasco A, Mane J, Santaolalla R, Pedrosa E, Mallolas J, et al. (2013) Comparison of lymphocyte isolation methods for endoscopic biopsy specimens from the colonic mucosa. J Immunol Methods 389: 29–37.
58. Smith PD, Janoff EN, Mosteller-Barnum M, Merger M, Orenstein JM, et al. (1997) Isolation and purification of CD14-negative mucosal macrophages from normal human small intestine. J Immunol Methods 202: 1–11.
59. Weigmann B, Tubbe I, Seidel D, Nicolaev A, Becker C, et al. (2007) Isolation and subsequent analysis of murine lamina propria mononuclear cells from colonic tissue. Nat Protoc 2: 2307–2311.

2

Intestinal Anti-Inflammatory Activity of Lentinan: Influence on IL-8 and TNFR1 Expression in Intestinal Epithelial Cells

Yosuke Nishitani[1], Ling Zhang[2], Masaru Yoshida[3,4], Takeshi Azuma[3], Kazuki Kanazawa[2], Takashi Hashimoto[2], Masashi Mizuno[2]*

1 Team of Health Bioscience, Organization of Advanced Science and Technology, Kobe University, Kobe, Japan, **2** Department of Agrobioscience, Graduate School of Agricultural Science, Kobe University, Kobe, Japan, **3** Gastroenterology Division, Department of Internal Medicine, Graduate School of Medicine, Kobe University, Kobe, Japan, **4** The Integrated Center for Mass Spectrometry, Graduate School of Medicine, Kobe University, Kobe, Japan

Abstract

Inflammatory bowel disease (IBD) is characterized by chronic inflammation of the gastrointestinal tract. It is unknown whether β-1,3;1,6-glucan can induce immune suppressive effects. Here, we study intestinal anti-inflammatory activity of *Lentinula edodes*-derived β-1,3;1,6-glucan, which is known as lentinan. Dextran sulfate sodium (DSS)-induced colitis mice were used to elucidate effects of lentinan *in vivo*. In the cellular level assessment, lentinan was added into a co-culture model consisting of intestinal epithelial Caco-2 cells and LPS-stimulated macrophage RAW264.7 cells. Ligated intestinal loop assay was performed for assessing effects of lentinan on intestinal epithelial cells (IECs) *in vivo*. Oral administration of lentinan (100 µg/mouse) significantly ameliorated DSS-induced colitis in body weight loss, shortening of colon lengths, histological score, and inflammatory cytokine mRNA expression in inflamed tissues. Lentinan reduced interleukin (IL)-8 mRNA expression and nuclear factor (NF)-κB activation in Caco-2 cells without decreasing of tumor necrosis factor (TNF)-α production from RAW264.7 cells. Flow cytometric analysis revealed that surface levels of TNF receptor (TNFR) 1 were decreased by lentinan treatment. A clathrin-mediated endocytosis inhibitor, monodansylcadaverine, canceled lentinan inhibition of IL-8 mRNA expression. Moreover, lentinan inhibited TNFR1 expression in Caco-2 cells in both protein and mRNA level. Lentinan also inhibited TNFR1 mRNA expression in mouse IECs. These results suggest that lentinan exhibits intestinal anti-inflammatory activity through inhibition of IL-8 mRNA expression associated with the inhibition of NF-κB activation which is triggered by TNFR1 endocytosis and lowering of their expression in IECs. Lentinan may be effective for the treatment of gut inflammation including IBD.

Editor: Benoit Foligne, Institut Pasteur de Lille, France

Funding: This research was supported by grants for project research (Development of fundamental technology for analysis and evaluation of functional agricultural products and functional foods) from the Ministry of Agriculture, Forestry and Fisheries of Japan. The funders had no role in study design, data collection and analysis, decision to publish, or preparation of the manuscript.

Competing Interests: The authors have declared that no competing interests exist.

* E-mail: mizuno@kobe-u.ac.jp

Introduction

The gastrointestinal tract of higher organisms is lined with a single layer of IECs. This physical barrier separates subepithelial mucosal immune cells such as lymphocytes, macrophages, and dendritic cells from a variety of antigenic substances present within the intestinal lumen including bacteria and food antigens [1,2]. The integrity of the epithelial barrier is essential for the maintenance of host homeostasis, as it prevents dysregulated uptake of luminal antigens. The incidence and prevalence of Crohn's disease and ulcerative colitis, collectively referred to as inflammatory bowel disease (IBD), have been increasing worldwide [3]. IBD is characterized by chronic inflammation of the gastrointestinal tract. The clinical features of Crohn's disease include diarrhea, pain, narrowing of the gut lumen leading to strictures and bowel obstruction, abscess formation, and fistulization of the skin and internal organs. Meanwhile, the clinical features of ulcerative colitis include severe diarrhea, blood loss, and progressive loss of peristaltic function [4]. While their precise etiology still remains unknown, understanding of the pathophysiology of IBD has advanced, and the typical features of these diseases have been shown in various studies, especially for intestinal immune cells and IECs of IBD patients. It has been reported that IECs, macrophages, and T cells secrete large amounts of chemokines such as IL-8 and pro-inflammatory cytokines including TNF-α, IL-6, IL-12, IL-17, IL-23, and interferon (IFN)-γ in the inflamed intestines of IBD patients [5]. IL-8 is a member of the C-X-C chemokines and is secreted excessively by a variety of cells at the site of inflammation, such as IECs, in IBD [6]. IL-8 causes excessive recruitment and transmigration of neutrophils into inflamed tissues followed by injury to the epithelia [7]. Lamina propria mononuclear cells (LPMCs) from patients with Crohn's disease spontaneously secreted TNF-α [8]. It is well-known that the secretion of inflammatory cytokines like IL-8 and TNF-α may be an important part of the immune response, and the dysregulation of these cytokines is implicated in the pathogenesis of IBD [9,10].

It has been reported that β-glucans derived from fungi and yeast possess immune modulating properties [11]. β-Glucans can enhance the functional activity of macrophages and activate the antimicrobial activity of mononuclear cells and neutrophils [12–14]. β-1,3-Glucans are major structural components of fungal cell walls which induce macrophage activation in mammals. Among the various β-1,3-glucans, lentinan possesses a structure composed of a backbone of β-1,3-linked glucose residues with side chains of β-1,6-glucose residues [15] and is an antitumor polysaccharide produced by *Lentinula edodes* [16]. Lentinan increases peritoneal macrophage cytotoxicity against metastatic tumors [17]. Lentinan can also activate the normal and alternative pathways of the complement system by splitting C3 into C3a and C3b, thereby enhancing macrophage activation [17]. Although a number of studies for the fascinating effect of β-1,3-glucans on the responsiveness or function of immune cells have been performed, their immune suppressive effects such as intestinal anti-inflammatory properties have not been studied sufficiently.

In our previous study, we established a gut inflammation *in vitro* model which is composed of intestinal epithelial Caco-2 cells and macrophage RAW264.7 cells [18]. When RAW264.7 cells were stimulated with lipopolysaccharide (LPS), IL-8 and TNF-α secretion increased. This gut inflammation model was used to search for anti-inflammatory factors that act against intestinal inflammation [18]. In the present study, we focused on the suppressive effect of lentinan on gut inflammation using an *in vivo* and an *in vitro* model and further examined its inhibitory mechanism.

Materials and Methods

Experimental Animals

Ethics statement. The care and use of the animals and experimental protocol were approved by the Guidelines for the Care and Use of Experimental Animals, of Rokkodai Campus, Kobe University, and were approved by the Animal Experiment Ethics Committee of Kobe University (Permission number: 22-05-06).

Female, 6-week-old C57BL/6CrSlc mice were purchased from SLC (Shizuoka, Japan). Mice were housed in an air-conditioned animal room at 23±2°C with a 12-h light/dark cycle, and acclimated for 7 days. Mice were fed with a laboratory diet (Nihon Nosan, Yokohama, Japan) and water ad libitum.

Reagents

Dulbecco's Modified Eagle Medium (DMEM) mixed with glutamine containing 1.0 g/l glucose, LPS from *E. coli* O127, and recombinant murine TNF-α (rmTNF-α) were purchased from Wako Pure Chemical Industries (Osaka, Japan). MEM (Eagle's Minimum Essential Medium) was purchased from Nissui Pharmaceutical (Tokyo, Japan). RPMI 1640 medium and MEM non-essential amino acids (NEAA) were purchased from Gibco BRL (Grand Island, NY). DMEM mixed with glutamine containing 4.5 g/l glucose, budesonide, cytochalasin D, and monodansylcadaverine were obtained from Sigma (St Louis, MO). Fetal bovine serum (FBS) was purchased from Biological Industries (Beit, Israel). Anti-human β-actin mouse monoclonal antibody (Ab) was purchased from Calbiochem (Darmstadt, Germany). Anti-human nuclear factor (NF)-κB p65 rabbit monoclonal antibody (Ab) and anti-human histone h1 mouse monoclonal Ab were obtained from Santa Cruz Biotechnology (Delaware Avenue, CA). Anti-human TNFR1 mouse monoclonal Ab was obtained from R&D Systems (Minneapolis, MN). Lentinan from *Lentinula edodes*, a dietary β-1,3;1,6-glucan used in this study, was gifted from Ajinomoto (Tokyo, Japan). Anti-lentinan rabbit polyclonal Ab has been reported in our previous study [19]. Other chemicals and reagents were ordinary commercial and guaranteed products.

Induction of DSS Colitis

Colitis was induced in 7-week-old mice by administration of 2% (w/v) DSS (molecular weight; 36,000–50,000) to drinking water for 7 days. Lentinan (50, 100, and 200 μg per mouse) or vehicle was administered daily via intragastric administration, starting 7 days before DSS treatment and continuing until sacrifice. Doses of lentinan were chosen according to various reasons, such as the estimated human intake of mushroom [20], the pharmaceutical dose of lentinan via i.p. or i.v. injection for gastric cancer treatment [21], as well as our trial test. Mice were killed on day 10 (initial DSS treatment as day 1). For histological examination, the degree of inflammation and epithelial damage on hematoxylin and eosin (HE)-stained sections (8 μm) of distal colon was graded according to the method of Hudert *et al.* [22].

Cell Culture

Cells from the human intestinal epithelial cell line Caco-2, obtained from American Type culture Collection (ATCC) (Manassas, VA, USA), were cultured in DMEM mixed with glutamine containing 4.5 g/l glucose, supplemented with 1% MEM-NEAA, 100 U/ml penicillin, 100 μg/ml streptomycin, and 10% decomplemented FBS (56°C, 30 min). Cell cultures were incubated in a humidified 5% CO_2 incubator at 37°C. When the cells reached subconfluence, Caco-2 cells were recovered from the culture flask by trypsin digestion after being washed with phosphate buffered saline (PBS). Cells from the murine macrophage cell line RAW264.7, obtained from ATCC, were cultured in DMEM mixed with glutamine containing 1.0 g/l glucose and supplemented with 10% (v/v) decomplemented FBS (56°C, 30 min), 100 U/ml penicillin, and 100 μg/ml streptomycin. Cell cultures were performed in a humidified 5% CO_2 incubator at 37°C and recovered in the same way as the Caco-2 cells described above. Cells from the murine fibrosarcoma cell line L929, obtained from ATCC, were cultured in MEM supplemented with 10% FBS, 2 mM L-glutamine, 100 U/ml penicillin, and 100 μg/ml streptomycin. Cell culturing was performed as for the Caco-2 cells described above.

Co-culture System

A co-culture experiment was performed as described in a previous report [18]. For inhibition of receptor internalization, endocytosis inhibitors, including cytochalasin D (2 μM) and monodansylcadaverine (100 μM), were used. Before co-culturing with RAW264.7 cells, Caco-2 cells on transwell membrane were treated with an inhibitor or vehicle at 37°C for 30 min. After incubation, cells were washed three times with PBS, and then used in a co-culture model.

For assessing the effect of anti-lentinan Ab on lentinan activity, a rabbit polyclonal anti-lentinan Ab was used. The Ab was diluted with PBS at ratios of 1:5 or 1:100, and then mixed with lentinan solution and incubated on ice for 30 min. A rabbit polyclonal isotype control Ab was used as control at the same protein concentration as anti-lentinan Ab (dilution ratio of 1:5).

TNF-α Content Measurement

TNF-α contents were quantified with a cytotoxicity assay involving L929 cells (an actinomycin D-treated murine fibroblast cell line) using rmTNF-α as the standard as described by Kerékgyártó *et al.* [23].

Western Blot Analysis

For Western blot analysis of NF-κB p65, nuclear protein was extracted as described by Zhang *et al.* [24]. For Western blot analysis of TNFR1, total protein was extracted with radioimmunoprecipitation (RIPA) buffer [1% Triton X-100, 0.5% deoxycholate, 0.1% sodium dodecyl sulfate (SDS), 2 mM PMSF, 2 mM ethylenediaminetetraacetic acid, and 2 mM orthovanadate] as described by Gaultier *et al.* [25]. The protein concentration was measured using the BCA™ Protein Assay Kit (Pierce, Rockford, IL). Equal amounts of the samples (5–30 μg) were mixed with sample buffer [125 mM Tris-HCl (pH 6.8), 4% SDS, 10% 2-mercaptoethanol, 0.2% bromophenol blue, and 20% glycerol] in a 1:1 ratio, boiled for 10 min, and subjected to electrophoresis on 12.5% acrylamide gel. The electrophoresed proteins were transferred from the gel onto a polyvinylidene fluoride membrane. The membrane was blocked with TBST (Tris-buffered saline containing 0.1% Tween 20) containing 7% skimmed milk for 1 h. After being blocked, the membrane was incubated with primary Ab against histone h1 (1:200), β-actin (1:15,000), NF-κB p65 (1:1,000), or TNFR1 (1:1,000) for 1 h. Then, the membrane was incubated with secondary Ab for 1 h at room temperature. Peroxidase conjugated anti-mouse IgM goat monoclonal Ab (1:1,500; Calbiochem) for β-actin primary Ab, peroxidase conjugated anti-rabbit IgG (H+L) goat Ab (1:1,000; Wako) for NF-κB primary Ab, and peroxidase conjugated anti-mouse IgG (H+L) goat Ab (1:10,000; Jacson Immuno Research Laboratories, West Grove, PA,) for TNFR1 and histone h1 primary Abs were used as secondary Ab. The ECL Plus™ Western blotting detection system (GE Healthcare) was used for blot detection according to the manufacturer's protocol. The reagent was drained, and the membrane was exposed to a hyper film in the film cassette.

RNA Isolation and Quantitative RT-PCR

Total RNA was isolated from cultured cells and colon tissues by using Sepasol RNA I super (Nacalai Tesque, Kyoto, Japan) and RNAqueous with Plant RNA Isolation Aid (Ambion, Austin, TX), respectively, according to the manufacturer's protocol. The reverse transcription of the RNA for quantitative PCR was performed using High-Capacity cDNA Reverse Transcription Kits (Applied Biosystems, Foster City, CA). Quantitative PCR was performed by the 7500 Fast Real Time PCR system (Applied Biosystems) using TaqMan® Fast Universal PCR Master Mix (Applied Biosystems), and Gene Expression Assays for mouse pro-inflammatory cytokines (TNF-α, IL-6, IL-1β, and IFN-γ), MIP-2 and β-actin, and human GAPDH and IL-8 (Applied Biosystems), according to the manufacturer's protocol. For all panels, the bars represent the ratio of target gene to endogenous gene expression, as determined by the relative quantification method (ΔΔCT) (mean ± S.E. of triplicate determination).

Flow Cytometry

Cells were harvested by scraping into medium and pelleted by centrifugation at 4°C. The subsequent fixing and staining steps were performed at 4°C. Pellets were washed twice in 0.5% bovine serum albumin in PBS and incubated in FB (2% FBS in PBS) for 10 min on ice. Cells were pelleted and resuspended in 100 μl of FB with mouse anti-human TNFR1 (1:50 dilution) or the isotype control and incubated for 30 min. Cells were washed twice in FB. Cells staining with anti-TNFR1 Ab were incubated with Alexa Fluor488-conjugated anti-mouse IgG (H+L) goat Ab (1:400 dilution; Molecular Probes, Eugene, OR) for 30 min, followed by washing twice in FB, and fixed with 4% paraformaldehyde in PBS. FACS analysis was performed with a FACSVerse (BD Biosciences) and FACSuite software (BD Biosciences). For quantitative analysis, the geometric mean fluorescence intensities (gMFIs) of samples were plotted as percentages of the gMFI obtained from medium treated cells, with the following fomula: % surface TNFR1 = (lentinan gMFI − isotype control gMFI)/(medium gMFI − isotype control gMFI) ×100.

Immunofluorescence Staining of NF-κB p65 in Caco-2 Cells

After the co-culture experiments, Caco-2 cells were fixed with methanol for 5 min, before being blocked for 30 min with 10% goat serum at room temperature. The cells were incubated with a 1:50 dilution of anti-NF-κB p65 antibody at room temperature for 2 h. The cells were stained with Alexa Fluor488-conjugated anti-rabbit IgG (H+L) goat antibody as secondary antibodies (1:400 dilution; Molecular Probes, Eugene, OR) for 1 h at room temperature. Nucleic acids were stained with propidium iodide (PI) (535/617) (1:500; Molecular Probes). Images were acquired using a fluorescence microscope (BZ-9000; Keyence, Osaka, Japan). PI staining appeared red and NF-κB p65 staining green. A quantitative imaging assay was performed as described previously [26].

Ligated Intestinal Loop Assay and Isolation of Epithelium

Mice were anaesthetized with avertin and kept warm with a 37°C warming pad during the assay. One hundred microliter of lentinan solution (1 mg/ml) or vehicle were injected into the separated two ligated intestinal loops which were located in ileum, respectively. After incubation for 1 h, the mice were killed and the ligated intestinal loops were excised from the intestine. IECs were isolated from mouse small intestine by modifying the method described by Hase *et al.* [27]. Briefly, intestinal loops were dissected from the mouse small intestine excluding Peyer's patches (PPs) and soaked in Hank's balanced salt solution (HBSS) containing 30 mM EDTA. After incubation on ice for 12 min, IECs were isolated by manipulation with a fine needle under stereomicroscopic monitoring. The isolated epithelial cell sheets were kept in ice-cold HBSS until RNA extraction.

Statistical Analysis

Data are expressed as the mean ± SE. Statistical analysis was performed using the Student's *t*-test. Statistical significance was defined as $P<0.05$. Statistical differences of colon lengths in DSS colitis mouse model were evaluated by analysis of variance (ANOVA) and Tukey-Kramer Multiple Comparisons Test to determine differences between groups. The results were considered significant when $P<0.05$.

See supplementary materials and methods for supporting information regarding lentinan content measurement (Text S1) and immunofluorescence staining of TNFR1 in Caco-2 cells (Text S2).

Results

Mouse Characteristics

To study the effect of lentinan on the innate immune response during colonic inflammation, an innate immune-mediated model of colitis induced by DSS was performed. DSS is a sulfated polysaccharide which can disrupt the mucosal epithelial barrier, thus exposing local macrophages to stimuli from the intestinal microflora [28]. Mice treated with DSS developed significant signs of IBD-like colitis, bloody diarrhea and wasting conditions with sluggish, weak movement, as well as a decrease in water and food uptake from day 4. In addition, a DSS-treated group decreased means of body weight in contrast to a vehicle-treated control group from day 5, and oral administration of 100 μg/mouse lentinan to DSS-induced colitis mice improved means of body weight (15.60±0.35 g on day 8, 15.08±0.44 g on day 9, and 14.82±0.62 g on day 10) which was significantly higher than that of DSS colitis mice (14.19±0.39 g, 13.33±0.33 g, and 12.86±0.29 g on corresponding day) ($P<0.05$) (Fig. 1A). Similar result was observed in the colon length. The colon length of DSS-treated mice with lentinan at the concentration of 100 μg/mouse (5.98±0.32 cm) was significantly longer than DSS-treated mice (4.87±0.22 cm) (Fig. 1B and 1C). These results suggest that oral administration of lentinan has inhibitory activity on body weight loss and shortening of the colon in DSS-induced colitis.

Histological Inflammation Characteristics

Histological examination of intestinal tissue of mice after DSS colitis was performed at day 10. As shown in Fig. 1D and 1E, mice treated with DSS induced a significant increase of histological score compared with the vehicle-treated control mice, and the oral administration of 100 and 200 μg/mouse lentinan to DSS-induced colitis mice significantly inhibited the increase of histological score ($P<0.05$). These results suggest that oral administration of lentinan has an intestinal anti-inflammatory activity through alleviating severity of inflammation, inflammatory cell infiltration to colonic mucosa, as well as the degree and extent of epithelial damage.

Cytokines and Chemokine Levels in the Colon

DSS-induced colitis model has been associated with increase in Th1 responses, therefore mRNA expression levels of several cytokines and chemokine in the whole colon tissue were analyzed by using real-time PCR. As shown in Fig. 2, compared with DSS-untreated mice, mRNA expression of pro-inflammatory cytokines such as TNF-α, IFN-γ, IL-6, and IL-1β increased dramatically in DSS-treated mice, and the treatment with lentinan improved the aberrant mRNA expression induced by DSS with significant reduction in Th1 type pro-inflammatory cytokine IFN-γ (100 and 200 μg/mouse of lentinan) and IL-1β (200 μg/mouse of lentinan) mRNA expression ($P<0.05$). These results suggest that oral administration of lentinan may exhibit anti-inflammatory activity via modulation of pro-inflammatory cytokines mRNA expression in the gut of DSS-induced colitis mice.

Anti-inflammatory Effect of Lentinan on IL-8 mRNA Expression in the gut Inflammation Model of Caco-2 Cells and LPS-activated RAW264.7 Cells

In order to determine the inhibitory mechanism of lentinan, we used a previously established *in vitro* gut inflammation model [18]. In our previous study, treatment with lentinan (500 μg/ml) significantly reduced the IL-8 mRNA expression in Caco-2 cells ($P<0.05$) [29]. In the presence of rmTNF-α in the basolateral compartment, the IL-8 mRNA expression was increased (Fig. S1A). We could not detect TNF-α secretion in the apical compartment of this model (data not shown), and a previous study showed that anti-mouse TNF-α Ab treatment of the basolateral compartment in this model completely suppressed IL-8 mRNA expression [18]. In addition, when the gut inflammation model were performed with Caco-2 cells grown as monolayers on the underside of the transwell inserts (inverted position), addition of LPS into the lower chamber did not induce IL-8 mRNA expression in Caco-2 cells despite that TNF-α production from RAW264.7 cells was relatively normal (Fig. S1B and S1C). These results suggested that TNF-α in the basolateral compartment is essential for the up-regulation of the IL-8 mRNA expression of Caco-2 cells in this model. In our previous study, lentinan did not reduce the secretion of TNF-α when RAW264.7 cells were stimulated by LPS [29]. These results suggest that lentinan suppresses IL-8 mRNA expression in IECs without a reduction in TNF-α production. An ELISA inhibition technique using an anti-lentinan Ab was carried out to verify whether lentinan could penetrate a Caco-2 monolayer. Lentinan was not detected in the basolateral supernatant (data not shown), ascertaining that lentinan was not able to penetrate the Caco-2 monolayer in this model. These results indicate that the inhibitory activity of lentinan on IL-8 mRNA expression acted through the interaction between lentinan and Caco-2 cells, but not between lentinan and RAW264.7 cells in this model.

Inhibitory Effect of Lentinan on NF-κB Translocation into the Nucleus of Caco-2 Cells

The transcriptional activity of the human IL-8 promoter is known to be regulated by various transcriptional factors such as NF-κB [30]. In Caco-2/RAW264.7 gut inflammation model, an increase in IL-8 mRNA expression in Caco-2 cells was observed in association with TNF-α production from LPS-stimulated RAW264.7 cells [29]. Therefore, we examined the NF-κB p65 level in the nucleus of Caco-2 cells. As expected, the NF-κB p65 level in the nucleus peaked at 5 h incubation in association with TNF-α production (Fig. S2A and S2B). Subsequently, we assessed the effect of lentinan on NF-κB activation in Caco-2 cells. Western blot and immunofluorescence analysis showed that treatment with lentinan (500 μg/ml) significantly lessened the increase in NF-κB p65 level (Fig. 3A and 3B). These results suggest that the addition of lentinan into the apical compartment suppresses the NF-κB activation of Caco-2 cells in the gut inflammation model.

Lentinan Reduces Surface Levels of TNFR1 in Caco-2 Cells

TNF-α transduces signals via specific receptors, and two TNFR isotypes, TNFR1 and TNFR2, are known. It has been reported that TNFR1 mediates TNF-α-induced NF-κB activation [31,32], and TNFR1 signaling in IECs is crucial for the disease pathogenesis of inflammatory colitis in intestinal epithelial IκB kinase-γ (IKKγ) knockout mice [33]. We hypothesized that the ability of lentinan to regulate the TNFR1 level in Caco-2 cells accounts for the decrease in IL-8 mRNA expression, which is a downstream event of TNFR1-dependent cell signaling. To test this hypothesis, cell surface levels of TNFR1 in Caco-2 cells was determined by flow cytometric analysis. As expected, lentinan reduced surface TNFR1 in Caco-2 cells (Fig. 4A). The geometric mean fluorescence intensities (gMFI) of lentinan-treated cells were decreased approximately 60% compared with vehicle-treated cells (Fig. 4B). These results are consistent with the hypothesis that lentinan inhibits TNF-α-induced NF-κB activation by down-regulating cell surface TNFR1. The subsequent experiments are performed to study the mechanism involved in TNFR1 down-regulation by lentinan.

Endocytosis Inhibitor Cancels Lentinan Inhibition of IL-8 mRNA Expression in Caco-2 Cells

We hypothesized that down-regulation of the cell surface TNFR1 by lentinan treatment may occur via receptor endocytosis. It has been reported that endocytosis of TNF receptor superfamily is dependent on actin or clathrin polymerization [34]. We therefore utilized inhibitors to target these specific pathways and evaluate their relative contributions to lentinan inhibition of IL-8 mRNA expression in Caco-2. As shown in Fig. 5A, cytochalasin D, an antagonist of actin polymerization, did not affect lentinan

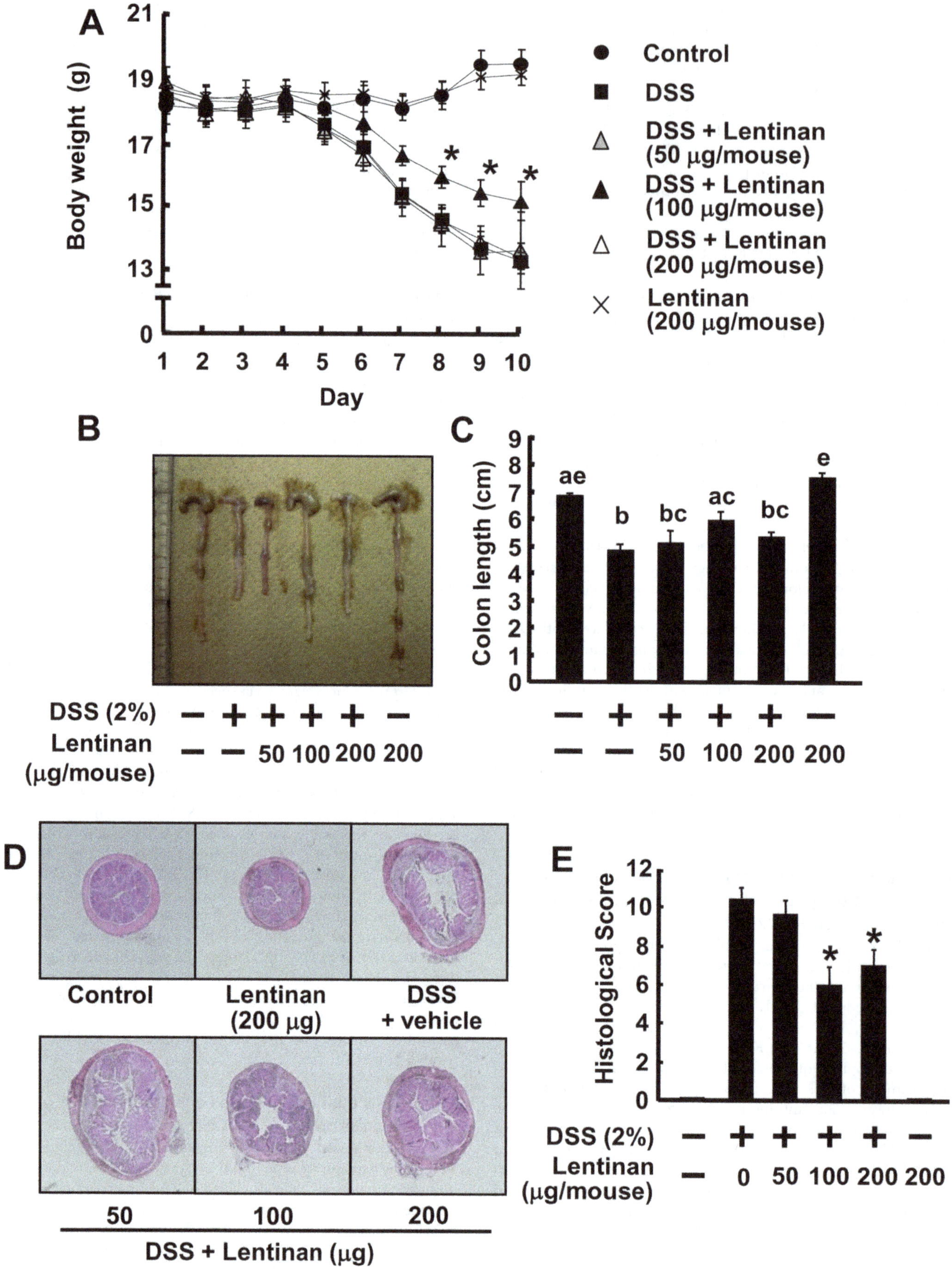
A
Body weight (g)
Day
Control
DSS
DSS + Lentinan (50 μg/mouse)
DSS + Lentinan (100 μg/mouse)
DSS + Lentinan (200 μg/mouse)
Lentinan (200 μg/mouse)
B
DSS (2%)
Lentinan (μg/mouse)
C
Colon length (cm)
ae
b
bc
ac
bc
e
D
Control
Lentinan (200 μg)
DSS + vehicle
50
100
200
DSS + Lentinan (μg)
E
Histological Score
DSS (2%)
Lentinan (μg/mouse)

Figure 1. Lentinan treatment ameliorates DSS-induced colitis in mice. Oral administration of lentinan was started 7 days prior to DSS treatment. (A) Body weight changes of DSS-induced colitis mice with or without lentinan treatment according to the protocol described in materials and methods. Difference between 100 μg/mouse of lentinan-treated mice and non-treated DSS colitis mice was significant at $P<0.05$ (*). (B) Macroscopic appearance of a representative colon from wild-type (WT) and DSS-colitis mice with or without administration of lentinan. (C) Mean colon lengths were plotted. Items with different letter were significantly different ($P<0.05$). (D) Photograph (×40) of HE-stained paraffin sections of a representative colon from WT mice and DSS-colitis mice with or without administration of lentinan. (E) Histological scores of the colon sections of DSS-colitis mice with or without administration of lentinan. Significance compared to a DSS-treated group, *$P<0.05$. Values represent the means ± SE ($n=6$). Experiments were repeated for three times.

inhibition of IL-8 mRNA expression in Caco-2 cells. In contrast, monodansylcadaverine, a hydrophobic amine which inhibits clathrin-dependent endocytosis by affecting the function of clathrin and clathrin-coated vesicles [35,36], canceled lentinan inhibition of IL-8 mRNA expression to LPS control level. However, TNF-α production from LPS-stimulated RAW264.7 cells was not affected by these endocytosis inhibitors compared to non-treatment LPS control (Fig. 5B). These results indicate that lentinan stimulation induce a clathrin-mediated endocytosis of TNFR1 in Caco-2 cells, resulting in inhibition of IL-8 mRNA expression.

Inhibitory Effect of Lentinan on TNFR1 Expression in Caco-2 Cells

Next, we investigated the expression of TNFR1 in Caco-2 cells after lentinan-induced endocytosis. As shown in Fig. 6A, western blot analysis revealed that the level of TNFR1 protein in whole cell extracts from Caco-2 cells was significantly decreased to approximately 60% of its control level by lentinan (500 μg/ml) treatment ($P<0.01$) for 5 h. Moreover, quantitative RT-PCR analysis revealed that 2 h of lentinan treatment also suppressed TNFR1 mRNA expression in Caco-2 cells ($P<0.01$). The inhibition rate reached approximately 30% (Fig. 6B). In this model, Caco-2 cells only expressed IL-8 when the cells were stimulated by rmTNF-α from basolateral side (Fig. S1). We hypothesized that the ability of lentinan to decrease TNFR1 expression in Caco-2 cells involves alteration of the receptor distribution. To determine the distribution of TNFR1 in Caco-2 cells, immunofluorescent analysis was performed. As expected, z-stack image scanning revealed that TNFR1 on the basolateral side of the cells was remarkably decreased by lentinan treatment while it was uniformly distributed from apical to basolateral side in the absence of lentinan (Fig. S3). These results indicate that lentinan exerts a suppressive effect on TNFR1 expression after inducing the receptor endocytosis, resulting in the absence of TNFR1 on the basolateral side of Caco-2 cells.

Inhibitory Effect of Lentinan on TNFR1 mRNA Expression *in vivo*

To investigate the effect of lentinan on TNFR1 mRNA expression *in vivo*, intestinal ligated loop assay was performed. As shown in Fig. 7, lentinan treatment significantly decreased TNFR1 mRNA expression in mouse IECs compared to vehicle control ($P<0.01$). The inhibition rate reached approximately 30% (Fig. 7). This result suggests that modulation of TNFR1 expression in IECs may be involved in gut anti-inflammatory activity of lentinan *in vivo*.

Effect of Anti-lentinan Polyclonal Ab on Lentinan Inhibition of IL-8 mRNA Expression in Caco-2 Cells

Although we showed that lentinan exhibits intestinal anti-inflammatory activity by inducing TNFR1 endocytosis in IECs, it remains unclear how these cells recognize lentinan. In order to assess the mechanism of how Caco-2 cells recognize lentinan, the effect of anti-lentinan rabbit polyclonal Ab on lentinan inhibition of IL-8 mRNA expression in Caco-2 cells was investigated. Treatment of anti-lentinan Ab did not have a significant effect on TNF-α production from RAW264.7 cells in an *in vitro* gut inflammation model (Fig. 8B). However, treatment of anti-lentinan Ab at a dilution ratio of 1:5, but not isotype control Ab, canceled lentinan inhibition of IL-8 mRNA expression in Caco-2 cells (Fig. 8A). These results suggest that Caco-2 cells may recognize the structure of lentinan via the cell surface receptor, followed by the subsequent TNFR1 endocytosis.

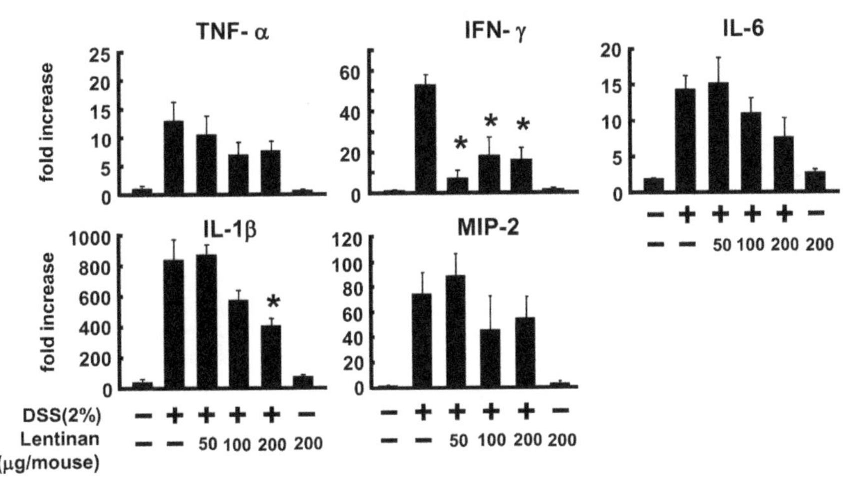

Figure 2. Lentinan improves inflammatory cytokines mRNA expression in colon tissues of DSS-induced colitis. Total RNA was extracted from the colon tissues of untreated and DSS-treated mice on day 10. TNF-α, IFN-γ, IL-6, IL-1β, and MIP-2 mRNA expression were measured by quantitative RT-PCR. Values represent the means ± SE ($n=6$). Significance compared with a DSS-treated group, *$P<0.05$.

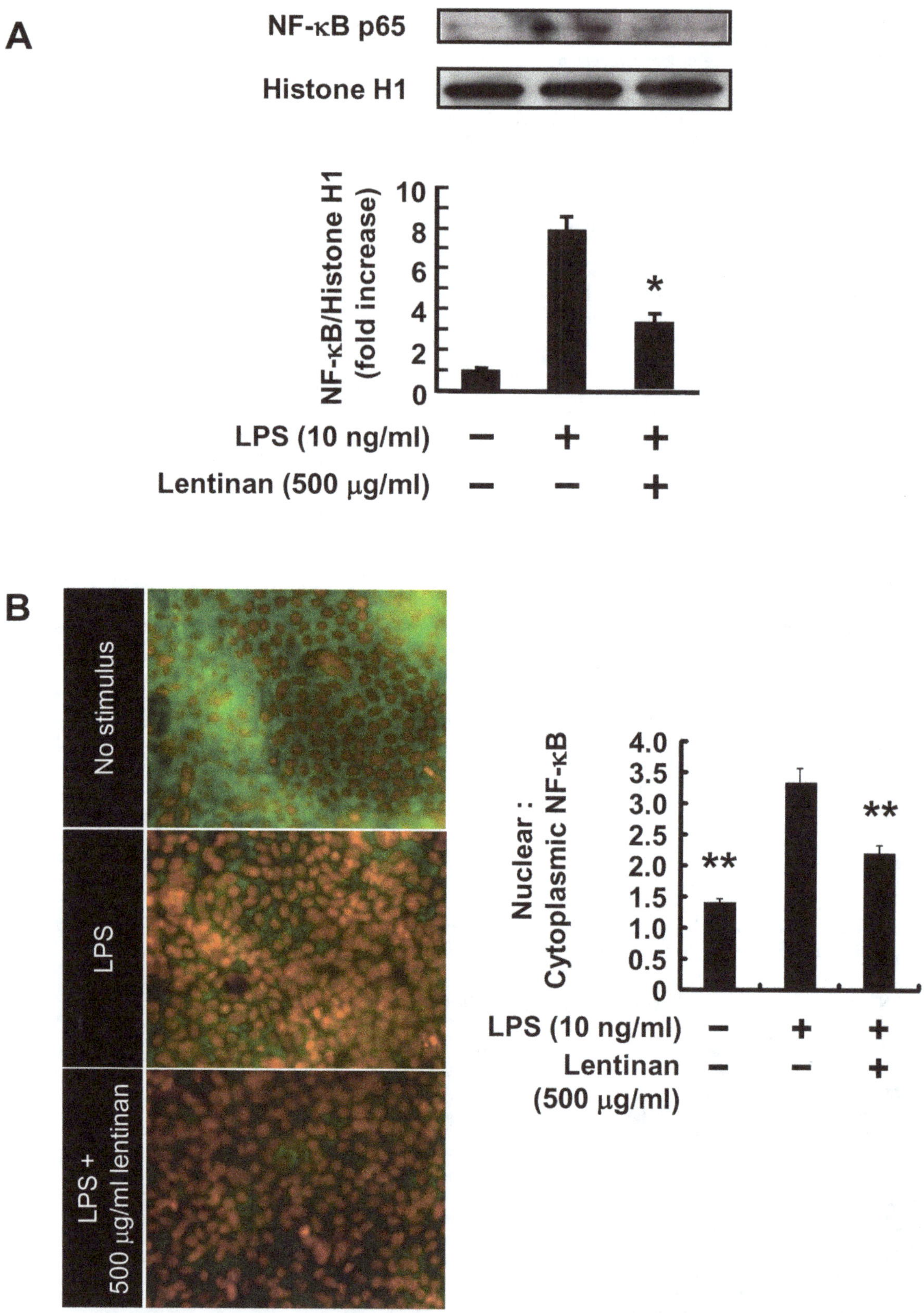

Figure 3. Lentinan inhibits NF-κB p65 nuclear translocation in Caco-2 cells. Lentinan (500 μg/ml) was added into the apical compartment of Caco-2/RAW264.7 co-culture model for 3 h. Subsequently, LPS was added to the basolateral compartment at a concentration of 10 ng/ml, followed by incubation for an additional 2 h. (A) Western blot analysis of the NF-κB p65 subunit was performed on nuclear extracts from Caco-2 cells. (B) Image analysis was performed according to the method described previously [26]. The values represent the means ± SE. Experiments were repeated for two times in triplicate. *$P<0.05$, **$P<0.01$ vs. LPS control.

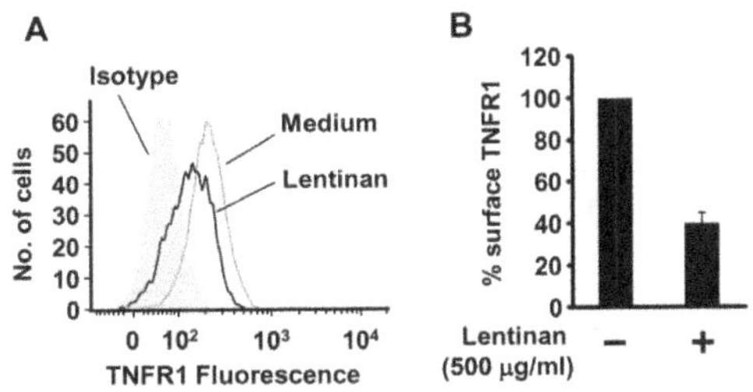

Figure 4. Lentinan suppresses cell surface levels of TNFR1 in Caco-2 cells. Lentinan (500 μg/ml) was added into the apical compartment of Caco-2/RAW264.7 co-culture model for 30 min. Subsequently, Caco-2 cells were harvested, fixed, and stained according to the method described in materials and methods. (A) Surface levels of TNFR1 were analyzed by flow cytometry. (B) The resulting gMFIs were plotted as percentages of the gMFI obtained from medium treated cells, with the following fomula: % surface TNFR1 = (lentinan gMFI – isotype control gMFI)/(medium gMFI – isotype control gMFI) ×100. The values represent the means ± SE. Experiments were repeated for three times in triplicate.

Discussion

The mainstream treatments used to manage IBD are largely based on immunosuppressive approaches with broad acting agents such as prednisone, cyclosporin A, and tacrolimus [37]. Although they are relatively effective, a number of patients develop significant side effects and/or become unresponsive to them. The perception that alternative medicine is healthier than classical therapeutic options, have led a growing segment of the population to seek alternative treatments to ameliorate various disorders including chronic intestinal inflammation [38]. However, the absence of empirical data showing their efficacy and mechanisms of action prevents their incorporation into mainstream medicine. Meanwhile, it has been reported that mushroom-derived β-glucan exhibits immune activating properties [11]. Although it has been reported that the yeast zymosan induces immunological tolerance and regulatory antigen presenting cells into secreting abundant IL-10 but little or no IL-6 or IL-12 p70 [39], it is unknown whether mushroom-derived β-glucan can also induce immunosuppressive effects such as anti-inflammatory effects. In the present study, we investigated whether lentinan, a dietary β-1,3;1,6-glucan derived from *Lentinula edodes*, exerts anti-inflammatory activities using an *in vivo* and an *in vitro* model of gut inflammation, and we provide evidences that lentinan inhibits gut inflammation through modulation of TNFR1 expression in IECs.

Plant polysaccharides have been previously shown to reduce the extensive colonic damage in experimental colitis [40–42], but little is known about the effect of supplementing edible mushroom glucans in intestinal inflammation. Lentinan significantly improved body weight loss, shortening of colon length, and histological scores which were used to assess the degree of gut inflammation. We also showed that lentinan treatment in DSS mice attenuated the increase in IL-1β and IFN-γ significantly in colon segments. Pro-inflammatory cytokines are known to play an important role in inflammation of the intestinal mucosa [43]. Specifically, increased levels of TNF-α, IL-1β, IFN-γ, IL-6, and IL-8 have been reported in ulcerative colitis patients [44,45]. IL-1β is a key cytokine involved in up-regulating the production of TNF-α, IL-6, and IL-8 [46], resulting in injury of intestinal epithelial tight junction barrier via up-regulating the production of myosin L chain kinase (MLCK) [47]. These results suggest that oral administration of lentinan exhibits anti-inflammatory activities in DSS-induced colitis mice through inhibition of pro-

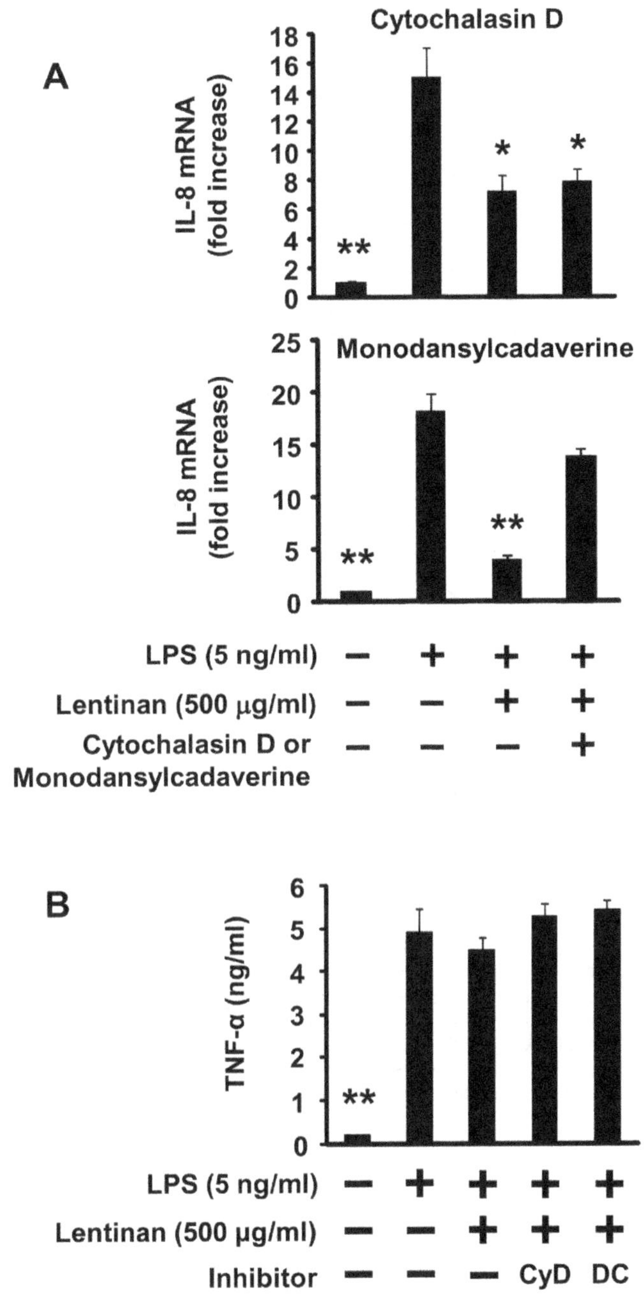

Figure 5. Effect of endocytosis inhibitors on lentinan inhibition of IL-8 mRNA expression in Caco-2 cells. Before co-culturing with RAW264.7 cells, Caco-2 cells on transwell membrane were treated with endocytosis inhibitors, cytochalasin D (2 μM) or monodansylcadaverine (100 μM), for 30 min. Caco-2 cells were washed three times with PBS, and then the cells were used in a co-culture model. Lentinan (500 μg/ml) was added into the apical compartment of a co-culture model for 3 h. Subsequently, LPS was added to the basolateral compartment at a concentration of 5 ng/ml, followed by incubation for an additional 3 h. IL-8 mRNA expression in Caco-2 cells was determined by quantitative RT-PCR. (B) TNF-α production in the basolateral compartment was determined by a L929 cytotoxicity assay. The values represent the means ± SE. Experiments were repeated for three times in triplicate. *P<0.05, **P<0.01 vs. LPS control.

inflammatory cytokines production. Furthermore, in order to unveil the mechanism of intestinal anti-inflammatory activity of

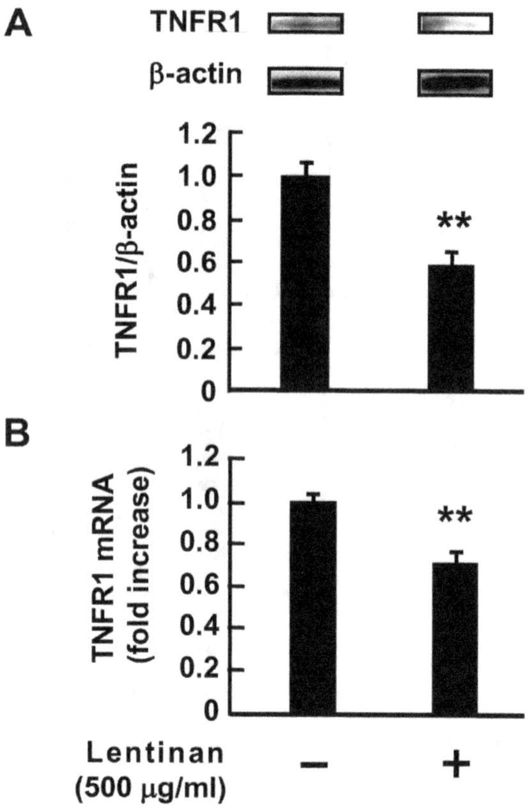

Figure 6. Lentinan inhibits TNFR1 protein and mRNA expression in Caco-2 cells. (A) Lentinan (500 μg/ml) was added into the apical compartment of Caco-2/RAW264.7 co-culture model for 3 h. Subsequently, LPS was added to the basolateral compartment at a concentration of 1 ng/ml, followed by incubation for an additional 2 h. Then, Western blot analysis of TNFR1 was performed on total cell extracts from Caco-2 cells. (B) Lentinan (500 μg/ml) was added into the apical compartment of Caco-2/RAW264.7 co-culture model for 2 h. The TNFR1 mRNA expression in Caco-2 cells was determined by quantitative RT-PCR. The values represent the means ± SE. Experiments were repeated for three times in triplicate. $^{**}P<0.01$.

lentinan exhibited *in vivo*, we used a gut inflammatory model with co-culture system as described in our previous study.

Lentinan suppressed IL-8 gene expression without affecting TNF-α production. Since lentinan was not detected in the basolateral compartment of this gut inflammation model (data not shown), it was ascertained that lentinan could not penetrate the Caco-2 monolayer. These results indicate that the inhibitory effect of lentinan on IL-8 mRNA expression is acted through the interaction between lentinan and Caco-2 cells. It has been reported that the transcriptional regulation of IL-8 genes is associated with the activation of such nuclear transcription factors as NF-κB, activator protein (AP)-1, and CCAAT/enhancer binding protein (C/EBP) [30,48,49]. Among these, the NF-κB binding site on genes has been found to be a functionally important regulatory element for IL-8 gene expression in human epithelial cells [50]. NF-κB is a complex composed of p65 and p50 and translocates to the nucleus in the presence of stimulations such as TNF-α and IL-1β [50]. As expected, the increase in the NF-κB p65 level in the nucleus was observed in this Caco-2/RAW264.7 gut inflammation model. Treatment of lentinan suppressed the increase of NF-κB level in the nucleus of Caco-2 cells. Since TNFR1 mediates TNF-α induced NF-κB activation [31,32] and is

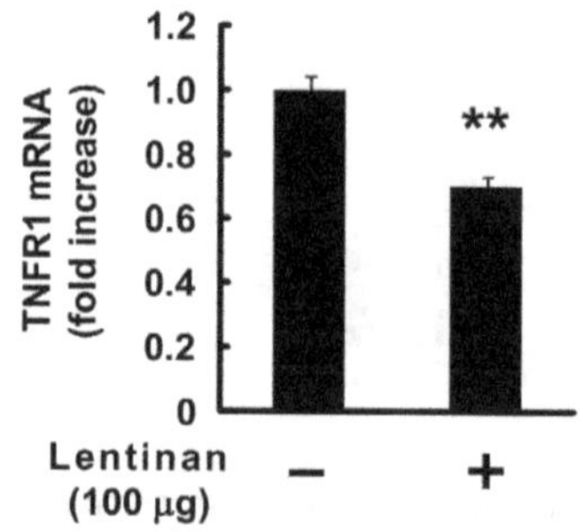

Figure 7. Lentinan suppresses TNFR1 mRNA expression in IECs *in vivo*. One hundred microliter of lentinan solution (1 mg/ml) or vehicle was injected into the separated two ligated intestinal loops which were located in mouse ileum, respectively. After incubation for 1 h, the mice were killed and the ligated intestinal loops were excised from the intestine. IECs were isolated and TNFR1 mRNA expression in the cells was determined by quantitative RT-PCR. The values represent the means ± SE. Experiments were repeated for three times in triplicate. $^{**}P<0.01$ vs. vehicle control.

crucial for murine colitis induction [33], subsequently we investigated the effect of lentinan on the receptor.

Upon ligand binding, TNFR1 initiates intracellular signal

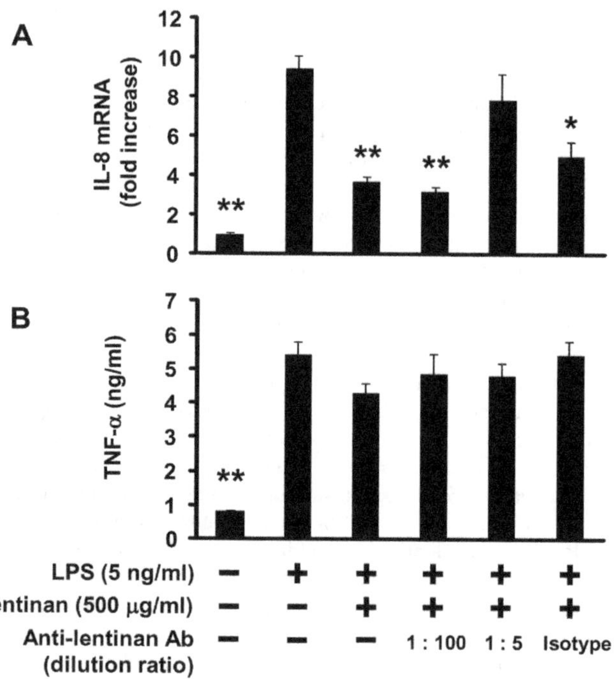

Figure 8. Effect of anti-lentinan polyclonal Ab on lentinan inhibition of IL-8 mRNA expression in Caco-2 cells. A rabbit polyclonal anti-lentinan Ab was diluted with PBS at ratios of 1:5 or 1:100, and then mixed with lentinan solution and incubated on ice for 30 min. A rabbit polyclonal isotype control Ab was used as control at the same protein concentration as anti-lentinan Ab (dilution ratio of 1:5). Antibody-treated lentinan (500 μg/ml) was added into the apical compartment of a co-culture model for 3 h. Subsequently, LPS was added to the basolateral compartment at a concentration of 5 ng/ml, followed by incubation for an additional 3 h. IL-8 mRNA expression in Caco-2 cells was determined by quantitative RT-PCR. (B) TNF-α production in the basolateral compartment was determined by a L929 cytotoxicity assay. The values represent the means ± SE. Experiments were repeated for three times in triplicate. $^{*}P<0.05$, $^{**}P<0.01$ vs. LPS control.

transduction. Two signaling pathways, leading to anti-apoptotic or pro-apoptotic responses, are known. First, ligand-activated TNFR1 promotes the activation of the transcription factor NF-κB via recruitment of TNFR-associated death domain (TRADD) protein, receptor-interacting protein-1 (RIP1) and TNFR-associated protein-2 (TRAF2) at the cell surface, leading to anti-apoptotic and pro-inflammatory responses [34]. Second, TNFR1 bound with ligand is internalized via clathrin-dependent endocytosis and TRADD recruits FAS-associated death domain protein (FADD) and caspase-8 to the internalized receptosomes, leading to cytotoxic and pro-apoptotic responses [34]. In this study, flow cytometric analysis revealed that surface levels of TNFR1 in Caco-2 cells were decreased by lentinan treatment. In addition, TNF-α-induced reduction of transepithelial electrical resistance (TER) of Caco-2 cell monolayer was not observed in lentinan-treated cells for 48 h though a significant reduction was observed in vehicle-treated cells (data not shown). It was reported that endocytosis of epidermal growth factor receptor (EGFR) in mouse colon epithelial cells resulted in desensitization because of reducing receptor accessible to its ligand [51]. These evidences indicate that TNFR1 endocytosis in Caco-2 cells by lentinan stimulation may lead to inhibit IL-8 mRNA expression via reduction of cell surface TNFR1 without inducing apoptosis. Since monodansylcadaverine altered lentinan inhibition of IL-8 mRNA expression in Caco-2 cells, it is thought that clathrin-mediated endocytosis may be involved in the pathway.

Chin *et al.* demonstrated that the receptor internalization and degradation (RID) complex, composed of two RIDα and one RIDβ protein subunits, of adenovirus plays an important role in modulating the immune response by down-regulating the surface levels of TNFR1, thereby inhibiting NF-κB activation [52]. They showed that RID is able to associate with TNFR1 on the cell surface, both RID and clathrin play an important role in mediating delivery of TNFR1 to intracellular sites that accelerate its degradation [53]. In this study, the treatment of lentinan exerted an inhibitory effect on epithelial TNFR1 expression in protein and mRNA level. In addition, lentinan also inhibited TNFR1 mRNA expression in IECs *in vivo*. These results suggest that the suppressive effect of lentinan on epithelial TNFR1 expression after the receptor endocytosis may be one of the key mechanisms for its anti-inflammatory activity on IECs. In order to obscure structure of lentinan, anti-lentinan polyclonal Ab was used in this study. As a result, treatment of anti-lentinan Ab canceled lentinan inhibition of IL-8 mRNA expression in Caco-2 cells. Although the direct interaction between lentinan and TNFR1 remains unclear, this evidence indicates that the structure of lentinan may be important for its effect on IECs. Further studies about the association between lentinan and TNFR1 or other cell surface receptors such as Dectin-1 which is known to recognize β-glucan are necessary to fully understand the mechanism of anti-inflammatory activity of lentinan.

In summary, a putative mechanism for the suppressive effect of lentinan on IL-8 mRNA expression in Caco-2 cells was demonstrated, as follows: 1) lentinan treatment induced TNFR1 endocytosis and exerted a suppressive effect on the TNFR1 expression of Caco-2 cells; 2) NF-κB translocation into the nucleus was decreased; 3) the increase in IL-8 mRNA expression was suppressed. Finally, elucidating the entire mechanism of the suppressive effect on intestinal inflammation induced by dietary β-1,3;1,6-glucan will provide valuable information toward the establishment of a new β-glucan therapy for treating patients with IBD.

Supporting Information

Figure S1 TNF-α stimulation from basolateral side is necessary for IL-8 mRNA expression in Caco-2 cells. (A) Caco-2 cells were treated with rmTNF-α (100 ng/ml) from the apical or basolateral side for 3 h. IL-8 mRNA expression in Caco-2 cells was detected by quantitative RT-PCR. $^{**}P<0.01$ vs. control. (B) Caco-2 cells were grown as monolayers in the upper chamber (normal) or on the underside of the transwell inserts (inverted) to form stable, polarized monolayers. The transwell inserts were added into multiple plate wells preloaded with RAW264.7 cells, and incubated for 3 h. Then, LPS was added into the lower chamber, followed by additional incubation for 3 h. IL-8 mRNA expression in Caco-2 cells was detected by quantitative RT-PCR. (C) TNF-α production in the basolateral compartment was determined by a L929 cytotoxicity assay. Black columns indicate normal and gray columns indicate inverted. The values represent the means ± SE ($n = 3$). $^{**}P<0.01$.

Figure S2 NF-κB p65 protein nuclear translocation in Caco-2 cells. (A) Caco-2 cells were incubated with RAW264.7 cells for 3 h. Subsequently, LPS was added to the basolateral compartment up to a final concentration of 10 ng/ml, followed by incubation for an additional 3 h. Western blot analysis of the NF-κB p65 subunit was performed on nuclear extracts from Caco-2 cells incubated for various times. (B) TNF-α production in the basolateral compartment was determined by a L929 cytotoxicity assay. The values represent the means ± SE ($n = 3$).

Figure S3 Lentinan induces alteration of TNFR1 distribution in Caco-2 cells. Lentinan (500 μg/ml) or vehicle was added into the apical compartment of Caco-2/RAW264.7 co-culture model for 5 h at 37°C. Then, immunofluorescent analysis of TNFR1 in Caco-2 cells was performed. Z-stack images of sample-treated Caco-2 cell monolayers were obtained by using a confocal laser scanning microscope. Immunofluorescent staining of TNFR1 (green) in Caco-2 cells, costained with phalloidin (red) for F-actin and TO-PRO-3 iodide (blue) for nuclei.

Text S1 Lentinan content measurement.

Text S2 Immunofluorescence staining of TNFR1 in Caco-2 cells.

Acknowledgments

We thank Yasuhito Shirai for helpful comments on the manuscript.

Author Contributions

Conceived and designed the experiments: YN MM. Performed the experiments: YN LZ. Analyzed the data: YN LZ. Contributed reagents/materials/analysis tools: MY TA KK TH MM. Wrote the paper: YN.

References

1. Haller D, Jobin C (2004) Interaction between resident luminal bacteria and the host: can a healthy relationship turn sour? J Pediatr Gastroenterol Nutr 38: 123–136.
2. Ley RE, Peterson DA, Gordon JI (2006) Ecological and evolutionary forces shaping microbial diversity in the human intestine. Cell 124: 837–848.

3. Loftus EV Jr, Sandborn WJ (2002) Epidemiology of inflammatory bowel disease. Gastroenterol Clin North Am 31: 1–20.
4. Bouma G, Strober W (2003) The immunological and genetic basis of inflammatory bowel disease. Nat Rev Immunol 3: 521–533.
5. Arai F, Takahashi T, Furukawa K, Matsushima K, Asakura H (1999) Mucosal expression of interleukin-6 and interleukin-8 messenger RNA in ulcerative colitis and Crohn's disease. Dig Dis Sci 43: 2071–2079.
6. Izutani R, Loh EY, Reinecker HC, Ohno Y, Fusunyan RD, et al. (1995) Increased expression of interleukin-8 mRNA in ulcerative colitis and Crohn's disease mucosa and epithelial cells. Inflamm Bowel Dis 1: 37–47.
7. Struyf S, Gouwy M, Dillen C, Proost P, Opdenakker G, et al. (2005) Chemokines synergize in the recruitment of circulating neutrophils into inflamed tissue. Eur J Immunol 35: 1583–1591.
8. Zareie M, Singh PK, Irvine EJ, Sherman PM, McKay DM, et al. (2001) Monocyte/macrophage activation by normal bacteria and bacterial products: implications for altered epithelial function in Crohn's disease. Am J Pathol 158: 1101–1109.
9. Murch SH, Braegger CP, Walker-Smith JA, MacDonald TT (1993) Location of tumour necrosis factor a by immunohistochemistry in chronic inflammatory bowel disease. Gut 34: 1705–1709.
10. Gerard C, Rollins BJ (2001) Chemokines and disease. Nat Immunol 2: 108–115.
11. Volman JJ, Ramakers JD, Plat J. (2008) Dietary modulation of immune function by beta-glucans. Physiol Behav 94: 276–284.
12. Williams DL (1997) Overview of (1→3)-beta-d-glucan immunobiology. Med Inflamm 6: 247–250.
13. Tzianabos AO (2000) Polysaccharide immunomodulators as therapeutic agents: structural aspects and biologic function. Clin Microbiol Rev 13: 523–533.
14. Zeković DB, Kwiatkowski S, Vrvić MM, Jakovljević D, Moran CA (2005) Natural and modified (1→3)-beta-d-glucans in health promotion and disease alleviation. Crit Rev Biotechnol 25: 205–230.
15. Sasaki T, Takasuka N (1976) Further study of the structure of lentinan, an anti-tumor polysaccharide from *Lentinus edodes*. Carbohydr Res 47: 99–104.
16. Chihara G, Hamuro J, Maeda YY, Shiio T, Suga T, et al. (1987) Antitumor and metastasis-inhibitory activities of lentinan as an immunomodulator: an overview. Cancer Detect Prev Suppl 1: 423–443.
17. Wasser SP (2002) Medicinal mushrooms as a source of antitumor and immunomodulating polysaccharides. Appl Microbiol Biotechnol 60: 258–274.
18. Tanoue T, Nishitani Y, Kanazawa K, Hashimoto T, Mizuno M (2008) In vitro model to estimate gut inflammation using co-cultured Caco-2 and RAW264.7 cells. Biochem Biophys Res Commun 374: 565–569.
19. Mizuno M, Minato K, Tsuchida H (1996) Preparation and specificity of antibodies to an anti-tumor beta-glucan, lentinan. Biochem Mol Biol Int 39: 679–685.
20. Zhang M, Huang J, Xie X, Holman CD (2009) Dietary intakes of mushrooms and green tea combine to reduce the risk of breast cancer in Chinese women. Int J Cancer 124: 1404–1408.
21. Horiguchi M, Saito A, Sonoda H (1988) A gastric cancer showing marked improvement (stage IV) with lentinan immunotherapy and 5-FU, MMC-chemotherapy. Gan To Kagaku Ryoho 15: 1973–1977.
22. Hudert CA, Weylandt KH, Lu Y, Wang J, Hong S, et al. (2006) Transgenic mice rich in endogenous omega-3 fatty acids are protected from colitis. Proc Natl Acad Sci USA 103: 11276–11281.
23. Kerékgyártó C, Virág L, Tankó L, Chihara G, Fachet J (1996) Strain differences in the cytotoxic activity and TNF production of murine macrophages stimulated by lentinan. Int J Immunopharmacol 18: 347–353.
24. Zhang L, Li N, Caicedo R, Neu J (2005) Alive and dead *Lactobacillus rhamnosus* GG decrease tumor necrosis factor-alpha–induced interleukin-8 production in Caco-2 cells. J Nutr 135: 1752–1756.
25. Gaultier A, Arandjelovic S, Niessen S, Overton CD, Linton MF, et al. (2008) Regulation of tumor necrosis factor receptor-1 and the IKK-NF-kappaB pathway by LDL receptor-related protein explains the antiinflammatory activity of this receptor. Blood 111: 5316–5325.
26. Noursadeghi M, Tsang J, Haustein T, Miller RF, Chain BM, et al. (2008) Quantitative imaging assay for NF-kappaB nuclear translocation in primary human macrophages. J Immunol Methods 329: 194–200.
27. Hase K, Ohshima S, Kawano K, Hashimoto N, Matsumoto K, et al. (2005) Distinct gene expression profiles characterize cellular phenotypes of follicle-associated epithelium and M cells. DNA Res 12: 127–137.
28. Kitajima S, Takuma S, Morimoto M (1999) Changes in colonic mucosal permeability in mouse in dextran sulfate sodium. Exp Anim 48: 137–143.
29. Mizuno M, Nishitani Y, Hashimoto T, Kanazawa K (2009) Different suppressive effects of fucoidan and lentinan on IL-8 mRNA expression in *in vitro* gut inflammation. Biosci Biotechnol Biochem 73: 2324–2325.
30. Li Q, Verma IM (2002) NF-kappaB regulation in the immune system. Nat Rev Immunol 2: 725–734.
31. Chen G, Goeddel DV (2002) TNF-R1 signaling: A beautiful pathway. Science 296: 1634–1635.
32. Chen NJ, Chio II, Lin WJ, Duncan G, Chau H, et al. (2008) Beyond tumor necrosis factor receptor: TRADD signaling in toll-like receptors. Proc Natl Acad Sci USA 105: 12429–12434.
33. Nenci A, Becker C, Wullaert A, Gareus R, van Loo G, et al. (2007) Epithelial NEMO links innate immunity to chronic intestinal inflammation. Nature 446: 557–561.
34. Schütze S, Tchikov V, Schneider-Brachert W (2008) Regulation of TNFR1 and CD95 signalling by receptor compartmentalization. Nat Rev Mol Cell Biol 9: 655–662.
35. Salisbury JL, Condeelis JS, Satir P (1980) Role of coated vesicles, microfilaments, and calmodulin in receptor-mediated endocytosis by cultured B lymphoblastoid cells. J Cell Biol 87: 132–141.
36. Wang LH, Rothberg KG, Anderson RG (1993) Mis-assembly of clathrin lattices on endosomes reveals a regulatory switch for coated pit formation. J Cell Biol 123: 1107–1117.
37. Hibi T, Inoue N, Ogata H, Naganuma M (2003) Introduction and overview: recent advances in the immunotherapy of inflammatory bowel disease. J Gastroenterol 38: 36–42.
38. Bent S, Ko R (2004) Commonly used herbal medicines in the United States: a review. Am J Med 116: 478–485.
39. Dillon S, Agrawal S, Banerjee K, Letterio J, Denning TL, et al. (2006) Yeast zymosan, a stimulus for TLR2 and dectin-1, induces regulatory antigen presenting cells and immunological tolerance. J Clin Invest 116: 916–928.
40. Rolandeli RH, Saul SH, Settle RG, Jacobs DO, Trerotola SO, et al. (1988) Comparison of parenteral nutrition and enteral feeding with pectin in experimental colitis in the rat. Am J Clin Nutr 47: 715–721.
41. Lim BO, Lee SH, Park DK, Choue RW (2003) Effect of dietary pectin on the production of immunoglobulins and cytokines by mesenteric lymph node lymphocytes in mouse colitis induced with dextran sulfate sodium. Biosci Biotechnol Biochem 67: 1706–1712.
42. Liu L, Wang ZP, Xu CT, Pan BR, Mei QB, et al. (2003) Effect of *Rheum tanguticum* polysaccharide on TNBS-induced colitis and $CD4^+$ T cells in rats. World J Gastroenterol 9: 2284–2288.
43. Nakamura M, Saito H, Kasanuki J, Tamura Y, Yoshida S (1992) Cytokine production in patients with inflammatory bowel disease. Gut 33: 933–937.
44. O'Shea JJ, Ma A, Lipsky P (2002) Cytokines and autoimmunity. Nat Rev Immunol 2: 37–45.
45. Pullman WE, Elsbury S, Kobayashi M, Hapel AJ, Doe WF (1992) Enhanced mucosal cytokine production in inflammatory bowel disease. Gastroenterology 102: 529–537.
46. Akira S, Hirano T, Taga T, Kishimoto T (1990) Biology of multifunctional cytokines: IL-6 and related molecules (IL 1 and TNF). FASEB J 4: 2860–2867.
47. Al-Sadi R, Ye D, Dokladny K, Ma TY (2008) Mechanism of IL-1β-induced increase in intestinal epithelial tight junction permeability. Immunology 180: 5653–5661.
48. Rahman I, Gilmour PS, Jimenez LA, Biswas SK, Antonicelli F, et al. (2003) Ergothioneine inhibits oxidativestress- and TNF-alpha-induced NF-kappaB activation and interleukin-8 release in alveolar epithelial cells. Biochem Biophys Res Commun 302: 860–864.
49. Zhu YM, Bradbury DA, Pang L, Knox AJ (2003) Transcriptional regulation of interleukin (IL)-8 by bradykinin inhuman airway smooth muscle cells involves prostanoid-dependent activation of AP-1 and nuclear factor (NF)-IL-6 and prostanoidindependent activation of NF-kappaB. J Biol Chem 278: 29366–29375.
50. Mukaida N, Okamoto S, Ishikawa Y, Matsushima K (1994) Molecular mechanism of interleukin-8 gene expression. J Leukoc Biol 56: 554–558.
51. McElroy SJ, Frey MR, Yan F, Edelblum KL, Goettel JA, et al. (2008) Tumor necrosis factor inhibits ligand-stimulated EGF receptor activation through a TNF receptor 1-dependent mechanism. Am J Physiol Gastrointest Liver Physiol 295: G285–293.
52. Chin YR, Horwitz MS (2006) Adenovirus RID complex enhances degradation of internalized tumour necrosis factor receptor 1 without affecting its rate of endocytosis. J Gen Virol 87: 3161–3167.
53. Chin YR, Horwitz MS (2005) Mechanism for removal of tumor necrosis factor receptor 1 from the cell surface by the adenovirus RIDα/β complex. J Virol 79: 13606–13617.

3

Reduced Intestinal Tumorigenesis in APCmin Mice Lacking Melanin-Concentrating Hormone

Jutta M. Nagel, Brenda M. Geiger, Apostolos K. A. Karagiannis, Beatriz Gras-Miralles, David Horst, Robert M. Najarian, Dimitrios C. Ziogas, XinHua Chen, Efi Kokkotou*

Division of Gastroenterology, Beth Israel Deaconess Medical Center, Harvard Medical School, Boston, Massachusetts, United States of America

Abstract

Background: Melanin-concentrating hormone (MCH) is an evolutionary conserved hypothalamic neuropeptide that in mammals primarily regulates appetite and energy balance. We have recently identified a novel role for MCH in intestinal inflammation by demonstrating attenuated experimental colitis in MCH deficient mice or wild type mice treated with an anti-MCH antibody. Therefore, targeting MCH has been proposed for the treatment of inflammatory bowel disease. Given the link between chronic intestinal inflammation and colorectal cancer, in the present study we sought to investigate whether blocking MCH might have effects on intestinal tumorigenesis that are independent of inflammation.

Methodology: Tumor development was evaluated in MCH-deficient mice crossed to the APCmin mice which develop spontaneously intestinal adenomas. A different cohort of MCH−/− and MCH+/+ mice in the APCmin background was treated with dextran sodium sulphate (DSS) to induce inflammation-dependent colorectal tumors. In Caco2 human colorectal adenocarcinoma cells, the role of MCH on cell survival, proliferation and apoptosis was investigated.

Results: APCmin mice lacking MCH developed fewer, smaller and less dysplastic tumors in the intestine and colon which at the molecular level are characterized by attenuated activation of the wnt/beta-catenin signaling pathway and increased apoptotic indices. Form a mechanistic point of view, MCH increased the survival of colonic adenocarcinoma Caco2 cells via inhibiting apoptosis, consistent with the mouse studies.

Conclusion: In addition to modulating inflammation, MCH was found to promote intestinal tumorigenesis at least in part by inhibiting epithelial cell apoptosis. Thereby, blocking MCH as a therapeutic approach is expected to decrease the risk for colorectal cancer.

Editor: Michelina Plateroti, University Claude Bernard Lyon 1, France

Funding: This work was supported by National Institutes of Health Grant DK080058, by an American Gastroenterological Association Foundation Bridging Grant and by IBD-0165 grant from the Broad Medical Research Program of The Broad Foundation (EK). The funders had no role in study design, data collection and analysis, decision to publish, or preparation of the manuscript.

Competing Interests: The authors have declared that no competing interests exist.

* E-mail: ekokkoto@bidmc.harvard.edu

Introduction

Melanin-concentrating hormone (MCH) is an evolutionarily conserved 17- to 19-amino-acid cyclic neuropeptide which was first recognized for its role in the aggregation of skin melanosomes in teleost fish in response to an environmental threat. In the last decade, important functions for MCH in mammals have emerged including the regulation of food intake, sleep, anxiety and glucose metabolism [1]. However, as of today, the focus on MCH research has been on its centrally mediated effects and, among one thousand publications concerning MCH, only twenty address aspects of its peripheral actions, an area which remains largely unexplored. This is despite reports documenting the presence of MCH in peripheral tissues and organs, including the intestine and colon [2,3,4]. Our own data also demonstrate MCH immunoreactivity in rat myenteric and submucosal plexus [5].

We have recently reported that mRNA expression of MCH and MCHR1 are upregulated in the afflicted mucosa of patients with inflammatory bowel disease (IBD) [5]. Most importantly, mice lacking MCH were found to be protected from acute experimental colitis [5] and *C. difficile* toxin-A mediated ileitis [6], suggesting a proinflammatory role of MCH. At the molecular level, we discovered that in colonic epithelial cells, MCHR1 expression is upregulated in response to an inflammatory milieu [5,6]. In turn, in the same cells activation of MCHR1 stimulated the expression of various proinflammatory cytokines and chemokines [5,6], most likely by activating erk1/2 and NFkB, as has been described for the neuropeptides substance P and neurotensin [7,8].

In the present study, we investigated whether MCH might play a role in intestinal tumorigenesis based on a) the expression of MCHR1 on colonocytes, b) our previous studies indicating the proinflammatory properties of MCH in the intestine, [5,6], and c) the well-established link between inflammation and cancer [9]. We first examined expression of MCHR1 on human colonic adenocarcinomas and in mouse LGR5 positive intestinal stem cells. Subsequently, we tested the effects of MCH on the survival and proliferation of Caco2 colonic epithelial cells. The impact of MCH ablation in intestinal tumor development was interrogated using APCmin mice, a model which shares genetic and phenotypic similarities to human colorectal neoplasia [10,11]. Notably in humans, mutations in the APC gene represent an initiating factor in the process of colon carcinogenesis and can be detected in the vast majority of familial adenomatous polyposis (FAP) patients, and in 60–80% of sporadic colorectal tumors [12].

In APCmin mice, a mutation in the *apc* gene prevents the APC complex from binding to and phosphorylating beta-catenin, a downstream effector of the wnt signalling pathway [10,13]. As a consequence, beta-catenin, instead of being marked for proteosomal degradation, is transported to the nucleus where it activates transcription of target genes, including the oncogene c-myc [14,15]. Depending on the genetic background and additional environmental factors, APCmin mice develop 30–50 intestinal adenomas, predominantly in the distal part of the small intestine [16,17,18]. However, in response to a colonic irritant like DSS, which triggers an inflammatory response, these mice develop large colonic tumors, in particular close to the rectum, well in advance of the development of tumors in their small intestine [19]. In our study we used both of these models and we obtained consistent results suggesting an inflammation-independent tumor promoting effect of MCH.

Materials and Methods

Ethics Statement

All studies were carried out according to the recommendations in the Guide for the Care and Use of Laboratory Animals of the National Institutes of Health and approved by the Beth Israel Deaconess Medical Center's Institutional Animal Care and Use Committee. To minimize suffering, mice were euthanized prior to tissue harvesting.

Mice

MCH+/− mice were crossed with APCmin/+ mice (Jackson Laboratories, Bar Harbour, Maine), both of the C57BL6 background, to yield the following compound genotypes: MCH+/+APCmin/+ and MCH−/−APCmin/+, (described herein for simplicity as WT and MCH-KO, respectively). Genotyping for MCH was performed as previously described[10]. Genotyping of APCmin mice was performed using the standard PCR protocol provided by Jackson Laboratory. LGR5 (leucine-rich-repeat-containing G-protein-coupled receptor 5)-labeled mice (Lgr5tm1(cre/ERT2)Cle/J) were purchased from Jackson Laboratories. Mice were maintained in a controlled environment with a 12 h light/dark cycle, and unlimited access to food (standard rodent chow) and water.

Intestinal Tumor Development in APCmin Mice Lacking MCH

Male MCH+/+APCmin/+ (WT) (n = 15) and MCH−/−APCmin/+ (MCH-KO) mice (n = 18) were sacrificed at 14 weeks of age and the small intestine was divided in three equal segments: proximal, medial and distal. After cleaning the small intestines by briefly washing with ice-cold PBS, tumors in each segment were counted and measured macroscopically by the same investigator using an electronic calliper (VWR). If necessary, lesions were verified using a dissecting microscope (Bausch & Lomb, Stereozoom 5, zoom range 0.8–4.0). Tissues were fixed overnight in 10% buffered formalin and the distal third of the small intestine was prepared as Swiss rolls. Paraffin-embedded H&E stained tissue sections were used for histological analysis.

DSS-induced Colorectal Tumor Development in APCmin Mice Lacking MCH

Colitis was induced in 6-week old female MCH+/+APCmin/+ (WT) (n = 24) and MCH−/−APCmin/+ (MCH-KO) mice (n = 32) by 7 days of treatment with 2% (w/v) Dextran Sulfate Sodium (DSS, MP Biomedicals, Solon, OH, USA) dissolved in their drinking water [9]. Mice were evaluated for colonic tumor development at 11 weeks of age. Colons were briefly rinsed with ice-cold PBS. Lesions were counted and measured macroscopically as described above. Tissues were then fixed overnight in 10% buffered formalin and prepared as modified Swiss rolls. Paraffin-embedded specimens were cut to 5-micrometer sections and stained with hematoxylin and eosin (H&E) for histological analyses.

Immunostaining

Immunostaining was performed in paraffin sections by the Specialized Histopathology Core at the Dana-Farber/Harvard Cancer Center. Antigen retrieval was achieved by EDTA in all cases except p-erk1/2 where citrate was used. Following endogenous peroxidase and protein blocking (Dako), the primary antibodies for Ki67 (Vector Labs cat#VP-RM04 Rabbit polyclonal, 1:250 dilution), beta-catenin (BD Pharmingen cat#610154 Mouse Monoclonal, 1:150 dilution), c-myc (Epitomics cat#1472-1 Rabbit monoclonal, 1:1000 dilution with TSA kit from PerkinElmer) and p-erk1/2 (Cell Signaling Technologies cat#4370, 1:150 dilution) were added for 1 hour followed by incubation with secondary labeled anti-mouse or anti-rabbit antibodies and color visualization (En Vision kit, DAKO). Apoptotic cells were labeled with TdT (1:16 dilution) using the ApopTag peroxidase *in situ* apoptosis detection kit (Millipore cat#S7100). Images were taken using a Zeiss Imager 1 at 10× magnification and scoring of the staining was performed by an investigator blinded to the group assignments.

In studies involving analysis of MCHR1 expression, we used a rabbit polyclonal anti-MCHR1 antibody. This antibody was raised against a conserved epitope in human, rat and mouse sequences and in an *in vitro* functional assay was found to block MCH-mediated inhibition of intracellular cAMP levels [6]. In immunohistochemical studies, the MCHR1 positive neurons identified using this antibody in brain and the enteric nervous system had the expected distribution [5]. Most importantly, treatment of mice with this anti-MCHR1 antibody resulted in attenuation of intestinal inflammation [6]. MCHR1 expression was examined in formalin-fixed intestinal frozen sections of patients with colorectal adenocarcinoma and controls (n = 4 per group, obtained from Origene), of APCmin mice with intestinal tumors, and of Lgr5tm1(cre/ERT2)Cle/J mice. MCHR1 expression was also evaluated in human (Caco2) and murine (MCA-38) colon adenocarcinoma cells grown in coverslips. Slides were incubated with anti-MCHR1 or pre-immune IgG serving as a negative control (1:200 in Protein Block-Dako) for 30 min at room temperature, followed by incubation with an Alexa Fluor-488 (green) or Alexa Fluor-546 (red) anti-rabbit secondary antibody (Invitrogen), 1:2000 in Protein Block, for 30 min at room temperature. Slides were mounted using Prolong Gold antifade with DAPI (Invitrogen). Images were taken using a Zeiss LSM510 META confocal system at 40× magnification.

Cell Treatments

Caco2 human colorectal adenocarcinoma cells were obtained from American Type Culture Collection. Cells growing in complete media (20% FBS) at 60–70% confluence were serum starved (2% FBS) overnight and then incubated for 48 hrs in media containing 2% FBS in the presence of various treatments: MCH (2.4 μg/ml, Bachem Bioscience), IGF-1(10 nM), MCH plus IGF-1, or 20% FBS as a positive control. Cell viability was measured using the MTT cell proliferation assay (ATCC). Cell proliferation was measured by BrdU incorporation using a commercially available kit (Cell Proliferation Elisa, BrdU; Roche Diagnostics). Cell apoptosis was evaluated using the Apo-One Homogenous Caspase3−/7 kit (Promega). Each experiment was performed in six replicas and was repeated twice. MCA-38 murine colon cancer cells were obtained from Dr Nicholas P. Restifo (National Cancer Institute) and cultured in RPMI 1640 media supplemented with 10% fetal calf serum and 1% antibiotic/antimycotic (Invitrogen).

Western Blot Analysis

NCM460 non-transformed human colonic epithelial cells stably expressing MCHR1 (NCM460/MCHR1) were maintained in M3D media (INCELL) supplemented with 10% fetal bovine serum and 1% antibiotic/antimycotic (Invitrogen). At 80% confluence, cells were serum starved for 16 hrs and then treated with MCH (2.4 μg/ml) for the indicated time points. Cells were harvested in 3× SDS sample buffer (Cell Signalling Technology) and protein concentration in the cell lysates was determined using the DC protein assay (Biorad). Thirty microgram of cell extracts were separated by SDS-PAGE and transferred to a PVDF membrane (Millipore). After blocking, membranes were incubated with anti-phospho erk1/2 ((Thr202/Tyr204)(Cell Signaling Technology) antibody or anti-GAPDH antibody (Santa Cruz Biotechnology) overnight at 4°C, followed by incubation with a peroxidase labeled secondary antibody (Santa Cruz Biotechnology). Specific bands were visualized in film after incubation with the SuperSignal West Pico chemiluminescent substrate (Pierce).

Statistical Analysis

Results are expressed as group mean +/− S*EM*. Data were analyzed by StatView, using unpaired t-test, ANOVA factorial followed by Fisher's PLSD analysis for multiple comparisons or a chi-square test where appropriate. A level of $p<0.05$ was considered statistically significant.

Results

MCHR1 is Expressed by Intestinal Epithelial Cells, Colonic Adenocarcinoma and Intestinal Crypt Stem Cells

In humans, we detected expression of MCHR1 in normal colonic epithelial cells as well as in colonic adenocarcinoma cells (fig 1A). Furthermore, according to the Human Protein Atlas project, among the 11 colorectal cancer samples examined, 7 showed strong MCHR1 staining of tumor cells and the remaining a moderate staining (http://www.proteinatlas.org/ENSG00000128285/cancer/colorectal+cancer). Likewise, MCHR1 was expressed in the normal mouse intestinal epithelium as well as in tumors developed in the APCmin mice (fig 1B). MCHR1 expression was also detected in a human (Caco2) and mouse (MCA-38) colon cancer cell line by immunofluorescence (fig 1, lower panels) as well as by RT-PCR (data not shown).

It has been suggested that intestinal adenomas arise from undifferentiated crypt base stem cells [20]. We thus investigated whether these stem cells are also MCHR1 positive. Intestinal crypt stem cells were labeled using a transgenic mouse that expresses eGFP under the LGR5 promoter as previously described [20]. Using an antibody against MCHR1, we demonstrated colocalization of MCH-R1 (red) with GFP-labeled LGR5- positive (green) intestinal stem cells (fig 2).

MCH Promotes Survival of Colon Adenocarcinoma Cells by Inhibiting Apoptosis

Because we had detected MCHR1 in human carcinomas, we next measured the *in vitro* effects of MCH on Caco2 cells. Treatment of these cells with MCH for 48 hours substantially increased cell viability as determined by the MTT dye conversion assay (100±7.2 vs 140.6±8.4, vehicle vs MCH treatment, respectively, $p=0.0029$; fig 3A). Two potential mechanisms may account for this observation, namely increased cell proliferation or inhibition of cell death. Indeed, MCH had a strong effect on inhibiting apoptosis in these cells (100±4.9 vs 67.6±2.5, vehicle versus MCH treatment, respectively; $p=0.0004$; fig 3B). Under the experimental conditions tested, MCH was not found to independently increase cell proliferation. However, MCH in combination with IGF-1 significantly enhanced cell proliferation (127.6+5.9 vs 166.4+11.8; IGF-1 vs IGF-1/MCH, respectively, $p=0.0026$; fig 3C). We can therefore speculate that IGF-1 and other growth factors released in the *in vivo* situation may synergize with MCH to add to their pro-proliferative effect. Treatment with MCH also increased cell survival by inhibiting apoptosis in HT-29 human colon adenocarcinoma cells and in MCA-38 murine colon carcinoma cells (data not shown).

It has been previously demonstrated that signaling via MCHR1 activates erk1/2 in HEK293 cells stably expressing MCHR1 and in 3T3L1 preadipocytes [21,22]. To test whether MCH had similar effects in colonic epithelial cells, we used a non-transformed human colonic cell line (NCM460). In these cells endogenous MCHR1 expression at baseline is very low, but it can be significantly upregulated in response to inflammation [6]. Thus these cells were stably transfected with human MCHR1 (NCM460/MCHR1), which resulted in a 5–10 fold increase in MCHR1 expression levels. Indeed, treatment of NCM460/MCHR1 cells with MCH induced erk1/2 phosphorylation in a time-dependent manner (fig. 3D).

MCH-deficiency Protects APCmin Mice Against Intestinal Adenoma Development and Progression

To determine the *in vivo* role of MCH in colorectal cancer, we evaluated spontaneous tumor development in WT ($n=15$) and MCH-KO ($n=18$) mice of the APCmin genetic background. As shown in fig 4A, WT mice started losing weight around 12 weeks of age, whereas MCH-KO mice continued to gain weight ($p=0.0355$ at sacrifice; fig 4A). At 14 weeks of age, MCH-KO mice had significantly fewer tumors in their small intestine than WT mice (51.0±4.9 vs. 76.87±7.4 tumors per mouse, respectively; $p=0.0054$, fig 4B). Differences in the number of tumors between genotypes were most pronounced in the medial (16.83±1.91 vs. 27.87±3.6 tumors per mouse; $p=0.0081$) and distal (27.06±2.77 vs. 40.83±4.55 tumors per mouse; $p=0.0122$) segments of the small intestine (fig 4C). Moreover, MCH-KO mice had smaller lesions than WT mice, especially in the groups of larger polyps (fig 4D). Supporting the macroscopic analysis at sacrifice, histologic analysis of small intestinal adenomas in the medial and distal segments of the small intestine confirmed the macroscopic results. Importantly, the number of high-grade adenomas was significantly lower in MCH-KO mice compared to WT mice (14.44±2.19 vs. 23.53±3.46, respectively; $p=0.0289$; fig 4E and 4F).

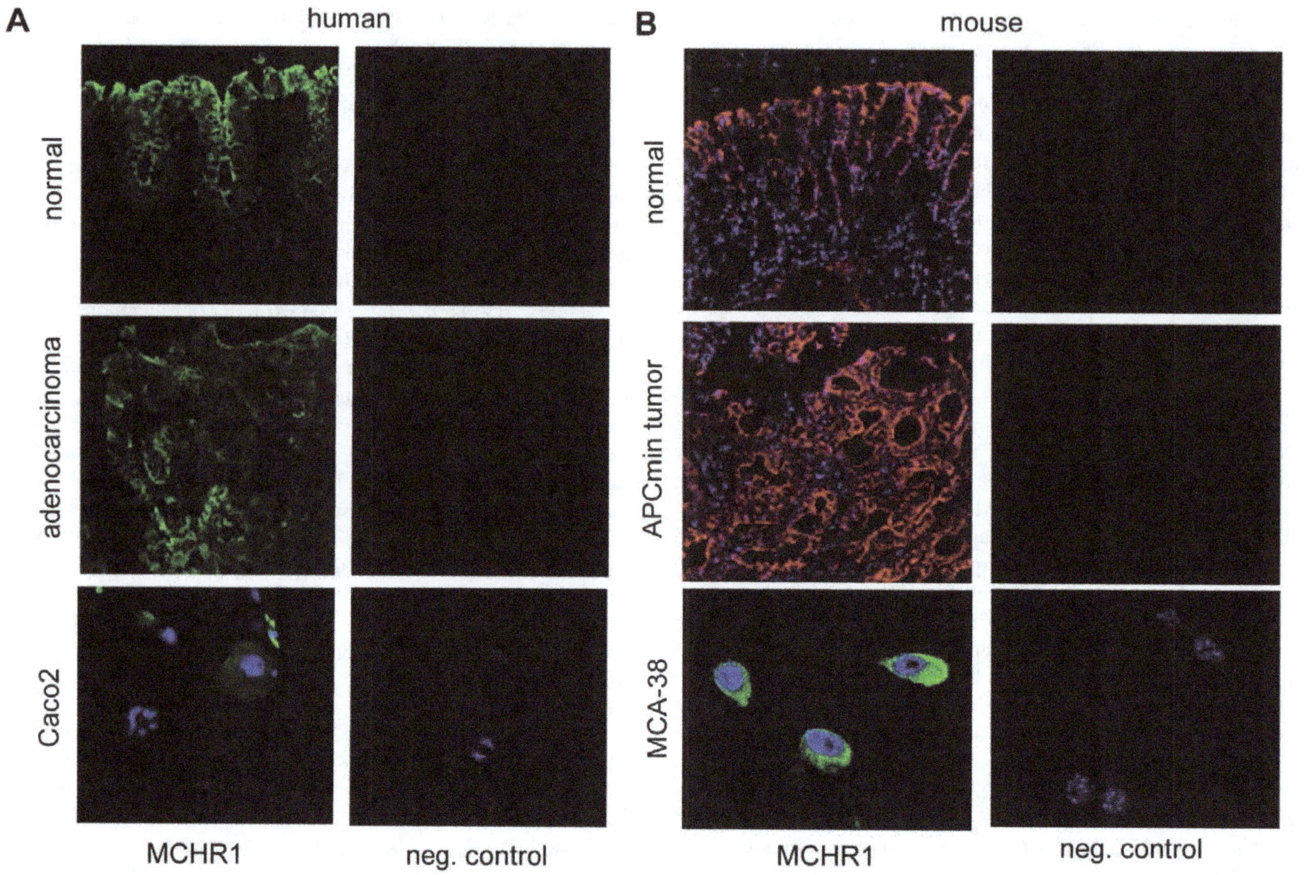

Figure 1. MCHR1 expression in normal colonic epithelial cells and colon adenocarcinoma. (A) In human colonic biopsies, normal epithelium as well as adenocarcinoma cells were positive for MCHR1 staining. Moreover, Caco2 cells, a human colon adenocarcinoma cell line, showed MCHR1 immunoreactivity. (B) Likewise, MCHR1 was found to be expressed by mouse intestinal epithelial cells, intestinal tumors developed in APCmin mice and the MCA-38 murine colon cancer cell line. Incubation with pre-immune serum was used as a negative control.

MCH-deficiency is Associated with Increased Apoptosis in Intestinal Adenomas

There are several potential mechanisms by which MCH could influence tumor development in the APCmin mice. The fact that MCH-KO mice developed fewer and smaller adenomas prompted us to examine the effects of MCH on pathways regulating cell growth and survival. Indeed, TUNEL analysis revealed that intestinal adenomas developed in MCH deficient mice had 5-fold as many apoptotic cells compared to WT mice (0.092±0.28 vs 0.458±0.117; MCH-KO vs WT, respectively; $p = 0.021$; fig 5A). These results are consistent with our *in vitro* findings of MCH increasing cell apoptosis in Caco2 colonic adenocarcinoma cells (fig 3C).

Furthermore, there was a trend of reduced cell proliferation in the adenomas developed in the MCH-KO mice, as revealed by Ki67 staining (77.2±2.2 vs 82.1±1.9; MCH-KO vs WT, respectively; $p = 0.12$; fig 5B), again consistent with our in vitro studies (fig 3D).

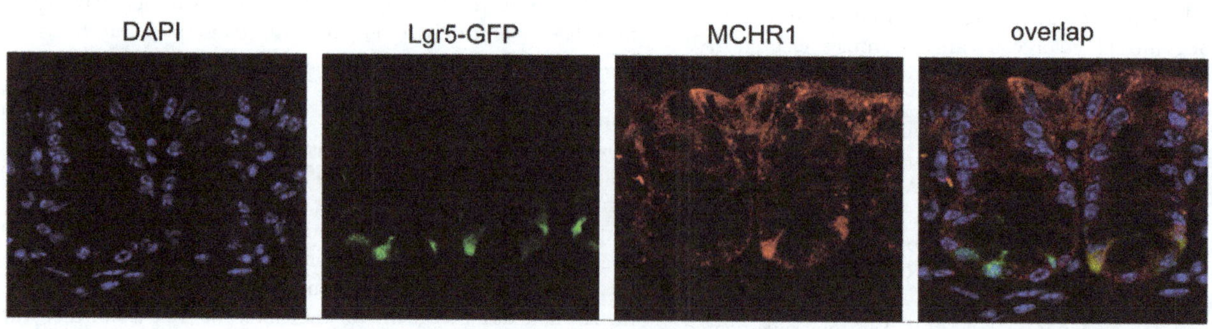

Figure 2. MCHR1 is expressed in LGR5 positive intestinal stem cells. For this experiment we used Lgr5-EGFP-IRES-creERT2 knock-in mice in which expression of EGFP was under the endogenous lgr5 promoter. Colonic biopsies from the above mice were stained with an anti-MCH antibody and co-localization (yellow) of MCHR1 (red) and LGR5 (green) was detected under a fluorescent microscope.

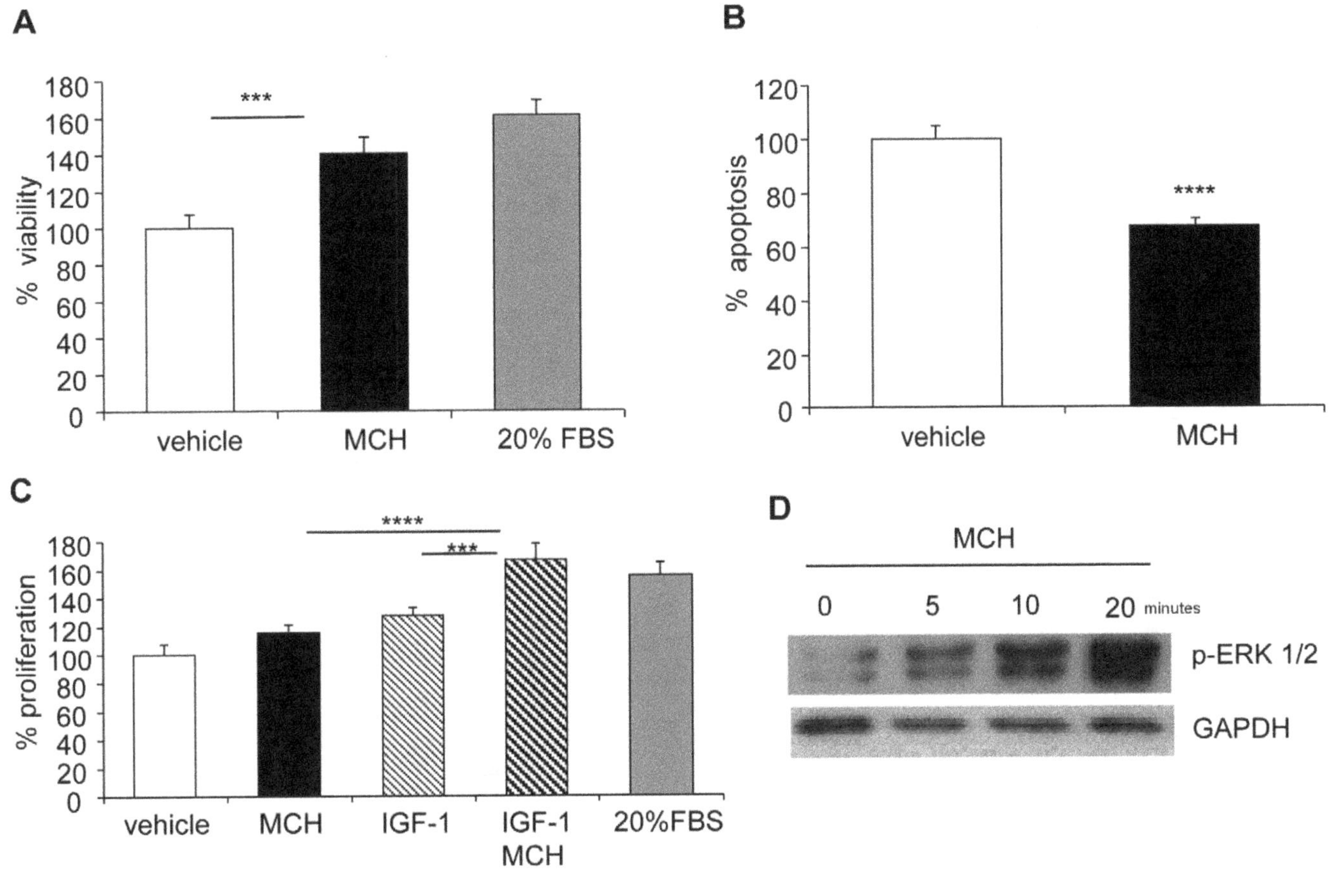

Figure 3. MCH increases cell viability *in vitro* by suppressing apoptosis. Caco2 human colonic adenocarcinoma cells were serum starved overnight (2% FBS) and treated for 48 hrs with MCH (2.4 μg/ml). (A) Cell viability was measured using the MTT assay. Treatment with 20% FBS served as a positive control. (B) Cell apoptosis was measured by the Apo-One Homogenous Caspase3−/7 assay. (C) Cells were treated with MCH (2.4 μg/ml), IGF-1 (10 nM) or their combination and cell proliferation was assessed by measuring BrdU incorporation using a colorimetric assay. Results are expressed relatively to vehicle treated cells (100). Graphs depict mean±sem of 6 replicates and are representative of 2 independent experiments. ***$p<0.005$; ****$p<0.001$ (D) NCM460 non-transformed human colonic epithelial cells stably expressing human MCHR1 (NCM460/MCHR1) were treated with MCH and erk1/2 phosphorylation at different time points was analyzed by western blot. Expression of GAPDH serves as a control for equal loading.

Attenuated Activation of the wnt/beta-catenin and erk1/2 Signaling Pathways in APCmin Mice Lacking MCH

Nuclear accumulation of beta-catenin and expression of its downstream target c-myc [14], were determined by immunohistochemistry, and were found to be more pronounced in the WT mice compared to MCH-KO mice. Specifically, in the WT mice, on average 85.9±1.2% of cells per adenoma showed nuclear accumulation of beta-catenin, while only 42.3±3.3% in MCH-KO mice ($p<0.0001$, fig 6A). This difference was apparent in adenomas, but not the surrounding normal tissue. In line with this finding, 71.9±1.7% of cells in adenomas from WT mice expressed c-myc but only 58.3±3.7% in MCH-KO mice ($p=0.0011$, fig 6B).

A recent report indicates that p-erk1/2 plays a critical role in stabilizing c-myc and promoting tumorigenesis through decreased apoptosis and increased proliferation [23]. Hence, we examined by immunohistochemistry erk1/2 phosphorylation in tumors from WT and MCH-KO mice. In WT mice, the majority of tumors had strong nuclear staining for p-erk within small parts of the adenoma, whereas MCH-KO mice often lacked p-erk1/2 staining or showed very few cells with nuclear staining in an adenoma ($p=0.0472$, fig 6C). These results are consistent with the direct activation of erk1/2 in colonocytes in response to MCH treatment, as shown in fig. 3D.

MCH-deficiency Attenuates DSS-induced Colorectal Tumor Development in APCmin Mice

In the presence of dextran sodium sulphate (DSS), an irritant that causes colonic inflammation, APCmin mice develop in a short period of time multiple colonic neoplasms [19]. We induced colitis in six-week-old MCH-KO mice and their WT littermates by treating them with DSS for 7 consecutive days. Colonic tumor development was evaluated when mice were 11 weeks of age. At this point, and compared to their initial body weight, WT mice lost slightly more weight compared to MCH-KO mice (110.52±1.79 vs. 102.25±2.19% respectively, $p=0.0132$; fig 7A). The majority of WT mice showed multiple individual lesions with clustering in the middle of the colon and near the rectum. In these mice, the rectal tumors were so dense and big that they became indistinguishable from one another (fig 7B). However, only a few of the MCH-KO mice developed confluent rectal tumors (23/32 vs. 4/24, respectively, $p=0.00004$; fig 7C). Moreover, in those MCH-KO mice with confluent rectal tumors, the length of the tumor occupied area was shorter than in WT mice

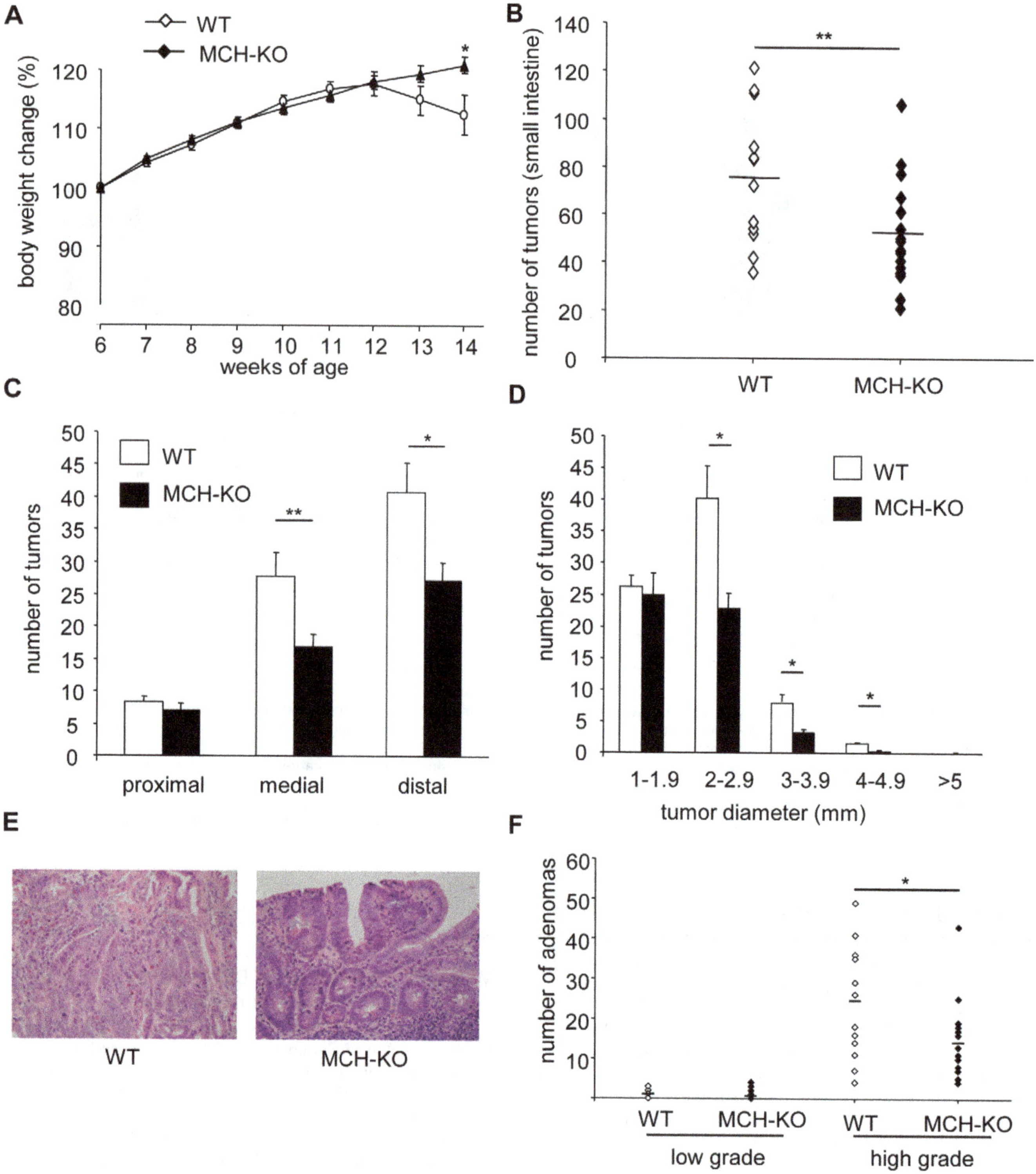

Figure 4. Reduced incidence and size of intestinal adenomas in APCmin mice lacking MCH. Mice of a compound genotype were generated, and were wild type (WT; n = 15) or deficient for MCH (MCH-KO; n = 18), all in the APCmin genetic background. At 14 weeks of age, mice were sacrificed and intestinal tumors were evaluated macroscopically and by histology. (A) Changes in body weight were expressed as % of body weight at 6 weeks of age. (B) Incidence of intestinal tumors in WT and MCH-KO mice. Horizontal bars represent the mean number of tumors per genotype. (C) Incidence of adenomas according to their location in the small intestine. (D) Distribution of intestinal tumors in WT and MCH-KO mice according to their diameter. (E) Representative H&E stained sections of a high grade adenoma in a WT mouse, and a low grade adenoma in a MCH-KO mouse. (F) Incidence of low and high grade adenomas in WT and MCH-KO mice as evaluated in H&E stained sections by a pathologist (RMN). *$p<0.05$; **$p<0.01$.

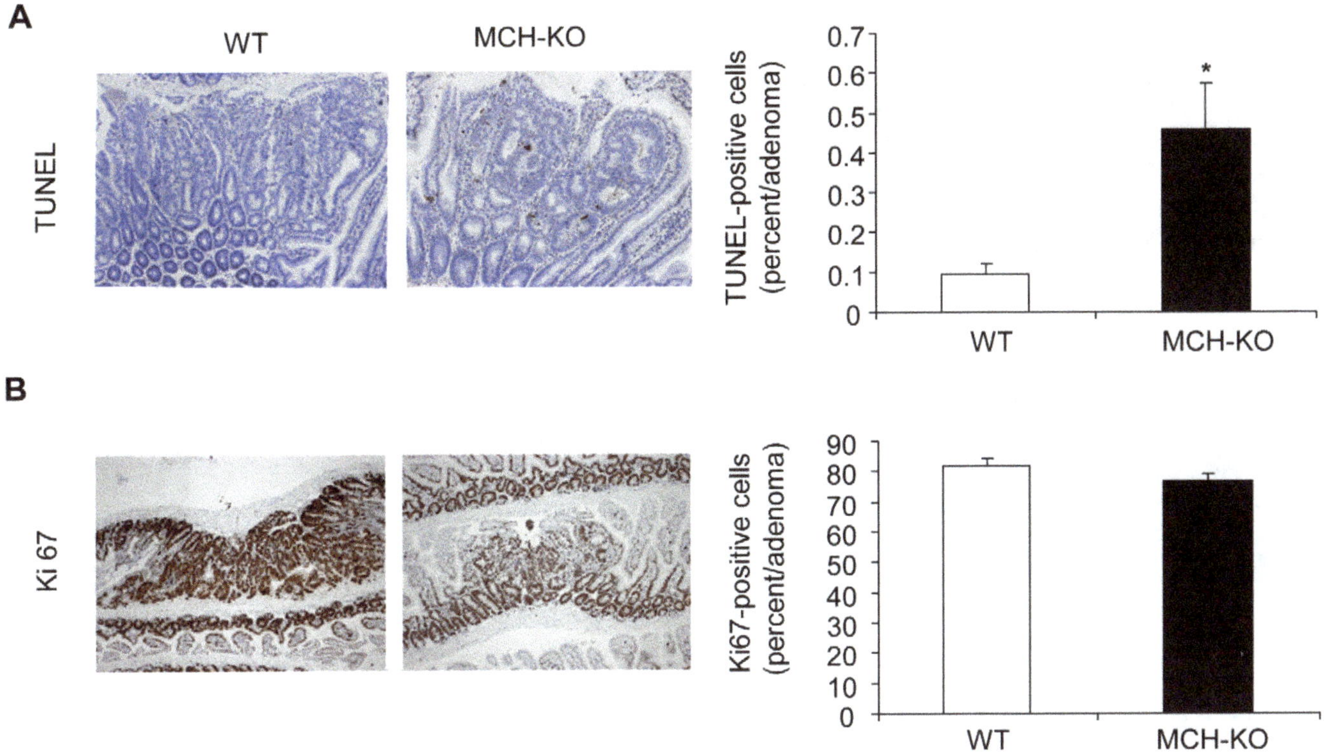

Figure 5. Increased apoptosis in intestinal adenomas developed in MCH-deficient APCmin mice. Paraffin sections of intestinal adenomas from WT and MCH-KO mice, both of the APCmin background, were stained for (A) TUNEL, a marker of apoptosis; and (B) Ki67, a marker of proliferation. Quantification of differences between the groups (percentage of positive cells per adenoma) is shown in graphs on the right of each picture. $^*p<0.05$.

(1.15 ± 0.58 mm vs. 5.34 ± 0.68 mm; $p<0.0001$; fig 7D). Since no individual tumors could be clearly distinguished in some of the cases, the percentage of colon covered by adenomas was evaluated. MCH-deficient APCmin mice had a significant increase in tumor-free area in their colon, compared to their wild-type littermates ($73.54\pm11.27\%$ vs. $58.75\pm4.81\%$, respectively, $p=0.0077$; fig 7E). Histologically, all adenomas showed high-grade dysplasia, but no invasive carcinoma was detected in either group. Furthermore, the adenomas from both groups showed mild infiltration of inflammatory cells, but no active colitis was detected. Thus, we found no indication of differences in the resolution of colitis between MCH-KO and WT mice at sacrifice. Additionally, at this time point, no differences in tumor development between WT and MCH-KO mice were apparent in the small intestine.

Discussion

The role of MCH beyond the central nervous system has not yet been fully investigated. Studies from our group and others have identified the intestine as a significant source of MCH as well as a target site for its actions [3,5,6]. In the present study, using a compound genetic model of spontaneous intestinal tumorigenesis, we describe for the first time that mice lacking MCH in the APCmin genetic background, develop fewer and smaller adenomas in their intestine and colon. The significance of this observation is corroborated by our observation of MCH receptor positive human colonic adenocarcinomas.

One intriguing and unexpected finding in the present study is the demonstration of MCHR1 expression in LGR5-positive crypt stem cells, which are considered to play a key role in the development of intestinal tumors [20]. The implications of this observation remain to be seen. In particular for the APC model, it has been shown that deletion of APC specifically in LGR5-positive cells is sufficient to give rise to adenomas within 3–5 weeks. In contrast, deletion of APC in short lived transit amplifying cells does not promote tumorigenesis [20].

Overall, our analysis of tumor development in APCmin mice lacking MCH suggests that MCH ablation affects primarily tumor growth rather than tumor formation. Several points of evidence support this conclusion. The most pronounced difference in tumor development in the MCH-KO mice was a reduction in the number of larger adenomas, whereas the number of small tumors remained comparable between the MCH-KO and WT mice as shown in fig. 4D. Furthermore, only the number of high-grade adenomas was lower in the MCH-KO mice (fig. 4F). These observations are consistent with a direct role for MCH in promoting cell survival, as our in vitro studies also indicate (fig. 3). Indeed, this is the first report demonstrating that MCH directly inhibits cell apoptosis. The exact signaling pathways leading to this effect need to be further elucidated. However, a previous study from our group has demonstrated increased levels of the tumor suppressor p53 in the liver and spleen of MCH knockout mice [24], which is consistent with the reduced size of adenomas in the MCH deficient mice reported in the current study. Moreover, it has previously been shown that in APCmin mice, deficiency of p53 enhances the number and invasiveness of the intestinal tumors [25].

We also report here that adenomas developed in MCH-deficient mice had lower expression of c-myc, compared to wild-type mice, most likely due to reduced activation of the wnt/beta-

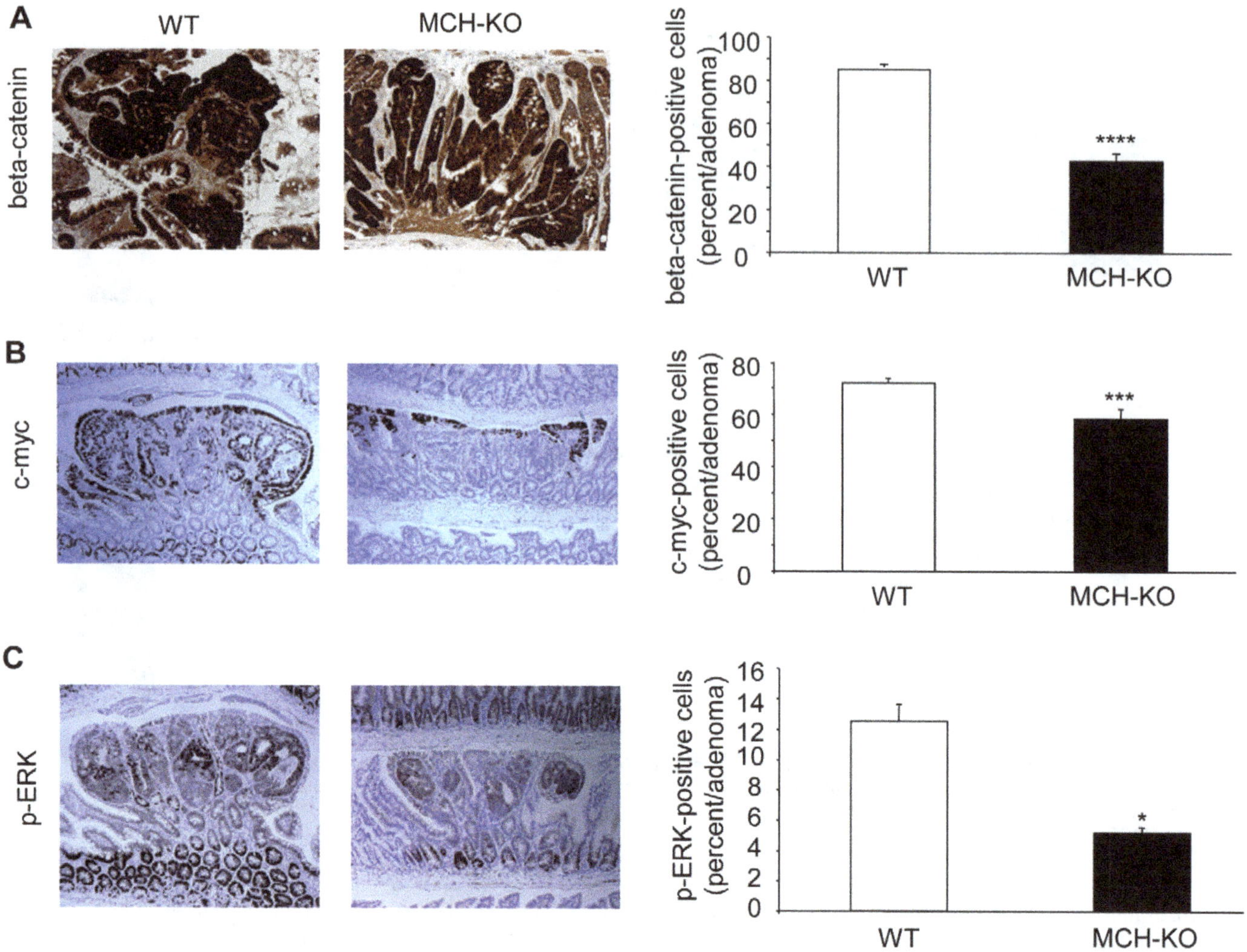

Figure 6. Attenuated activation of the wnt/beta-catenin and ERK signaling pathways in APCmin mice lacking MCH. Paraffin sections of intestinal adenomas from WT and MCH KO mice, both of the APCmin background, were stained for (A) beta-catenin, a downstream effector of the wnt signaling pathway; (B) c-myc, a target of beta-catenin; and (C) p-erk. Quantification of differences between the groups (percentage of positive cells per adenoma) is shown in graphs on the right of each picture. Results are expressed as mean±sem. ***$p<0.005$; ****$p<0.001$.

catenin pathway. C-myc is an oncogene that plays a critical role in the early stages of carcinogenesis following inactivation of APC. Besides transcriptional upregulation of c-myc by beta-catenin, it has been shown that c-myc deficiency can rescue the phenotype of mice with APC loss, even in the presence of high levels of nuclear beta-catenin [15]. Moreover, a recent study underscores the role of erk signaling in the APCmin model of intestinal tumorigenesis by demonstrating that erk can phosphorylate and stabilize c-myc, thus preventing its ubiquitination and proteasomal degradation [23]. Indeed, it has been previously shown in different cell types that activation of MCHR1 results in erk1/2 phosphorylation [21,22].

Previous studies have shown that MCH can act in combination with additional factors, for example forskolin or isoproterenol, to synergistically activate erk [21]. This might explain why in our *in vitro* experiments we were able to detect an MCH-mediated increase in cell proliferation only in the presence of IGF-1. The significance of this observation is underscored by epidemiologic and experimental evidence suggesting that IGF-1 signaling is critical in the pathogenesis of intestinal carcinogenesis [26]. It has been suggested that one of the mechanisms by which IGF-1 contributes to cell transformation is the phosphorylation of beta-catenin [27]. As such, agents targeting IGF-1 are currently under development for the treatment of colorectal cancer [28], and perhaps could be used in combination with anti-MCH treatments.

From a mechanistic point of view, this report has focused on the role of MCH on colonic epithelial cells. However, additional cell types might mediate the effects of MCH in tumorigenesis. For instance, the presence of MCHR1 on monocytes and T-cells has been previously recognized, though the biological significance of such findings remains elusive [29]. Interestingly, in activated lymphocytes, MCH appears to inhibit cell proliferation [29,30]. MCH is also produced by human microvascular endothelial cells, which might be of importance in tumor angiogenesis [31].

The concept of gut neuropeptides and hormones like MCH, modulating carcinogenesis does not appear to be unique for MCH. It has been previously shown that, like MCH, gastrin-deficient APCmin mice exhibited significant decrease in the number and proliferative capacity of intestinal adenomas [32]. On the other hand, neuropeptides known to regulate cell growth, differentiation and survival, like GLP-2, do not necessarily modify intestinal tumor growth [33].

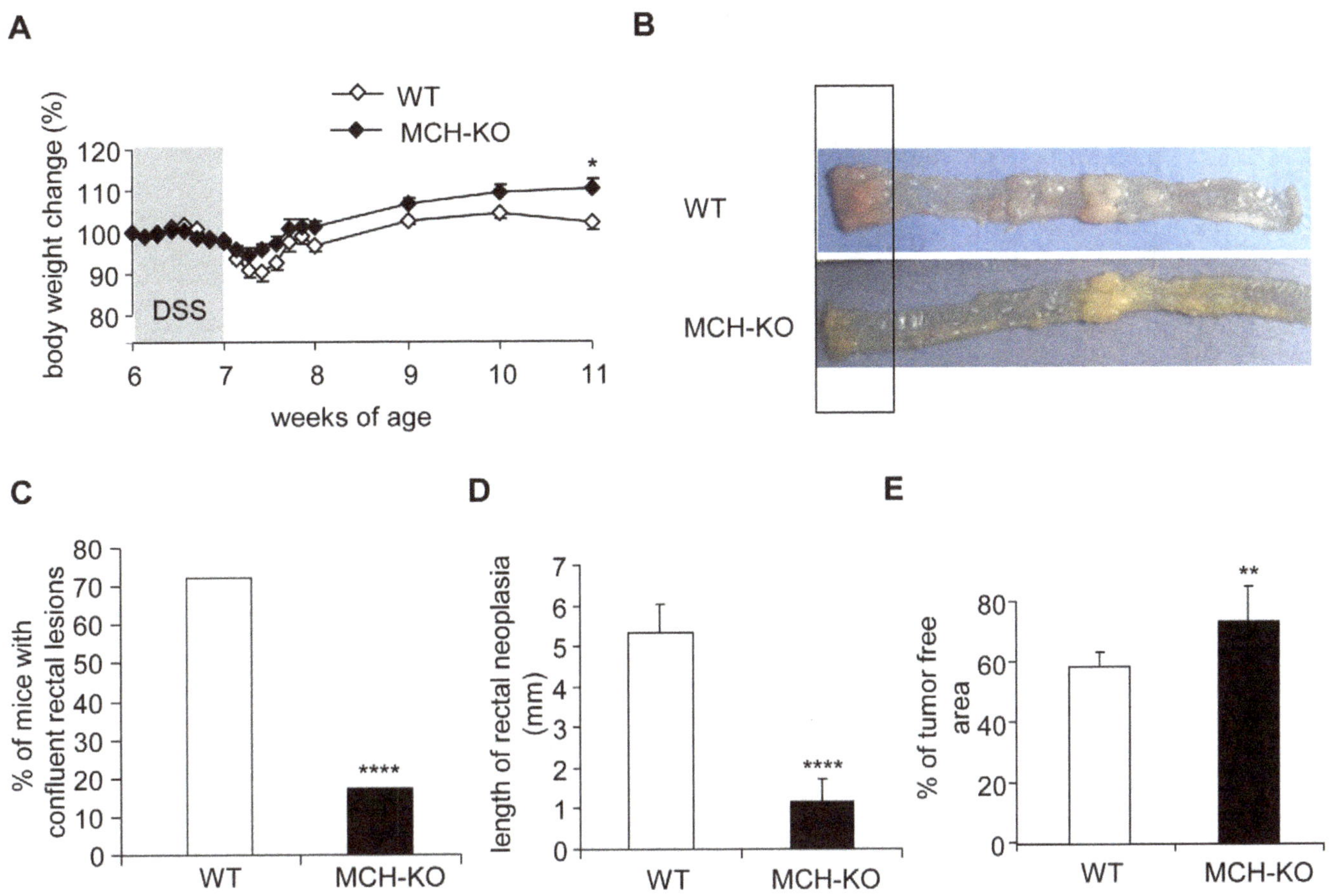

Figure 7. Reduced incidence and size of colorectal adenomas in DSS-treated APCmin lacking MCH. To induce colitis, six week old WT (n = 24) and MCH-KO (n = 32) mice, both of the APCmin background, were treated with 2% DSS in their drinking water for 7 days. At 11 weeks of age, mice were evaluated for colonic tumor development. (A) Changes in body weight over time in mice treated with DSS are expressed as % of their body weight at 6 weeks of age. (B) Representative pictures of tumor development patterns in the colon of WT and MCH-KO mice. Striking differences in tumor development between the two genotypes were noted in the rectal area. (C) Not only a lower percentage of MCH KO mice developed colorectal lesions, but (D) also the size of these lesions was smaller in the MCH-KO mice. (E) Percentage of adenoma-free area in the colon of WT and MCH-KO mice. *$p<0.05$; **$p<0.01$; ****$p<0.001$.

Often, chronic inflammation predisposes to cancer development via multiple mechanisms [34] and epidemiological evidence suggests that patients with inflammatory bowel disease (IBD) are at increased risk for colorectal cancer. A recent report estimated that incidence rates of cancer in patients with IBD was 75 per 100,000 person years compared to 47 per 100,000 person-years in patients without IBD [35]. Notably, in patients with IBD we have found a significant upregulation of MCH and its receptor, which correlated positively with the severity of the disease [5]. In this context, MCH not only promotes intestinal inflammation as we have previously demonstrated [5,6], which is a predisposing factor for tumorigenesis, but also, based on the present study, it contributes to intestinal tumor growth independently of inflammation. Combined, these properties render MCH an attractive target for the treatment of inflammatory bowel disease, which will also reduce the risk of subsequent cancer development. Indeed, during the last decade there is an ongoing investigation by many pharmaceutical companies on MCH antagonists, primarily for the treatment of obesity [1]. The fields of IBD and cancer therapeutics are likely to benefit in the foreseeable future by taking advantage of this momentum.

Acknowledgments

We thank Dr. Eleftheria Maratos-Flier for kindly providing us with MCH knockout breeding pairs and Dr Simon Robson for sharing with us the MCA-38 cells.

Author Contributions

Conceived and designed the experiments: JN DZ XC EK. Performed the experiments: JN BG AK BGM. Analyzed the data: JN BG AK DH RN EK. Wrote the paper: JN BG EK. Revised the manuscript: EK JN BG AK BGM DH RN DZ XC.

References

1. Chung S, Parks GS, Lee C, Civelli O (2011) Recent updates on the melanin-concentrating hormone (MCH) and its receptor system: lessons from MCH1R antagonists. J Mol Neurosci 43: 115–121.
2. Hervieu G, Nahon JL (1995) Pro-melanin concentrating hormone messenger ribonucleic acid and peptides expression in peripheral tissues of the rat. Neuroendocrinology 61: 348–364.

3. Hervieu G, Volant K, Grishina O, Descroix-Vagne M, Nahon JL (1996) Similarities in cellular expression and functions of melanin-concentrating hormone and atrial natriuretic factor in the rat digestive tract. Endocrinology 137: 561–571.
4. Burdyga G, Varro A, Dimaline R, Thompson DG, Dockray GJ (2006) Feeding-dependent depression of melanin-concentrating hormone and melanin-concentrating hormone receptor-1 expression in vagal afferent neurones. Neuroscience 137: 1405–1415.
5. Kokkotou E, Moss AC, Torres D, Karagiannides I, Cheifetz A, et al. (2008) Melanin-concentrating hormone as a mediator of intestinal inflammation. Proc Natl Acad Sci U S A 105: 10613–10618.
6. Kokkotou E, Espinoza DO, Torres D, Karagiannides I, Kosteletos S, et al. (2009) Melanin-concentrating hormone (MCH) modulates C difficile toxin A-mediated enteritis in mice. Gut 58: 34–40.
7. Zhao D, Zhan Y, Zeng H, Koon HW, Moyer MP, et al. (2005) Neurotensin stimulates interleukin-8 expression through modulation of I kappa B alpha phosphorylation and p65 transcriptional activity: involvement of protein kinase C alpha. Mol Pharmacol 67: 2025–2031.
8. Koon HW, Zhao D, Na X, Moyer MP, Pothoulakis C (2004) Metalloproteinases and transforming growth factor-alpha mediate substance P-induced mitogen-activated protein kinase activation and proliferation in human colonocytes. J Biol Chem 279: 45519–45527.
9. Coussens LM, Werb Z (2002) Inflammation and cancer. Nature 420: 860–867.
10. White BD, Chien AJ, Dawson DW (2012) Dysregulation of Wnt/beta-Catenin Signaling in Gastrointestinal Cancers. Gastroenterology 142: 219–232.
11. Taketo MM, Edelmann W (2009) Mouse models of colon cancer. Gastroenterology 136: 780–798.
12. Powell SM, Zilz N, Beazer-Barclay Y, Bryan TM, Hamilton SR, et al. (1992) APC mutations occur early during colorectal tumorigenesis. Nature 359: 235–237.
13. Korinek V, Barker N, Morin PJ, van Wichen D, de Weger R, et al. (1997) Constitutive transcriptional activation by a beta-catenin-Tcf complex in APC−/− colon carcinoma. Science 275: 1784–1787.
14. He TC, Sparks AB, Rago C, Hermeking H, Zawel L, et al. (1998) Identification of c-MYC as a target of the APC pathway. Science 281: 1509–1512.
15. Sansom OJ, Meniel VS, Muncan V, Phesse TJ, Wilkins JA, et al. (2007) Myc deletion rescues Apc deficiency in the small intestine. Nature 446: 676–679.
16. Su LK, Kinzler KW, Vogelstein B, Preisinger AC, Moser AR, et al. (1992) Multiple intestinal neoplasia caused by a mutation in the murine homolog of the APC gene. Science 256: 668–670.
17. Dietrich WF, Lander ES, Smith JS, Moser AR, Gould KA, et al. (1993) Genetic identification of Mom-1, a major modifier locus affecting Min-induced intestinal neoplasia in the mouse. Cell 75: 631–639.
18. Wasan HS, Novelli M, Bee J, Bodmer WF (1997) Dietary fat influences on polyp phenotype in multiple intestinal neoplasia mice. Proc Natl Acad Sci U S A 94: 3308–3313.
19. Tanaka T, Kohno H, Suzuki R, Hata K, Sugie S, et al. (2006) Dextran sodium sulfate strongly promotes colorectal carcinogenesis in Apc(Min/+) mice: inflammatory stimuli by dextran sodium sulfate results in development of multiple colonic neoplasms. Int J Cancer 118: 25–34.
20. Barker N, Ridgway RA, van Es JH, van de Wetering M, Begthel H, et al. (2009) Crypt stem cells as the cells-of-origin of intestinal cancer. Nature 457: 608–611.
21. Pissios P, Trombly DJ, Tzameli I, Maratos-Flier E (2003) Melanin-concentrating hormone receptor 1 activates extracellular signal-regulated kinase and synergizes with G(s)-coupled pathways. Endocrinology 144: 3514–3523.
22. Bradley RL, Mansfield JP, Maratos-Flier E, Cheatham B (2002) Melanin-concentrating hormone activates signaling pathways in 3T3-L1 adipocytes. Am J Physiol Endocrinol Metab 283: E584–592.
23. Lee SH, Hu LL, Gonzalez-Navajas J, Seo GS, Shen C, et al. (2010) ERK activation drives intestinal tumorigenesis in Apc(min/+) mice. Nat Med 16: 665–670.
24. Jeon JY, Bradley RL, Kokkotou EG, Marino FE, Wang X, et al. (2006) MCH−/− mice are resistant to aging-associated increases in body weight and insulin resistance. Diabetes 55: 428–434.
25. Halberg RB, Katzung DS, Hoff PD, Moser AR, Cole CE, et al. (2000) Tumorigenesis in the multiple intestinal neoplasia mouse: redundancy of negative regulators and specificity of modifiers. Proc Natl Acad Sci U S A 97: 3461–3466.
26. Guo YS, Narayan S, Yallampalli C, Singh P (1992) Characterization of insulinlike growth factor I receptors in human colon cancer. Gastroenterology 102: 1101–1108.
27. Playford MP, Bicknell D, Bodmer WF, Macaulay VM (2000) Insulin-like growth factor 1 regulates the location, stability, and transcriptional activity of beta-catenin. Proc Natl Acad Sci U S A 97: 12103–12108.
28. Adachi Y, Yamamoto H, Ohashi H, Endo T, Carbone DP, et al. (2010) A candidate targeting molecule of insulin-like growth factor-I receptor for gastrointestinal cancers. World J Gastroenterol 16: 5779–5789.
29. Lakaye B, Coumans B, Harray S, Grisar T (2009) Melanin-concentrating hormone and immune function. Peptides 30: 2076–2080.
30. Verlaet M, Adamantidis A, Coumans B, Chanas G, Zorzi W, et al. (2002) Human immune cells express ppMCH mRNA and functional MCHR1 receptor. FEBS Lett 527: 205–210.
31. Orihara K, Morita H, Yagami A, Kajiwara N, Nakae S, et al. (2009) TH2 cytokines potently induce an appetite-stimulating peptide, melanin-concentrating hormone, in human vascular endothelial cells. J Allergy Clin Immunol 124: 612–614, 614 e611–612.
32. Koh TJ, Bulitta CJ, Fleming JV, Dockray GJ, Varro A, et al. (2000) Gastrin is a target of the beta-catenin/TCF-4 growth-signaling pathway in a model of intestinal polyposis. J Clin Invest 106: 533–539.
33. Koehler JA, Harper W, Barnard M, Yusta B, Drucker DJ (2008) Glucagon-like peptide-2 does not modify the growth or survival of murine or human intestinal tumor cells. Cancer Res 68: 7897–7904.
34. O'Connor PM, Lapointe TK, Beck PL, Buret AG (2010) Mechanisms by which inflammation may increase intestinal cancer risk in inflammatory bowel disease. Inflamm Bowel Dis 16: 1411–1420.
35. Herrinton LJ, Liu L, Levin TR, Allison JE, Lewis JD, et al. (2012) Incidence and Mortality of Colorectal Adenocarcinoma in Persons with Inflammatory Bowel Disease from 1998 to 2010. Gastroenterology.

4

Deoxynivalenol as a new Factor in the Persistence of Intestinal Inflammatory Diseases: An Emerging Hypothesis through Possible Modulation of Th17-Mediated Response

Patricia M. Cano[1,2]☯, Julie Seeboth[1,2]☯, François Meurens[3,6], Juliette Cognie[4], Roberta Abrami[1,2,5], Isabelle P. Oswald[1,2]*, Laurence Guzylack-Piriou[1,2]*

1 INRA, UMR1331, Toxalim, Research Centre in Food Toxicology, Toulouse, France, **2** Université de Toulouse, INPT, UMR1331, Toxalim, Toulouse, France, **3** INRA, UMR1282 Infectiologie et Santé Publique, Nouzilly, France, **4** INRA, Physiologie de la Reproduction et des Comportements, Nouzilly, France, **5** Universidade Estadual de Londrina, Lab Patologia Animal, Londrina, Brazil, **6** Vaccine and Infectious Disease Organization, University of Saskatchewan, Saskatoon, Saskatchewan, Canada

Abstract

Background/Aims: Deoxynivalenol (DON) is a mycotoxin produced by *Fusarium* species which is commonly found in temperate regions worldwide as a natural contaminant of cereals. It is of great concern not only in terms of economic losses but also in terms of animal and public health. The digestive tract is the first and main target of this food contaminant and it represents a major site of immune tolerance. A finely tuned cross-talk between the innate and the adaptive immune systems ensures the homeostatic equilibrium between the mucosal immune system and commensal microorganisms. The aim of this study was to analyze the impact of DON on the intestinal immune response.

Methodology: Non-transformed intestinal porcine epithelial cells IPEC-1 and porcine jejunal explants were used to investigate the effect of DON on the intestinal immune response and the modulation of naive T cells differentiation. Transcriptomic proteomic and flow cytometry analysis were performed.

Results: DON induced a pro-inflammatory response with a significant increase of expression of mRNA encoding for IL-8, IL-1α and IL-1β, TNF-α in all used models. Additionally, DON significantly induced the expression of genes involved in the differentiation of Th17 cells (STAT3, IL-17A, IL-6, IL-1β) at the expenses of the pathway of regulatory T cells (Treg) (FoxP3, RALDH1). DON also induced genes related to the pathogenic Th17 cells subset such as IL-23A, IL-22 and IL-21 and not genes related to the regulatory Th17 cells (rTh17) such as TGF-β and IL-10.

Conclusion: DON triggered multiple immune modulatory effects which could be associated with an increased susceptibility to intestinal inflammatory diseases.

Editor: Niels Olsen Saraiva Câmara, Universidade de Sao Paulo, Brazil

Funding: Patricia Cano, Julie Seeboth and Roberta Abrami were supported by a doctoral fellowships financed by INRA and ANSES (France), the Ministry for Education and Research (France), CAPES-COFECUB (Brazil) respectively. This study was supported by the EU projects INTERPLAY (FP7-KBBE-KBBE-2008–2B), MycoRed (FP7-KBBE-2007–2A) and by a grant for newly recruited scientist from INRA-Division of animal health. The funders had no role in study design, data collection and analysis, decision to publish, or preparation of the manuscript.

Competing Interests: The authors have declared that no competing interests exist.

* E-mail: laurence.guzylack@toulouse.inra.fr (LGP); isabelle.oswald@toulouse.inra.fr (IPO)

☯ These authors contributed equally to this work.

Introduction

Mycotoxins are fungal secondary metabolites that commonly contaminate human food and animal feed. Given their global and frequent occurrence, their stability through the food processing chain [1] as well as their known toxic effects, mycotoxins have become a major concern in Europe and North America. Their effects on humans and domestic animals range from decreased resistance to infectious diseases and growth impairment, to cancer induction and death [2,3,4].

Deoxynivalenol (DON) is a mycotoxin of the trichothecenes family mainly produced by *Fusarium graminearum* and *F. culmorum.* Although it is not the most acutely toxic trichothecene, DON is regarded as an important food safety issue since it is the most prevalent trichothecene in wheat, corn, barley and their by-products in Europe and North America [5,6]. Toxicity of DON has been largely demonstrated for humans and all animal species tested [7] but swine, which are readily exposed to this toxin through their cereal-rich diet, are the most sensitive [8]. Therefore they make an excellent research model for animal and even human exposure to DON due to higher similarities concerning the digestive and the immune system than other animal models [9,10]. Acute exposure to high doses of DON results in diarrhea, vomiting, leukocytosis, gastrointestinal hemorrhage and ultimately death whereas chronical exposure to low doses of this toxin induces anorexia, reduced weight gain and altered nutritional efficiency [7].

This toxin specifically targets dividing cells such as intestinal epithelial cells and immune cells [11]. It can alter the expression of transcription factors by readily binding to the ribosomes and rapidly activating mitogen-activated protein kinases (MAPKs), thus possibly affecting cytokines production and membrane receptors [12].

The intestinal tract is the first physical barrier against food contaminants, chemicals and intestinal pathogens and as such, it plays an important role in the regulation of the immune response to these intrusions. Previous studies have demonstrated that intestinal absorbance of DON takes mainly place in the jejunum both directly from the intestinal lumen to the apical side of the intestinal epithelium and also indirectly through already absorbed toxin reaching the intestinal epithelial cells (IECs) from the blood stream to the basolateral side [13]. Low doses of this toxin can induce morphological and histological impairments of IECs such as atrophy and fusion of the villi [14,15]. It can also decrease the number of goblet cells [14] and alter the intestinal permeability by repressing the expression of tight junction proteins such as claudins 3-4, ZO-1 and occludin [14,16,17,18]. Basolateral exposure to DON recently showed to have a more severe impact on the intestinal barrier integrity and DNA fragmentation than apical exposure [19].

As a defense mechanism, the intestinal epithelial cells are able to produce several pro-inflammatory cytokines such as the tumor necrosis factor-alpha (TNF-α), interleukin (IL)-6 and different chemokines such as IL-8 and the CC-chemokine ligand (CCL)-20 that are crucial for the recruitment and activation of the underlying immune cells of the *lamina propria* [20]. IECs also have a particularly close interaction with dendritic cells (DCs) that play an essential role in the initiation of the adaptive immune response mediated for the most part by $CD4^+$ T helper (Th) cells. Depending on the local intestinal environment, different populations of DCs shape the immune response by activating naive T cells and inducing their differentiation into specific effector T cell populations [21]. Against intracellular infections, Th1 cells are induced to secrete interferon-gamma (IFN-γ) and IL-12 and regulate cellular immunity. DCs are also strongly implicated in the maintenance of tolerance by inducing T regulatory cells (Tregs) that secrete IL-10 and the tumor growth factor beta (TGF-β). Another subset of T helper lymphocytes, the Th17, was recently described as an important mediator of mucosal immunity, defense against extracellular pathogens and autoimmunity [22]. Interestingly, Th17 cells have been related to both pathogenic and regulatory responses, which are generated by two distinct populations of Th17 with a common signature cytokine, IL-17A [23,24]. The dichotomy of Th17 cells results from different stimuli: IL-6, IL-1β and IL-23 promote the expression of pro-inflammatory cytokines by the so-called pathogenic Th17 whereas IL-6 and TGF-β restrain the pathogenic potential of these cells by inducing the production of IL-10 by regulatory Th17 (rTh17) [23,24]. The same plasticity allows induced Tregs to reverse their phenotype and acquire the functions of pathogenic Th17 when cultured with IL-6 [25]. Plasticity of T lymphocytes ensures the adequacy of the immune response to an offensive situation and is critical to maintain the balance between protection and homeostasis. All of this relies on a well-established communication between IECs, DCs and the different T helper cell subsets. The damages caused to the intestinal epithelium by exposure to DON could disrupt these interactions and thus lead to severe disturbances of the intestinal immune system. Taken together, all of this could lead to persistent tissue inflammation and eventually, to chronic intestinal inflammatory diseases such as intestinal bowel disease (IBD) characterized by a dysfunctional intestinal barrier and autoimmune responses. DON could play a role in the induction and/or persistence of such inflammatory diseases [26]. However it is noteworthy that few publications have paid attention to the intestinal effects of DON, and even less to the effect of DON on the above mentioned balance between T cells populations.

The aim of this study was to analyze the influence of a low but relevant concentration of DON on the cytokines levels produced by the different subsets of intestinal T lymphocytes using three methodological approaches: *in vitro*, a non transformed porcine intestinal epithelial cell line (IPEC-1) [16,17] and *ex vivo* porcine intestinal explants [27].

Materials and Methods

Chemicals

Purified DON stock (Sigma Aldrich, Ayshire, UK) was dissolved in dimethylsulfoxide (DMSO) and stored at −20°C before dilution in complete cell culture media. Control samples were treated with equivalent concentrations of DMSO, which were non cytotoxic.

Treatment of the Intestinal Epithelial Cell Line IPEC-1

The Intestinal Porcine Epithelial cell line (IPEC-1) was derived from the small intestine of a newborn unsuckled piglet [28]. IPEC-1 cells are capable of differentiating into mature enterocytes to form a uniform and polarized epithelial layer that suitably mimics the intestinal epithelial barrier and its apico-basolateral discrimination. They have been largely previously used to study bacterial infections, intestinal epithelial integrity, and trans-epithelial transport [18,29,30].

IPEC-1 cells were grown and differentiated as previously described [31]. Briefly, cells were seeded into 4.2 cm^2 polyethylene terephtalate membrane inserts with 0.4 µm pore size (Beckon Dickinson, Pont de Claix, France) at 2 x 10^5 cells per well in 2 ml of growth media. Treatments were applied to the apical compartments of the inserts.

IPEC-1 cells were incubated for 1.5 h, 4 h, 8 h, 12 h or 24 h in the presence of 10 µM of DON or DMSO at 39°C in a humidified atmosphere of 5% CO_2. After treatment, supernatants were collected to evaluate cytokine production and cells were harvested for transcriptional analysis.

Treatment of Explants Cultures

All animal experiments were carried out in accordance with European Guidelines for the Care and Use of Animals for Research Purposes. Jejunal tissue was obtained from six piglets which were 5 week-old, 7–days after weaning. Animals were fed ad libitum prior to the experiment. A 5 cm middle jejunum segment was collected in pre-warmed Williams media (Sigma) supplemented with 200 U/mL penicillin and 200 µg/mL streptomycin (Eurobio, Courtaboeuf, France). It was washed twice and opened longitudinally. Then, the external *tunica muscularis* was removed and explants were made with punch trocards (centravet, Lapalisse, France) and were placed in Williams culture media supplemented with 1% of penicillin/streptomycin, 0.5% of gentamycine (Eurobio), 4.5 g/L of glucose (Sigma), 10% FBS (Eurobio) and 30 mM of amino acid (Ala/Glu) (Eurobio). Pig jejunal explants were incubated with 10 µM of DON or DMSO for 4 h, 8 h or 12 h at 39°C in a humidified atmosphere of 5% CO_2. After treatment, tissues were collected for transcriptional analysis.

IL-8, IL-1 Alpha and IL-17 Cytokine Assays

Concentrations of IL8 and IL-1 alpha were measured by enzyme linked immuno-absorbent assays (ELISA) using specific kits for porcine IL8 and IL-1 alpha (R&D Systems, Minneapolis, MN, USA). Plates were washed with PBS/Tween 20 and then blocked with PBS containing 1% BSA (w/v) for 1 h at room temperature (RT). Supernatant samples were added to the ELISA plate in duplicate and incubated for 2 h at RT. After washing, wells were incubated with biotinylated specific detection antibodies for porcine IL8 and porcine IL1-alpha (R&D Systems) for 2 h at RT. Then, streptavidin-HRP-conjugated antibody (Thermo Fisher Scientific, Courtaboeuf, France) was added for 30 min at 37°C. Positive reactions were revealed by 3,3′,5,5′-tetramethylbenzidine (TMB) (Thermo Fisher Scientific) and reactions were stopped with H_2SO_4 2 N. The optical density (OD) was read at 450 nm.

Cytokine IL-17 was measured using the swine IL-17A VetSet™ ELISA Development kits (Kingfisher biotech, St.Paul, MN, USA).

RNA Extraction and Quantitative Real-Time Polymerase Chain Reaction (qRT-PCR) Analysis

Quantitative real-time PCR (qPCR) was performed to determine the relative mRNA expression levels of chemokines, interleukins, chemokines receptors, enzymes, and several transcription factors involved in the modulation of the intestinal immune response. Total RNA from IPEC-1 cultures and jejunal explants was extracted with Trizol Reagent (Extract all, Eurobio). RNA concentration, integrity and quality were determined spectrophotometrically using Nanodrop ND1000 (Labtech International, Paris, France). RIN of these mRNA fluctuated between 6.80 and 4.70 for 4 hours and 12 hours of culture times, respectively. Then, reverse transcription and real-time qPCR steps were performed as previously described [32]. Non-reverse transcripted RNA was used as non-template control for verification of genomic DNA amplification signal. Specificity of qPCR products was assessed at the end of the reactions by analyzing dissociation curves. Primers were purchased from Invitrogen (Invitrogen, Life Technologies Corporation, Paisley, UK). Specific sequences were specified in tableô 1. Amplification efficiency and initial fluorescence were determined by the ΔΔCt method, then obtained values were normalized using two reference genes, ribosomal protein L32 (RPL32) and cyclophilline A [33]. Stability of these genes was demonstrated previously in intestinal tissues [34]. mRNA expression levels were expressed relative to the mean of the control group at 4 h of exposure to DMSO alone.

Analysis of T Regulatory Cells Phenotype in Lamina Propria Cultured With DON

Leucocytes were isolated from jejunal lamina propria harvested from two pigs by collagenase digestion as described previously [35]. Briefly, pieces of small intestine were incubated for 2 times 45 min in several changes of calcium and magnesium-free Hank's balanced salt solution (HBSS), containing 1 mM of ethylenediamine tetra-acetic acid (EDTA) at 37°C on a shaking platform. This procedure largely removed the epithelial layer. The remaining tissue was then digested in RPMI-1640 containing 0.36 g/ml of collagenase (Collagenase Grade V, Sigma), 10% of FBS, 20 mM of Hepes (Eurobio, Paris, France) and 2000 U/ml of Dnase1 (Roche diagnostics, Mannheim, Germany) at 37°C for 1 h on a shaking platform. Cells were suspended in a 40% Percoll in RPMI solution and underlaid with a 80% Percoll solution (Pharmacia, Uppsala, sweden). Low-density cells were recovered from the 40%/80% gradient interface. Cell suspensions isolated from lamina propria were cultured with different concentration of DON: 0.1 to 10 mM for 48 h at 39°C.

Following 2 days of culture, lymphocytes were evaluated for their expression of CD4, CD25, and FoxP3 using flow cytometry. Briefly, cells were first stained with mouse anti-porcine CD4 (clone MIL17, ACRIS, Herford, Germany) and mouse anti-porcine CD25 (AbD Serotec, Colmar, France). As secondary antibodies isotype-specific fluorochrome- or biotin-labelled goat anti-mouse antibodies (αIgG1-Alexa 488, αIgG2b-biotin (Invitrogen) were used. Biotin-labelled secondary antibodies were further marked with APC-Cy7 streptavidin conjugate (Invitrogen). For intracellular staining, cells were permeabilized with a FoxP3 permeabilization/fixation buffer kit followed by staining with anti-mouse/rat FoxP3-PE that reacts with porcine FoxP3 (eBioscience Inc., San Diego, CA). Flow cytometric analysis was conducted on the lymphocytes using a MACSQuant analyser (Miltenyi biotech, Paris, France) and Venturi solfware. Dendritic cells were excluded based on forward and side scatter.

Statistics

After checking of normal distribution of data, we performed Fisher test and Student's t-test to compare values between multiple groups. The statistical analysis of the data was carried out with Statview software (Statistical Analysis System; SAS for Windows 98; SAS Institute Inc., Cary, NC, USA). Differences were considered to be statistically significant when the p-value was lower than 0.05.

Results

DON potentiated the expression of immune genes and increased protein concentration in differentiated IPEC-1 cells in a time-dependent manner.

We initially aimed to investigate the effects of DON on gene expression and protein production involved in the inflammatory immune response. Characterization of DON immune modulatory effects was first assessed by mRNA expression analysis in intestinal epithelial cells (IPEC-1) (Fig.ô 1). In untreated cells, no statistical difference in mRNA expression was measured between the different times of exposure, reflecting the absence of spontaneous inflammation caused by extended culture time. Exposure to DON significantly increased the expression of pro-inflammatory and regulatory cytokines, chemokines and of the enzyme RALDH (Fig.ô 1A). Early up-regulation in response to DON treatment was observed for IL-8, IL-1α and CCL20. Expression of these genes reached a maximum level after 4 h of DON exposure (100, 14 and 18 fold increase, respectively). mRNA expression levels of these three cytokines decreased in the course of time but remained significantly up-regulated until 24 h of DON exposure. These responses were correlated with IL-8 and IL-1α protein levels which were significantly up-regulated after 8 h of DON exposure (Fig.ô 1B). In addition to these early expressed genes, TGF-β, CX3CL1 and RALDH1 were also significantly increased but only after 8 h of exposure to DON (Fig.ô 1A).

Differentiated IPEC-1 cells were cultured in presence (black squares/bars) or absence (white diamonds/gray bars) of 10 μM of DON for 1.5 h, 4 h, 8 h, 12 h or 24 h. Gene expression was analyzed by RT-qPCR and protein levels by ELISA. Gene expressions were normalized by the mean of two reference genes (Cyclophilin A and RPL32). Data are presented as means +/− SEM of values obtained with three independent experiments. mRNA values are expressed relative to the control group at 4 h. Asterisks denote significant differences between groups: * $P<0.05$; ** $P<0.01$; *** $P<0.001$.

Table 1. List of genes, primers sequences (F: Forward; R: Reverse) and accession numbers and references.

Gene Symbol	Gene name	Primer sequence	References
IL1-α	Interleukin 1 - alpha	F: TCAGCCGCCCATCCAA	NC_010445.3
		R: AGCCCCGGTGCCATGT	
IL1-β	Interleukin 1 - beta	F: GAGCTGAAGGCTCTCCACCTC	NM_001005149
		R: ATCGCTGTCATCTCCTTGCAC	
TNF-α	Tumor necrosis factor - alpha	F: ACTGCACTTCGAGGTTATCGG	NM_214022
		R: GGCGACGGGCTTATCTGA	[32]
IL6	Interleukin 6	F: GGCAAAAGGGAAAGAATCCAG	NM_214399
		R: CGTTCTGTGACTGCAGCTTATCC	[68]
IL8	Interleukin 8	F: GCTCTCTGTGAGGCTGCAGTTC	NM_213867
		R: AAGGTGTGGAATGCGTATTTATGC	[14]
IL10	Interleukin 10	F: GGCCCAGTGAAGAGTTTCTTTC	NM_214041
		R: CAACAAGTCGCCCATCTGGT	[14]
IL12-p40	Interleukin 12 p40	F: GGTTTCAGACCCGACGAACTCT	NM_214013
		R: CATATGGCCACAATGGGAGATG	
IL17α	Interleukin 17 - alpha	F: CCAGACGGCCCTCAGATTAC	AB102693
		R: CACTTGGCCTCCCAGATCAC	[69]
IL21	Interleukin 21	F : GGCACAGTGCCCCATAAATC	MN_214415
		R: GCAGCAATTCAGGGTCCAAG	[70]
IL22	Interleukin 22	F: AAGCAGGTCCTGAACTTCAC	AY937228
		R: CACCCTTAATACGGCATTGG	[69]
IL23A	Interleukin 23 - alpha	F: GAGAAGAGGGAGATGATGAGACTACA	[66]
		R: GGTGGATCCTTTGCAAGCA	
TGF-β	Transforming growth factor - beta	F: GAAGCGCATCGAGGCCATTC	X54859
		R: GGCTCCGGTTCGACACTTTC	[69]
CCL20/MIP3 alpha	Chemokine (CCL20)	F: GCTCCTGGCTGCTTTGATGTC	NM_001024589
		R: CATTGGCGAGCTGCTGTGTG	[66]
IFN-γ	Interferon - gamma	F: TGGTAGCTCTGGGAAACTGAATG	NM_213948
		R: GGCTTTGCGCTGGATCTG	[66]
ROR-γ like	Nuclear receptor ROR-gamma-like	F: CCTGGCCCTGGGCATGT	NC_010446.3
		R: TGTTCTAGCAGCGTCCGAAGT	
FoxP3	Forkhead box P3	F: GGTGCAGTCTCTCTGGAACAA	AY669812
		R: GGTGCCAGTGGCTACAATAC	[66]
CX3CL1/Fractalkine	Chemokine (CX3CL1)	F: GCAGCTCCTAGTCCATTAC	EST CK464144
		R: CACCATTCTGACCCAAAG	[66]
XCR1	Chemokine (XCR1)	F: TCTTCTGCAAGCTTCTCAACATC	[66]
		R: GGCTGACCACGGACAGGTA	
CCR6	Chemokine (CCR6)	F: CCTGCACTGCTGCCTCAA	[71]
		R: TTCAGAAAGTAGCTCCGGAA	
STAT3	Signal transducer and activator of transcription 3	F: TGCAGCAGAAAGTGAGCTAC	MN_001044580
		R: CCGGTCTTGATGACTAATGG	[22]
RALDH1	Retinaldehyde deshydrogenase 1	F: TGGAGTGTGTGGCCAGATCA	N-010460-3
		R: GCAGGCCCTATCTTCCAAATG	[72]
T-bet	T-cell beta chain Th17-Th22 like	F: TTTGTGGCCTTTTGCATCCT	Present study
		R: CCTGTGTTTGTGATCTTGTTCCTT	
Cyclo A	Cyclophilin A	F: CCCACCGTCTTCTTCGACAT	MN_214353
		R: TCTGCTGTCTTTGGAACTTTGTCT	[22]
RPL32	Ribosomal Protein L32	F: AGTTCATCCGGCACCAGTCA	MN_001001636
		R: GAACCTTCTCCGCACCCTGT	[16]

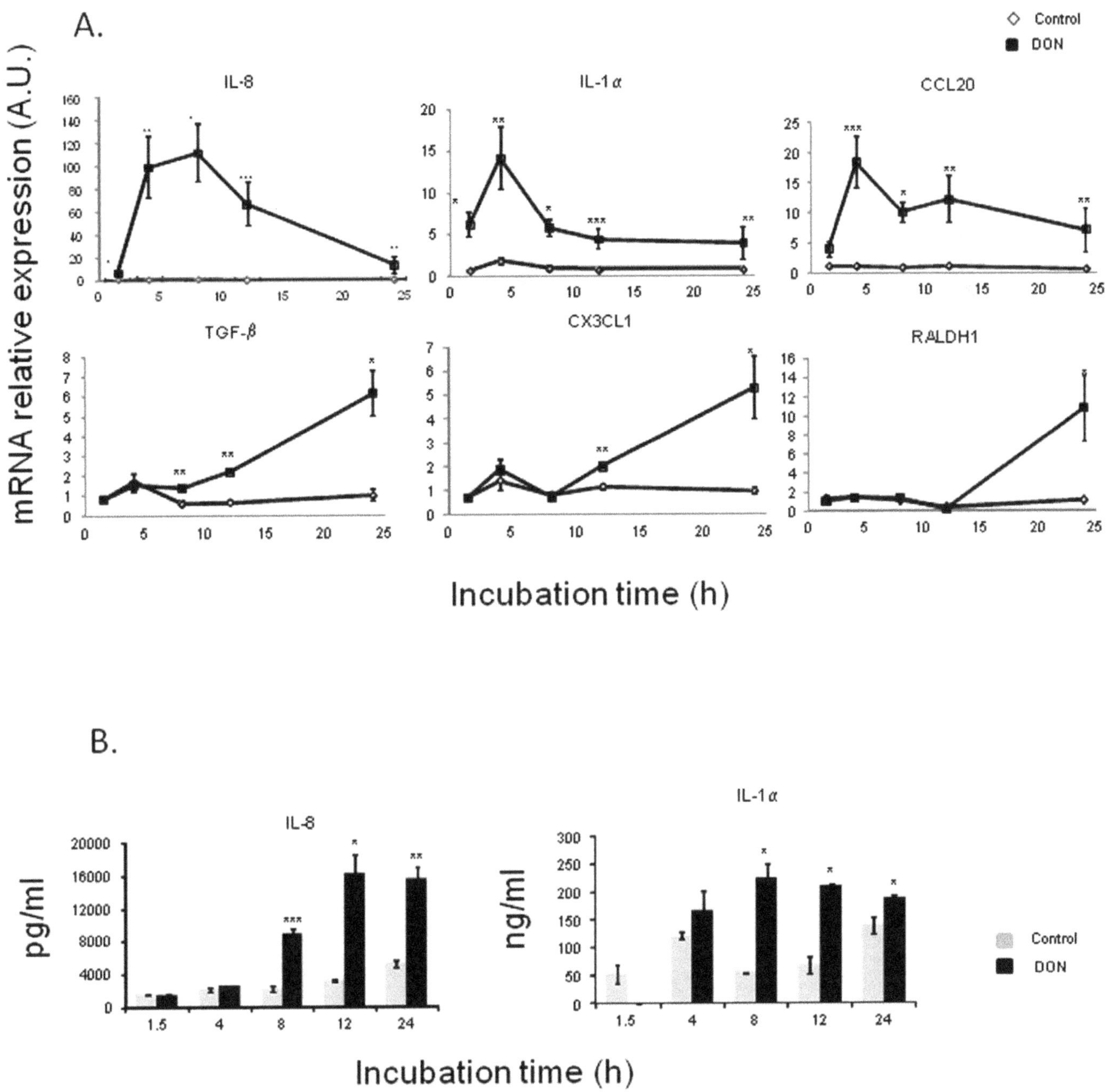

Figure 1. Deoxynivalenol induced cytokines and chemokines mRNA relative expression (A) and protein concentration (B) in IPEC-1 cells.

DON increased relative mRNA Expression Levels of Both pro-Inflammatory Cytokines and DC-Recruiting Chemokines in an *ex vivo* Model of Porcine jejunal Explants

In order to get an insight on the impact of DON on the cross-talk between epithelial cells and immune cells and its impact on the emergence of the mucosal immune response, porcine jejunal explants were exposed to 10 μM of DON. After 4 h, DON exposure induced an up-regulation of mRNA expression of pro-inflammatory cytokines (IL-8, IL-1α and TNF-α) as well as DC-recruiting chemokines (CCL20, CCR6, CX3CL1 and XCR1) (Fig.ô 2). Concerning pro-inflammatory cytokines, two different kinetics appeared again. The increase of both IL-8 and IL-1α was progressive in a time dependent manner and these cytokines reached their highest expression levels after 12 h (12 and 13 fold induction, respectively) (Fig.ô 2A). On the contrary, the significant up-regulation of TNF-α kept more or less steady along the different time points. An additional experiment involving jejunal loops of a 5 week-old pig *in vivo* to 10 μM of DON, suggested a decrease in the expression of these pro-inflammatory cytokines after 24 h of exposure (Fig. S1).

The expression of DC-recruiting chemokines was also measured in our explants model to analyze the effect of DON on CCL20/CCR6-mediated signals which can induce chemotaxis of CCR6-

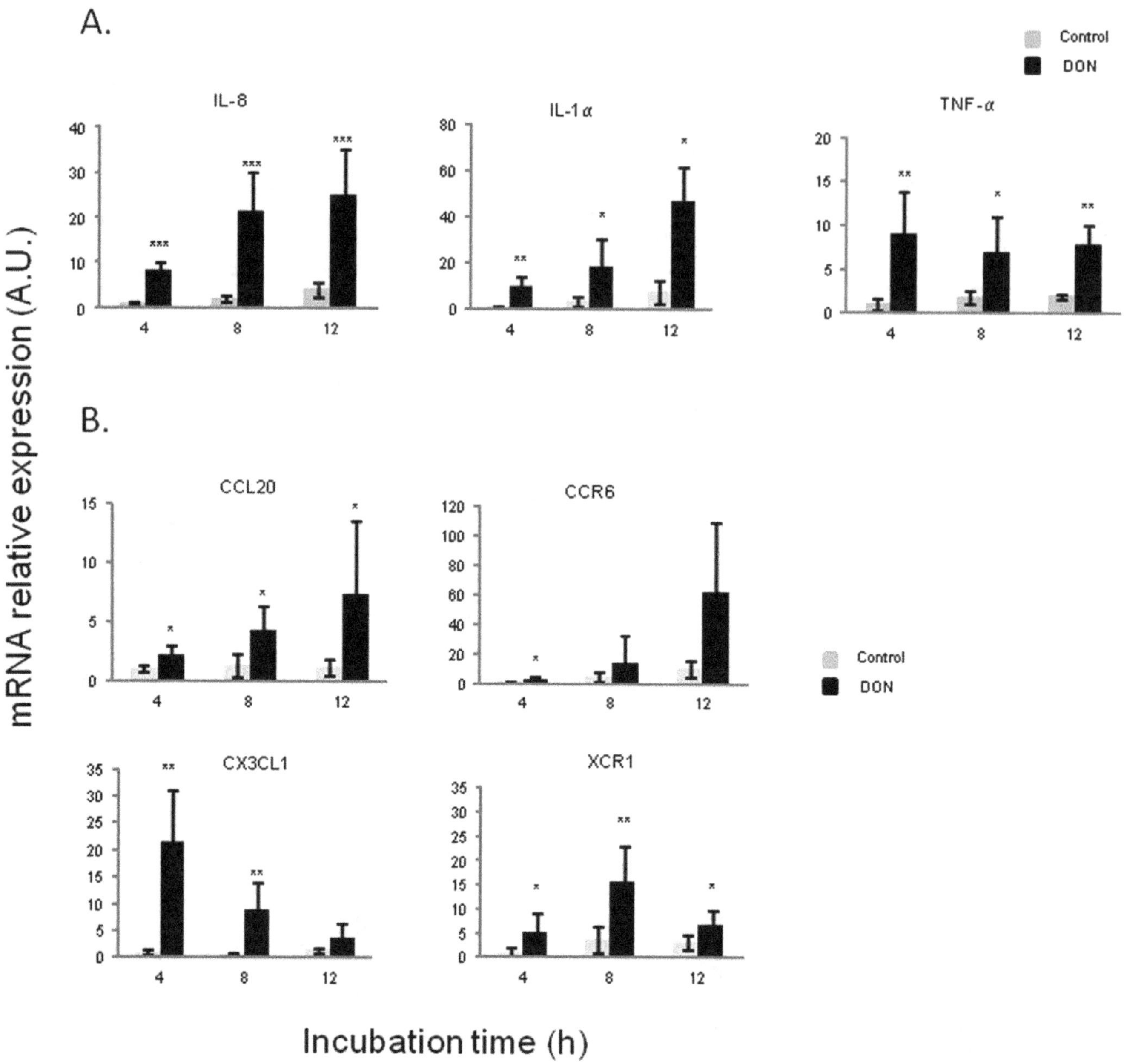

Figure 2. Deoxynivalenol up-regulated pro-inflammatory cytokines (A) and DCs-recruiting chemokines mRNA relative expression (B) in jejunal explants.

expressing DCs and macrophages to sites of tissue damage, driving preferentially the differentiation of naive T-cells towards Th1 or Th17 (Fig.ô 2B). The exposure of jejunal explants to DON significantly increased the expression of CCL20 and CCR6 with a peak after 12 h of exposure (7 and 12 fold induction, respectively). Secondly, we analyzed the expression of CX3CL1 which is known to inhibit Th1 and Th17 differentiation. Opposite to CCL20 and CCR6, CX3CL1 exhibited a maximum peak at 4 h (22 fold induction) and decreased progressively after 8 h and 12 h of DON exposure. XCR1, which is also implicated in DC recruitment, was significantly induced by DON at all exposure times but its maximum level was reached at 8 h of DON exposure (7 fold increase). The expression of both CX3CL1 and XCR1 decreased after their maximal induction peak (after 4 h and 8 h respectively) and this tendency was maintained in the loops experiment after 24 h of exposure (Fig. S1).

Explants were exposed or not with 10 μM of DON for 4 h, 8 h or 12 h. Gene expressions were evaluated by RT-qPCR and normalized with two reference genes (Cyclophilin A and RPL32). Data are presented as means +/− SEM of values obtained with intestinal explants from six different piglets and expressed relative to the control group at 4 h. Asterisks denote significant differences between untreated (gray bars) and DON-treated explants (black bars): * $P<0.05$; ** $P<0.01$; *** $P<0.001$.

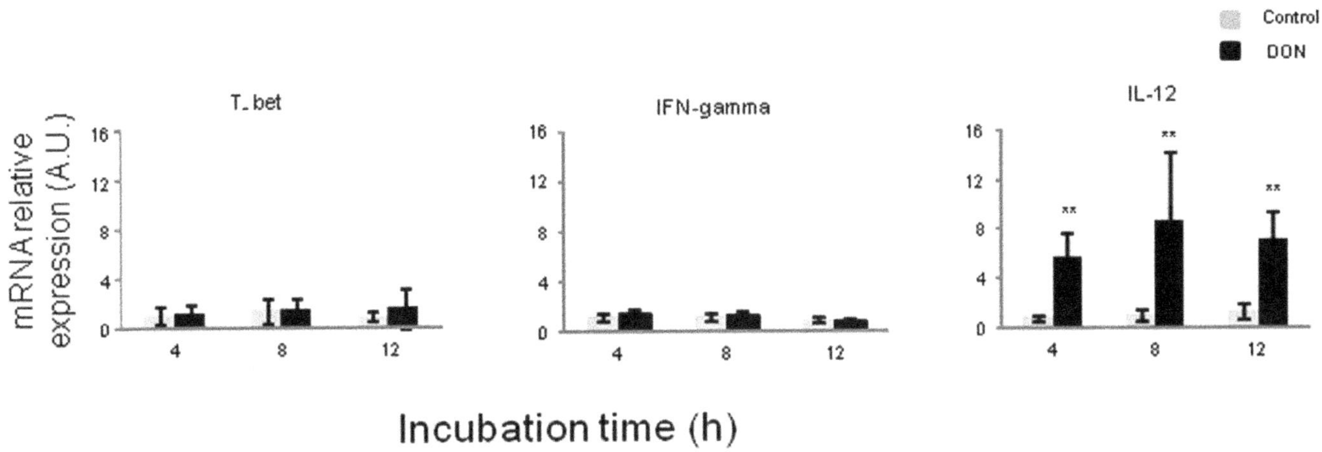

Figure 3. Deoxynivalenol increased IL-12 but not IFN-γ gene expression in jejunal explants.

DON Triggered Th17 Signature genes in Porcine jejunal Explants

In order to examine the effects of DON on naive Th cells differentiation, we analyzed mRNA expression levels of transcription factors and cytokine genes related to Th1 cells (Fig.ô 3), Th17 cells (Fig.ô 4) and Treg cells (Fig.ô 5). DON treatment did not affect expression of T-bet transcription factor nor IFN-γ mRNA levels (Fig.ô 3). Significant increase of IL-12 expression levels was observed at all exposure times (between 6 and 8 fold induction) (Fig.ô 3). DON treatment also induced a time-dependent increase of expression of mRNA encoding for IL-17 A, IL-6 and STAT3 (Fig.ô 4A). Accordingly the protein expression of IL-17A was significantly increased after 12 h of exposure to DON (Fig.ô 4B). IL-1β expression levels were also significantly up-regulated but its levels did not did not vary much in a time dependent manner (16 to 12 fold induction) (Fig.ô 4A). Surprisingly, RORγ-like, an important Th17 transcription factor was negatively regulated by DON treatment (Fig.ô 4A). A different expression profile was observed in genes related to Treg cells. FoxP3 and RALDH1 were not affected by DON treatment after 4 h and 8 h of culture and they were down regulated after 12 h of toxin exposure (Fig.ô 5A). This decrease of Treg cells was also found when analyzing the effect of DON on $CD4^+$ $CD25^+$ $FoxP3^+$ leukocytes extracted from the intestinal lamina propria (Fig.ô 5B). 10 μM of DON significantly reduced the $CD4^+$ $CD25^+$ $FoxP3^+$ cell population of 40%. On the contrary, the preliminary *in vivo* results using the loops experiment suggest an increase of expression of Treg cells related genes (Fig. S1).

Relative mRNA expression of transcription factors and cytokines related to Th1 cells were assessed by RT-qPCR. Explants were exposed or not with 10 μM of DON for 4 h, 8 h or 12 h. Values were normalized with two reference genes (Cyclophilin A and RPL32). Data are presented as means +/− SEM of values obtained with intestinal explants from six different piglets and expressed relative to the control group at 4 h. Asterisks denote significant differences between untreated (gray bars) and DON-treated explants (black bars): * $P<0.05$; ** $P<0.01$; *** $P<0.001$.

Relative mRNA expression of transcription factors and cytokines related to Th17 cells (A) and IL-17 A protein concentration (B) were assessed by RT-qPCR and ELISA. Explants were exposed or not with 10 μM of DON for 4 h, 8 h or 12 h. Values were normalized with two reference genes (Cyclophilin A and RPL32). Data are presented as means +/− SEM of values obtained with intestinal explants from six different piglets and expressed relative to the control group at 4 h. Asterisks denote significant differences between untreated (gray bars) and DON-treated explants (black bars): * $P<0.05$; ** $P<0.01$; *** $P<0.001$.

(A) Relative mRNA expression of transcription factors related to T reg cells were assessed by RT-qPCR. Explants were exposed or not with 10 μM of DON for 4 h, 8 h or 12 h. Values were normalized with two reference genes (Cyclophilin A and RPL32). Data are presented as means +/− SEM of values obtained with intestinal explants from six different piglets and expressed relative to the control group at 4 h. (B) The frequency of $CD4^+CD25^+FoxP3^+$ Treg cells were evaluated by flow cytometry after 2 days of co-culture with different concentration of DON (0.1 to 10 μM). Graphs show the mean ± SEM from duplicates from immune cells of jejunal lamina propria isolated 2 different pigs. Data were calculated as relative percentage to control without toxin. Asterisks denote significant differences between untreated (gray bars) and DON-treated explants (black bars): * $P<0.05$; ** $P<0.01$; *** $P<0.001$.

DON Triggered Pathogenic Th17 Cells Subset in Detriment of Regulatory Th17 (rTh17) Cells in Porcine jejunal Explants

To understand which subset of Th17 cells is preferentially induced by DON, pathogenic Th17-related genes (IL-23 A, IL-22 and IL-21) and rTh17-related genes (TGF-β and IL-10) were analyzed (Fig.ô 6). DON significantly increased IL-23A mRNA expression in a time-dependent manner (3, 17 and 31 fold induction at 4, 8 and 12 hours respectively) (Fig.ô 6A). mRNA expression levels of both IL-22 and IL-21 were also significantly induced but to a lesser extent (maximum levels of 10 and 3.5 fold induction respectively) (Fig.ô 6A). Interestingly, upregulation of these genes did not show after 24 h of DON exposure (Fig. S1). On the contrary, TGF-β mRNA expression was not induced by DON treatment (Fig.ô 6B). Interestingly, IL-10 which is produced by both rTh17 and Treg cells showed a significant induction in the presence of DON (6 fold increase) (Fig.ô 6B).

Discussion

Mycotoxins have become an issue of major concern given their global and frequent occurrence as well as their known toxic effects. Among all, DON is of particular interest because it is one of the most prevalent mycotoxins in Europe and North America. The intestinal tract represents the first barrier against DON-contam-

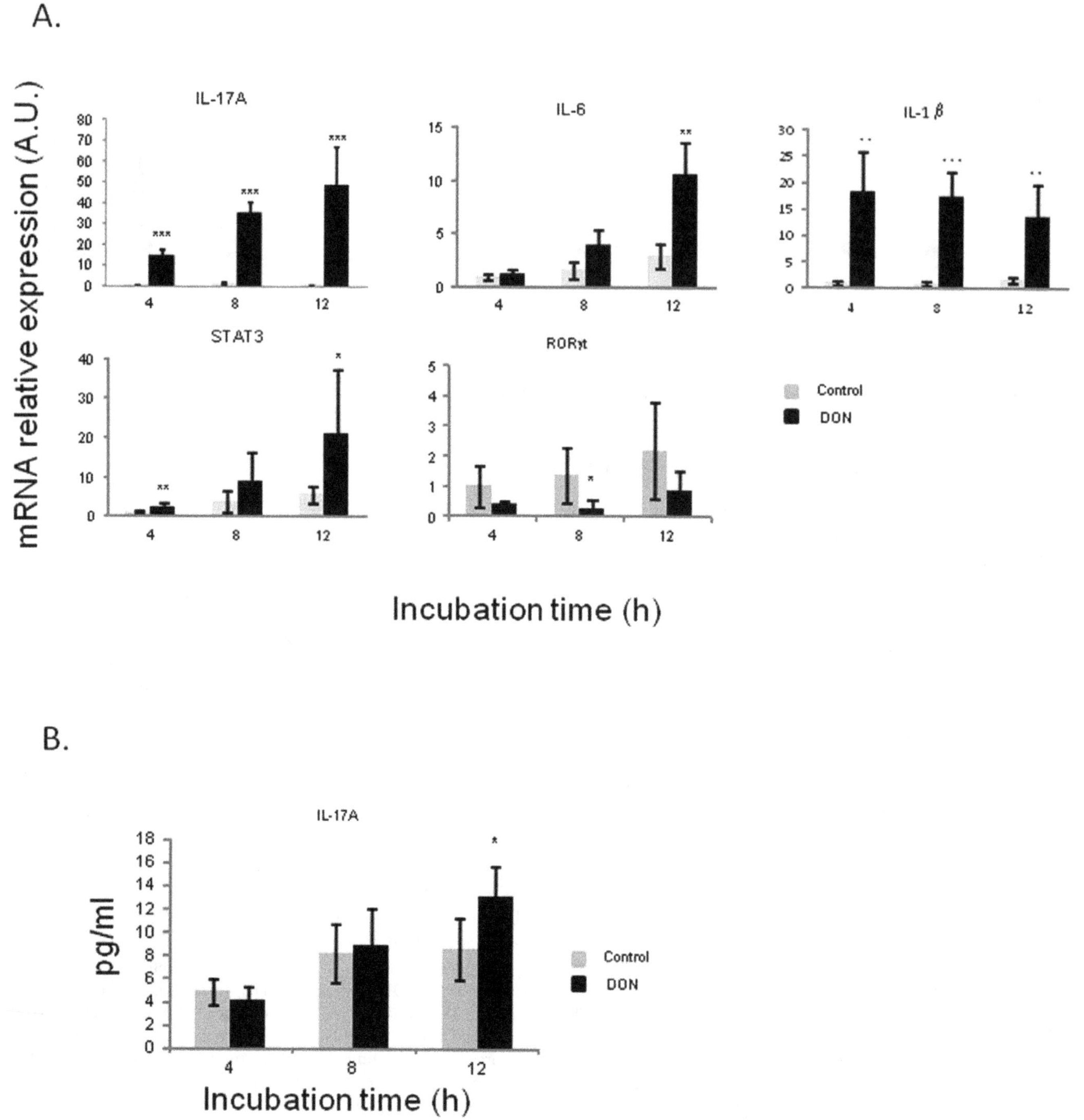

Figure 4. Deoxynivalenol triggered Th17 response in jejunal explants.

inated food and feed. Many authors have already reported Th17 cells to be critical for protection against microbial infections like bacteria, virus and fungi at mucosal surfaces [36,37,38]. The aim of our work was to assess the impact of DON exposure onto the intestinal homeostasis controlled by pro-inflammatory Th17 and the regulatory Treg response. To the best of our knowledge this is the first study showing that DON disrupts the intestinal homeostasis and promotes the Th17 response over the Th1 and T regulatory responses.

Intestinal epithelial cells and jejunal explants were used to investigate the modulation of the intestinal immune response by DON. The choice of using 10 μM of DON was based mainly on the US Federal Grain Inspection Service and the European Union surveys [6,39,40] which evaluated the naturally occurring concentration of this mycotoxin to range between 19 and 50 mg/kg in grain cereals. Assuming that DON would be ingested in one meal, diluted in 1 L of gastrointestinal fluid and would be totally bioaccessible, 10 μM correspond approximately to 3 mg/kg [39,40]. In addition to that, a previous study of our group

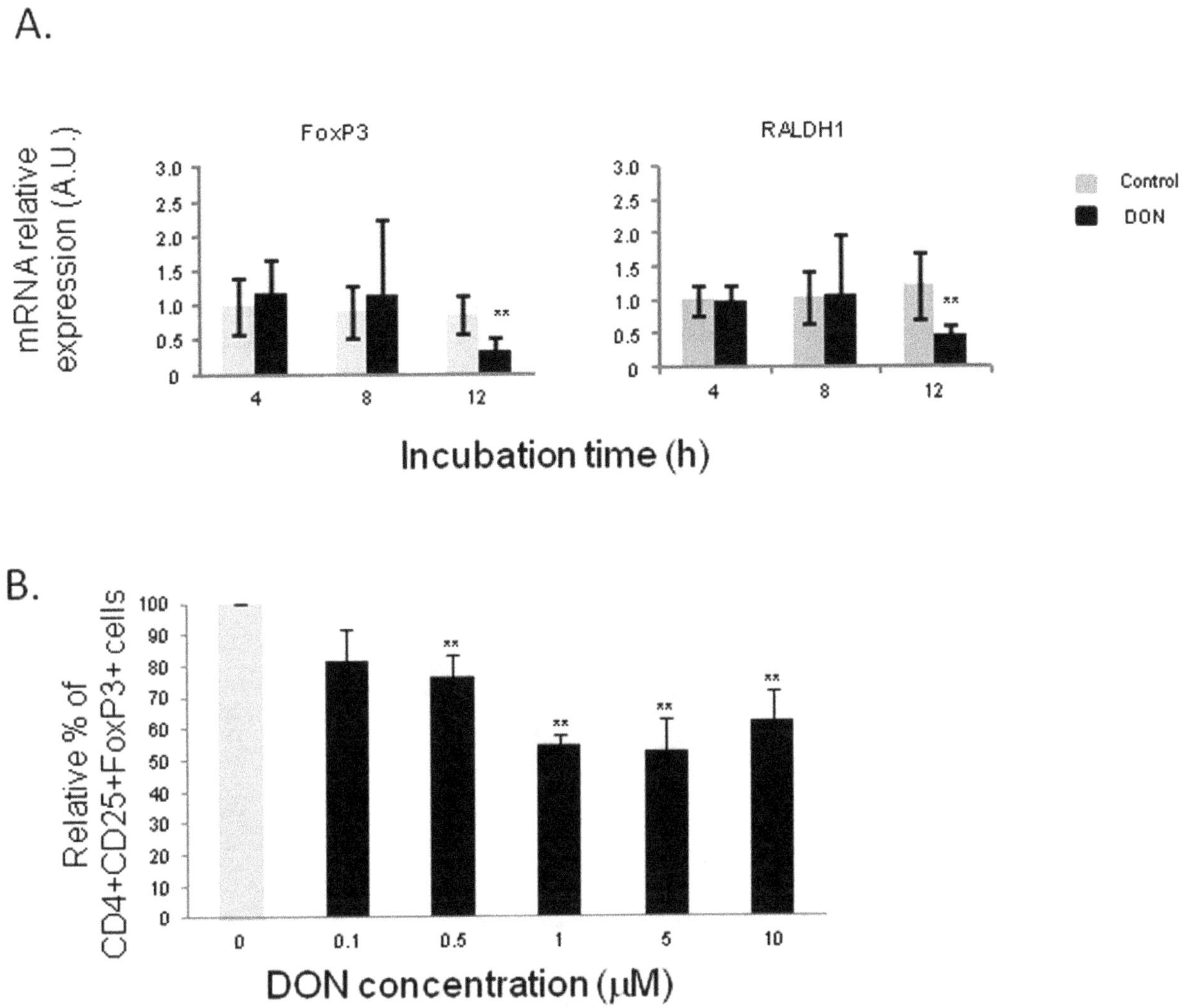

Figure 5. Deoxynivalenol decreased T regulatory response in jejunal explants.

showed that this concentration does not affect cell viability up to 48 h after treatment in the porcine intestinal cell line, IPEC-1 [17] but it does affect the morphology of the epithelial barrier according to another study [27].

In the present experiment, *in vitro* and *ex vivo* exposure to DON led to an early general state of inflammation depicted by mRNA expression increase of IL-8, IL-1α and TNF- α, which is in agreement with previous results of similar studies [41,42]. The inflammation generated at the epithelial level could elicit the activation of the population of Th17 cells by triggering further communication with immune cells of the *lamina propria*. The mode of action by which DON induces such inflammatory response has been described by several authors and it was not the purpose of the present study. Indeed, it has already largely been demonstrated that DON activates ERK1/2 and p38 thus triggering MAPK signaling cascades which upregulate COX-2 and PGE-2, major inductors of the inflammatory response [11]. This molecular mechanism most likely occurs in all immune cellular types, including IECs. Therefore we can also soundly hypothesize that DON-induced MAPK activation in IECs induces chemokine secretion which then stimulates intestinal DCs, thus initiating the classical immune response cascade and lymphocyte activation.

In this study, the exposure to DON induced IL-6, IL-23 and IL-1β expression but did not affect the expression of TGF-β and strongly repressed FoxP3 and RALDH1. These data suggest that in our model DON mainly drives the intestinal immune system towards a Th17 response. In agreement with that, DON strongly induced IL-17 A which is the signature cytokine of these T helper cells, but which can also be produced by other immune cells. However to our knowledge, there is no available antibody for of porcine IL-17 A intracellular labeling which would allow to clarify the source of this cytokine. Despite that, the fact that STAT3, a transcription factor expressed by Th17 cells, was also upregulated in the intestinal explants is a strong indication of the increase of this population in the intestinal tissues. Nevertheless, ROR-γt like, which has been described as the other major transcription factor governing Th17 differentiation in mice [23,43], was not induced but repressed by the presence of DON in explants model. Although this result is surprising, it could be possible that, unlike in the mouse model, in the porcine specie the transcription factor STAT3 plays a more important role than ROR-γt in Th17 differentiation. It would be very interesting to further investigate this point.

The two lineages, Th17 and Tregs share a co-evolutionary origin [44,45] which could explain why they share similarities at

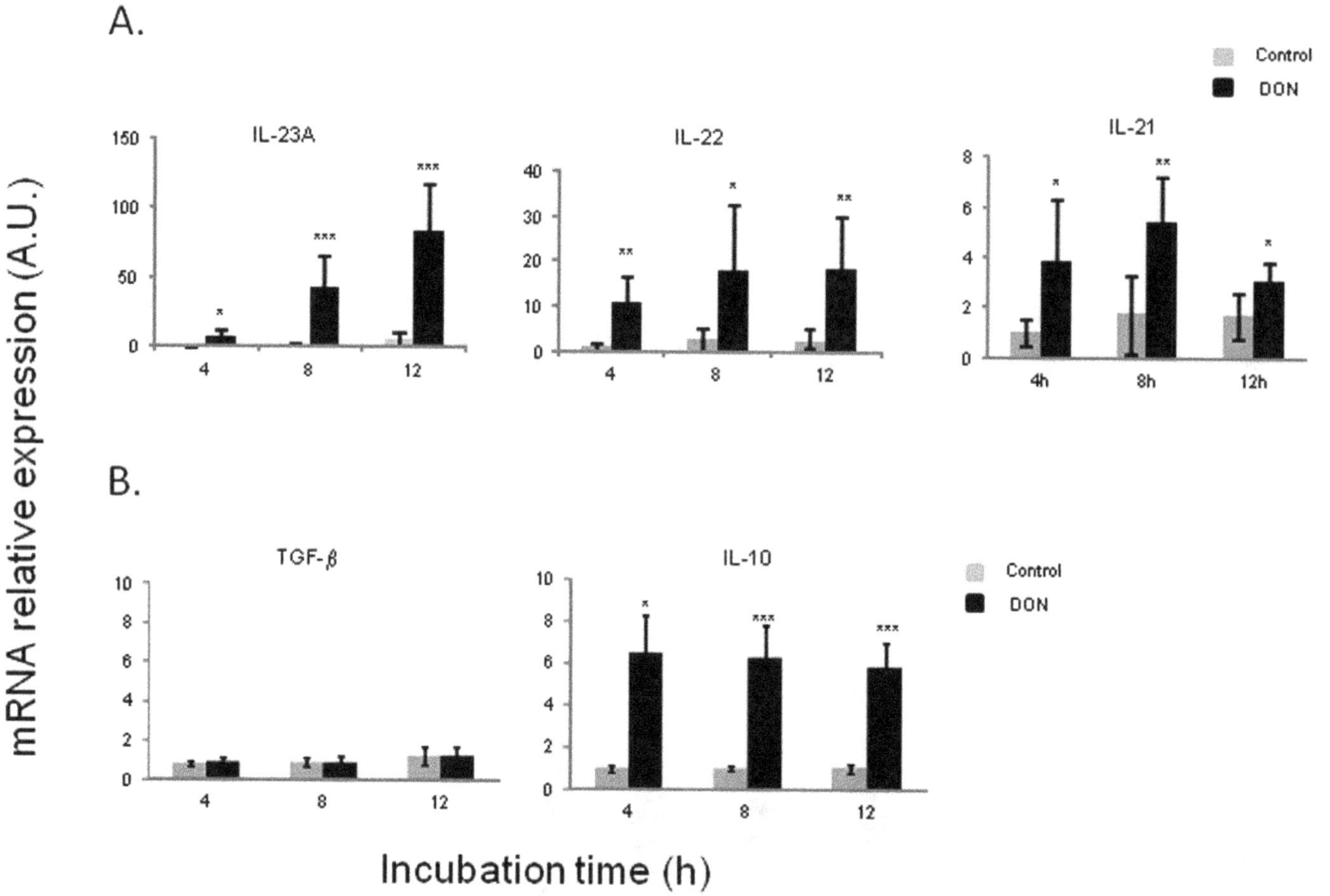

Figure 6. Deoxynivalenol triggered pathogenic Th17 cells subset but not regulatory Th17 (rTh17) cells in porcine jejunal explants.

many levels [46,47,48,49]. In this way, CCR6 appears to be the only chemokine receptor essentially implicated in driving Th17 migration *in vivo* but it is also highly expressed by Tregs [50]. CCL20, the ligand of this receptor drives the conversion of the pathogenic Th17 into the regulatory subsets [23,51]. Our results showed that CCR6 and CCL20 were induced by DON in a time-dependent manner in the intestinal explants. It is therefore tempting to speculate that along the overall pro-inflammatory response both in the intestinal epithelial cells and the intestinal explants, there is a regulatory rTh17 response setting up-rather than the Treg response.

Plasticity of T cells is also reflected in the similarities between rTh17 and Treg cells. Besides their common regulatory action, these two populations share the importance of TGF-β and IL-10 [23,24,51]. TGF-β is involved in the differentiation of these two populations. In this study, there was no significant effect of DON on the expression of this cytokine in the intestinal explants. TGF-β was however secreted by the intestinal epithelial cells after 8, 12 and 24 h of exposure to DON. Further studies will be important to understand the exact role of TGF-β in the differentiation of Tregs in swine but also the impact of DON on the intestinal secretion of this cytokine. However, previous studies have also showed that TGF-β presents minor or absent changes after PMA/Ionomycin or CD3 stimulation [52,53] which might be an indication of the fact that TGF-β might be of less importance in the regulatory response compared to humans and mice. IL-10 is produced by both Tregs and rTh17 to regulate inflammation and has the ability of reversing the pathogenic phenotype of Th17 into rTh17 [24]. In this study, this cytokine was up-regulated in a time independent manner by the presence of DON on explants, which is in contradiction with the absence of increase of FoxP3 and TGF-β. However it is well described that many cells of the innate and adaptive immune system other than Tregs and rTh17 cells express IL-10, such as DCs, macrophages, Th1, Th2 and B cells [54]. Given our results in the intestinal explants on Th1 and Treg, it is most likely for IL-10 to be produced by DCs, macrophages or B cells in that experiment

Taken together, all these results suggest that DON preferentially induces a pro-inflammatory response directed by pathogenic Th17, when CCR6, CCL20 and IL-10 results point to a concomitant protective response most likely lead by rTh17. Supplementary *in vivo* data seems to indicate an increase in the protective response after 24 h of exposure.

Determining whether immune activation or suppression should occur in response to a given pathogen is a critical decision to be taken by the adaptive immune system. Indeed, there is a fine line between inflammation and pathogen elimination and excessive inflammation and tissue damage. Numerous diseases such as rheumatoid arthritis and multiple sclerosis arise from a failure to restore the state of equilibrium [55]. In the intestine, inflammatory bowel diseases (IBD) like ulcerative colitis (UC) and Crohn's disease (CD) are triggered by excessive inflammation of the colon and/or the small bowel leading to recurrent diarrhea and pain [56]. Until recently only excessive Th1 and Th2 responses were accounted for these diseases. Nevertheless, the discovery of the Th17 subset gave a new insight on the causes of these disorders as

IL-17 producing cells were shown to be of major importance in IBD [57]. Besides IL-17, IL-21, IL-22 and IL-23 have also been reported to play an important role in the onset of these diseases [57,58]. Interestingly, all of these cytokines were up-regulated by the presence of DON in our experiments which could imply that chronic exposure to this toxin could be a triggering or enhancing factor of IBD. This hypothesis is supported by a recent study [26] which draws a strong parallel between the alterations caused by exposure to several mycotoxins including DON and the symptoms observed during IBD. In addition to the induction of the above-mentioned cytokines, intestinal permeability is also related to both DON exposure and IBD. This mycotoxin specifically targets claudin expression [16,17] which directly leads to an increase of permeability of the intestinal barrier which could result in increased bacterial translocation, one of the main causes of IBD [56]. The same applies for toll-like receptors (TLRs) impairment, associated with DON exposure [59]. Over activation of dendritic cells (DCs) drawn by abnormal TLR activity could lead to inability to detect bacterial components which is another major source of IBD. Notably, TLR activation disruption has been detected after exposure to T-2 toxin, another member of the trichothecene family [60].

As depicted above, bacterial interactions with the immune cells of the *lamina propria* are a central component of IBD, since inflammation might arise from lack of tolerance to antigens present in commensal bacteria [61]. Besides, loss of the transcription factor T-bet, which regulates TNF-α production, influences bacterial homeostasis by favoring colitogenic microbial populations. The resulting increase of TNF-α production by DCs could trigger breakdown of the intestinal epithelium and facilitate bacterial translocation to the *lamina propria*, increasing risks of IBD [62]. It has already been demonstrated that DON alters the intestinal microbiota of pigs [63]. It thus comes as no surprise that in this study, exposure to DON could possibly lead to induction of colitogenic populations and to strong impairment of the epithelial barrier by the lack of effect on T-bet and significant increase of the expression levels of TNF-α. It is noteworthy that colonization of the small intestine by segmented filamentous bacteria (SFB) of the intestinal microbiota is directly associated with the appearance of Th17 cells and that SFB promote the expression of inflammatory genes linked to IBD [64].

In conclusion, exposure to the mycotoxin DON clearly induced an early intestinal inflammatory response resulting from the interplay of different intestinal cell types and leading to the activation of Th17 cells. These results together with previous observations strengthen the idea that chronical exposure to deoxynivalenol could impair intestinal homeostasis and trigger the appearance of IBD. However, the molecular mechanisms by which this toxin specifically activates Th17 remain unclear. Further research should therefore address the link between MAP kinases activation by DON [11,12] and the herein presented effects on lymphocyte populations. In addition to that, the cellular interplay that takes play among immune cells (IECs – DCs – T cells) upon DON exposure should be better characterized by analyzing for instance cellular migration of DCs, macrophages and T lymphocytes. Finally, more insight should be gained on the role of commensal and pathogenic bacteria on modulating the Th17 response and the impact of DON on such modulation.

Supporting Information

Figure S1 Fold mRNA expression increase of cytokines and transcription factors after DON exposure in an *in vivo* model of jejunal loops. Following the guidelines provided by the French Council for Animal Care (permit number 2011–07–1) and previous published protocols [65,66,67], loops were performed in a 5 week-old pig. Very briefly, 6 consecutive loops (10-–0 cm long) were made by surgical ligation in a 2–4 m long segment of the jejunum which was previously thoroughly washed with a solution of metrodinazole, a common antibiotic. PBS was injected in 3 loops as negative control and 10 μM of DON were injected in 3 other loops. The pig was euthanized by barbiturate overdose 24 h post surgery. Jejunal tissues were then collected and snap-frozen in liquid nitrogen before RNA extraction. Relative mRNA expression levels of immune genes related to pro-inflammatory cytokines (A), DC-recrutment chemokines (B), Th1 (C), Th17 (D) and Treg (E) signature and pathogenic/regulatory Th17 cytokines (F) were assessed by RT-qPCR. Gene expressions were normalized by the mean of two reference genes (Cyclophilin A and RPL32). Data are presented as mean +/− SEM of values obtained with three different loops and expressed relative to the control group. Significant differences between untreated loops (gray bars) and treated loops (black bars) with 10 μM of DON are marked with asterisks (* $P<0.05$).

Acknowledgments

The authors are also grateful to Philippe Pinton, Anne-Marie Cossalter, Sophie Ausset and Claire Loiseau for their excellent technical assistance.

Author Contributions

Conceived and designed the experiments: LGP IPO. Performed the experiments: PMC JS JC RA. Analyzed the data: PMC JS FM JC RA. Contributed reagents/materials/analysis tools: JC. Wrote the paper: PMC JS.

References

1. Doll S, Danicke S (2011) The *Fusarium* toxins deoxynivalenol (DON) and zearalenone (ZON) in animal feeding. Prev Vet Med 102: 132–145.
2. Bryden WL (2007) Mycotoxins in the food chain: human health implications. Asia Pacô Jô Clin Nutr 16 Suppl 1: 95–101.
3. Oswald IP, CC (1998) Immunotoxicity of mycotoxins. Revue Med Vet 149: 585–590.
4. Oswald IP, Marin DE, Bouhet S, Pinton P, Taranu I, et al. (2005) Immunotoxicological risk of mycotoxins for domestic animals. Food Addit Contam 22: 354–360.
5. CAST (2003) Mycotoxins: riks in plant, animal and human systems. Council Agr Sc Technol Task Force Rep. 138: 136–142.
6. SCOOP (2003) Collection of occurrence data of *Fusarium* toxins in food and assessment of dietary intake by the population of EU member states. Directorate-General Health and Cosummer Protection.
7. Pestka JJ, AT S (2005) Deoxynivalenol: Toxicology and Potential effects on Humans. Jô Toxicol Environ Health 8: 39–69.
8. Rotter BA, Prelusky DB, JJ P (1996) Toxicology of deoxynivalenol (vomitoxin). Jô Toxicol Environ Health 48: 1–34.
9. Meurens F, Summerfield A, Nauwynck H, Saif L, Gerdts V (2011) The pig: a model for human infectious diseases. Trends in Microbiology 20: 50–57.
10. Patterson JK, Lei XG, Miller DD (2008) The Pig as an Experimental Model for Elucidating the Mechanisms Governing Dietary Influence on Mineral Absorption. Exp Biol Med 233: 651–664.
11. Pestka JJ, Zhou H-R, Moon Y, Chung YJ (2004) Cellular and molecular mechanisms for immune modulation by deoxynivalenol and other trichothecenes: unraveling a paradox. Toxicology Letters 153: 61–73.
12. Zhou HR, Islam Z, Pestka JJ (2003) Rapid, sequential activation of mitogen-activated protein kinases and transcription factors precedes proinflammatory cytokine mRNA expression in spleens of mice exposed to the trichothecene vomitoxin. Toxicol Sci 72: 130–142.
13. Avantaggiato G, Havenaar R, Visconti A (2004) Evaluation of the intestinal absorption of deoxynivalenol and nivalenol by an in vitro gastrointestinal model, and the binding efficacy of activated carbon and other adsorbent materials. Food Chem Toxicol 42: 817–824.
14. Bracarense A-PFL, Lucioli J, Grenier B, Drociunas Pacheco G, Moll W-D, et al. (2012) Chronic ingestion of deoxynivalenol and fumonisin, alone or in

interaction, induces morphological and immunological changes in the intestine of piglets. Brô Jô Nutr: 107: 1776–1786.
15. Maresca M, Mahfoud R, Garmy N, Fantini J (2002) The Mycotoxin Deoxynivalenol Affects Nutrient Absorption in Human Intestinal Epithelial Cells. Jô Nutr 132: 2723–2731.
16. Pinton P, Braicu C, Nougayrede JP, Laffitte J, Taranu I, et al. (2010) Deoxynivalenol impairs porcine intestinal barrier function and decreases the protein expression of claudin-4 through a mitogen-activated protein kinase-dependent mechanism. Jô Nutr 140: 1956–1962.
17. Pinton P, Nougayrède J-P, Del Rio J-C, Moreno C, Marin DE, et al. (2009) The food contaminant deoxynivalenol, decreases intestinal barrier permeability and reduces claudin expression. Toxicol Appl Pharmacol 237: 41–48.
18. Pinton P, Tsybulskyy D, Lucioli J, Laffitte J, Callu P, et al. (2012) Toxicity of deoxynivalenol and its acetylated derivatives on the intestine: differential effects on morphology, barrier function, tight junctions proteins and MAPKinases. Toxicol Sci 130: 180–190.
19. Diesing A-K, Nossol C, Dänicke S, Walk N, Post A, et al. (2011) Vulnerability of Polarised Intestinal Porcine Epithelial Cells to Mycotoxin Deoxynivalenol Depends on the Route of Application. PLoS ONE 6: e17472.
20. Oswald IP (2006) Role of intestinal epithelial cells in the innate immune defence of the pig intestine. Veterinary Research 37: 359–368.
21. Coombes JL, Powrie F (2008) Dendritic cells in intestinal immune regulation. Nat Rev Immunol 8: 435–446.
22. Curtis MM, Way SS (2009) Interleukin-17 in host defence against bacterial, mycobacterial and fungal pathogens. Immunology 126: 177–185.
23. Ghoreschi K, Laurence A, Yang XP, Tato CM, McGeachy MJ, et al. (2010) Generation of pathogenic T(H)17 cells in the absence of TGF-beta signalling. Nature 467: 967-U144.
24. McGeachy MJ, Bak-Jensen KS, Chen Y, Tato CM, Blumenschein W, et al. (2007) TGF-beta and IL-6 drive the production of IL-17 and IL-10 by T cells and restrain TH-17 cell-mediated pathology. Nature Immunol 8: 1390–1397.
25. Zhu J, Paul WE (2009) Heterogeneity and plasticity of T helper cells. Cell Res 20: 4–12.
26. Maresca M, Fantini J (2010) Some food-associated mycotoxins as potential risk factors in humans predisposed to chronic intestinal inflammatory diseases. Toxicon 56: 282–294.
27. Kolf-Clauw M, Castellote J, Joly B, Bourges-Abella N, Raymond-Letron I, et al. (2009) Development of a pig jejunal explant culture for studying the gastrointestinal toxicity of the mycotoxin deoxynivalenol: Histopathological analysis. Toxicol in Vitro 23: 1580–1584.
28. Gonzalez-Vallina R, Wang H, Zhan R, Berschneider HM, Lee RM, et al. (1996) Lipoprotein and apolipoprotein secretion by a newborn piglet intestinal cell line (IPEC-1). Amô Jô Physiol 271: G249–259.
29. Zanello G, Berri M, Dupont J, Sizaret P-Y, D'Inca R, et al. (2011) *Saccharomyces cerevisiae* Modulates Immune Gene Expressions and Inhibits ETEC-Mediated ERK1/2 and p38 Signaling Pathways in Intestinal Epithelial Cells. PLoS ONE 6: e18573.
30. Gonzalez-Vallina R, Wang H, Zhan R, Berschneider HM, Lee RM, et al. (1996) Lipoprotein and apolipoprotein secretion by a newborn piglet intestinal cell line (IPEC-1). Amô Jô Physiol 271: G249–G259.
31. Bouhet S, Hourcade E, Loiseau N, Fikry A, Martinez S, et al. (2004) The mycotoxin fumonisin B1 alters the proliferation and the barrier function of porcine intestinal epithelial cells. Toxicol Sci 77: 165–171.
32. Meissonnier GM, Pinton P, Laffitte J, Cossalter AM, Gong YY, et al. (2008) Immunotoxicity of aflatoxin B1: impairment of the cell-mediated response to vaccine antigen and modulation of cytokine expression. Toxicol Appl Pharmacol 231: 142–149.
33. Bruel T, Guibon R, Melo S, Guillen N, Salmon H, et al. (2010) Epithelial induction of porcine suppressor of cytokine signaling 2 (SOCS2) gene expression in response to *Entamoeba histolytica*. Dev Comp Immunol 34: 562–571.
34. Delgado-Ortega M, Melo S, Meurens F (2011) Expression of SOCS1–7 and CIS mRNA in porcine tissues. Vet Immunol Immunopathol 144: 493–498.
35. Haverson K, Singha S, Stokes CR, Bailey M (2000) Professional and non-professional antigen-presenting cells in the porcine small intestine. Immunology 101: 492–500.
36. Zelante T, Bozza S, De Luca A, D'Angelo C, Bonifazi P, et al. (2009) Th17 cells in the setting of *Aspergillus* infection and pathology. Med Mycol 47: S162–S169.
37. Khader SA, Gaffen SL, Kolls JK (2009) Th17 cells at the crossroads of innate and adaptive immunity against infectious diseases at the mucosa. Mucosal Immunol 2: 403–411.
38. Kolls JK, Khader SA (2010) The role of Th17 cytokines in primary mucosal immunity. uCytokine Growth Factor Rev 21: 443–448.
39. Trucksess MW, Thomas F, Young K, Stack ME, Fulgueras WJ, et al. (1995) Survey of deoxynivalenol in U.S. 1993 wheat and barley crops by enzyme-linked immunosorbent assay. Jô AOAC Int 78: 631–636.
40. Abouzied MM, Azcona JI, Braselton WE, Pestka JJ (1991) Immunochemical assessment of mycotoxins in 1989 grain foods: evidence for deoxynivalenol (vomitoxin) contamination. Appl Environ Microbiol 57: 672–677.
41. Pestka JJ, Amuzie CJ (2008) Tissue distribution and proinflammatory cytokine gene expression following acute oral exposure to deoxynivalenol: comparison of weanling and adult mice. Food Chem Toxicol 46: 2826–2831.
42. Amuzie CJ, Shinozuka J, Pestka JJ (2009) Induction of suppressors of cytokine signaling by the trichothecene deoxynivalenol in the mouse. Toxicol Sci 111: 277–287.
43. Manel N, Unutmaz D, Littman DR (2008) The differentiation of human T(H)-17 cells requires transforming growth factor-beta and induction of the nuclear receptor RORgammat. Nat Immunol 9: 641–649.
44. Weaver CT, Harrington LE, Mangan PR, Gavrieli M, Murphy KM (2006) Th17: An Effector CD4 T Cell Lineage with Regulatory T Cell Ties. Immunity 24: 677–688.
45. Weaver CT, Hatton RD (2009) Interplay between the TH17 and TReg cell lineages: a co-evolutionary perspective. Nat Rev Immunol 9: 883–889.
46. Kaser T, Gerner W, Saalmuller A (2011) Porcine regulatory T cells: mechanisms and T-cell targets of suppression. Dev Comp Immunol 35: 1166–1172.
47. Kaser T, Gerner W, Mair K, Hammer SE, Patzl M, et al. (2011) Current knowledge on porcine regulatory T cells. Vet Immunol Immunopathol 148: 136–138.
48. Kaser T, Gerner W, Hammer SE, Patzl M, Saalmuller A (2008) Detection of Foxp3 protein expression in porcine T lymphocytes. Vet Immunol Immunopathol 125: 92–101.
49. Kaser T, Gerner W, Hammer SE, Patzl M, Saalmuller A (2008) Phenotypic and functional characterisation of porcine CD4(+)CD25(high) regulatory T cells. Vet Immunol Immunopathol 122: 153–158.
50. Comerford I, Bunting M, Fenix K, Haylock-Jacobs S, Litchfield W, et al. (2010) An immune paradox: how can the same chemokine axis regulate both immune tolerance and activation?: CCR6/CCL20: a chemokine axis balancing immunological tolerance and inflammation in autoimmune disease. Bioessays 32: 1067–1076.
51. Esplugues E, Huber S, Gagliani N, Hauser AE, Town T, et al. (2011) Control of TH17 cells occurs in the small intestine. Nature 475: 514–518.
52. Ledger TN, Pinton P, Bourges D, Roumi P, Salmon H, et al. (2004) Development of a Macroarray To Specifically Analyze Immunological Gene Expression in Swine. Clin Diagn Lab Immunol 11: 691–698.
53. Käser T, Müllebner A, Hartl RT, Essler SE, Saalmüller A, et al. (2012) Porcine T-helper and regulatory T cells exhibit versatile mRNA expression capabilities for cytokines and co-stimulatory molecules. Cytokine 60: 400–409.
54. Paul G, Khare V, Gasche C (2011) Inflamed gut mucosa: downstream of interleukin-10. Eurô Jô Clin Invest 42: 95–109.
55. Miossec P (2009) Diseases that may benefit from manipulating the Th17 pathway. Eurô Jô Immunol 39: 667–669.
56. Matricon J, Barnich N, Ardid D (2010) Immunopathogenesis of inflammatory bowel disease. Self Nonself 1: 299–309.
57. Caprioli F, Pallone F, Monteleone G (2008) Th17 immune response in IBD: A new pathogenic mechanism. Jô Crohns Colitis 2: 291–295.
58. Ouyang W, Valdez P (2008) IL-22 in mucosal immunity. Mucosal Immunol 1: 335–338.
59. Pestka J, Zhou HR (2006) Toll-like receptor priming sensitizes macrophages to proinflammatory cytokine gene induction by deoxynivalenol and other toxicants. Toxicol Sci 92: 445–455.
60. Seeboth J, Solinhac R, Oswald I, Guzylack-Piriou L (2012) The fungal T-2 toxin alters the activation of primary macrophages induced by TLR-agonists resulting in a decrease of the inflammatory response in the pig. Vet Res 43: 35.
61. Chassaing B, Darfeuille-Michaud A (2011) The commensal microbiota and enteropathogens in the pathogenesis of inflammatory bowel diseases. Gastroenterology 140: 1720–1728.
62. Garrett WS, Lord GM, Punit S, Lugo-Villarino G, Mazmanian SK, et al. (2007) Communicable ulcerative colitis induced by T-bet deficiency in the innate immune system. Cell 131: 33–45.
63. Waché YJ, Hbabi-Haddioui L, Guzylack-Piriou L, Belkhelfa H, Roques C, et al. (2009) The mycotoxin Deoxynivalenol inhibits the cell surface expression of activation markers in human macrophages. Toxicol 262: 239–244.
64. Ivanov, II, Atarashi K, Manel N, Brodie EL, Shima T, et al. (2009) Induction of intestinal Th17 cells by segmented filamentous bacteria. Cell 139: 485–498.
65. Gerdts V, Uwiera RRE, Mutwiri GK, Wilson DJ, Bowersock T, et al. (2001) Multiple intestinal "loops" provide an in vivo model to analyse multiple mucosal immune responses. Jô Immunol Methods 256: 19–33.
66. Meurens F, Berri M, Auray G, Melo S, Levast B, et al. (2009) Early immune response following *Salmonella enterica* subspecies enterica serovar *Typhimurium* infection in porcine jejunal gut loops. Vet Res 40: 05.
67. Vandenbroucke V, Croubels S, Martel A, Verbrugghe E, Goossens J, et al. (2011) The Mycotoxin Deoxynivalenol Potentiates Intestinal Inflammation by *Salmonella Typhimurium* in Porcine Ileal Loops. PLoS ONE 6: e23871.
68. Grenier B, Loureiro-Bracarense AP, Lucioli J, Pacheco GD, Cossalter AM, et al. (2011) Individual and combined effects of subclinical doses of deoxynivalenol and fumonisins in piglets. Mol Nutr Food Res 55: 761–771.
69. Levast B, de Monte M, Chevaleyre C, Melo S, Berri M, et al. (2010) Ultra-early weaning in piglets results in low serum IgA concentration and IL17 mRNA expression. Vet Immunol Immunopathol 137: 261–268.
70. Kiros TG, van Kessel J, Babiuk LA, Gerdts V (2011) Induction, regulation and physiological role of IL-17 secreting helper T-cells isolated from PBMC, thymus, and lung lymphocytes of young pigs. Vet Immunol Immunopathol 144: 448–454.
71. Royaee AR, Husmann RJ, Dawson HD, Calzada-Nova G, Schnitzlein WM, et al. (2004) Deciphering the involvement of innate immune factors in the development of the host response to PRRSV vaccination. Vet Immunol Immunopathol 102: 199–216.
72. Saurer L, McCullough KC, Summerfield A (2007) In vitro induction of mucosa-type dendritic cells by all-trans retinoic acid. Jô Immunol 179: 3504–3514.

5

Regulation and Migratory Role of P-Selectin Ligands during Intestinal Inflammation

Ute Hoffmann[1]☯, Matthias Pink[1]☯, Uta Lauer[1], Markus M. Heimesaat[2], Caroline Winsauer[1], Andrei Kruglov[1], Kerstin Schlawe[1], Claudia Leichsenring[1], Oliver Liesenfeld[2], Alf Hamann[1], Uta Syrbe[1,3]*

1 Deutsches Rheumaforschungszentrum, Berlin, Germany, **2** Institut für Mikrobiologie und Hygiene, Campus Benjamin Franklin, Universitätsmedizin Charité, Berlin, Germany, **3** Klinik für Gastroenterologie, Infektiologie und Rheumatologie, Campus Benjamin Franklin, Universitätsmedizin Charité, Berlin, Germany

Abstract

Dendritic cells from mesenteric lymph nodes (MLN) can convert retinal to retinoic acid (RA), which promotes induction of the gut-specific homing receptor α4β7. In contrast, priming within peripheral lymph nodes leads to upregulation of E- and P-selectin ligands (E- and P-lig). Apart from its α4β7 promoting effect, RA was shown to suppress E- and P-lig induction in vitro. However, enhanced frequencies of P-lig$^+$ CD4$^+$ T cells were reported during intestinal inflammation. To understand this contradiction, we first determined whether location of intestinal inflammation, that is, ileitis or colitis, affects P-lig induction. Both conditions promoted P-lig expression on CD4$^+$ T cells; however, P-lig expressed on T cells facilitated Th1 cell recruitment only into the inflamed colon but not into inflamed small intestine induced by oral *Toxoplasma gondii* infection. A majority of P-lig$^+$CD4$^+$ T cells found within MLN during intestinal inflammation co-expressed α4β7 confirming their activation in the presence of RA. Mesenteric P-lig$^+$CD4$^+$ cells co-expressed the 130 kDa isoform of CD43 which requires activity of core 2 (beta)1,6-N-acetyl-glycosaminyltransferase-I (C2GlcNAcT-I) suggesting that C2GlcNAcT-I contributes to P-lig expression under these conditions. To test whether inflammatory mediators can indeed overrule the inhibitory effect of RA on P-lig expression we stimulated CD4$^+$ T cells either polyclonal in the presence of IL-12 and IFNγ or by LPS-activated MLN-derived dendritic cells. Both conditions promoted P-lig induction even in the presence of RA. While RA impeded the induction of fucosyltransferase-VII it did not affect IL-12-dependent C2GlcNAcT-I induction suggesting that C2GlcNAcT-I can support P-lig expression even if fucosyltransferase-VII mRNA upregulation is dampened.

Editor: Ari Waisman, Johannes Gutenberg University of Mainz, Germany

Funding: This work was supported by the Deutsche Forschungsgemeinschaft (TR 52, SFB 633) and BMBF (CIPP). The funders had no role in study design, data collection and analysis, decision to publish, or preparation of the manuscript.

Competing Interests: The authors have declared that no competing interests exist.

* E-mail: Uta.Syrbe@charite.de

☯ These authors contributed equally to this work.

Introduction

Effector/memory T lymphocytes recirculate through peripheral tissues and by that provide immune surveillance of the body. Homing receptors required for their recruitment into peripheral tissue are induced upon effector cell differentiation. *In vivo* experiments using ovalbumin-TCR-transgenic CD4$^+$ T cells and systemic administration of ovalbumin with LPS as adjuvant showed that the priming location of the naive T cells dictates the induced homing molecule pattern: T cells activated within peripheral lymph nodes (PLN) upregulate E- and P-selectin ligands (E- and P-lig), whereas T cells activated within mesenteric lymph nodes (MLN) express α4β7 and CCR9 [1]. E- and P-selectin are displayed by skin vessels and function as skin-specific gate keepers whereas mucosal addressin cell adhesion molecule (MAdCAM) and the chemokine CCL25 are displayed by vessels within the intestine where they control T cell entry into the gut [2].

Tissue-specific antigen-presenting cells (APC), in particular CD103$^+$ dendritic cells (DCs), but also stromal cells are instrumental for the tissue-specific induction of homing receptors [3–5]. In contrast to PLN-derived DCs, MLN-derived DCs have the capacity to convert retinal to retinoic acid (RA) which promotes induction of the gut-homing receptor α4β7 and, in cooperation with IL-4, also induction of CCR9 [6,7].

E- and P-lig are induced by IL-12 *in vitro* resulting in high expression of selectin ligands in Th1 cells [8,9]. *In vivo*, additional pathways seem to exist as P-lig is also expressed on Th2 cells as well as on subsets of Tregs [1,10,11]. Vitamin D which controls CCR10 expression in the skin has no inducing effect on P-lig expression [12].

E- and P-lig are composed of a carrier protein which requires appropriate glycosylation in order to bind to E- and P-selectin. Generation of these epitopes mainly depends on induction of core 2 (beta)1,6-N-acetyl-glycosaminyltransferase I (C2GlcNAcT-I) and, specifically in T cells, on fucosyltransferase-VII (FucT-VII) [13–15]. RA, apart from its promoting effect on the gut-homing molecule expression, counteracts E- and P-lig induction and was shown to suppress FucT-VII induction in T cells [4,6,12].

Functional binding epitopes serving as E- and P-lig are generated by specific glycosylation of several carrier proteins upon activation and differentiation of T cells. P-selectin glycoprotein ligand-1 (PSGL-1), a dimeric glycoprotein expressed constitutively on all T cells, is the predominant carrier of functional P-lig

[16]. In contrast, E-lig are displayed on both PSGL-1 and alternative carrier proteins such as CD43 and CD44 [17–19].

Generation of P-selectin binding epitopes depends on the induction of fucosyltransferase (FucT)-VII and core 2 (beta)1,6-N-acetyl-glycosaminyltransferase I (C2GlcNAcT-I) [13–15]. Thus, Chinese hamster ovary (CHO) cells expressing PSGL-1 bind to P-selectin only if co-transfected with fucosyltransferases and C2GlcNAcT-I [20]. Fucosylation is required for synthesis of both, E- and P-lig. In T cells, E- and P-lig expression requires fucosyltransferase (FucT)-VII activity while FucT-IV is dispensable [15]. C2GlcNAcT-I is particularly important for P-lig generation, since leukocytes of C2GlcNAcT-I$^{-/-}$ mice display impaired P-selectin binding while binding to E-selectin is less affected [13,14,21]. RA, apart from its promoting effect on the gut-homing molecule expression, counteracts E- and P-lig induction and was shown to suppress FucT-VII induction in T cells [4,6,12].

In line with the opposing effect of RA on the induction of $\alpha4\beta7$ and E- and P-lig, an almost mutual exclusive expression of E- and P-lig and $\alpha4\beta7$ is indeed observed under homeostatic conditions on CD4$^+$ T cells [1,10]. However, during experimental colitis enhanced frequencies of P-lig expressing CD4$^+$ T cells were reported within intestinal sites, such as the MLN and the lamina propria [22]. Also during immunization with OVA and CFA injected intraperitoneally an IL-12-dependent upregulation of P-lig was observed on antigen-reactive T cells in the draining lymph nodes suggesting that inflammatory stimuli can overrule the tissue-specific induction pattern of selectin ligands [23].

To analyze whether P-lig induction is a common feature of intestinal inflammation we analyzed P-lig expression on CD4$^+$ T cells within MLN during inflammation either of the small intestine induced by oral infection with the protozoan parasite *Toxoplasma gondii* (*T. gondii*) which induces a strong Th1 cytokine-driven pathology within the small intestine [24,25] or during colitis. We show that under both conditions increased frequencies of P-lig$^+$ T cells are present and a large proportion of these cells co-expressed $\alpha4\beta7$.

Also *in vitro* we found that activation of MLN-derived DCs by Toll-like receptor (TLR) ligands such as LPS increased their capacity to induce P-lig, while induction of $\alpha4\beta7$ was partially impaired. Upon polyclonal activation of CD4$^+$ T cells in the absence of APCs, IL-12 and IFNγ increased P-lig induction even in the presence of RA suggesting that inflammatory mediators, like LPS, rather act via induction of IL-12 than by modulating the retinol-converting capacity of the DCs. RA impeded the activation-induced FucT-VII expression, however, it did not impair the IL-12-dependent C2GlcNAcT-I induction which apparently supports P-lig generation even in the presence of low FucT-VII mRNA expression.

Materials and Methods

Mice

6–12 weeks old, female BALB/c, C57BL/6, RAG-1$^{-/-}$ and DO11.10 purchased from the Bundesinstitut fuer Risikobewertung (BfR, Berlin, Germany) were housed under specific pathogen free (SPF) conditions. C.B-17 severe combined immunodeficient (SCID) mice were obtained from Charles River Breeding Laboratories (Sulzfeld, Germany) and used at an age of 4–6 weeks. *Fut7*$^{-/-}$ mice on C57BL6 background provided by J. Lowe were backcrossed to BALB/c at least seven times. All animal experiments were performed in accordance with German animal protection laws after approval by the LaGeSo (G0227-98, G0331-08).

Antibodies, Staining and Sorting Reagents

The following antibodies were produced in our laboratory: anti-FcR II/III (2.4G2), anti-CD4-FITC (GK1.5), anti-CD8 (53–672), anti-CD25 (PC/6), anti-Mac-1 (M1/70), anti-CD3 (145.2C11), anti-CD28 (37.51), and anti-IL4 (11B11), anti-IFN-γ (AN18.17.24), anti-IL12 (C17.8), anti $\alpha4\beta7$-Bio (DATK32). The following antibodies were purchased from BD Pharmingen (Heidelberg, Germany): anti-CD4-FITC or anti-CD4-PerCP (RM4-5), anti-CD62L-PE (Mel-14), anti-CD45RB-PE (16A), IgG1-FITC (R3-34) and SA-PerCP. The anti-CD43-PECy7 (1B11) and isotype control were purchased from BioLegend (London, UK). The recombinant P-selectin human IgG fusion protein was kindly provided by D. Vestweber (Munster, Germany). PE-labeled anti-human IgG antibodies were obtained from Jackson Immuno Research (Suffolk, UK). All microbeads were obtained from Miltenyi Biotec (Bergisch-Gladbach, Germany).

Induction of Intestinal Inflammation

To induce inflammation of the small intestine female C57BL/6 mice were infected per os with 10 or 100 cysts of *Toxoplasma gondii* (ME49 strain) which were obtained from NMRI mice infected 2–3 months prior. Migration studies were performed on day 3, 5 and 7 after oral infection with 100 cysts. For T cell analysis from MLN animals were orally infected with 10 cysts of Toxoplasma and sacrificed on day 9.

For induction of large intestinal inflammation (experimental colitis) either 3×10^5 CD4$^+$CD45Rb^{high} T cells from BALB/c or from C57BL/6 were transferred i.p. into SCID (BALB/c background) or RAG mice (C57BL/6 background) as described [26]. SCID mice developed colitis within 10 to 12 weeks, whereas in RAG-1$^{-/-}$ mice disease onset was accelerated and occurred already after 3 to 4 weeks.

Cell Isolation and Purification

For analysis of homing receptor expression single cell suspensions were produced from MLN and spleen by teasing the cut organs through stainless steel meshes. After washing erythrocytes were lysed by hypotonic lyses.

For CD4 T cell isolation, cells were purified either by panning using anti-CD8 (53–672), anti-CD25 (PC/6), anti-Mac-1 (M1/70) and anti-FcR II/III (2.4G2) antibodies or by direct isolation of CD4$^+$ cells by anti-CD4-FITC (GK1.5) and anti-FITC multisort-MACS beads to a purity of $\geq$ 98%. Naive CD4$^+$CD62L$^+$ cells were MACS-sorted with anti-CD62L microbeads to a purity of $\geq$ 98%. In some experiments CD25$^+$ T cells were depleted before further enrichment of naive T cells.

MLN-derived DCs were prepared by positive selection of CD11c$^+$ cells using anti-CD11c-MACS beads reaching a purity of about 95% of CD11c$^+$ DCs.

For induction of SCID or RAG-1$^{-/-}$ colitis CD4$^+$CD45Rb^{high} T cells were enriched by CD4-FITC and anti-FITC-MACS beads. The CD45Rb^{high} population was sorted after staining with CD45Rb-PE by the Fluorescent activated cell sorter (FACS-DIVA; BD Biosciences, Heidelberg, Germany) to a purity of >95–99%.

In vitro Stimulation of Naïve T Cells

For DC-dependent stimulation naive OVA-TCR^{tg} T cells from DO11.10 mice were activated by 0.5 μM OVA$_{323-339}$ peptide (Biochemistry department, Charité, Berlin) in the presence of CD11c$^+$ DCs at a T cell/DC cell ratio of 10:1 and total cell number of 2×10^6 cells/ml in complete RPMI 1640, containing

10% FCS and 10 μM 2-ME (Life Technologies). 1 μg/ml LPS (Sigma-Aldrich, Muenchen, Germany) from *E. coli* strain 055:B5 was added. Homing receptor expression was determined on day 5 after stimulation. Retinal (Sigma- Aldrich) was added at a concentration of 10 nM.

For polyclonal activation, sorted naive T cells from BALB/c mice were cultured on plates coated with anti-CD3 and anti-CD28 mAbs at 1×10^6 cells/ml in the presence or absence of retinoic acid (10 nM). For Th1 polarizing conditions cultures were supplemented with recombinant murine IL-2 at 5 ng/ml, IL-12 at 5 ng/ml, IFNγ at 20 ng/ml (all recombinant cytokines: R&D Systems, Wiesbaden, Germany) and neutralizing anti-IL-4 mAb at 5 μg/ml. For Th0 conditions recombinant murine IL-2 at 5 ng/ml and neutralizing anti-IL-12 mAb, anti-IFNγ and anti-IL-4 mAb were added to the culture. Cells were removed from the stimulus after 72 h and rested for 2 days before analysis.

For homing studies, Th1 cells were generated from wild type and *Fut7*$^{-/-}$ mice by polyclonal activation by plate-bound anti-CD3/anti-CD28 stimulation in the presence of IL-12, IFNγ and anti-IL-4. After 72 h cells were removed from the stimulus and rested for 2 further days. On day 5 the cells were used for migration studies.

Flow Cytometric Analysis

Cytometric analysis was performed using a FACSCalibur and the CellQuest software (BD Biosciences). P-selectin ligands were detected by P-selectin human IgG chimeric protein stained in HBSS containing Ca^{2+} and $Mg^{2+}$and PE-conjugated anti-human IgG antibody. OVA-TCR^{tg} CD4$^+$ T cells were identified using the clonotype-specific antibody KJ1.26.

For intracellular cytokine detection cells were stimulated with phorbol myristate acetate (PMA)/ionomycin (10 ng/ml; 500 ng/ml; Sigma-Aldrich) for 4 h with addition of Brefeldin A (10 μg/ml; Sigma-Aldrich) for the last 2 h. Afterwards, cells were surface stained for CD4 and selectin ligands, fixed in 2% paraformaldehyde (Sigma-Aldrich), permeabilized by 0.5% saponin (Sigma) and stained intracellularly for IFNγ. To prevent unspecific staining, anti FcRII/II (2.4G2) and whole rat IgG (Jackson Immuno Research) were added.

Quantitative PCR

Total RNA was isolated with RNeasy Mini Kit and QiaShredder (Qiagen) and DNA removed with RNase-Free DNase Set (Qiagen). RNA was reverse transcribed by Superscript II Reverse Transcriptase (Invitrogen) using oligo(dT) and random hexamer primer (Qiagen). Quantitative PCR was performed on a Mx3000P or Mx3005P qPCR system (Agilent Technologies, Santa Clara, USA). Platinum SYBR Green qPCR Super-Mix-UDG (Invitrogen) was used together with the primers previously described for FucT-VII and C2GlcNAcT-I [27]. For detection of CCR9, PSGL-1 and FucT-IV mRNA the following primers were used: CCR9: forward: 5′-TGCCATGTTCATCTCCAACTG-3′, reverse: 5′-GAACTGGGTTCAGACAACTGTGG-3; PSGL-1: forward: 5′-GGGATGACGATTTTGAGGAC-3′, reverse: 5′-TCCTGTACCTGGGGCAGTAG-3′; FucT-IV: forward: 5′-GAGGTGGGTGTGGATGAACT-3′, reverse: 5′-TCGCTCCTGGAATAGAGGAA-3′.

In vivo Homing Assay

The homing assay was performed as previously described [28]. In brief, Th1 cells were labeled with 20 μCi/ml ^{51}Cr (Amersham Buchler) followed by incubation at 37°C for two hours in fresh medium and removal of dead cells with gradient centrifugation (17.1% isotonic Nycodenz, Nyegaard, Norway). 1–4$\times10^6$ labeled cells were injected into tail vein of mice. After three hours mice were sacrificed, several organs were removed and radioactivity of these organs and the remaining body was counted using a γ-counter (Wallac, Turku, Finland).

Results

Enhanced Frequency of P-lig$^+$ CD4$^+$ T Cells in MLN during Small and Large Intestinal Inflammation

Induction of P-lig has been described during inflammation of the large intestine [22] and also within the small intestine after intraperitoneal immunization [23]. To analyze whether P-lig is commonly induced during intestinal inflammation we determined the P-lig expression of Th1 effector cells in MLN during inflammation of either the large or the small intestine. Large intestinal inflammation was induced by transfer of naive T cells into SCID mice [29] while small intestinal inflammation, i.e. a pan-ileitis, was induced by oral infection of wildtype (WT) mice with *T. gondii* [30,31]. During colitis but also during ileitis, more than 25% of the CD4$^+$ T cells in MLN expressed P-lig which was significantly higher than under homeostatic conditions (Figure 1A). Also if we determined specifically the percentage of P-lig$^+$ cells among Th1 effector cells identified by IFNγ-expression a drastic increase in the frequency of P-lig$^+$ cells was observed during both, colitis and ileitis, compared to homeostatic conditions (Figure 1A). This suggests that during intestinal inflammation P-lig is strongly induced on newly generated Th1 effector cells.

P-lig and α4β7 are Co-expressed on MLN CD4$^+$ T Cells

RA, the main inducer of α4β7, was shown to inhibit the expression of E- and P-lig *in vitro* [6]. To analyze whether P-lig induction under intestinal inflammation occurs in parallel to α4β7 induction and hence in the presence of RA, we analyzed P-lig and α4β7 expression simultaneously in MLN of RAG-1$^{-/-}$ mice after induction of colitis by transfer of CD45Rb^{high} T cells in comparison to healthy C57BL/6 mice. In addition to the enhanced frequencies of P-lig$^+$ CD4$^+$ T cells we observed a dramatic increase in the frequency of α4β7 CD4$^+$ T cells in the colitis mice indicating indirectly that the majority of effector cells had been exposed to RA during priming (Figure 1B). Also among P-lig$^+$ CD4$^+$ T cells, the majority, i.e. about 60%, co-expressed α4β7 suggesting that these cells have been exposed to RA during priming as well. Among the few P-lig$^+$ CD4$^+$ T cells found in healthy C57/Bl6 mice more than 40% co-expressed α4β7 showing that co-induction of α4β7 and P-lig can also occur under non-lymphopenic conditions (Figure 1B). Among the enlarged fraction of α4β7$^+$ CD4$^+$ T cells found during colitis a significant percentage, i.e. about 35% co-expressed P-lig (Figure 1B).

This suggests that P-lig and α4β7 are co-induced under inflammatory conditions within the intestine. To determine whether the P-selectin-binding activity of CD4$^+$ effector cells generated during intestinal inflammation depends on C2GlcNAcT-I activity we analyzed the expression of the 130 kDa isoform of CD43 – a C2GlcNAcT-I-dependent epitope which is specifically recognized by the mAb 1B11 and used as a surrogate marker of C2GlcNAcT-I activity [32,33]. As shown in Figure 1C, essentially all P-lig$^+$ CD4$^+$ cells within MLN of colitis mice co-expressed the 130 kDa isoform of CD43 indicating C2GlcNAcT-I activity in these cells.

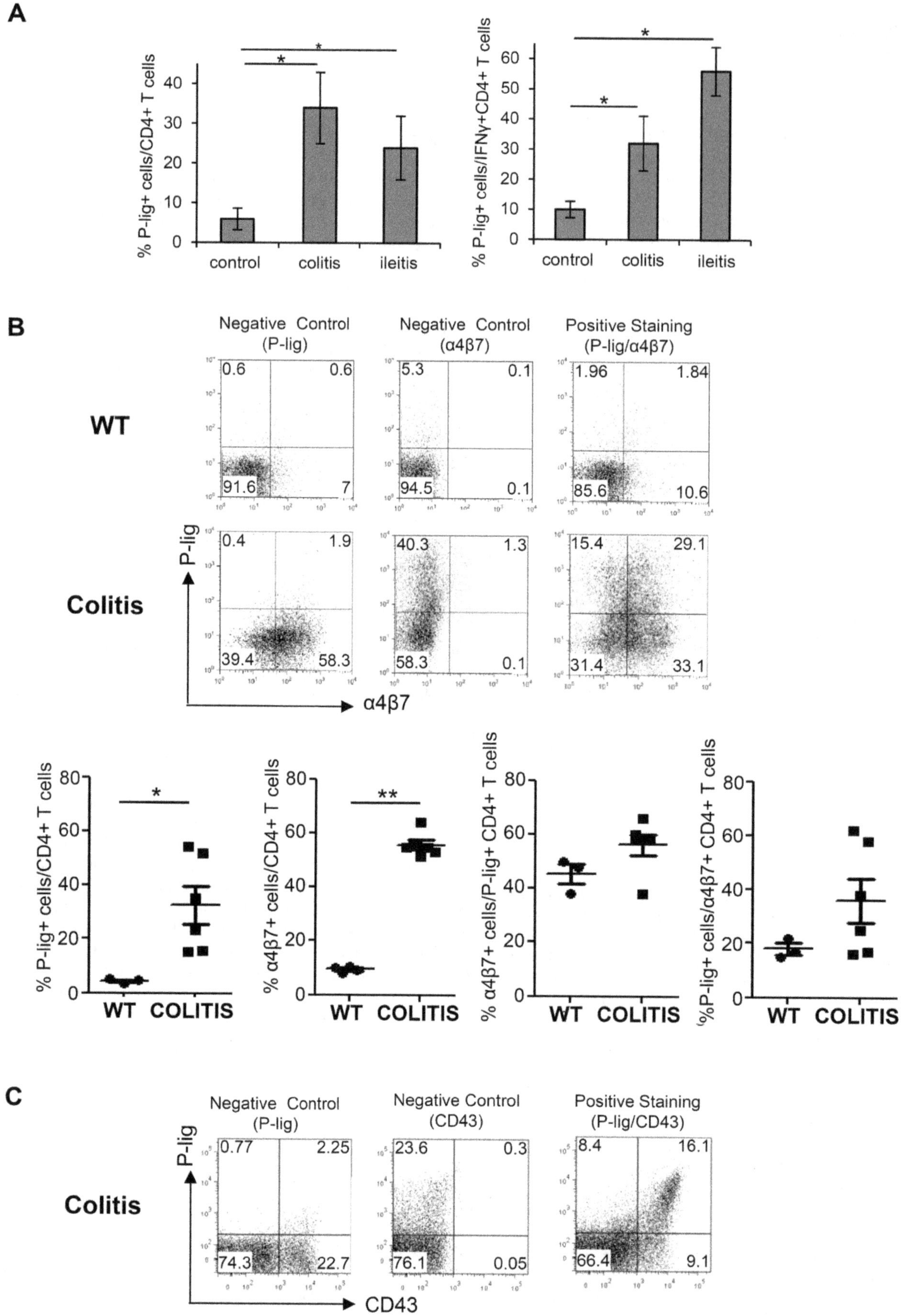
A
% P-lig+ cells/CD4+ T cells
control
colitis
ileitis
% P-lig+ cells/IFNγ+CD4+ T cells
control
colitis
ileitis
B
Negative Control (P-lig)
Negative Control (α4β7)
Positive Staining (P-lig/α4β7)
WT
0.6 0.6 91.6 7
5.3 0.1 94.5 0.1
1.96 1.84 85.6 10.6
Colitis
0.4 1.9 39.4 58.3
40.3 1.3 58.3 0.1
15.4 29.1 31.4 33.1
P-lig
α4β7
% P-lig+ cells/CD4+ T cells
% α4β7+ cells/CD4+ T cells
% α4β7+ cells/P-lig+ CD4+ T cells
%P-lig+ cells/α4β7+ CD4+ T cells
WT COLITIS
C
Negative Control (P-lig)
Negative Control (CD43)
Positive Staining (P-lig/CD43)
Colitis
0.77 2.25 74.3 22.7
23.6 0.3 76.1 0.05
8.4 16.1 66.4 9.1
P-lig
CD43

Figure 1. Coexpression of P-lig and α4β7 on a major subset of CD4⁺ T cells in MLN during intestinal inflammation. A) The percentage of P-lig⁺ cells/CD4⁺ T cells (left panel) and the percentage of P-lig⁺ cells/IFNγ⁺CD4⁺ T cells (right panel) in MLN of healthy mice (control), SCID mice after induction of colitis (colitis) and mice orally infected with 10 cysts of *T. gondii* (ileitis) is shown. Mean ± SD of four to six mice per group from two independent experiments is shown. B) In the upper panel, examples of control and positive stainings of P-lig⁺ and α4β7⁺ cells among CD4⁺ T cells from MLN of wildtype mice (WT) and RAG-1$^{-/-}$ mice after induction of colitis (colitis) is shown. Lower panel shows the mean and individual measurements of the frequencies of P-lig⁺ cells/CD4⁺ T cells and α4β7⁺ cells/CD4⁺ T cells acquired in two independent experiments. Among P-lig⁺ cells the frequency of α4β7⁺ co-expressing cells was determined as well as the frequency of P-lig⁺ cells among α4β7⁺ T cells. C) Control and positive stainings of the 130 kDa isoform of CD43 and P-lig gated on CD4⁺ T cells from pooled cells of MLN of four mice with colitis induced as in B (one representative example of two independent experiments). *$p<0.05$; **$p<0.01$; Mann Withney U test.

P-lig Expression on T Cells Supports Recruitment of CD4⁺ Effector T Cells into the Inflamed Large Intestine but not into the Inflamed Small Intestine

Now, we aimed to analyze whether selectin ligand expression is at all required for Th1 cells to enter inflamed intestinal sites. Therefore, we generated Th1 cells from wildtype (WT) or *Fut7*$^{-/-}$-deficient mice. In *Fut7*$^{-/-}$ Th1 cells P-lig [15]) expression is abolished while effector functions, such as IFNγ production, are unaffected (Figure 2A). To study the impact of P-lig for T cell recruitment into small intestinal inflammation WT or *Fut7*$^{-/-}$ Th1 cells were radioactively labeled and transferred into untreated recipient mice or mice orally infected with *T. gondii* either three, five or seven days before. *Toxoplasma gondii* infected mice were randomly assigned at the day of the homing experiment to the groups either receiving Th1 cells from WT or *Fut7*$^{-/-}$ mice. Infection of mice with *T. gondii* elicited a strong immigration of Th1 cells into the small intestine on day 7 after infection, the day when inflammatory responses and development of small intestinal pathology peak [30,31] as indicated by increased recovered radioactivity compared to non-infected gut (Figure 2B). However, *Fut7*$^{-/-}$ Th1 cells lacking P-lig expression entered the small intestine equally well as WT Th1 cells suggesting that P-lig expression on T cells is dispensable for the recruitment of Th1 cells to the inflamed small intestine. To analyze whether P-lig can support recruitment into the inflamed colon WT and *Fut7*$^{-/-}$ Th1 cells were transferred into SCID mice in which colitis was induced before by transfer of CD45Rb^{high} T cells from WT mice. Migration of *Fut7*$^{-/-}$ Th1 cells into the inflamed colon was reduced by about 50% compared to WT Th1 cells (Figure 2C) suggesting that the interaction of P-lig with its ligand P-selectin can indeed support immigration of Th1 cells into the inflamed colon.

Treatment with LPS Enhances the Induction of P-lig on CD4⁺ T Cells by MLN-derived DCs

To clarify the mechanism of P-lig induction within the gut environment, i.e. in the presence of RA, we first analyzed whether bacterial stimuli affect the capacity of MLN-DCs to induce P-lig on T cells. Therefore, we isolated CD11c⁺ DCs from MLN and used those for activation of OVA-transgenic T cells by OVA in the presence or absence of LPS. LPS significantly enhanced the induction of P-lig on CD4⁺ T cells cultured in the presence of MLN-derived DCs but slightly reduced induction of α4β7 (Figure 3A). Addition of retinal which is metabolized by MLN-DCs to retinoic acid was accompanied by a strongly increased induction of α4β77 on CD4⁺ T cells whereas P-lig induction was only slightly reduced. The additional inducing effect of LPS on P-lig expression was retained in cultures containing retinal.

LPS treatment of MLN-derived DCs could affect the capability of the DCs to convert retinal or it could induce production of inflammatory cytokine, in particular IL-12, which is known to induce P-lig. To determine if Th1 polarizing cytokines can induce P-lig expression even in the presence of RA, we activated naïve T cells by anti-CD3/CD28 in the presence or absence of RA and in the absence or presence of Th1-polarizing cytokines, i.e. IL-12, IFNγ and anti-IL-4 (Figure 3B). In the absence of polarizing cytokines, i.e. under Th0 conditions, no matter whether RA was present or not, low induction of P-lig was seen. α4β7, expressed at intermediate levels in the absence of RA, increased upon exposure to 10 nM RA. Similarly, presence of RA increased CCR9 mRNA expression under non-polarizing Th0 and Th1-polarizing conditions. In the presence of Th1 cytokines, high levels of P-lig were induced even in the presence of RA. α4β7 induction was slightly reduced under these conditions. The frequency of P-lig/ α4β7 double positive CD4⁺ T cells increased to about 40% in the presence of RA and Th1-polarizing conditions. Analysis of FucT-VII and C2GlcNAcT-I mRNA levels showed that although RA almost completely abrogated FucT-VII induction, C2GlcNAcT-I mRNA induction was not significantly reduced by RA and reached similar levels as under Th1 conditions in the absence of RA (Figure 3C). PSGL-1 levels were unaffected by RA treatment. Also expression levels of FucT-IV induced under Th1 conditions were unchanged upon RA treatment. This suggests that unimpaired C2GlcNAcT-I expression determines P-lig expression under these conditions even in the presence of low FucT-VII induction.

Discussion

In this study we confirm that P-ligs are induced on a significant proportion of CD4⁺ T cells during inflammation within the intestine. During small and large intestinal inflammation we observed a high frequency of P-lig expressing T cells in the draining MLN excluding a major impact of the specific intestinal location on this induction. As during intestinal inflammation the majority of P-lig⁺ T cells found within the MLNs co-expressed α4β7, intestinal priming of these cells is very likely. This suggests that induction of P-ligs is effective under inflammatory conditions even in the intestinal environment which primarily supports induction of gut-specific homing molecules [1].

The functional role of P-selectin-P-lig interactions for mucosal inflammation is controversially discussed [34]. Bonder et al. showed E- and P-selectin-dependent interactions of Th1 and Th2 cells within small intestine in response to intraperitoneal TNF and IL-4 treatment by intravital microscopy [35]. In models of chronic ileitis like the SAMP/Yit model, administration of a mAb directed against P-selectin-glycoprotein-1 (PSGL-1, 2PH1), which primarily affects P-selectin-dependent adhesion, attenuated disease [36]. Interestingly, PSGL-1 is displayed in this model by the small intestinal vasculature and only vascular expression was critical for disease development whereas it was dispensable on hematopoetic cells [37].

In accordance with this latter study, deficiency in selectin-ligand expression on Th1 cells did not abrogate recruitment of the Th1 cells into the inflamed small intestine during oral infection with *T. gondii* as tested here. In addition to the proposed interaction of leukocytes with vascular PSGL-1, immigration of the *in vitro* generated Th1 cells could also be guided by interaction of α4β7

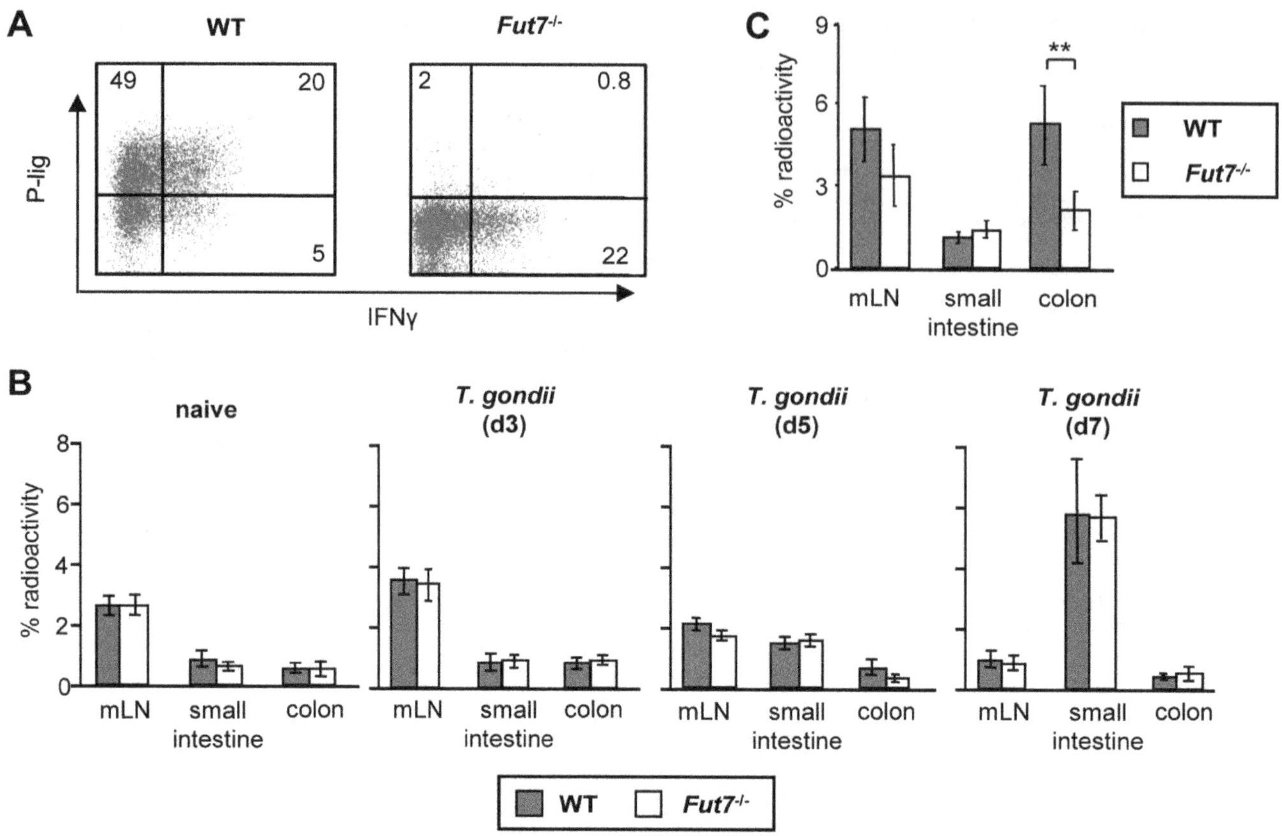

Figure 2. P-lig expression can support recruitment of Th1 cells into the inflamed colon but not into the inflamed small intestine. A) Naive T cells from wiltype (WT) and $Fut7^{-/-}$ mice were differentiated in vitro under Th1 polarizing conditions in the absence of RA. P-lig and PMA/ionomycin-induced IFNγ expression of Th1 cells generated from $Fut7^{-/-}$ and WT mice is shown. B) ^{51}Cr-labeled Th1 cells generated from WT or $Fut7^{-/-}$ mice were transferred into naive mice or mice infected orally with 100 cysts of *T. gondii* three, five or seven days before. Radioactivity (mean ± SD) per organ was determined three hours after transfer of radioactive T cells and is given as the percentage of total recovered radioactivity (n = 5 animals/group). The experiment was repeated on d7 with 5 animals/group with similar results. C) ^{51}Cr-labeled Th1 cells from WT or $Fut7^{-/-}$ mice were injected into SCID mice with established colitis induced by transfer of CD4^{+}CD45Rb^{high} cells. The percentage (mean and SD) of recovered radioactivity per organ of one representative experiment out of 3 independent experiments with 4–6 mice/ group is shown. **$p<0.01$; Mann Whitney U test.

with MAdCAM as these cells also express α4β7 (Figure 3B). In conclusion, both the SAMP/Yit model, a mixed Th1/Th2 model [38] and the Th1 model of *Toxoplasma gondii*-induced ileitis [24], do not require T cell-expressed selectin ligands for entry of Th1 cells into the inflamed small intestine. This might suggest that selectin ligands on T cells are in general dispensable for their entry into the small intestine in T cell-dependent ileitis.

In contrast to the small intestine, we found about 50% impairment of the recruitment of $Fut7^{-/-}$ Th1 cells into the inflamed colon. Thus, P-selectin-dependent homing mechanisms contribute to recruitment into the inflamed colon.

In a DTH model we found that immigration of $Fut7^{-/-}$ Th1 is reduced by more than 90% compared to WT Th1 cells [39]. This suggests that within the inflamed skin, entry of Th1 cells almost completely depends on E- and P-selectin-dependent adhesion whereas in colitis, P-lig-dependent migration accounts only partially for inflammatory T cell recruitment. In line with our study, blockade of P-selectin dependent interaction with the PSGL-1 mAb can reduce leukocyte recruitment in the acute dextran sodium sulfate (DSS) colitis model which also attenuates disease [40]. In contrast, PSGL-1 deficient CD4^{+} T cells were able to induce colitis in the transfer colitis model as used here [41]. This suggests that P-selectin dependent adhesion mechanisms rather complement or synergize during inflammation with the α4β7-dependent adhesion system of the intestine. Thus, transfer of naive T cells from $Itgb7^{-/-}$ mice results in strongly delayed, although not complete prevention of colitis confirming the importance of the α4β7-dependent adhesion for rapid and efficient localization of T cells in intestinal tissues [42].

By analyzing the frequency of P-lig^{+} T cells among cytokine producing cells within the spleen and lung during influenza virus and *Nippostrongylus* infection and within the liver during oral *T. gondii* infection we have previously found, that P-lig expression is particularly high among cytokine producing cells at the site of inflammation [10]. Similar to that, we found a high proportion, i.e. about 50%, of P-lig^{+} T cells among IFNγ-producing T cells within the MLN during *T. gondii* infection. This suggests that the local inflammatory mediators present during ileitis and colitis not only promote Th1 differentiation but also induction of P-lig expression, even in the intestine. In this line, Haddad et al. showed that P-lig expression on T cells primed within MLN after antigen-specific i.p.-immunization in the presence of CFA, a strong trigger of Th1 immunity, is abrogated by IL-12 blockade [23]. Innate, in particular dendritic cells are activated by bacterial structures and there is a debate whether Toll like receptor (TLR) triggering can modulate the retinal-converting capacity of DCs. In fact, a de-

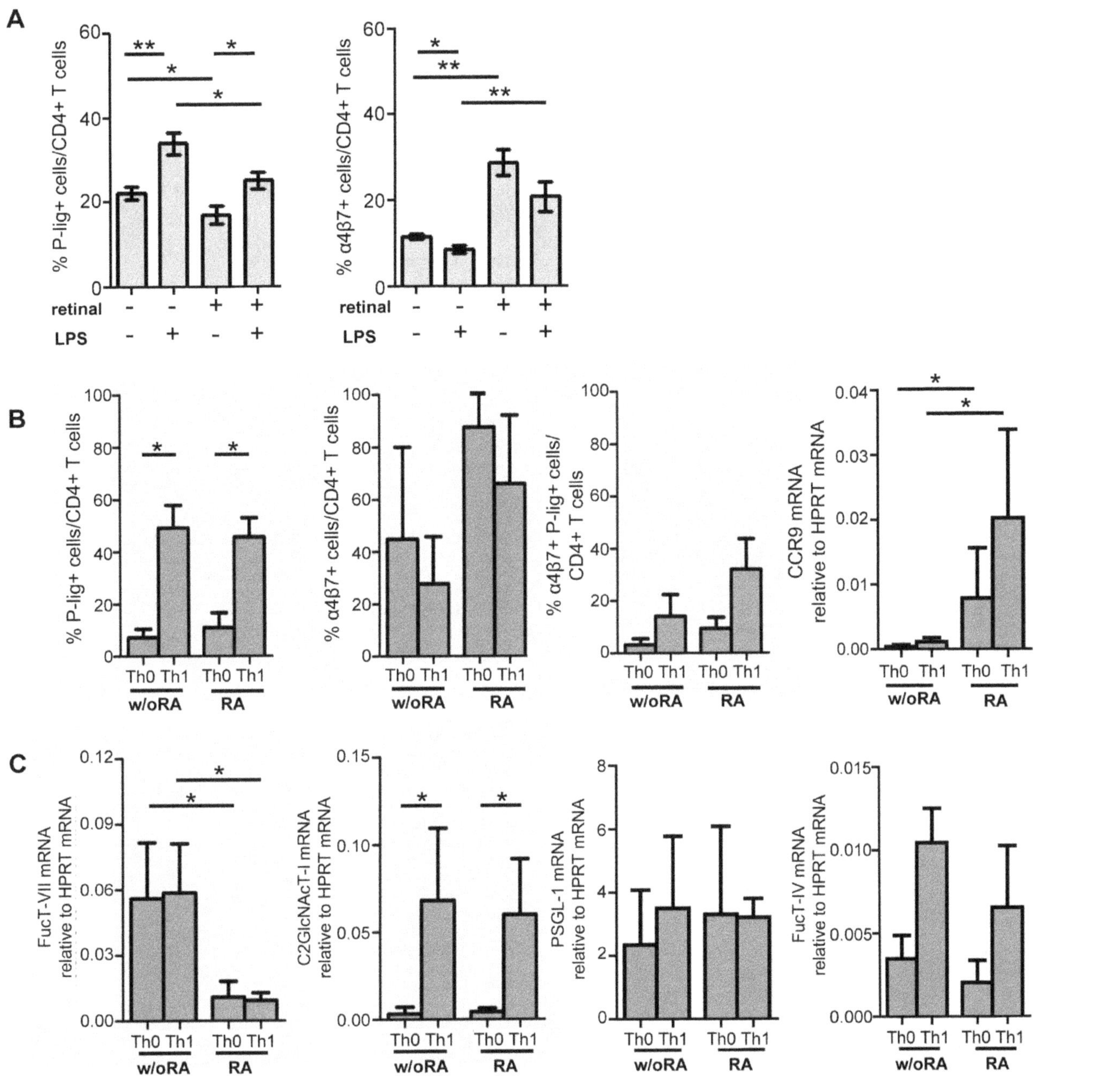

Figure 3. Inflammatory stimuli increase P-lig but reduce α4β7induction on CD4⁺ T cells even in the presence of RA. A) Naive OVA-TCR^{tg} CD4$^+$ T cells were activated with OVA$_{323-339}$ peptide and CD11c$^+$ DCs from MLN in the presence or absence of LPS and presence or absence of 10 nM retinal. Percentage of P-lig$^+$/CD4$^+$ T cells and α4β7$^+$/CD4$^+$ T cells (mean + SD of n = 6 from two independent experiments) was determined on d5 after activation. B) Naive CD4$^+$ T cells were activated by plate bound antiCD3/antiCD28 in the presence or absence of polarizing cytokines and 10 nM retinoic acid. The frequency of P-lig$^+$, α4β7$^+$ as well as double-positive CD4$^+$ T cells was determined on day 4 by FACS while CCR9 expression was determined on mRNA level (mean + SD, n = 4 from four independent experiments). C) FucT-VII and C2GlcNAcT-I mRNA as well as PSGL-1 and FucT-IV mRNA expression were determined on day 4 after activation (mean + SD of four independent experiments). $^*p<0.05$; $^{**}p<0.01$; Mann Whitney U test (for A–C).

crease in the aldehyde dehydrogenase (ALDH) activity has been described in MLN DCs from *Myd88*$^{-/-}$ *Trif*$^{-/-}$ mice and from germfree mice suggesting that bacterial stimuli promote expression of ALDH [43]. However, among several TLR ligands only TLR 1/2 ligand Pam$_3$CSK$_4$ but not LPS strongly upregulated ALDH activity of mucosal DCs from mice housed under specific pathogen-free conditions [44]. Our results suggest that LPS might even suppress ALDH activity since expression α4β7 was slightly reduced upon LPS exposure of MLN-DCs. However, as we observed a strong increase in the frequency of α4β7 CD4$^+$ cells during colitis this effect seems to be negligible in vivo. The high percentage of P-lig$^+$ T cells in MLN co-expressing α4β7 rather suggests that inflammatory stimuli promoted P-lig induction despite the presence of RA. In line with this, we observed strong induction of P-lig under Th1-polarizing conditions in vitro even in the presence of retinoic acid. Thus, this suggests that enhanced P-lig expression upon intestinal inflammation is primarily stimulated by enhanced local cytokine production rather than by modulation of the retinal-converting capacity.

The generation of P-lig epitopes in CD4⁺ T cells depends on induction of FucT-VII and C2GlcNAcT-I [14,15]. In accordance with published data, we found strong inhibition of FucT-VII mRNA expression by RA [4,6]. However, IL-12-induced C2GlcNAcT-I expression was almost unaffected by retinoic acid and obviously promoted P-lig expression even in the presence of low FucT-VII expression. Involvement of C2GlcNAcT-I is also suggested by our in vivo data, as we found high expression of the core-2-dependent 130 kDa isoform of CD43. However, as *Fut7*$^{-/-}$ Th1 cells lack P-lig expression (Figure 3) residual, low level expression of FucT-VII is required for P-lig generation.

Altogether our data suggest that inflammatory stimuli can overrule tissue-specific homing pathways in the gut. P-lig expression is achieved under these conditions by unimpaired induction of C2GlcNAcT-I by IL-12 even though FucT-VII induction is suppressed in a retinoic acid-dependent way.

Acknowledgments

P-selectin-human IgG chimeric protein was kindly provided by D. Vestweber. *Fut7*$^{-/-}$ mice were from J. Lowe. We thank H. Schliemann, H. Hecker, and T. Geeske for providing mAbs and T. Kayser for assistance in FACSorting.

Author Contributions

Conceived and designed the experiments: OL AH US. Performed the experiments: UH MP UL MMH CW AK KS CL. Analyzed the data: UH MP CL US UL. Wrote the paper: AH OL US .

References

1. Campbell DJ, Butcher EC (2002) Rapid acquisition of tissue-specific homing phenotypes by CD4+ T cells activated in cutaneous or mucosal lymphoid tissues. J Exp Med 195: 135–141.
2. Sigmundsdottir H, Butcher EC (2008) Environmental cues, dendritic cells and the programming of tissue-selective lymphocyte trafficking. Nat Immunol 9: 981–987.
3. Dudda JC, Lembo A, Bachtanian E, Huehn J, Siewert C, et al. (2005) Dendritic cells govern induction and reprogramming of polarized tissue-selective homing receptor patterns of T cells: important roles for soluble factors and tissue microenvironments. Eur J Immunol 35: 1056–1065.
4. Mora JR, Cheng G, Picarella D, Briskin M, Buchanan N, et al. (2005) Reciprocal and dynamic control of CD8 T cell homing by dendritic cells from skin- and gut-associated lymphoid tissues. J Exp Med 201: 303–316.
5. Edele F, Molenaar R, Gutle D, Dudda JC, Jakob T, et al. (2008) Cutting edge: instructive role of peripheral tissue cells in the imprinting of T cell homing receptor patterns. J Immunol 181: 3745–3749.
6. Iwata M, Hirakiyama A, Eshima Y, Kagechika H, Kato C, et al. (2004) Retinoic acid imprints gut-homing specificity on T cells. Immunity 21: 527–538.
7. Elgueta R, Sepulveda FE, Vilches F, Vargas L, Mora JR, et al. (2008) Imprinting of CCR9 on CD4 T cells requires IL-4 signaling on mesenteric lymph node dendritic cells. J Immunol 180: 6501–6507.
8. Austrup F, Vestweber D, Borges E, Löhning M, Bräuer R, et al. (1997) P-and E-selectin mediate recruitment of T helper 1 but not T helper 2 cells into inflamed tissues. Nature 385: 81–83.
9. Wagers AJ, Waters CM, Stoolman LM, Kansas GS (1998) Interleukin 12 and interleukin 4 control T cell adhesion to endothelial selectins through opposite effects on alpha1, 3-fucosyltransferase VII gene expression. J Exp Med 188: 2225–2231.
10. Kretschmer U, Bonhagen K, Debes GF, Mittrucker HW, Erb KJ, et al. (2004) Expression of selectin ligands on murine effector and IL-10-producing CD4(+) T cells from non-infected and infected tissues. Eur J Immunol 34: 3070–3081.
11. Huehn J, Siegmund K, Lehmann J, Siewert C, Haubold U, et al. (2004) Developmental stage, phenotype and migration distinguish naive- and effector/memory-like CD4+ regulatory T cells. J Exp Med 199: 303–313.
12. Sigmundsdottir H, Pan J, Debes GF, Alt C, Habtezion A, et al. (2007) DCs metabolize sunlight-induced vitamin D3 to 'program' T cell attraction to the epidermal chemokine CCL27. Nat Immunol 8: 285–293.
13. Sperandio M, Thatte A, Foy D, Ellies LG, Marth JD, et al. (2001) Severe impairment of leukocyte rolling in venules of core 2 glucosaminyltransferase-deficient mice. Blood 97: 3812–3819.
14. Snapp KR, Heitzig CE, Ellies LG, Marth JD, Kansas GS (2001) Differential requirements for the O-linked branching enzyme core 2 beta1-6-N-glucosaminyltransferase in biosynthesis of ligands for E- selectin and P-selectin. Blood 97: 3806–3811.
15. Smithson G, Rogers CE, Smith PL, Scheidegger EP, Petryniak B, et al. (2001) Fuc-TVII is required for T helper 1 and T cytotoxic 1 lymphocyte selectin ligand expression and recruitment in inflammation, and together with Fuc-TIV regulates naive T cell trafficking to lymph nodes. J Exp Med 194: 601–614.
16. Yang J, Hirata T, Croce K, Merrill Skoloff G, Tchernychev B, et al. (1999) Targeted gene disruption demonstrates that P-selectin glycoprotein ligand 1 (PSGL-1) is required for P-selectin-mediated but not E-selectin-mediated neutrophil rolling and migration. J Exp Med 190: 1769–1782.
17. Matsumoto M, Atarashi K, Umemoto E, Furukawa Y, Shigeta A, et al. (2005) CD43 functions as a ligand for E-Selectin on activated T cells. J Immunol 175: 8042–8050.
18. Alcaide P, King SL, Dimitroff CJ, Lim YC, Fuhlbrigge RC, et al. (2007) The 130-kDa glycoform of CD43 functions as an E-selectin ligand for activated Th1 cells in vitro and in delayed-type hypersensitivity reactions in vivo. J Invest Dermatol 127: 1964–1972.
19. Katayama Y, Hidalgo A, Chang J, Peired A, Frenette PS (2005) CD44 is a physiological E-selectin ligand on neutrophils. J Exp Med 201: 1183–1189.
20. Kumar R, Camphausen RT, Sullivan FX, Cumming DA (1996) Core2 beta-1,6-N-acetylglucosaminyltransferase enzyme activity is critical for P-selectin glycoprotein ligand-1 binding to P-selectin. Blood 88: 3872–3879.
21. Ellies LG, Tsuboi S, Petryniak B, Lowe JB, Fukuda M, et al. (1998) Core 2 oligosaccharide biosynthesis distinguishes between selectin ligands essential for leukocyte homing and inflammation. Immunity 9: 881–890.
22. Thoma S, Bonhagen K, Vestweber D, Hamann A, Reimann J (1998) Expression of selectin-binding epitopes and cytokines by CD4+ T cells repopulating scid mice with colitis. Eur J Immunol 28: 1785–1797.
23. Haddad W, Cooper CJ, Zhang Z, Brown JB, Zhu Y, et al. (2003) P-selectin and P-selectin glycoprotein ligand 1 are major determinants for Th1 cell recruitment to nonlymphoid effector sites in the intestinal lamina propria. J Exp Med 198: 369–377.
24. Liesenfeld O, Kosek J, Remington JS, Suzuki Y (1996) Association of CD4+ T cell-dependent, interferon-gamma-mediated necrosis of the small intestine with genetic susceptibility of mice to peroral infection with Toxoplasma gondii. J Exp Med 184: 597–607.
25. Vossenkamper A, Struck D, Alvarado-Esquivel C, Went T, Takeda K, et al. (2004) Both IL-12 and IL-18 contribute to small intestinal Th1-type immunopathology following oral infection with Toxoplasma gondii, but IL-12 is dominant over IL-18 in parasite control. Eur J Immunol 34: 3197–3207.
26. Powrie F, Correa Oliveira R, Mauze S, Coffman RL (1994) Regulatory interactions between CD45RBhigh and CD45RBlow CD4+ T cells are important for the balance between protective and pathogenic cell-mediated immunity. J Exp Med 179: 589–600.
27. Syrbe U, Jennrich S, Schottelius A, Richter A, Radbruch A, et al. (2004) Differential regulation of P-selectin ligand expression in naïve versus memory T cells: evidence for epigenetic regulation of involved glycosyltransferase genes. Blood 104: 3243–3248.
28. Siegmund K, Hamann A (2005) Use of Labeled Lymphocytes to Analyze Trafficking In Vivo. In: Hamann A, Engelhardt B, editors. Leukocyte Trafficking. Weinheim: Wiley-VCH Verlag GmbH & Co.KGaA. 497–508.
29. Powrie F, Leach MW, Mauze S, Caddle LB, Coffman RL (1993) Phenotypically distinct subsets of CD4+ T cells induce or protect from chronic intestinal inflammation in C. B-17 scid mice. Int Immunol 5: 1461–1471.
30. Munoz M, Heimesaat MM, Danker K, Struck D, Lohmann U, et al. (2009) Interleukin (IL)-23 mediates Toxoplasma gondii-induced immunopathology in the gut via matrixmetalloproteinase-2 and IL-22 but independent of IL-17. J Exp Med 206: 3047–3059.
31. Munoz M, Liesenfeld O, Heimesaat MM (2011) Immunology of Toxoplasma gondii. Immunol Rev 240: 269–285.
32. Jones AT, Federspiel B, Ellies LG, Williams MJ, Burgener R, et al. (1994) Characterization of the activation-associated isoform of CD43 on murine T lymphocytes. J Immunol 153: 3426–3439.
33. Barran P, Fellinger W, Warren CE, Dennis JW, Ziltener HJ (1997) Modification of CD43 and other lymphocyte O-glycoproteins by core 2 N-acetylglucosaminyltransferase. Glycobiology 7: 129–136.
34. Rivera-Nieves J, Gorfu G, Ley K (2008) Leukocyte adhesion molecules in animal models of inflammatory bowel disease. Inflamm Bowel Dis 14: 1715–1735.
35. Bonder CS, Norman MU, Macrae T, Mangan PR, Weaver CT, et al. (2005) P-selectin can support both Th1 and Th2 lymphocyte rolling in the intestinal microvasculature. Am J Pathol 167: 1647–1660.
36. Inoue T, Tsuzuki Y, Matsuzaki K, Matsunaga H, Miyazaki J, et al. (2005) Blockade of PSGL-1 attenuates CD14+ monocytic cell recruitment in intestinal mucosa and ameliorates ileitis in SAMP1/Yit mice. J Leukoc Biol 77: 287–295.
37. Rivera-Nieves J, Burcin TL, Olson TS, Morris MA, McDuffie M, et al. (2006) Critical role of endothelial P-selectin glycoprotein ligand 1 in chronic murine ileitis. J Exp Med 203: 907–917.

38. Bamias G, Martin C, Mishina M, Ross WG, Rivera-Nieves J, et al. (2005) Proinflammatory effects of TH2 cytokines in a murine model of chronic small intestinal inflammation. Gastroenterology 128: 654–666.
39. Doebis C, Siegmund K, Loddenkemper C, Lowe JB, Issekutz AC, et al. (2008) Cellular players and role of selectin ligands in leukocyte recruitment in a T-cell-initiated delayed-type hypersensitivity reaction. Am J Pathol 173: 1067–1076.
40. Rijcken EM, Laukoetter MG, Anthoni C, Meier S, Mennigen R, et al. (2004) Immunoblockade of PSGL-1 attenuates established experimental murine colitis by reduction of leukocyte rolling. Am J Physiol Gastrointest Liver Physiol 287: G115–124.
41. Ostanin DV, Furr KL, Pavlick KP, Gray L, Kevil CG, et al. (2007) T cell-associated CD18 but not CD62L, ICAM-1, or PSGL-1 is required for the induction of chronic colitis. Am J Physiol Gastrointest Liver Physiol 292: G1706–1714.
42. Sydora BC, Wagner N, Lohler J, Yakoub G, Kronenberg M, et al. (2002) beta7 Integrin expression is not required for the localization of T cells to the intestine and colitis pathogenesis. Clin Exp Immunol 129: 35–42.
43. Guilliams M, Crozat K, Henri S, Tamoutounour S, Grenot P, et al. (2010) Skin-draining lymph nodes contain dermis-derived CD103(−) dendritic cells that constitutively produce retinoic acid and induce Foxp3(+) regulatory T cells. Blood 115: 1958–1968.
44. Wang S, Villablanca EJ, De Calisto J, Gomes DC, Nguyen DD, et al. (2011) MyD88-dependent TLR1/2 signals educate dendritic cells with gut-specific imprinting properties. J Immunol 187: 141–150.

6

Constitutive TL1A (TNFSF15) Expression on Lymphoid or Myeloid Cells Leads to Mild Intestinal Inflammation and Fibrosis

David Q. Shih[1], Robert Barrett[1], Xiaolan Zhang[1,2], Nicole Yeager[1], Hon Wai Koon[3], Piangwarin Phaosawasdi[1], Yahui Song[3], Brian Ko[1], Michelle H. Wong[1], Kathrin S. Michelsen[1], Gislaine Martins[1], Charalabos Pothoulakis[3], Stephan R. Targan[1]*

1 Inflammatory Bowel and Immunobiology Research Institute, Cedars-Sinai Medical Center, Los Angeles, California, United States of America, **2** Department of Gastroenterology, The Second Hospital of Hebei Medical University, Shijianzuang, China, **3** Division of Digestive Diseases, Inflammatory Bowel Disease Center, David Geffen School of Medicine, University of California Los Angeles, Los Angeles, California, United States of America

Abstract

TL1A is a member of the TNF superfamily and its expression is increased in the mucosa of inflammatory bowel disease patients. Moreover, a subset of Crohn's disease (CD) patients with the risk *TL1A* haplotype is associated with elevated TL1A expression and a more severe disease course. To investigate the *in vivo* role of elevated TL1A expression, we generated two transgenic (*Tg*) murine models with constitutive Tl1a expression in either lymphoid or myeloid cells. Compared to wildtype (WT) mice, constitutive expression of Tl1a in either lymphoid or myeloid cells showed mild patchy inflammation in the small intestine, which was more prominent in the ileum. In addition, mice with constitutive Tl1a expression exhibited enhanced intestinal and colonic fibrosis compared to WT littermates. The percentage of T cells expressing the gut homing chemokine receptors CCR9 and CCR10 was higher in the *Tl1a Tg* mice compared to WT littermates. Sustained expression of Tl1A in T cells also lead to increased Foxp3+ Treg cells. T cells or antigen presenting cells (APC) with constitutive expression of Tl1a were found to have a more activated phenotype and mucosal mononuclear cells exhibit enhanced Th1 cytokine activity. These results indicated an important role of TL1A in mucosal T cells and APC function and showed that up-regulation of TL1A expression can promote mucosal inflammation and gut fibrosis.

Editor: Markus M. Heimesaat, Charité, Campus Benjamin Franklin, Germany

Funding: USPHS grant DK056328. The funders had no role in study design, data collection and analysis, decision to publish, or preparation of the manuscript.

Competing Interests: The authors have declared that no competing interests exist.

* E-mail: targans@cshs.org

Introduction

Inflammatory bowel disease (IBD), encompassing CD and ulcerative colitis (UC), is a chronic inflammatory disorder caused by dysregulated immune responses in a genetically predisposed individual (reviewed in [1]). CD is a chronic inflammatory condition that predominately affects the gut with distinctive pathological features such as patchy transmural intestinal inflammation, relative sparing of inflammation in the rectum, intestinal fibrostenosis and a dysregulated T helper (Th) 1 and Th17 immune response [1,2]. Accumulating data, including genome-wide association studies (GWAS), demonstrate that more than 80 distinct genetic loci confer CD susceptibility, and are being used to define critical molecules and pathways that converge in physiologic processes that lead to mucosal inflammation [2,3]. Among the several recently discovered IBD associated gene variants, only those in the tumor necrosis factor superfamily member 15 (*TNFSF15*) have been shown to be associated with CD in all ethnic and age groups [1].

TL1A plays an important role in modulating the adaptive immune response. In the Th1 effector immune response, binding of TL1A to its receptor (death domain receptor 3, DR3, TNFRSF25) enhances IFN-γ production from peripheral and mucosal T cells [4,5]. Studies have shown that TL1A can be induced in APC by FcγR signaling [6,7] and microbial antigen/organisms [8] suggesting that augmentation of the Th1 immune response by TL1A may occur through APC-T cell interactions. In murine models of chronic mucosal inflammation, TL1A enhanced Th1 and Th17 effector function by up-regulating IFN-γ and IL17 production, respectively, in gut-associated lymphoid tissue (GALT) $CD4^+$ cells under Th1/Th17 polarizing conditions, indicating that TL1A is an important modulator in the development of gut mucosal inflammation [9]. In addition to mediating Th1 responses, TL1A also promotes Th2 and Th17 effector cell function [10,11,12].

Several studies implicate the TL1A/DR3 signaling pathway in mucosal inflammation. The expression of TL1A and DR3 is up-regulated in the inflamed gut mucosa of two distinct murine models of ileal inflammation [13]. Neutralizing anti-mouse TL1A Ab attenuated inflammation in both the dextran sulfate sodium induced chronic colitis and a G protein αi2-/- ($G\alpha i2^{-/-}$) T cell transfer colitis model [9]. In humans, TL1A can enhance IFN-γ production in $CD4^+$ T cells expressing the gut-homing receptor CCR9 [14]. Increased expression of both TL1A and DR3 was found in gut mucosal biopsies and lamina propria (LP) T cells of both UC and CD patients [4,15]. Furthermore, TL1A and DR3 expression are correlated with severity of gut mucosal inflammation as their transcripts were several times more abundant in RNA from mucosal biopsies taken from inflamed CD lesions than in those taken from uninvolved areas [4,15].

To determine the *in vivo* consequence of increased TL1A expression, we generated two *Tg* murine models that constitutively express Tl1A in either lymphoid or myeloid cells. We found that constitutive expression of Tl1A in either lymphoid or myeloid cells induced mild spontaneous patchy intestinal inflammation by 10 months of age. We showed that a higher percentage of T cells and APC from the mesenteric lymph nodes (MLN) have an activated phenotype and express the gut homing chemokine receptors CCR9 and CCR10, associated with increased production of IFN-γ. Consistent with previous reports [16,17], we observed goblet cell hyperplasia and an increased number of Paneth cells in the ileum of *Tl1a* transgenic (*Tg*) mice. We also showed enhanced intestinal and colonic fibrosis in mice that constitutively express Tl1a. These 2 novel murine *Tl1A Tg* models have patterns of site directed mucosal inflammation and fibrosis seen in human CD and may be useful models to study the pathogenesis of IBD.

Results

Generation of *in vivo* constitutive Tl1a expression in the myeloid and T cell lineage

To investigate the contribution of sustained APC or T cell Tl1a expression on gut mucosal homeostasis and inflammation, we generated *Tg* mice that constitutively express Tl1a in either T cells or myeloid cells. We used the proximal *lck* promoter and *CD2* enhancer to drive T cell lineage-specific expression and the *c-fms* promoter to mediate myeloid specific expression in APC such as macrophages and DC [18,19]. We also cloned an *IRES-GFP* element downstream of the murine *Tl1a* so that *Tg* Tl1a expressing cells could be identified by GFP. The cloning strategies and schematic of the *Tg* construct are described in Materials and Methods section and figure 1A, respectively. The *Tg* constructs were injected into C57BL/6 pronuclei to ensure genetic homogeneity except for the *Tl1a* transgene.

Expression of the transgene was determined in myeloid *Tg* mice (named *FMS-Tl1a-GFP Tg*) and T-cell lineage specific expression of Tl1a (named *LCK-CD2-Tl1a-GFP Tg*) by the expression of GFP. We found that in the *FMS-Tl1a-GFP Tg* mice, GFP was present in over 70% of CD11c and F4/80 positive cells, and the expression of the Tl1a transgene persisted as the mice aged (Fig. 1B). The specificity of the *c-fms* promoter was illustrated by the fact that we did not detect GFP expression in CD3, CD4 or CD8 positive T cells (Fig. 1C). In the *LCK-CD2-Tl1A-GFP Tg* mice, GFP was present in over 90% of CD3, CD4 and CD8 positive cells (Fig. 1C). Similar to the *FMS-Tl1a-GFP Tg*, the expression of the transgene in the lymphoid *Tl1a Tg* mice also persisted as the mice got older (Fig. 1C). Less than 10% GFP expression was detected in F4/80 or CD11c positive cells (Fig. 1B), indicating that the *Lck* promoter and *Cd2* enhancer element drives T cell lineage-specific expression. We directly showed that Tl1a mRNA is higher in the spleen, mesenteric lymph nodes (MLN), colon and ileum of both *Tg* mice compared to WT mice (Fig. 1D). Together, these data demonstrate that we generated tissue specific constitutive *in vivo* expression of Tl1a in APC and T cells.

Mice with constitutive Tl1a expression do not develop gross tissue inflammation

Both *FMS-Tl1a-GFP* and *LCK-CD2-Tl1a-GFP Tg* mice are fertile, but are born at less than Mendelian frequency. Mendelian expectation is 50% transmission of the transgene. When *Tg* hemizygous mice are mated to WT mice, the frequency of *FMS-Tl1a-GFP Tg* mice born is 42% (58/138) and in *LCK-CD2-Tl1aTg* mice, the frequency is 40% (51/126). Both the *FMS* and *LCK Tl1a Tg* mice appeared healthy and gained weight at similar rates (Fig. 2A). There were no differences in the disease activity index (DAI) [20] between *Tg* and WT for up to 10 months (Fig. 2B). We also did not observe differences in the splenic cell number, MLN cell number, lamina propria mononuclear cell (LPMC) number in the small bowel or colon, colon length, small bowel (SB) length or spleen size between WT and *Tl1a Tg* mice at 2 or 10 months (Fig. 2C and data not shown). There was a trend toward higher cell numbers in the MLN and SB LPMC in *Tl1a Tg* mice but they did not reach statistical significance (Fig. 2B and data not shown).

Tl1a expression in APC and T cells induce mild histologic small bowel inflammation

Elevated Tl1a expression is implicated in gut mucosal inflammation. We therefore investigated whether mice with elevated Tl1a expression develop spontaneous colitis at 2 months and 10 months of age. The colon and small intestine did not show gross inflammation between WT and *Tg* mice using a standard macroscopic scoring system (Fig. 3A) [21]. Another measure for gut inflammation is to determine myeloperoxidase (MPO) activity [22]. We found significantly increased MPO activity in the small intestine of *LCK-CD2-Tl1a Tg* mice than WT mice (Fig. 3B). MPO activity was similar in the colon of WT and *Tl1a Tg* mice (Fig. 3B). Histological examination of the colon did not reveal increased inflammatory infiltrates, mucin depletion, epithelial cell hyperplasia, abnormal crypt artchitecture, crypt abscess or erosions in either WT or *Tg* mice at 2 or 10 months of age (Fig. 3C and data not shown). As elevated TL1A production in IBD patients is associated with fibrostenotic disease [23,24], we assessed whether the *Tl1a Tg* mice had increased histologic fibrosis. Notably, we observed increased fibrosis in the colonic mucosa and submucosa of both *LCK-CD2-* and *FMS-Tl1a Tg* mice as compared to WT littermate mice by 10 months of age using the Masson Trichrome stain (Fig. 3D).

At 2 months of age, histological examination of the small intestine revealed a significant increase in the number of goblet cells and Paneth cells (Fig. 4A and 4B). There was blunting of the villi and increased LPMC in the ileum of both the *LCK-CD2-* and *FMS-Tl1a Tg* mice compared to WT mice (Fig. 4A). These histological changes were reflected by a significant increase in the inflammatory score in the ileum of *Tl1a Tg* mice using a standard quantitative scoring system (Fig. 4B) [21]. We did not observe villus blunting nor increased mononuclear cells in the LP of the duodenum and jejunum between WT and *Tl1a Tg* mice at 2 months of age (Fig. 4A).

At 10 months, we similarly observed Paneth cell hyperplasia in both *LCK-CD2-* and *FMS-Tl1a Tg* compared to WT mice (Fig. 5A and 5B). In contrast to younger mice (2 months of age), there were no detectable differences in the number of goblet cells between WT and *Tg* mice at 10 months of age (Fig. 5A and 5B). The inflammatory changes in the small intestine such as increased mononuclear cell infiltrate of the LP and blunting of the villi was more prominent and progressive, involving the duodenum, jejunum and ileum (Fig. 5A and 5B). The increased inflammation in both *LCK-CD2-* and *FMS-Tl1a Tg* mice was associated with increased histologic fibrosis by the more extensive Masson Trichrome stain in the small intestine (Fig. 6). Together, these results indicated that constitutive expression of Tl1a in T cells and myeloid cells lead to progressive spontaneous intestinal inflammation and fibrosis.

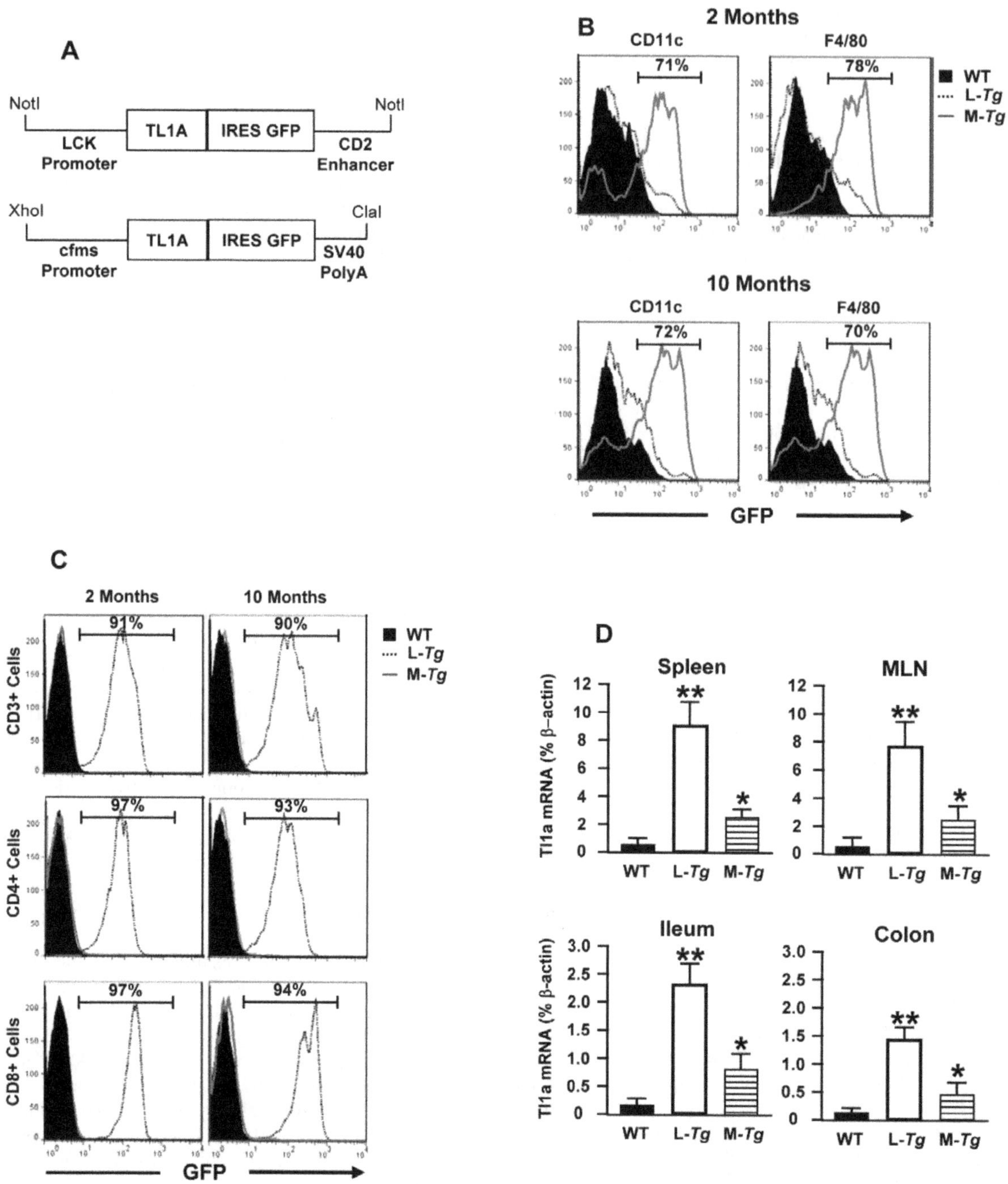

Figure 1. Generation of constitutive *in vivo* expression of Tl1a in T- and antigen presenting cells. (A) Schematic of *LCK-CD2-Tl1a* and *FMS-Tl1a* transgenic construct. An internal ribosomal entry site (IRES) element is used for both transgenic constructs so that a bi-cistronic message can be made from the transgene and the Tl1a expressing cells are tagged by GFP. (B) Flow cytometric analysis of the transgene marker GFP on either CD11c or F4/80 gated splenocytes from WT (black filled), *LCK-CD2-Tl1a Tg* mice (L-*Tg*, dotted line) or *FMS-Tl1a Tg* mice (M-*Tg*, solid grey line). Representative histograms are shown. (C) Representative analysis of the transgene marker GFP on either CD3, CD4 or CD8 gated splenocytes from WT (black filled), *LCK-CD2-Tl1a Tg* mice (L-*Tg*, dotted line) or *FMS-Tl1a Tg* mice (solid grey line). (D) Tl1a mRNA expression was determined in the spleen, MLN, ileum or colon by real-time polymerase chain reaction. Data are expressed as mean percent of β-actin ± standard deviation (SD). *$P<0.05$, **$P<0.01$. $n=6$ independent littermate mice per group were used for B-D.

Mice with constitutive Tl1a expression develop extra-intestinal pathology

At a low frequency, we observed extra-intestinal pathology in both the *FMS-Tl1a-* and *LCK-CD2-Tl1a Tg* mice. One such feature was an erythematous ulcerated skin lesion that was observed in 1 out of 58 *FMS-Tl1a Tg*, 2 of 51 *LCK-CD2-Tl1a Tg* and 1 out of 155 WT littermate mice (Fig. 7). Another observed pathology was joint erythema and swelling (Fig. 7) that caused movement difficulties and resultd in mice not able to feed. Arthropathy was observed in 2 out of 58 *FMS Tg*, 2 out of 51 *LCK-CD2 Tl1a Tg* mice and 0 out of 155 WT mice. Three out of 4 *Tg* mice with arthropathy had monoarticular and 1 *LCK-CD2-Tl1a Tg* mice had polyarticular

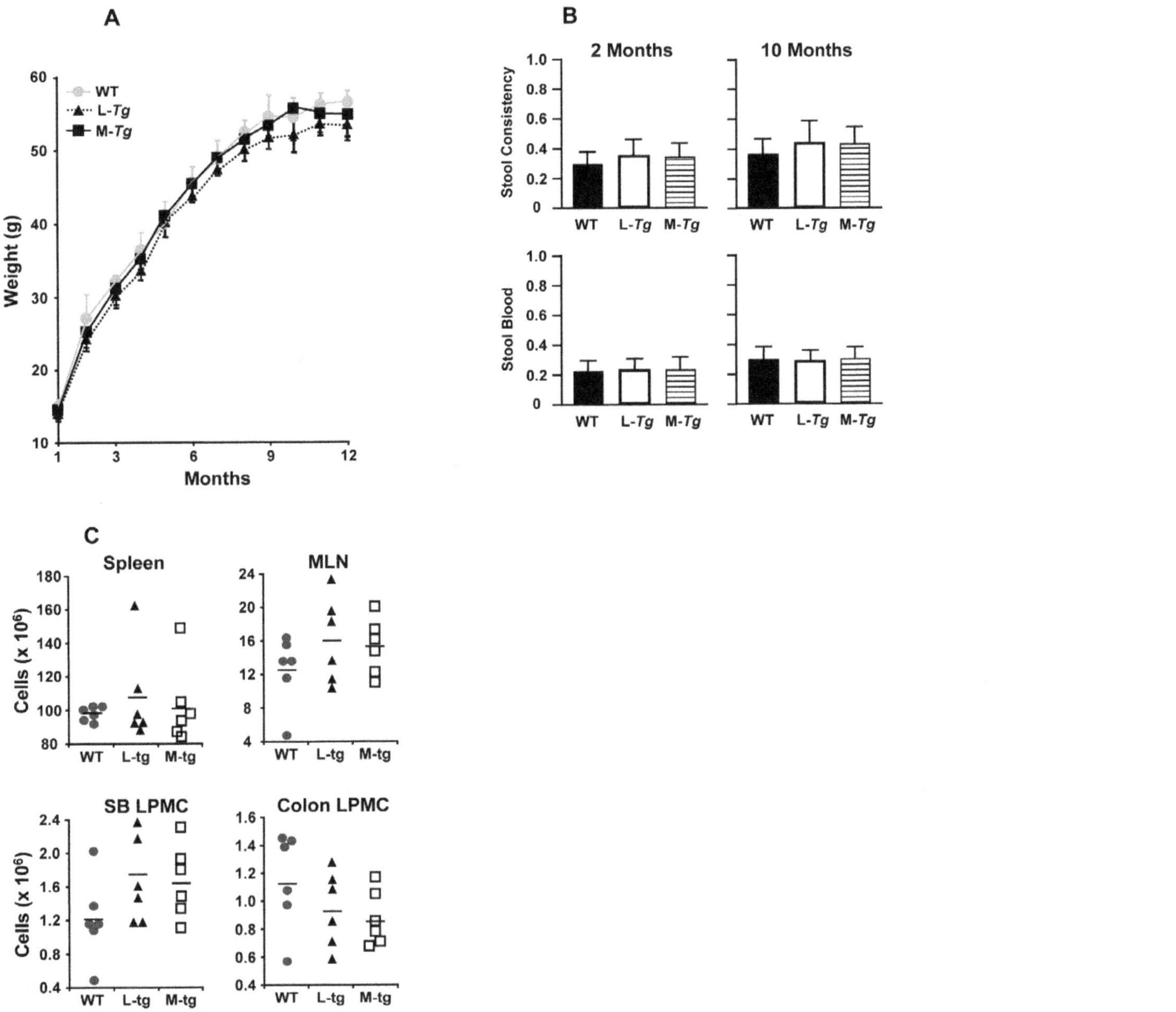

Figure 2. Phenotypic characterization of *Tl1a Tg* mice. (A) Body weights for WT (grey circle), *LCK-CD2-Tl1a Tg* mice (L-*Tg*, black filled triangle) or *FMS-Tl1a Tg* mice (M-*Tg*, black filled square) are shown n = 20 per group. Data are expressed as mean weight in grams (g) ± SD. (B) Stool consistency (top panels) and fecal blood (bottom panels) were determined using standard methods from WT, *LCK-CD2-Tl1a Tg* (L-*Tg*) or *FMS-Tl1a Tg* mice (M-*Tg*) mice [20]. Data are expressed as mean ± SD. N = 20 per group. (C) Total number of cells were isolated from spleen, MLN and lamina propria mononuclear cells (LPMC) from the colon and distal 10 cm of small intestine isolated from 10 months old WT (grey circle), *LCK-CD2-Tl1a Tg* (L-*Tg*, black triangle) or FMS-*Tl1a Tg* mice (M-*Tg*, open square) and represented as absolute cell number x 10^6. Each data point represents an independent mouse.

disease. Our data suggested these novel murine models with constitutive expression of Tl1a in APC and T cells develop extra-intestinal pathology such as ulcerated skin lesion and arthropathy.

Accelerated T- and antigen presenting cell activation in LCK-CD2- and FMS-Tl1a *Tg* mice

To assess whether constitutively expressed Tl1a can co-stimulate T cells *in vivo*, we compared the expression of an activation marker on $CD4^+$ and $CD8^+$ cells between *Tg* and WT littermate controls. $CD4^+CD45RB^{low}CD25^+$ Treg cells were gated out in order to examine the expression of activation markers on conventional T cells. At 2 months, there were almost 2 fold higher $CD4^+CD44^+$ T cells from the spleen but not MLN of *LCK-CD2-Tl1a Tg* mice (Fig. 8A). There was also no difference in the expression of the activation marker CD44 on $CD8^+$ T cells in the MLN and spleen at 2 months of age between *Tl1a Tg* mice and WT littermates (Fig. 8A). By 10 months of age, a higher percentage of *Tl1a Tg* $CD4^+$ cells in both the spleen and MLN expressed the activation marker CD44, particularly in the *LCK-CD2-Tl1a Tg* mice (Fig. 8B). In contrast, only $CD8^+$ cells from the *LCK-CD2-Tl1a Tg* (not *FMS-Tl1a Tg*) spleen and MLN exhibited an increased expression of the activation marker CD44 (Fig. 8B).

To assess the effect of constitutive Tl1a expression on the activation state of DC and macrophages, the expression of the

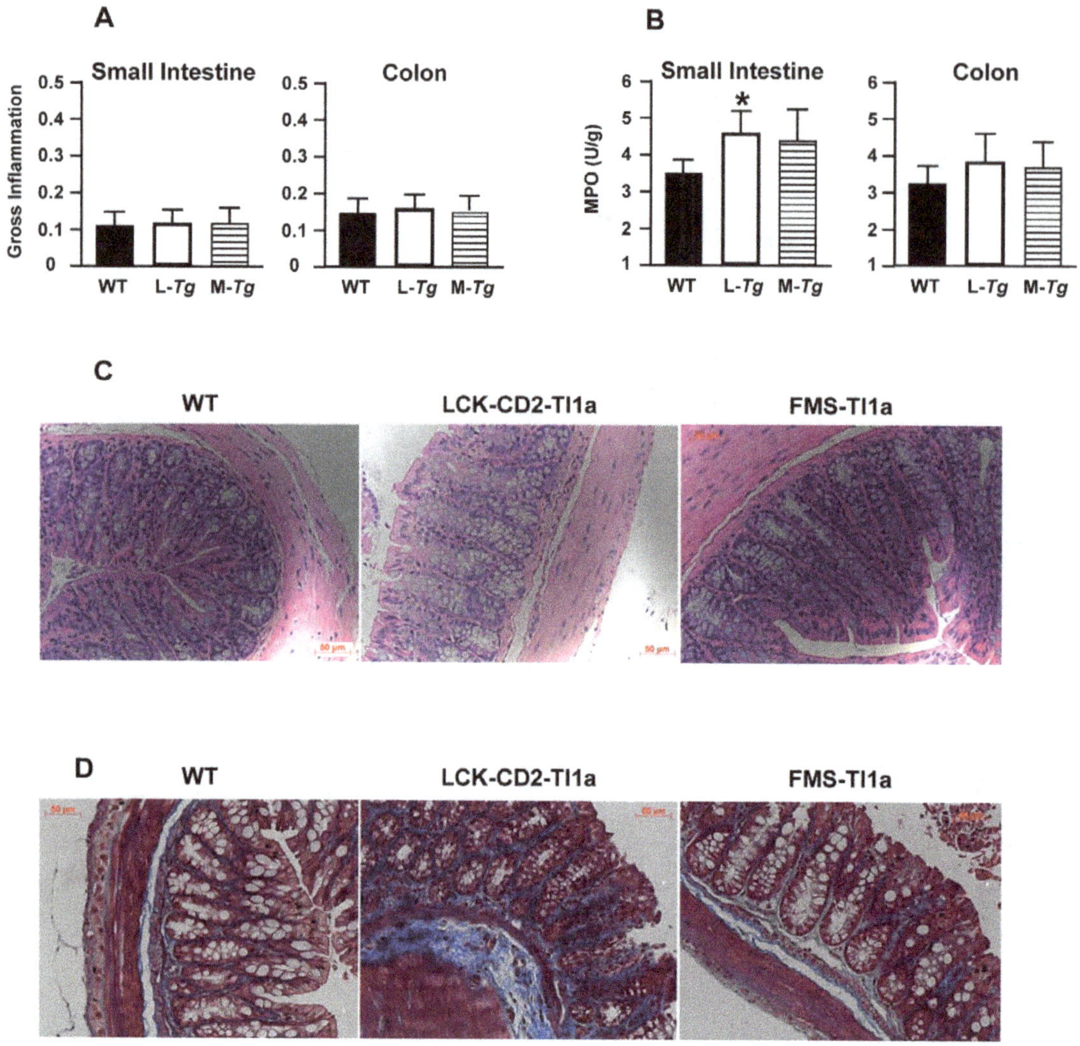

Figure 3. *Tl1a Tg* mice do not develop gross intestinal inflammation but exhibit enhanced colonic fibrosis. (A) Gross appearance (wall thickening, hyperemia, rigidity or adhesions) of small intestine and colon are measured from 10 months old WT, *LCK-CD2-Tl1a Tg* (L-*Tg*) or *FMS-Tl1a Tg* (M-*Tg*) mice using a standard scoring system [21]. Data are expressed as mean ± SD. (B) Myeloperoxidase (MPO) activity is measured on the distal 3 cm of ilea and mid-colon and data are expressed as arbitrary unit (U) per gram (g) of protein. **P*<0.05 (C) Representative hematoxylin and eosin (H&E) stained colon section obtained from mid-colon of 10 months old WT, *LCK-CD2-Tl1a Tg* or *FMS-Tl1a Tg* mice are shown. (D) Masson Trichrome staining of collagen deposition in tissue sections of mouse mid-colon. Collagen is stained blue versus red background. There are increased blue collagen stain in *LCK-CD2-Tl1a Tg* and *FMS-Tl1a Tg* compared to WT littermate mice. Magnification 200X. Results are representative of six mice per group for A–D.

activation marker CD86 was compared between *Tl1a Tg* and WT littermate controls. Flow cytometric (FACS) analysis revealed increased $CD86^+$ expression on DC (CD11c+) and macrophages (F4/80+) in both the spleen and MLN of Tl1a *Tg* mice compared to WT mice (Fig. 9A). In contrast to *LCK-CD2-Tl1a Tg* mice, there was a negligible further increase in the percentage of activated DC and macrophages over time (compare 2 and 10 months, Fig. 9A and B). These data demonstrated that sustained Tl1a expression could result in enhanced activation of $CD4^+$, $CD8^+$, DC and macrophages *in vivo*.

Constitutive *in vivo* Tl1a expression leads to an increased number of T cells expressing Treg and gut homing markers

FACS analysis did not reveal any differences in the frequencies of $CD3^+$, $CD4^+$, $CD8^+$, $MHCII^+$, $CD11c^+$ or $F4/80^+$ cells in the spleen and MLN between *FMS-Tl1a Tg*, *LCK-CD2-Tl1a Tg* or WT littermate mice (data not shown). There was an increase in the frequency of Foxp3 positive cells in the spleen and MLN of *LCK-CD2-Tl1a Tg* mice (Fig. 10A and B). The percentage of $Foxp3^+$ cells further increased as the *LCK-CD2-Tl1a Tg* mice aged (Fig. 10A and B). In contrast, there was no difference in the frequency of $Foxp3^+$ cells in the spleen or MLN of *FMS-Tl1a Tg* mice at both 2 and 10 months (Fig. 10A and B).

A trend toward a higher cell number in the MLN and small bowel LPMC was noted in older (Fig. 2C and 5A). To determine whether this finding was due to increased trafficking to the gut immune compartment, we assessed the expression of the gut homing markers CCR9 and CCR10 in the MLN and spleen of *Tl1a Tg* and WT littermate mice. In the spleen, there was no difference in $CCR9^+$ or $CCR10^+$ cells at 2 or 10 months between either *Tl1a Tg* or WT mice (data not shown). Notably, we found an increase in the percentage of cells expressing CCR9 and CCR10 in the MLN of *LCK-CD2-Tl1a Tg* mice compared to WT

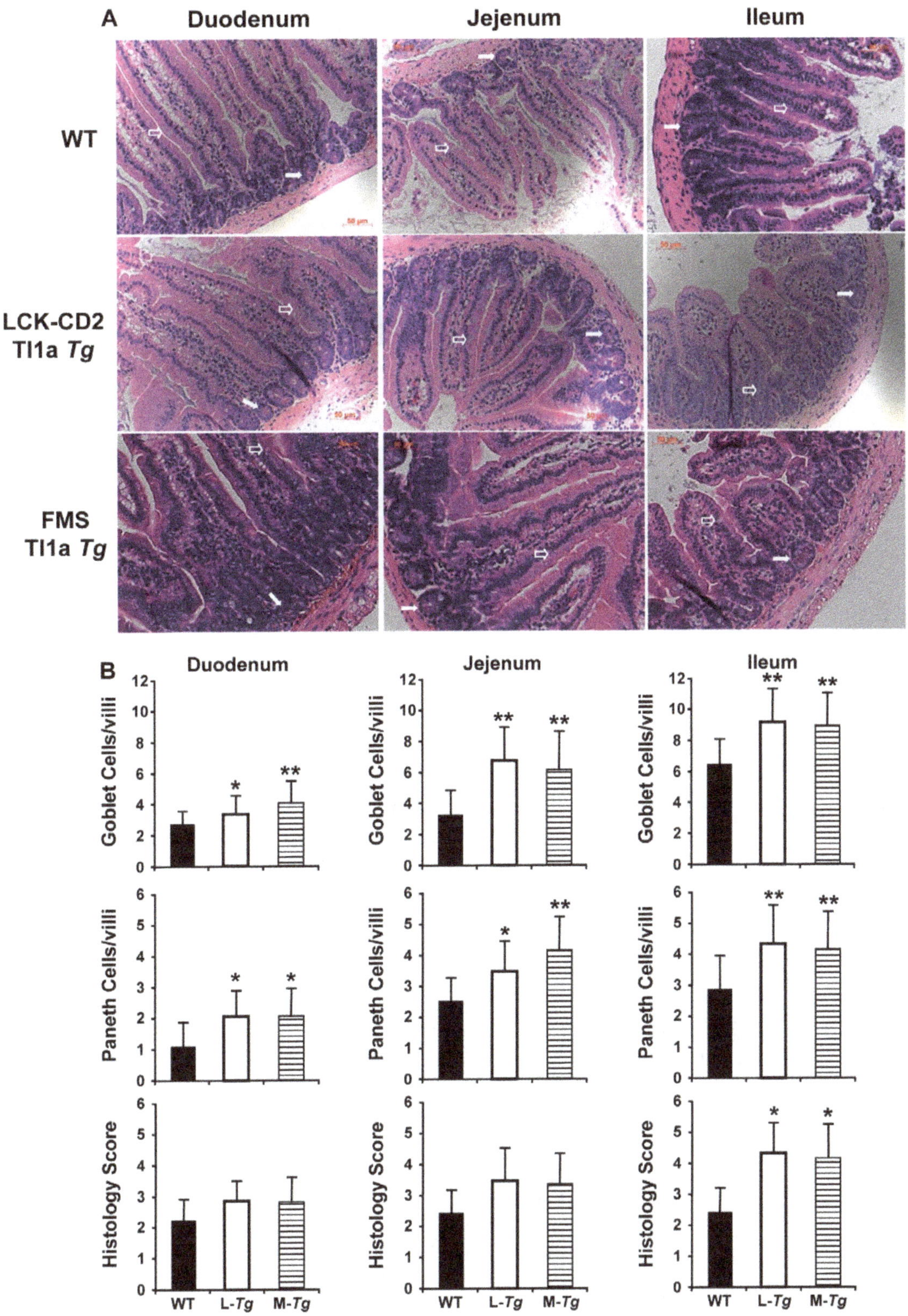

Figure 4. Constitutive Tl1a expression leads to increased numbers of goblet and Paneth cells in the small intestine and ileal histological inflammation. (A) Representative H&E stained sections obtained from the indicated portions of small intestine from 2 months old WT, *LCK-CD2-Tl1a Tg* (L-*Tg*) or *FMS-Tl1a Tg* (M-*Tg*) mice are shown. Goblet cells are denoted by an open arrow. Paneth cells are denoted by a filled arrow. Results are representative of six mice per group. Magnification 200X. (B) The numbers of goblet (top panel) and Paneth cells (middle panel) were determined by examining at least 80 individual villi at the indicated portions of the small intestine from six mice (2 months old) per group by 2 observers blinded to mouse genotype. Data are expressed as mean (SD. Histologic scores (bottom panel) were determined by 2 observers blinded to mice using standard methods [21]. Data are expressed as mean (SD. At least 36 fields from 6 mice per group at 200x magnification were scored. $^{*}P<0.05$, $^{**}P<0.01$.

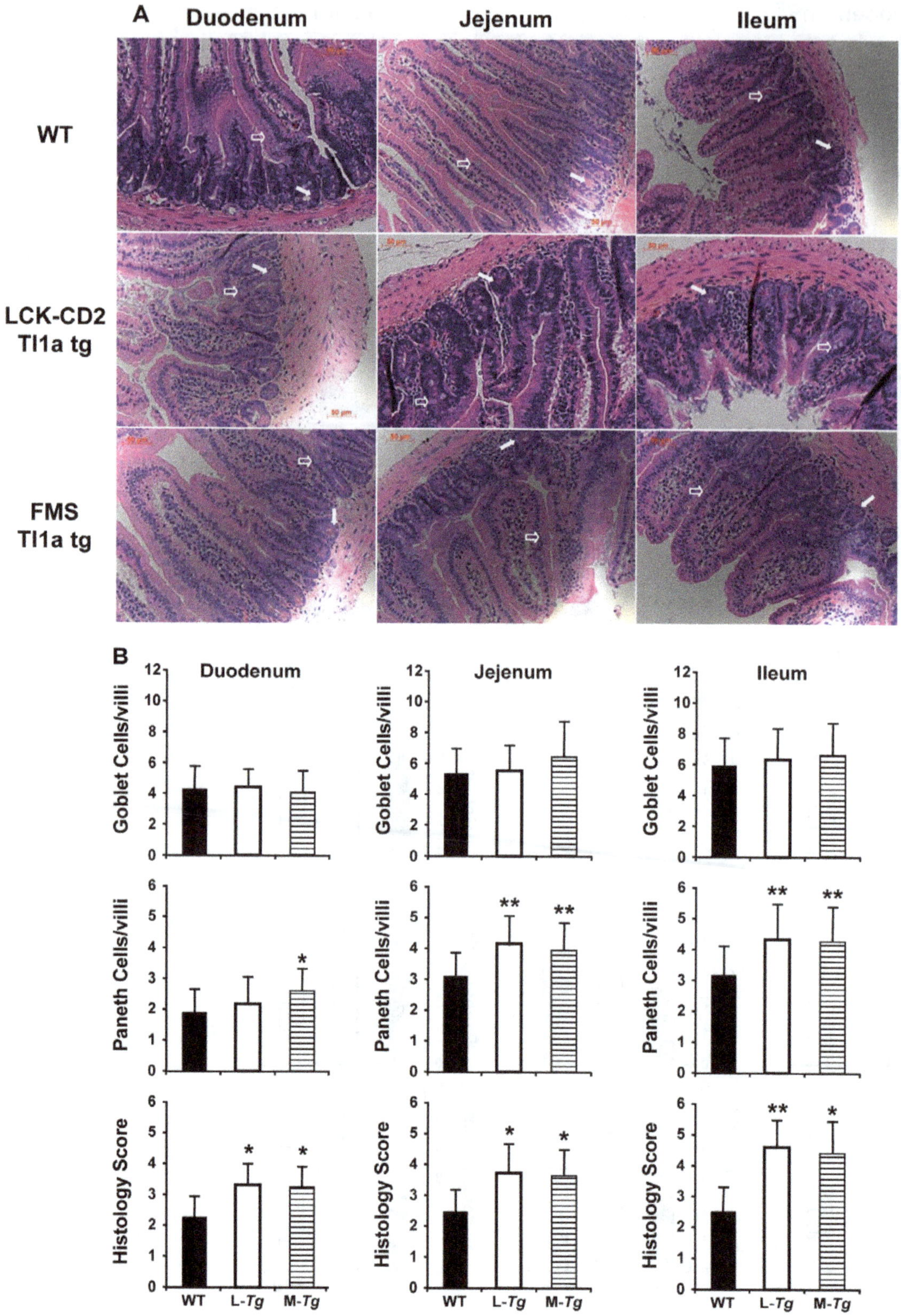

Figure 5. Persistent Paneth cell hyperplasia and worsened small intestinal inflammation as the *Tl1a Tg* mice aged. (A) Representative H&E stained section obtained from the indicated portions of small intestine from 10 months old WT, *LCK-CD2-Tl1a Tg* (L-*Tg*) or *FMS-Tl1a Tg* (M-*Tg*) mice are shown. Goblet cells are denoted by an open arrow. Paneth cells are denoted by a filled arrow. Results are representative of six mice per group. Magnification 200X. (B) The numbers of goblet (top panel) and Paneth cells (middle panel) were determined by 2 observers blinded to mice genotype. Histologic scores (bottom panel) were determined from 10 months old WT, *LCK-CD2-Tl1a Tg* (L-*Tg*), or *FMS-Tl1a Tg* (M-*Tg*) mice using standard methods [21]. Quantification of goblet and Paneth cells was determined by examining at least 80 individual villi and histological scores were determined by examining at least 36 fields at 200X magnification. Six independent mice per group were used (A–B). Data are expressed as mean (SD. $^{*}P<0.05$, $^{**}P<0.01$.

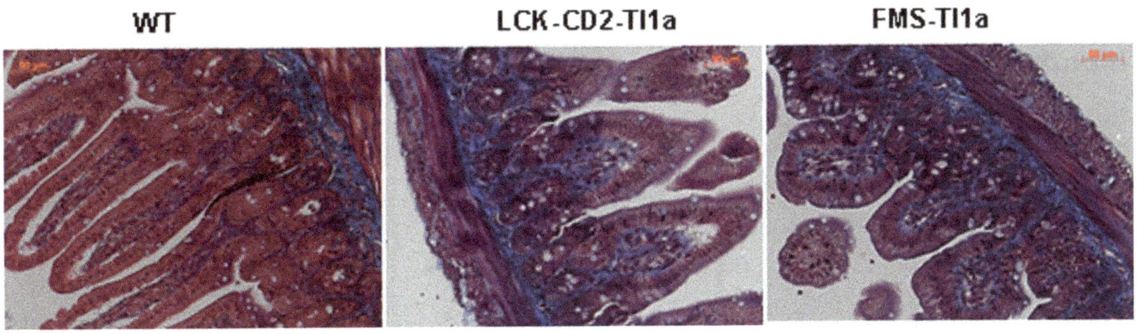

Figure 6. Increased fibrosis in the small intestine of *Tl1a Tg* mice. Masson Trichrome staining was performed on mice ileal sections (distal 3 cm of small intestine). There is increased blue collagen stain in *LCK-CD2-Tl1a Tg* and *FMS-Tl1a Tg* compared to WT littermate mice. Magnification 200X. Six independent mice per group were used.

mice at 2 months and the difference became even greater as the mice aged (Fig. 11A). For the *FMS-Tl1a Tg* mice, a higher percentage of CCR9$^+$ and CCR10$^+$ cells was observed at 10 months (but not at 2 months) (Fig. 11A).

Tl1a Tg mice have an enhanced proinflammatory cytokine profile in the MLN and small intestine

To assess the molecular consequences of increased expression of activation and gut homing marker, we measured the expression of IFN-γ, IL-13 and IL-17 by FACS analysis and ELISA. There was no difference in the expression of CD4$^+$IFN-γ$^+$, CD4$^+$IL-13$^+$, CD4$^+$IL-17$^+$ T cells by either intracellular stain or ELISA at 2 months of age between *FMS-Tl1a Tg*, *LCK-CD2-Tl1a Tg* or WT littermate mice (data not shown). By 10 months of age, the frequency of CD4$^+$IFN-γ$^+$ and CD4$^+$IL-17$^+$ T cells increased by approximately 3- and 2- fold respectively, in the MLN of *LCK-CD2-Tl1a Tg* mice (Fig. 11B). In the *FMS-Tl1a Tg* mice, the percentage of CD4$^+$IFN-γ$^+$ cells increased by approximately 2-fold (Fig. 11B). We did not observe any differences in the CD4$^+$IL-13$^+$ T cells in both of the *Tl1a Tg* mice and only a negligible difference in the CD4$^+$IL-17$^+$ T cells in *FMS-Tl1a Tg* mice (Fig. 11B).

To confirm the FACS findings, we isolated cells from the spleen, MLN and LPMC from the colon and small intestine and assessed their ability to produce cytokines following stimulation with anti-CD3 and anti-CD28. Similar to the intracellular stain, we found significantly higher IFN-γ production in the MLN and small intestine LPMC of *LCK-CD2-Tl1a Tg* mice (Fig. 12A). *FMS-Tl1a Tg* mice also exhibited significantly increased IFN-γ production in MLN and a trend toward a higher level in the LPMC from the small intestine (Fig. 12A). There was also a trend toward higher IL-17 and IL-13 production in the MLN and small intestine LPMC of both *LCK-CD2-Tl1a* and *FMS-Tl1a Tg* mice, but this did not reach statistical significance (Fig. 12B and C). Interestingly, the expression of the anti-inflammatory cytokine IL-10 appeared to be higher in both the *Tl1a Tg* mice and reached statistical significance in the splenic cells of *LCK-CD2-Tl1a Tg* as compared to WT mice (Fig. 12D). These data suggested that constitutive expression of Tl1a *in vivo* resulted in enhanced IFN-γ and IL-10 production and potentially enhanced IL-17 and IL-13 production.

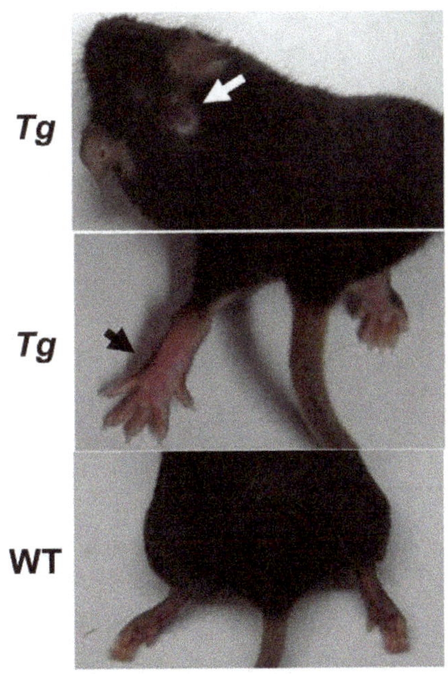

Figure 7. Tl1a transgenic mice develop ulcerated skin lesions and arthropathy. A typical ulcerated skin lesion is illustrated (white arrow, top). Erythematous arthropathy found in the transgenic (*Tg*) mice is shown (black arrow, middle). A WT joint is shown in the bottom panel for comparison.

Discussion

This study shows that constitutive expression of Tl1a on either T- or APC cells leads to progressive histological inflammation in the small intestine and worsened fibrosis in both the small intestine and colon over time. Even though sustained expression of Tl1a in T- or APC did not result in gross macroscopic gut inflammation or colitis symptoms as measured by DAI (weight loss, fecal occult blood or loose stool) for up to 1 year, there were histologically determined inflammation as evidenced by blunting of the small intestinal villi, hyperplasia of goblet and Paneth cells and increased LPMC infiltrate. These histological changes are markers of early gut inflammation that are also found in other murine models of colitis and ileitis [25,26]. As the small bowel inflammation worsened with age, there was no difference in the goblet cell number between *Tl1a Tg* and WT littermate mice (Fig. 4 and 5). This was likely due to the fact that goblet cell number decreased with worsened inflammation in older *Tl1a Tg* mice [26,27,28]. This histologic inflammation was only detected in the small intestine (not colon) and was particularly evident in the ileum. The degree of inflammation in the small intestine was similar between *Tg* mice with sustained Tl1a expression in T- and myeloid cells (Fig. 4).

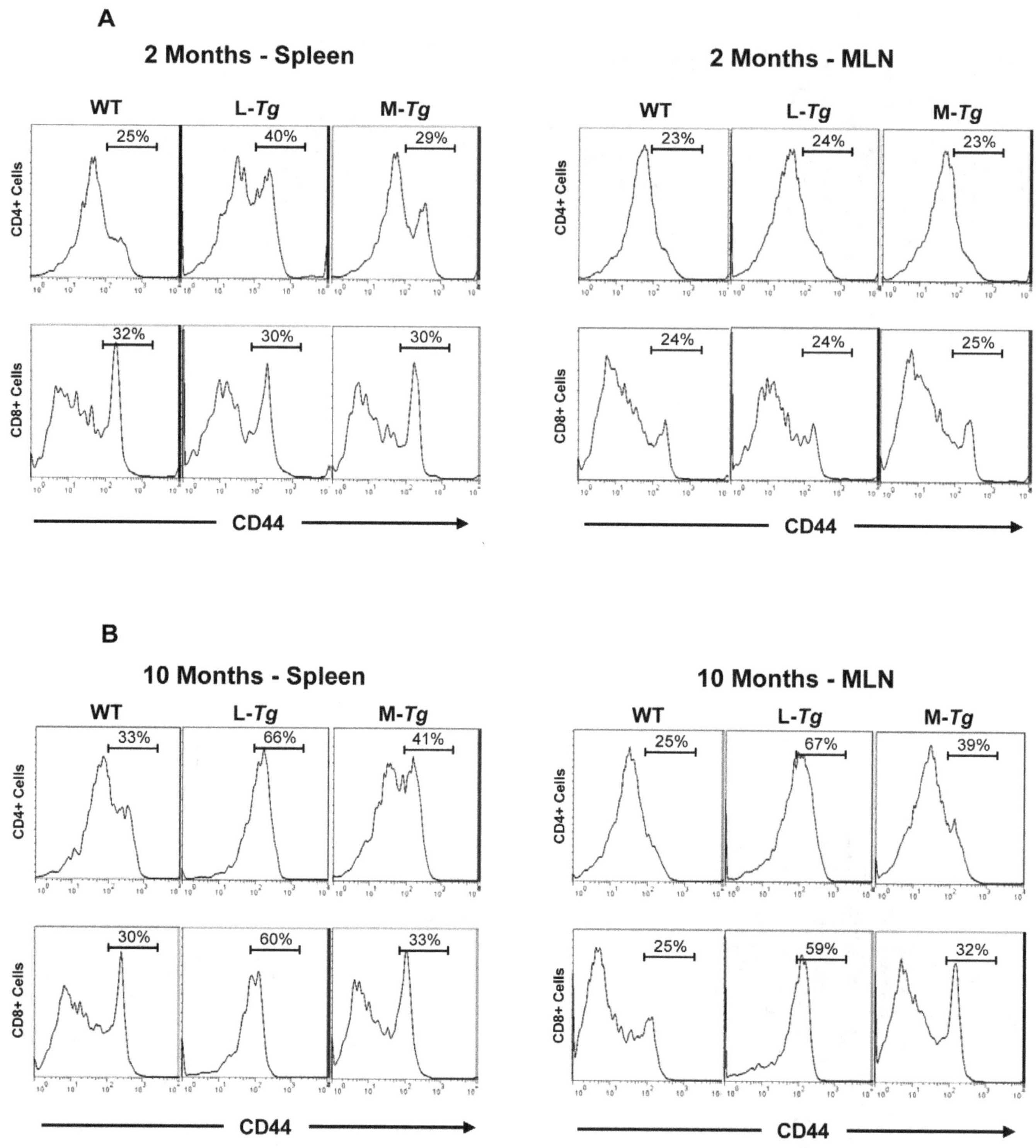

Figure 8. Sustained Tl1a expression leads to an increased percentage of activated T cells. FACS plot of 2 month (A) and 10 month (B) splenocytes and MLN cells showing expression of activation markers CD44. Either $CD4^+$ or $CD8^+$ cells are gated as indicated. Data shown are representative of 4 mice per group. WT = wildtype, L-*Tg* = *LCK-CD2-Tl1a-GFP Tg* mice, M-*Tg* = *FMS-Tl1a Tg* mice.

Another histological finding was increased small intestinal and colonic fibrosis in *Tl1a Tg* compared to WT littermate mice by 10 months of age (Fig. 3D and 6). This could be due to the fact that there was higher transgene expression in the *LCK-CD2-Tl1a Tg* mouse (approximately 90% of T cells) compared to its expression in APC (approximately 70% of DC and macrophages). Alternatively, constitutive Tl1a expression in lymphocytes could be more fibrogenic than its expression on either DC or macrophages. The presence of colonic fibrosis in the absence of detectable histologic inflammation suggested that Tl1a may be a pro-fibrogenic factor in addition to its role in inflammation. Notably, *TL1A haplotype B* which is associated with increased secretion of soluble and

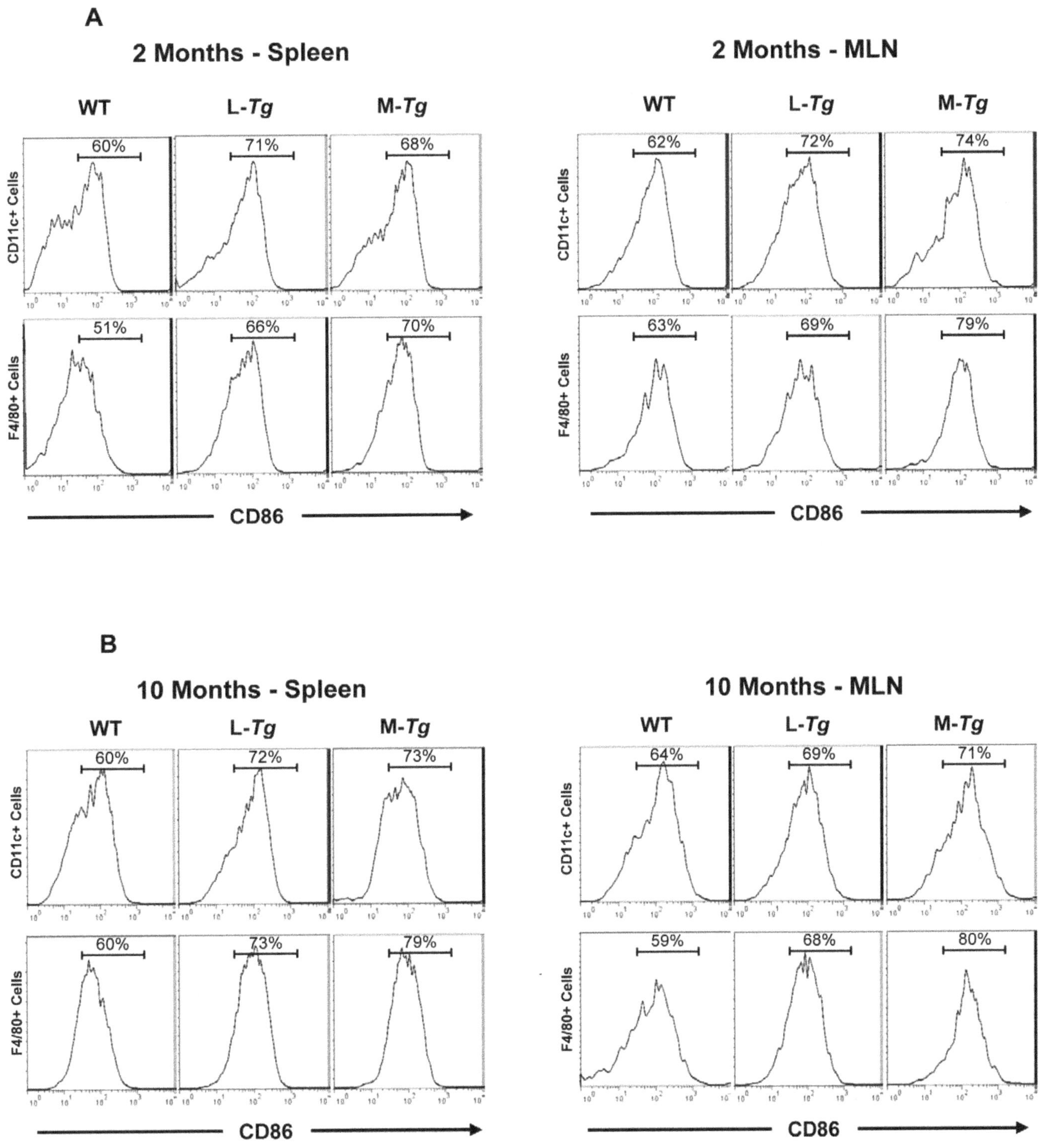

Figure 9. Sustained Tl1a expression leads to an increased percentage of activated DC and macrophages. FACS plot of 2 month (A) and 10 month (B) splenocytes and MLN cells showing expression of activation markers CD86. Either F4/80$^+$ or CD11c$^+$ cells were gated as indicated. Data shown are representative of 4 mice per group. WT = wildtype, L-*Tg* = *LCK-CD2-Tl1a-GFP Tg* mice, M-*Tg* = *FMS-Tl1a Tg* mice.

membrane TL1A is also characterized by increased need for surgery especially in Jewish patients [23,24]. Fibrostenotic disease was also more common in this group. It would be medically useful to determine whether downregulating the TL1A/DR3 pathway can prevent the progression of IBD-associated fibrosis since there is currently no effective medical therapy to treat established fibrostenotic disease in IBD patients. It would be interesting to study the interaction between TL1A and other known pro-fibrogenic factors such as transforming growth factor beta 1 (TGF-β1) and insulin-like growth factor 1 (IGF-1) using the chronic 2,4,6-trinitrobenzensulfonic acid (TNBS) colonic injury model which causes both colitis and intestinal fibrosis [29,30,31].

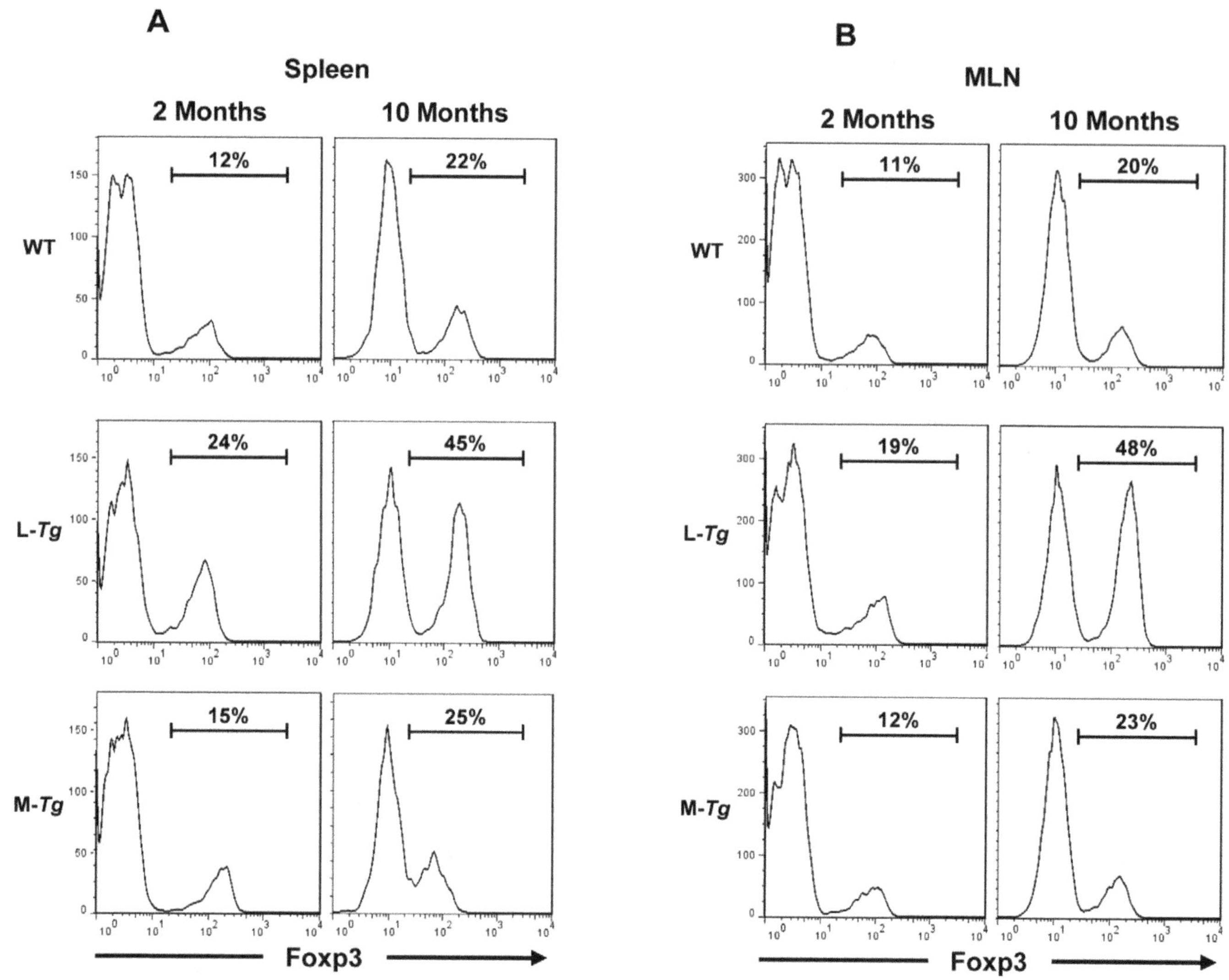

Figure 10. Increased numbers of regulatory T (Treg) cells in *Tl1a Tg* mice. FACS plot of CD4$^+$ Foxp3$^+$ splenocytes (A) or CD4$^+$ Foxp3$^+$ MLN cells (B) are shown. Data shown are representative of 4 mice per group at either 2 or 10 months of age. WT = wildtype, L-*Tg* = *LCK-CD2-Tl1a-GFP Tg* mice, M-*Tg* = *FMS-Tl1a-GFP Tg* mice.

We observed a low frequency of extra-intestinal pathology in both *LCK-CD2-Tl1a Tg* and *FMS-Tl1a Tg* mice. These included ulcerated skin lesions and erythematous swollen joints (fig. 7), which are similar to known extra-intestinal manifestations associated with human IBD. The cause of the extra-intestinal pathology in *Tl1a Tg* mice remains to be investigated, but may be related to the differential expression of CCR10 homing molecules in the *Tl1a Tg* mice. In addition to its function as a gut mucosal homing receptor [32], CCR10 is important in lymphocyte trafficking to the skin [33,34].

The chemokine receptors CCR9 and CCR10 play a major role in *in vivo* lymphocyte trafficking to portals of microbial entry, such as gut mucosal tissues and the skin [33,34,35,36,37]. The higher LPMC infiltrate in the small intestine as compared to the colon in *Tl1a Tg* mice may be due to the fact that CCR9 is preferentially found in the small intestine [38] and its ligand CCL25/TECK is expressed in both lamina propria venules and small intestine enterocytes [39,40]. In contrast, colonic expression of CCR9 and its ligand CCL25/TECK is limited [39,40]. The clinical importance of dysregulated immune trafficking in IBD is highlighted by the efficacious therapies such as natalizumab that blocks gut homing in inducing and maintaining remission in CD [41].

We found that constitutive expression of Tl1a resulted in a progressive activated phenotype over time in CD4$^+$ and CD8$^+$ T cells (Fig. 8), macrophages and DC (Fig. 9). Increased T cell and APC activation in *Tl1a Tg* mice may be a direct consequence of constitutive TL1a costimulation of DR3 expressing T cells and macrophages [11,42,43] or indirectly through failure of immunological tolerance leading to enhanced activation. In fact, recent studies have shown that the TL1A-DR3 pathway can attenuate the suppressive effect of Tregs on effector T cells [16,17]. The activated phenotype of T and APC in combination with the constitutive costimulation of TL1A-DR3 signaling pathway may lead to the significantly higher IFN-γ expression (Fig. 11B and 12A) that we saw in the *Tl1a Tg* mice, which is consistent with the previous observation that TL1A is involved in mediating the Th1 response [4,5,8,9,13,14,15,44,45]. There was also a trend toward increased IL-13 and IL-17 expression in mice with constitutive Tl1a expression (Fig. 12B and C), which was consistent with the

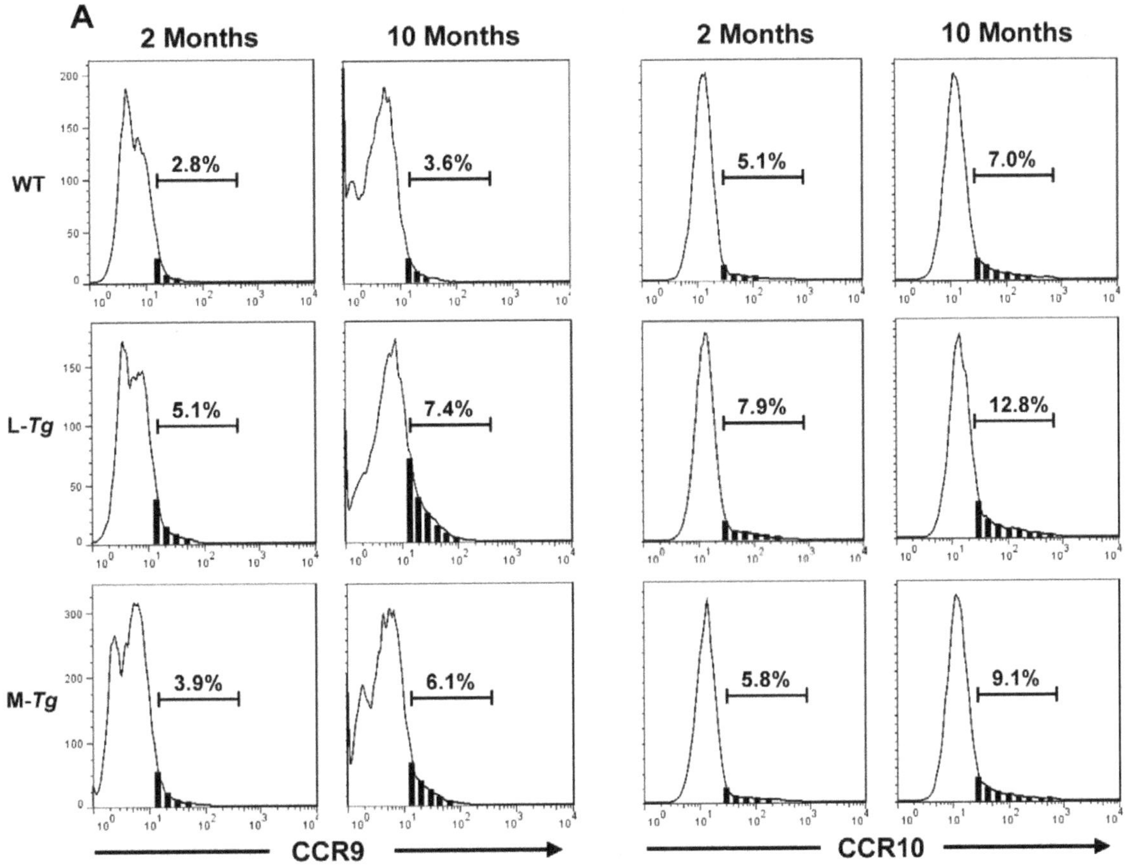
A
2 Months
10 Months
2 Months
10 Months
WT
L-Tg
M-Tg
2.8%
3.6%
5.1%
7.0%
5.1%
7.4%
7.9%
12.8%
3.9%
6.1%
5.8%
9.1%
CCR9
CCR10

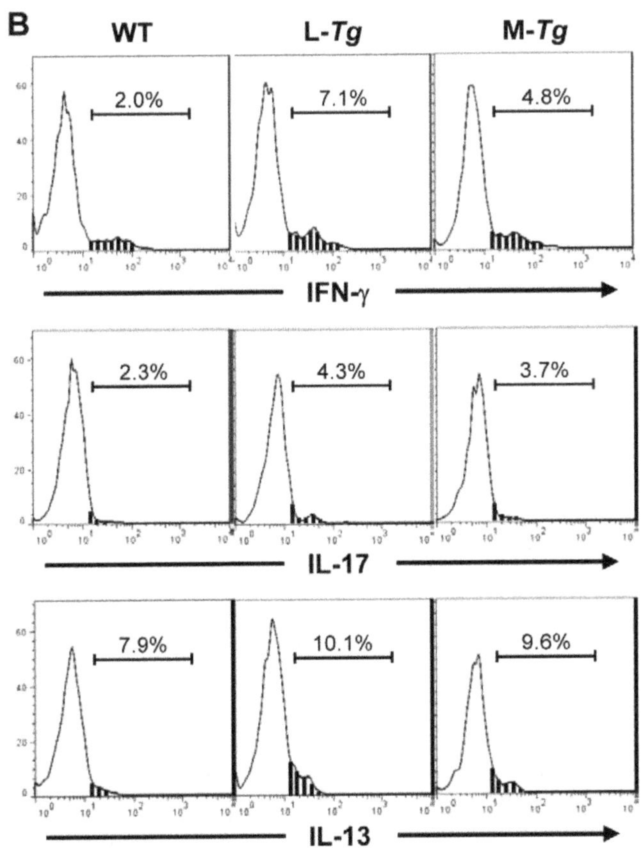
B
WT
L-Tg
M-Tg
2.0%
7.1%
4.8%
IFN-γ
2.3%
4.3%
3.7%
IL-17
7.9%
10.1%
9.6%
IL-13

Figure 11. Increased expression of gut homing markers and IFN-γ in *Tl1a Tg* mice. (A) FACS plots showing expression of gut homing markers CCR9 and CCR10 on CD4+ cells isolated from the MLN. (B) FACS plot of gated CD4+ cells from MLN and stained for intracellular IFN-γ, IL-17, and IL-13 expression from 10 months old WT, *LCK-CD2-Tl1a Tg* (L-*Tg*) or *FMS-Tl1a Tg* (M-*Tg*) mice. Data shown are representative of 4 mice per group (A and B). Black bars indicate area under the curve that is gated as CCR9 positive cells. WT = wildtype, L-*Tg* = *LCK-CD2-Tl1a-GFP Tg* mice, M-*Tg* = *FMS-Tl1a Tg* mice.

role of TL1A in Th2- and Th17- mediated functions in various mouse models [9,10,11,12,16,17]. Lastly, we found significantly increased IL-10 production in *LCK-CD2-Tl1a Tg* mice (Fig. 12D), which could be related to higher percentage of Foxp3+ Treg cells in *LCK-CD2-Tl1a Tg* as compared to *FMS-Tl1a Tg* or WT mice (Fig. 10A and B).

Recently, two groups independently reported the generation of transgenic mice with sustained TL1A expression in DC and T cells. Our results were similar to the constitutive Tl1a expressing *Tg* mice in Meylan et al. and Taraban et al., with the increased goblet, Paneth and Treg cells, ileitis and activated phenotype in T and APC cells [16,17]. However, a major difference was that the

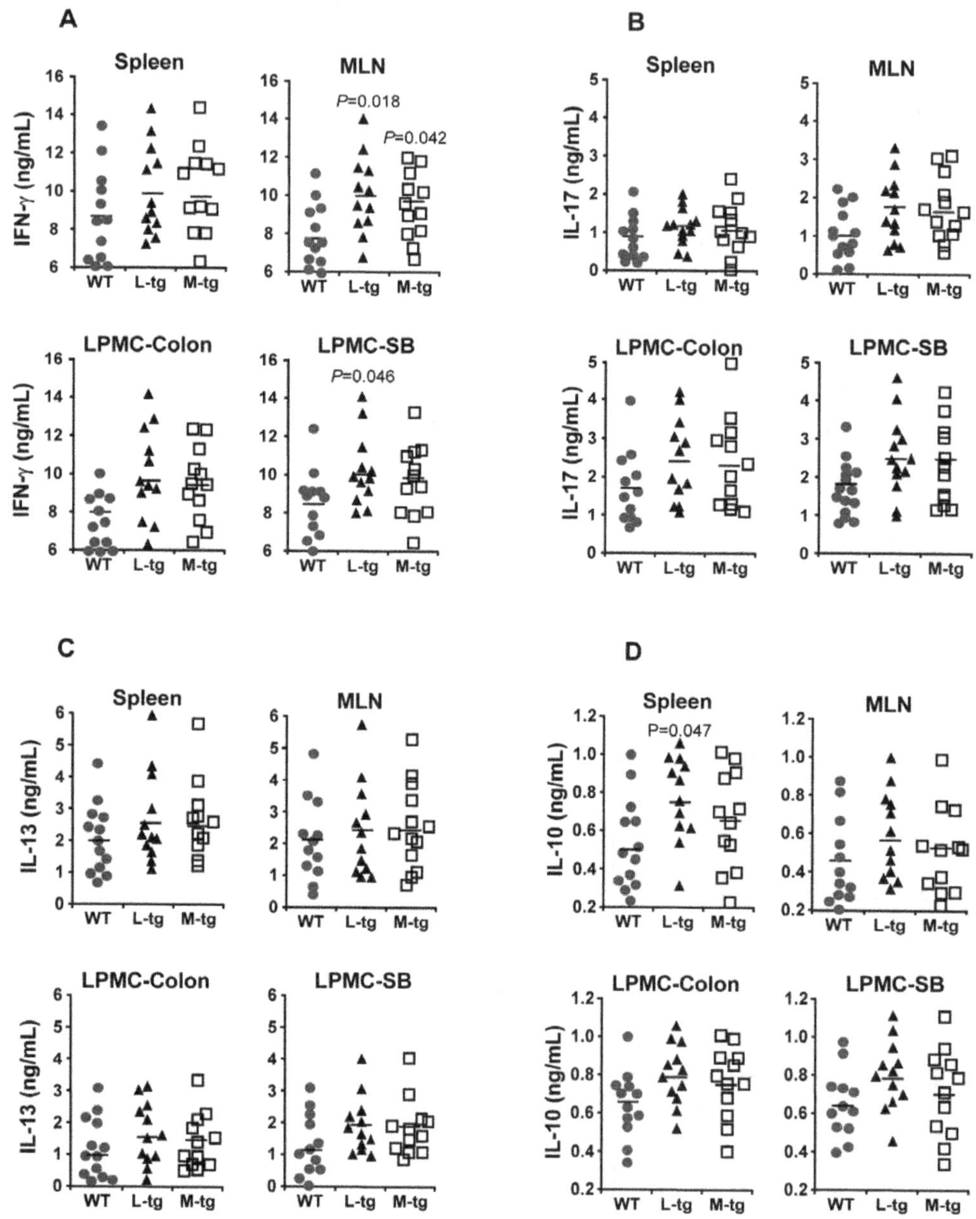

Figure 12. Cytokine profile of *Tl1a Tg* and WT littermate mice. IFN-γ (A), IL-17 (B), IL-13 (C) and IL-10 (D) secretion after stimulation with anti-CD3 and anti-CD28 were assessed by enzyme-linked immunosorbent assay (ELISA). Each data point (A-D) represents cytokine expression for either splenocytes, MLN cells or lamina propria mononuclear cells (LPMC) from either the colon or the distal 10 cm of small intestine isolated from an individual mouse. *p*-values are indicated the figure where significant. WT = wildtype, L-*Tg* = *LCK-CD2-Tl1a-GFP Tg* mice, M-*Tg* = *FMS-Tl1a Tg* mice.

ileitis found in the recently published *Tl1a Tg mice* appeared to be mainly attributed to Th2/IL-13 effector pathway [16,17], whereas we observed a higher production of IFN-γ from the *Tl1a Tg* mice generated in this study (Fig. 11B and 12A). In addition, we observed extra-intestinal pathology and increased gut fibrosis in the *Tl1a Tg* mice, which were not reported in the other *Tl1a Tg* mice. Several reasons may account for the phenotypical differences between the *Tl1a Tg* mice. One explanation may be methodological differences. For example, different promoter/enhancer elements were used to drive tissue specific expression of the different *Tl1a Tg* mice. We used the *LCK-CD2* promoter/enhancer element [19], whereas the CD2 promoter [46] was used to generate the T cell specific *Tl1a Tg* mice [16]. The *c-fms* promoter vector [18] was used to generate myeloid specific *Tl1a Tg* mice for this report whereas the *CD11c* promoter [47] was used for the recently published studies [16,17]. Differences in the phenotype of the transgenic mice using the different T cell promoter/enhancer element to drive transgene expression was observed previously in the T cell specific *LIGHT Tg* mice [19,48,49]. Another reason may lie in the mouse strain used. The *Tl1a Tg* mice used in this report were generated by direct microinjection into C57BL/6 pronuclei whereas the DC specific *Tl1a Tg* mouse [17] was generated by microinjecting into FVB/N zygotes and subsequently backcrossed 4–5 generations to the C57BL/6 strain. Alternatively, these phenotypical differences may be due to the different gut microflora between the animal housing facilities. Previous studies have demonstrated that genetically identical inbred mice strain raised in different facilities had different immune composition due to the different intestinal microbiota composition [50,51,52]. The potential immunomodulatory role of gut microbiota in the different *Tl1a Tg* mice highlights the previously described role of the TL1A-DR3 signaling pathway in bacteria recognition and microbial-host interactions [6,8,10,16].

In summary, we generated tissue specific, *in vivo* expression of Tl1a in T cells and APC and found that it lead to patchy small bowel inflammation and fibrosis in both the small intestine and the colon. Sustained expression of Tl1a leads to an activated immune phenotype, increased expression of gut homing molecules and Th1 (and possibly Th17 and Th2) responses. These novel Tl1a transgenic models of intestinal inflammation may be useful to study fibrotic response in inflammation and the pathogenesis of various disorders of immune dysregulation such as IBD.

Materials and Methods

Transgenic mice and genotype

Murine *Tl1A* cDNA (Open Biosystems, Clone ID 30740802) was digested by EcoRI/SmaI and inserted into the EcoRI/SmaI site of pIRES2-EGFP (Clontech). To generate lymphoid specific Tl1A transgenic mice, DNA fragment containing murine *Tl1A-IRES2-EGFP* was amplified by PCR using sense primer 5′-AATGGGGGCGCGCCGGGCTCTCTGGTCAGAAGGGATCAG-3′ and antisense primer 5′-TTTACGGGCGCGCCCCTTAAGATACATTGATGAGTTTGG-3′, digested with AscI, and cloned into AscI site of plck.E2 (generous gift from T. Hettmann, The University of Chicago), which contains the proximal *lck* promoter, human growth hormone gene (polyadenylation site), and locus control region elements from the human *CD2* gene to generate plasmid pLCK-Tl1a-IRES2-EGFP. The plck.E2 has been used to mediate T cell lineage specific expression [19]. The *Tl1A-IRES2-EGFP* fragment was sequenced to confirm that no mutations were generated during the cloning process. A 10-kb fragment was excised by NotI digest and used for microinjection into C57BL/6 pronuclei performed by Caliper Life Sciences. 8 independent murine lines containing genomic integration of the *Tl1a transgene* were identified by PCR using the following primers: 5′- GACTAACAAAGATGCCTGCCTGTGG-3′ and 5′-GCCATCCTTCTGCTGTCTTGGAGA-3′. Only 2 of the 8 lines showed T-cell lineage specific expression of TL1A (95% of T cells and 34% of T cells). We used the founder transgenic (*Tg*) mouse line with *Tl1A* transgene expression in 95% of T cells and called it *LCK-CD2-Tl1A-GFP Tg* mouse.

To generate myeloid specific *Tl1a Tg* mice, a XhoI/EcoRI fragment was blunt ended by klenow (NEB) and cloned to blunt ended MluI site of *c-fms* promoter vector (generous gift from D. Underhill, Cedars-Sinai Medical Center). Tl1A-IRES2-EGFP fragment was sequenced to confirm that no mutations were generated during the cloning process. The *c-fms* promoter vector has been used previously to drive expression for cells of the mononuclear phagocyte lineage including macrophages and dendritic cells [18]. A 10-kb fragment was excised by XhoI/ClaI digest and used for microinjection into C57BL/6 pronuclei performed by Caliper Life Sciences. 6 independent murine lines containing genomic integration of the *Tl1a* transgene were identified by PCR using the following primers: 5′-TTGGAAGCTGATTGAAGGGTCCA-3′ and 5′-AGCTCCTCTGCCATCCTTCTGCT-3′. Two of the six lines showed myeloid specific expression of the transgene in approximately 70% of macrophages and dendritic cells, but one has higher GFP level than the other founder line. We used the founder Tg line with the higher GFP expression and called this line *FMS-Tl1a-GFP Tg* mouse.

All mice were maintained under specific pathogen-free conditions in the Animal Care Facility at Cedars-Sinai Medical Center. Littermate control mice were used for all experiments. This study was carried out in strict accordance with the recommendations in the Guide for the Care and Use of Laboratory Animals of the NIH. Mice used in all experiments were specifically approved by Cedars-Sinai Medical Center Animal Care and Use Committee. Approved protocol 2269 was used for this study.

Disease activity index (DAI), macroscopic and histopathological analysis

Mice were weighed and inspected for diarrhea and rectal bleeding once a week for the first 2 months after weaning, then once a month thereafter. The DAI (combined score of weight loss, presence of blood in stool, and stool consistency) was determined according to a standard scoring system previously described [20]. Colon and small intestine were scored for macroscopic evidence of inflammation using the established classification [21]. Tissue was fixed in 10% neutral buffered formalin (Sigma). Samples were embedded, sectioned, and stained with hematoxylin and eosin by the Histology Core at Cedars-Sinai Medical Center. Masson Trichrome staining was performed as described previously [29]. Histopathological scores of colons and small intestine were assigned in a blinded manner by at least 2 trained pathologists (DQS and HWK) using previously established methods [21]. The histologic score is calculated from observation of at least 36 different fields of stained sections at 200X from 6 mice in each group. The numbers of goblet cells and Paneth cells were determined by examining at least 80 individual villi and crypts from each group.

Real-time PCR analysis

Total RNA was isolated as previously described [8]. Two micrograms of total RNA was used in each RT reaction using the

Omniscript kit (Qiagen), with oligo dT as primer. TL1A and β-actin transcripts were amplified by quantitative real-time RT-PCR as previously described [9]. Duplicates differing by less than one cycle were averaged and amount of transcript was analyzed and expressed as percentage of β-actin.

Cell isolation and culture

LPMC isolation, culture, and stimulation by anti-CD28 and anti-CD3ϵ were carried out as previously reported [9]. We used the whole colon for LPMC isolation. We used the distal 10 cm of the SB for LPMC isolation. Cytokine concentration was assayed by enzyme-linked immunosorbent assay (ELISA) using ELISA kits for IFN-γ, IL-17 IL-13, and IL-10 (eBioscience) per manufacture protocol and as previously described [9].

Flow cytometry and measurement of intracellular cytokine expression

Cells were stained with antibodies against murine CD4 (RM4-5), CD44 (IM7), CD86 (GL1) (BD Biosciences), CCR9 (242503), CCR10 (248918) (R&D systems), CD8 (53-6.7), CD11c (N418), F4/80 (BM8) (Biolegend) and FoxP3 (FJK-165) (eBiosciences). CD16/CD32 (clone 2.4G2) was used to block nonspecific FcR binding (eBiosciences). Intracellular staining was performed with antibodies against IFN-γ (XMG1.2), IL-17 (17B7) and IL13 (13a) (eBioSciences). For determination of intracellular cytokine production by leukocytes, cells were incubated for 5 hours at 37°C with BD Leukocyte Activation Cocktail with BD GolgiPlug (BD Biosciences). For FoxP3 staining, fixation and permeabilization buffers provided from the manufacturer (eBiosciences) were used. Data of the stained cells were acquired on a Cyan flow cytometer (Dako-Cytomation) and analyzed using FlowJo analysis software (Tree Star, Inc).

Statistical analysis

Data are presented as the mean ± standard deviation. Comparison between two groups was performed by a two tailed, Student's *t*-test. A value of $p<0.05$ was considered significant.

Acknowledgments

The authors thank Loren Karp for critical reading of the manuscript. We are grateful to Patricia Lin for help with flow cytometry.

Author Contributions

Conceived and designed the experiments: DQS SRT. Performed the experiments: DQS RB XZ NY HWK PP BK MHW GM. Analyzed the data: DQS RB XZ GM SRT. Contributed reagents/materials/analysis tools: DQS RB KSM HWK CP. Wrote the paper: DQS. Performed the Masson Trichrome staining of 3D and 6: YS.

References

1. Shih DQ, Targan SR (2009) Insights into IBD Pathogenesis. Curr Gastroenterol Rep 11: 473–480.
2. Shih DQ, Targan SR, McGovern D (2008) Recent advances in IBD pathogenesis: genetics and immunobiology. Curr Gastroenterol Rep 10: 568–575.
3. Stappenbeck TS, Rioux JD, Mizoguchi A, Saitoh T, Huett A, et al. (2010) Crohn disease: A current perspective on genetics, autophagy and immunity. Autophagy 7: Epub ahead of print.
4. Prehn JL, Mehdizadeh S, Landers CJ, Luo X, Cha SC, et al. (2004) Potential role for TL1A, the new TNF-family member and potent costimulator of IFN-gamma, in mucosal inflammation. Clin Immunol 112: 66–77.
5. Papadakis KA, Prehn JL, Landers C, Han Q, Luo X, et al. (2004) TL1A synergizes with IL-12 and IL-18 to enhance IFN-gamma production in human T cells and NK cells. J Immunol 172: 7002–7007.
6. Cassatella MA, Pereira-da-Silva G, Tinazzi I, Facchetti F, Scapini P, et al. (2007) Soluble TNF-like cytokine (TL1A) production by immune complexes stimulated monocytes in rheumatoid arthritis. J Immunol 178: 7325–7333.
7. Prehn JL, Thomas LS, Landers CJ, Yu QT, Michelsen KS, et al. (2007) The T cell costimulator TL1A is induced by FcgammaR signaling in human monocytes and dendritic cells. J Immunol 178: 4033–4038.
8. Shih DQ, Kwan LY, Chavez V, Cohavy O, Gonsky R, et al. (2009) Microbial induction of inflammatory bowel disease associated gene TL1A (TNFSF15) in antigen presenting cells. Eur J Immunol 39: 3239–3250.
9. Takedatsu H, Michelsen KS, Wei B, Landers CJ, Thomas LS, et al. (2008) TL1A (TNFSF15) regulates the development of chronic colitis by modulating both T-helper 1 and T-helper 17 activation. Gastroenterology 135: 552–567.
10. Meylan F, Davidson TS, Kahle E, Kinder M, Acharya K, et al. (2008) The TNF-family receptor DR3 is essential for diverse T cell-mediated inflammatory diseases. Immunity 29: 79–89.
11. Fang L, Adkins B, Deyev V, Podack ER (2008) Essential role of TNF receptor superfamily 25 (TNFRSF25) in the development of allergic lung inflammation. J Exp Med 205: 1037–1048.
12. Pappu BP, Borodovsky A, Zheng TS, Yang X, Wu P, et al. (2008) TL1A-DR3 interaction regulates Th17 cell function and Th17-mediated autoimmune disease. J Exp Med 205: 1049–1062.
13. Bamias G, Mishina M, Nyce M, Ross WG, Kollias G, et al. (2006) Role of TL1A and its receptor DR3 in two models of chronic murine ileitis. Proc Natl Acad Sci U S A 103: 8441–8446.
14. Papadakis KA, Zhu D, Prehn JL, Landers C, Avanesyan A, et al. (2005) Dominant role for TL1A/DR3 pathway in IL-12 plus IL-18-induced IFN-gamma production by peripheral blood and mucosal CCR9+ T lymphocytes. J Immunol 174: 4985–4990.
15. Bamias G, Martin C, 3rd, Marini M, Hoang S, Mishina M, et al. (2003) Expression, localization, and functional activity of TL1A, a novel Th1-polarizing cytokine in inflammatory bowel disease. J Immunol 171: 4868–4874.
16. Meylan F, Song YJ, Fuss I, Villarreal S, Kahle E, et al. (2010) The TNF-family cytokine TL1A drives IL-13-dependent small intestinal inflammation. Mucosal Immunol: Epub ahead of print.
17. Taraban VY, Slebioda TJ, Willoughby JE, Buchan SL, James S, et al. (2010) Sustained TL1A expression modulates effector and regulatory T-cell responses and drives intestinal goblet cell hyperplasia. Mucosal Immunol;Epub ahead of print.
18. Sasmono RT, Oceandy D, Pollard JW, Tong W, Pavli P, et al. (2003) A macrophage colony-stimulating factor receptor-green fluorescent protein transgene is expressed throughout the mononuclear phagocyte system of the mouse. Blood 101: 1155–1163.
19. Wang J, Lo JC, Foster A, Yu P, Chen HM, et al. (2001) The regulation of T cell homeostasis and autoimmunity by T cell-derived LIGHT. J Clin Invest 108: 1771–1780.
20. Rachmilewitz D, Karmeli F, Shteingart S, Lee J, Takabayashi K, et al. (2006) Immunostimulatory oligonucleotides inhibit colonic proinflammatory cytokine production in ulcerative colitis. Inflamm Bowel Dis 12: 339–345.
21. Ostanin DV, Pavlick KP, Bharwani S, D'Souza D, Furr KL, et al. (2006) T cell-induced inflammation of the small and large intestine in immunodeficient mice. Am J Physiol Gastrointest Liver Physiol 290: G109–119.
22. Katakura K, Lee J, Rachmilewitz D, Li G, Eckmann L, et al. (2005) Toll-like receptor 9-induced type I IFN protects mice from experimental colitis. J Clin Invest 115: 695–702.
23. Picornell Y, Mei L, Taylor K, Yang H, Targan SR, et al. (2007) TNFSF15 is an ethnic-specific IBD gene. Inflamm Bowel Dis 13: 1333–1338.
24. Michelsen KS, Thomas LS, Taylor KD, Yu QT, Mei L, et al. (2009) IBD-associated TL1A gene (TNFSF15) haplotypes determine increased expression of TL1A protein. PLoS One 4: e4719.
25. Vidrich A, Buzan JM, Barnes S, Reuter BK, Skaar K, et al. (2005) Altered epithelial cell lineage allocation and global expansion of the crypt epithelial stem cell population are associated with ileitis in SAMP1/YitFc mice. Am J Pathol 166: 1055–1067.
26. Kosiewicz MM, Nast CC, Krishnan A, Rivera-Nieves J, Moskaluk CA, et al. (2001) Th1-type responses mediate spontaneous ileitis in a novel murine model of Crohn's disease. J Clin Invest 107: 695–702.
27. Shinoda M, Shin-Ya M, Naito Y, Kishida T, Ito R, et al. (2010) Early-stage blocking of Notch signaling inhibits the depletion of goblet cells in dextran sodium sulfate-induced colitis in mice. J Gastroenterol 45: 608–617.
28. Kajino-Sakamoto R, Inagaki M, Lippert E, Akira S, Robine S, et al. (2008) Enterocyte-derived TAK1 signaling prevents epithelium apoptosis and the development of ileitis and colitis. J Immunol 181: 1143–1152.
29. Koon HW, Shih D, Karagiannides I, Zhao D, Fazelbhoy Z, et al. (2010) Substance P Modulates Chronic Inflammation-Induced Colonic Fibrosis. Am J Pathol 177: 2300–2309.
30. Di Sabatino A, Jackson CL, Pickard KM, Buckley M, Rovedatti L, et al. (2009) Transforming growth factor beta signalling and matrix metalloproteinases in the mucosa overlying Crohn's disease strictures. Gut 58: 777–789.
31. Simmons JG, Pucilowska JB, Keku TO, Lund PK (2002) IGF-I and TGF-beta1 have distinct effects on phenotype and proliferation of intestinal fibroblasts. Am J Physiol Gastrointest Liver Physiol 283: G809–818.

32. Hieshima K, Kawasaki Y, Hanamoto H, Nakayama T, Nagakubo D, et al. (2004) CC chemokine ligands 25 and 28 play essential roles in intestinal extravasation of IgA antibody-secreting cells. J Immunol 173: 3668–3675.
33. Reiss Y, Proudfoot AE, Power CA, Campbell JJ, Butcher EC (2001) CC chemokine receptor (CCR)4 and the CCR10 ligand cutaneous T cell-attracting chemokine (CTACK) in lymphocyte trafficking to inflamed skin. J Exp Med 194: 1541–1547.
34. Soler D, Humphreys TL, Spinola SM, Campbell JJ (2003) CCR4 versus CCR10 in human cutaneous TH lymphocyte trafficking. Blood 101: 1677–1682.
35. Wurbel MA, Malissen M, Guy-Grand D, Meffre E, Nussenzweig MC, et al. (2001) Mice lacking the CCR9 CC-chemokine receptor show a mild impairment of early T- and B-cell development and a reduction in T-cell receptor gammadelta(+) gut intraepithelial lymphocytes. Blood 98: 2626–2632.
36. Marsal J, Svensson M, Ericsson A, Iranpour AH, Carramolino L, et al. (2002) Involvement of CCL25 (TECK) in the generation of the murine small-intestinal CD8alpha alpha+CD3+ intraepithelial lymphocyte compartment. Eur J Immunol 32: 3488–3497.
37. Svensson M, Marsal J, Ericsson A, Carramolino L, Broden T, et al. (2002) CCL25 mediates the localization of recently activated CD8alphabeta(+) lymphocytes to the small-intestinal mucosa. J Clin Invest 110: 1113–1121.
38. Zabel BA, Agace WW, Campbell JJ, Heath HM, Parent D, et al. (1999) Human G protein-coupled receptor GPR-9-6/CC chemokine receptor 9 is selectively expressed on intestinal homing T lymphocytes, mucosal lymphocytes, and thymocytes and is required for thymus-expressed chemokine-mediated chemotaxis. J Exp Med 190: 1241–1256.
39. Kunkel EJ, Campbell JJ, Haraldsen G, Pan J, Boisvert J, et al. (2000) Lymphocyte CC chemokine receptor 9 and epithelial thymus-expressed chemokine (TECK) expression distinguish the small intestinal immune compartment: Epithelial expression of tissue-specific chemokines as an organizing principle in regional immunity. J Exp Med 192: 761–768.
40. Papadakis KA, Prehn J, Nelson V, Cheng L, Binder SW, et al. (2000) The role of thymus-expressed chemokine and its receptor CCR9 on lymphocytes in the regional specialization of the mucosal immune system. J Immunol 165: 5069–5076.
41. Targan SR, Feagan BG, Fedorak RN, Lashner BA, Panaccione R, et al. (2007) Natalizumab for the treatment of active Crohn's disease: results of the ENCORE Trial. Gastroenterology 132: 1672–1683.
42. Kang YJ, Kim WJ, Bae HU, Kim DI, Park YB, et al. (2005) Involvement of TL1A and DR3 in induction of pro-inflammatory cytokines and matrix metalloproteinase-9 in atherogenesis. Cytokine 29: 229–235.
43. McLaren JE, Calder CJ, McSharry BP, Sexton K, Salter RC, et al. (2010) The TNF-like protein 1A-death receptor 3 pathway promotes macrophage foam cell formation in vitro. J Immunol 184: 5827–5834.
44. Migone TS, Zhang J, Luo X, Zhuang L, Chen C, et al. (2002) TL1A is a TNF-like ligand for DR3 and TR6/DcR3 and functions as a T cell costimulator. Immunity 16: 479–492.
45. Biener-Ramanujan E, Gonsky R, Ko B, Targan SR (2010) Functional signaling of membrane-bound TL1A induces IFN-gamma expression. FEBS Lett 584: 2376–2380.
46. Zhumabekov T, Corbella P, Tolaini M, Kioussis D (1995) Improved version of a human CD2 minigene based vector for T cell-specific expression in transgenic mice. J Immunol Methods 185: 133–140.
47. Brocker T, Riedinger M, Karjalainen K (1997) Targeted expression of major histocompatibility complex (MHC) class II molecules demonstrates that dendritic cells can induce negative but not positive selection of thymocytes in vivo. J Exp Med 185: 541–550.
48. Shaikh RB, Santee S, Granger SW, Butrovich K, Cheung T, et al. (2001) Constitutive expression of LIGHT on T cells leads to lymphocyte activation, inflammation, and tissue destruction. J Immunol 167: 6330–6337.
49. Wang J, Anders RA, Wu Q, Peng D, Cho JH, et al. (2004) Dysregulated LIGHT expression on T cells mediates intestinal inflammation and contributes to IgA nephropathy. J Clin Invest 113: 826–835.
50. Ivanov II, Frutos Rde L, Manel N, Yoshinaga K, Rifkin DB, et al. (2008) Specific microbiota direct the differentiation of IL-17-producing T-helper cells in the mucosa of the small intestine. Cell Host Microbe 4: 337–349.
51. Ivanov II, Atarashi K, Manel N, Brodie EL, Shima T, et al. (2009) Induction of intestinal Th17 cells by segmented filamentous bacteria. Cell 139: 485–498.
52. Wu HJ, Ivanov II, Darce J, Hattori K, Shima T, et al. (2010) Gut-residing segmented filamentous bacteria drive autoimmune arthritis via T helper 17 cells. Immunity 32: 815–827.

7

Regional Neuroplastic Brain Changes in Patients with Chronic Inflammatory and Non-Inflammatory Visceral Pain

Jui-Yang Hong[1,3,6,8*], **Jennifer S. Labus**[1,2,3,5,6], **Zhiguo Jiang**[10,11], **Cody Ashe-Mcnalley**[1,2,3,6], **Ivo Dinov**[9], **Arpana Gupta**[1,2,3,6], **Yonggang Shi**[12], **Jean Stains**[1,3,6], **Nuwanthi Heendeniya**[1,3,6], **Suzanne R. Smith**[1,3,6], **Kirsten Tillisch**[1,2,3,6], **Emeran A. Mayer**[1,2,3,4,5,6,7]

1 Gail and Gerald Oppenheimer Family Center for Neurobiology of Stress, University of California Los Angeles, Los Angeles, California, United States of America, **2** Pain and Interoception Imaging Network (PAIN), University of California Los Angeles, Los Angeles, California, United States of America, **3** Department of Medicine, University of California Los Angeles, Los Angeles, California, United States of America, **4** Department of Psychiatry, University of California Los Angeles, Los Angeles, California, United States of America, **5** Brain Research Institute, University of California Los Angeles, Los Angeles, California, United States of America, **6** Division of Digestive Diseases, University of California Los Angeles, Los Angeles, California, United States of America, **7** Ahmanson Lovelace Brain Mapping Center, David Geffen School of Medicine, University of California, Los Angeles, California, **8** Department of Bioengineering, University of California Los Angeles, Los Angeles, California, United States of America, **9** University of Michigan School of Nursing, Ann Arbor, Michigan, United States of America, **10** Department of Biomedical Engineering, New Jersey Institute of Technology, Newark, New Jersey, United States of America, **11** Human Performance and Engineering Laboratory, Kessler Foundation Research Center, West Orange, New Jersey, United States of America, **12** Laboratory of Neuro-Imaging, University of Southern California, Los Angeles, California United States of America

Abstract

Regional cortical thickness alterations have been reported in many chronic inflammatory and painful conditions, including inflammatory bowel diseases (IBD) and irritable bowel syndrome (IBS), even though the mechanisms underlying such neuroplastic changes remain poorly understood. In order to better understand the mechanisms contributing to grey matter changes, the current study sought to identify the differences in regional alterations in cortical thickness between healthy controls and two chronic visceral pain syndromes, with and without chronic gut inflammation. 41 healthy controls, 11 IBS subjects with diarrhea, and 16 subjects with ulcerative colitis (UC) underwent high-resolution T1-weighted magnetization-prepared rapid acquisition gradient echo scans. Structural image preprocessing and cortical thickness analysis within the region of interests were performed by using the Laboratory of Neuroimaging Pipeline. Group differences were determined using the general linear model and linear contrast analysis. The two disease groups differed significantly in several cortical regions. UC subjects showed greater cortical thickness in anterior cingulate cortical subregions, and in primary somatosensory cortex compared with both IBS and healthy subjects. Compared with healthy subjects, UC subjects showed lower cortical thickness in orbitofrontal cortex and in mid and posterior insula, while IBS subjects showed lower cortical thickness in the anterior insula. Large effects of correlations between symptom duration and thickness in the orbitofrontal cortex and postcentral gyrus were only observed in UC subjects. The findings suggest that the mechanisms underlying the observed gray matter changes in UC subjects represent a consequence of peripheral inflammation, while in IBS subjects central mechanisms may play a primary role.

Editor: André Mouraux, Université catholique de Louvain, Belgium

Funding: This work was funded in part by the National Institutes of Health through Center for Neurobiology (CNS) grants: K08 DK071626, R03 DK084169, K23DK073451, R01 AT007137, P50 DK064539, R01 DK048351, and LONI grants: NIBIB 9P41EB015922-15, NCRR 2-P41-RR-013642-15, NCRR U54 RR021813, U24-RR025736, U24-RR021992. The funders had no role in study design, data collection and analysis, decision to publish, or preparation of the manuscript.

Competing Interests: The authors have declared that no competing interests exist.

* E-mail: usagilberthong@hotmail.com

Introduction

Inflammatory bowel diseases (IBD) such as ulcerative colitis (UC) are characterized by chronically recurring symptoms of abdominal pain associated with flares of mucosal inflammation. In contrast, in irritable bowel syndrome (IBS), chronically recurring symptoms of abdominal pain and discomfort occur in the absence of mucosal inflammation or other identifiable nociceptive triggers (therefore referred to as "functional" pain syndromes), and symptom flares are often triggered by psychosocial stressors. It is generally assumed that abdominal pain in UC results initially from inflammation induced peripheral and central sensitization of visceral afferent pathways [1], while symptoms in IBS may reflect primarily an alteration in central pain modulation, including alterations in endogenous descending pain modulation mechanisms [2]. On the other hand, several pieces of evidence support the concept that IBD patients effectively engage endogenous pain inhibition systems [3], including greater engagement of a cortico limbic-pontine pain modulation network compared to IBS subjects [4]. These differences in the engagement of endogenous pain modulation systems may explain the clinical observation that in uncomplicated UC, abdominal pain is not a prominent symptom even during flares.

Several studies have applied multimodal brain imaging to investigate the presence of grey matter changes in patients with various chronic pain conditions without known nociceptive drive [5–9], with presumed nociceptive drive [10–12], and with known inflammatory drive [13–18]. Reported abnormalities in these studies suggest some similarities in findings (e.g. gray matter reduction in insula [INS] and anterior cingulate cortex [ACC] subregions), and increases in CT in somatosensory regions regardless of pain syndrome, and no clear differences have emerged between the different pain categories, in particular between chronic visceral pain of "functional" and of inflammatory origin. The use of different analysis techniques by different groups, makes interpretive comparisons between studies and between different patient populations more difficult.

In the current study, we used the Laboratory of Neuroimaging (LONI) Pipeline [19,20] for image preprocessing, volumetric analysis and cortical thickness (CT) analysis. We focused on differences of local morphologic brain alterations between UC and healthy control subjects (HCs), and compared them to findings in IBS subjects. Specifically, we aimed to test the following hypotheses: 1) Both IBS and UC patients differ from HCs in terms of regional CT changes. 2) UC patients show CT changes in brain regions involved in somatosensory and viscerosensory processing and modulation. 3) IBS patients show CT changes in brain regions involved in the integration of affective, cognitive and interoceptive signals. 4) In UC patients, there are correlations between CT changes and duration of gut inflammation, reflecting the chronic influence of peripheral inflammation on the brain.

Materials and Methods

Subjects

A total 68 right-handed male and female subjects were recruited through the UCLA Digestive Disease Clinic and advertisements including HCs (n = 41; mean age = 28.2 years old, range = 19–48 years; 16 males), IBS with diarrhea (n = 11; mean age = 31.6 - years old, range = 21–47 years; 2 males), and UC subjects (n = 16; mean age = 28. 6 years old, range 18–48 years; 10 males). 15 HCs and 5 IBS subjects of the respective samples have been included in a previously published gray matter volume analysis [9]. Exclusion criteria for all subjects comprised pregnancy, postpartum or nursing females, current substance abuse or dependence, abdominal surgery, any past or present neurological illness or trauma, claustrophobia or learning disability, and current psychiatric diagnosis. A diagnosis of IBS was made by a gastroenterologist or nurse practitioner with expertise in functional GI disorders based on the ROME II or ROME III symptom criteria during a clinical assessment [21,22]. The diagnostic criteria include recurrent abdominal pain or discomfort associated with two or more of the following: 1) pain/discomfort is relieved/improved by defecation 2) the onset of pain/discomfort is related to a change in frequency of stool 3) the onset of pain/discomfort is related to a change in the form (appearance) of stool. In order to match the predominant bowel habit of UC patients, only IBS patients with diarrhea were used in this study. In addition, IBS subjects with current regular use of analgesic drugs (including narcotics, opioids and alpha2-delta ligands) were excluded. UC patients were diagnosed by a gastroenterologist, which was supported by biopsies obtained by endoscopy. During screening, all subjects completed the modified Mayo UCDAI (disease activity index for Stool frequency, rectal bleeding and physician rating of disease activity) to assess degree of current disease. A score of 0–1 is considered Remission, score of 2–4 mild disease, and >4 is considered active disease [23]. Exclusion criteria specific to the UC population were corticosteroid use within last 6 months, or use of any psychotropic medications. All procedures were approved by the UCLA Medical Institutional Review Board, and all subjects provided written informed consent. Questionnaires were completed before scanning to determine symptom type, severity, duration of symptoms, and abdominal sensation (UCLA Bowel Symptom Questionnaire, BSQ) [24], comorbid affective and mood disorders (Hospital Anxiety Depression Scale, HAD) [25], and IBS-related fears and anxiety (Visceral Sensitivity Index, VSI) [26,27]. Details are shown in Table 1.

Structural MRI Acquisition

All high-resolution T1-weighted brain images were collected at the UCLA Brain Mapping Center using a Siemens 3 Tesla Trio with magnetization prepared rapid gradient echo scanning parameters (TR = 2200 ms, TE = 3.26 ms, flip angle = 9°, duration = 9:03 mins, FOV = 256).

Data analysis

We employed the LONI pipeline for image preprocessing, cortical surface modeling and gray matter thickness analysis [19,20]. Following a de-identification step, the structural neuroimaging data were converted from Digital Imaging and Communications in Medicine to ANALYZE 7.5 format, skull-stripped using the LONI Skull-Stripping Meta Algorithm pipeline workflow [28] and cortical surface models were generated using FreeSurfer 4.0 [29] (http://surfer.nmr.mgh.harvard.edu/fswiki and http://ucla.in/xSQPqT). Cortical grey matter thickness was computed at each point of the surface using the distance from the pial surface to the nearest point on the white matter surface. For numerical implementation, we first built the signed distance function [30,31] of the white matter surface in 3D space and then computed the CT as the value on the signed distance function at those locations. The cortical surfaces and the corresponding CT maps were registered to the International Consortium for Brain Mapping (ICBM) brain surface [32] and then vertex-wise correspondences were established between all cortical surface models using a Conformal Metric Optimization method [33]. An experienced human brain researcher rated each brain surface reconstruction by visually inspecting the surfaces using LONI ShapeViewer (http://www.loni.ucla.edu/Software/ShapeViewer). The quality of surface reconstruction and accuracy of vertex labeling were assessed on the scale of 0 to 1 (0 = completely unacceptable; 1 = perfectly reconstructed and labeled). A threshold of 0.7 was selected as the criterion to reconstruct a subject's surface data to be included in the final analysis.

Region of interest analysis

We examined the CT change in several manually delineated regions of interest (ROIs) in each hemisphere based on previous studies [11,14,34–39]. These ROIs included insular subregions (anterior INS [aINS], mid INS [mINS], and posterior INS [pINS]), cingulate subregions (subgenual ACC [sgACC], pregenual ACC [pgACC], anterior midcingulate cortex [aMCC] and posterior MCC [pMCC]), orbitofrontal gyrus (OFG) (lateral OFG and medial OFG), pre- and postcentral gyri [32]. No subregions of pre- and postcentral gyri were drawn. The subregions of INS and cingulum were manually delineated on the 3D ICBM brain atlas [32] by two well-trained researchers with good command of neuroanatomical knowledge (Figure S1). The 3D ROI masks were transformed back onto the ICBM

Table 1. Clinical and behavioral characteristics.

	HCs			IBS subjects			UC subjects			F	Sig.
	N	Mean	SD	N	Mean	SD	N	Mean	SD		
Sex (Male/Female)	16/25			2/9			10/6				
Age	41	28.17	8.43	11	31.55	9.49	16	28.56	8.95	.66	.52
Anxiety symptoms[1]	41	2.8	2.33	11	6.91	3.67	16	7.31	3.55	18.29	<.01
Depression symptoms[1]	41	.85	1.22	11	2.64	2.73	16	3.44	3.54	7.77	<.01
Visceral Sensitivity Index [2]	40	2.83	5.17	11	37.45	12.94	15	26.13	14.09	61.68	<.01
Overall Bowel Symptoms[3]				11	11.91	2.74	13	4.69	2.46	54.12	<.01
Abdominal Pain[4]				11	10.55	4.3	14	4.14	3.61	18.01	<.01
Abdominal Discomfort[5]				11	11.91	4.21	16	4.06	3.86	49.63	<.01
Duration of symptoms[6]				10	8.5	6.13	16	9.81	9.35	1.67	.69

F = main effect of group from ANOVA and t-tests for four and two group comparisons, respectively.
1. HAD: Hospital Anxiety and Depression [25];
2. VSI: Visceral Sensitivity Index [26,27];
BSQ: Bowel Symptom Questionnaire [24].
3. BSQ Overall Symptoms in the Past week (0–20).
4. BSQ Abdominal Pain in the Past week (0–20).
5. BSQ Discomfort in the Past week (0–20).
6. BSQ Duration in years, derived from onset of symptom.
Statistically significant p<0.05.

surface space by resampling the atlas map based on masks' Euclidean coordinates [33].

Statistical analysis

To determine potential protocol differences in ROIs, a general linear model (GLM) was applied to examine differences in total gray matter volumes within HCs as a function of protocol. Group differences in CT within ROIs as a function of group, sex and group*sex were determined using the GLM and weighted linear contrast analysis controlling for total gray matter volume, and age in SPSS v19. The contrasts testing the interaction between group and sex were weighted to eliminate any bias caused by unbalanced representation of sexes. Although this was a hypothesis driven study, we implemented a conservative procedure to adjust for multiple comparisons in order to control for type I error. Specifically, the false-discovery rate (FDR) for the 66 contrasts (11 bilateral ROIs [n = 22] for each of three independent contrasts) was held at 5% [40–42]. GLM and linear contrast analysis controlling for sex and age were also applied to examine differences in BSQ between IBS and UC subjects as well as group differences in non-BSQ clinical and behavioral characteristics including VSI and HAD. Significance was determined after controlling FDR at 5% [40,41].

Correlation Analysis of Clinic Variables

Within group exploratory partial correlation analyses controlling for total gray matter volume, sex, and age were performed to characterize the association between subjects' clinic characteristics (BSQ, VSI, HAD and Mayo UCDAI) and regions showing significant group differences in CT. However, for the partial correlation between significant ROIs and symptom duration, we did not include age as a covariate, as these explanatory variables were significantly correlated, for IBS group (duration, r = .39, p = .036), and for UC group (duration, r = .67, p = .001) [43]. Significance was determined after controlling FDR at 5% [40,41].

Results

Subject Characteristics

Subjects' clinical data are summarized in Table 1. Compared to the HCs, the two disease groups showed significantly higher measures of symptom related anxiety (VSI scores: IBS>HCs, F = 126.28, p<.001; UC>HCs, F = 71.97, p<.001; IBS>UC, F = 10.61, p = .002), anxiety symptoms (HAD scores: IBS>HCs, F = 17.03, p<.001; UC>HCs, F = 28.02, p<.001), and depression symptoms (HAD scores: IBS>HCs, F = 4.88, p = .031; UC>HCs, F = 15.16, p<.001). IBS subjects had significantly higher overall bowel symptoms scores, more abdominal discomfort and pain than UC subjects. Using the Mayo UCDAI [23], 5 of the UC subjects were in remission, 7 had mild disease and 4 had active disease (mild flare). There were no differences in terms of age of subjects and duration of GI symptoms.

Regional Cortical Thickness Changes Using ROI Analysis

Regional CT differences were observed between UC, IBS and HCs. Mean CT values and statistical significance after FDR correction are shown in Table 2 and Table S1. As depicted in Figure 1A, compared to both IBS and HCs, UC subjects showed greater CT in left cingulate cortical subregions (aMCC, pMCC, pgACC and sgACC), and in left post central gyrus (statistically significant differences following FDR correction for multiple comparisons are shown in Figure 1A and marked with asterisks). As shown in Figure 1B, compared to both IBS and HCs, UC subjects had reduced CT in prefrontal regions (left medial and lateral OFG) and in left INS subregions (most significant in pINS). Following FDR correction for multiple comparisons, the results between HCs and UC remained significant even though some differences (OFG and INS) between IBS and UC groups were no longer significant (significant differences are shown in Figure 1B and marked with asterisks). All results remained significant after controlling for depression. However, after controlling for anxiety, the observed differences between HCs and UC subjects in left pMCC, aINS and mINS were no longer significant after FDR

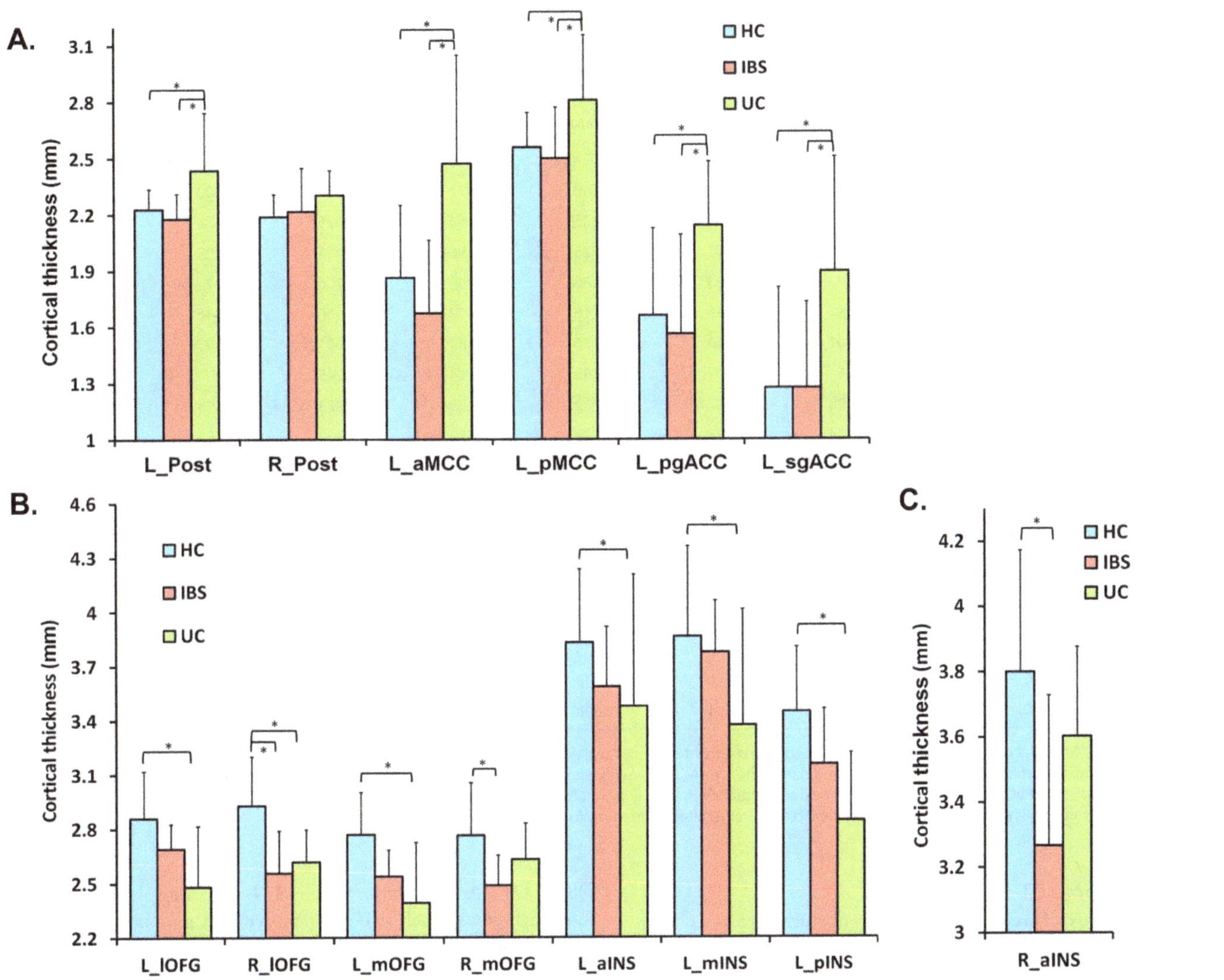

Figure 1. Mean cortical thickness of the ROIs showing significant group differences. (A) UC subjects showed the greatest CT in the regions of somatosensory and cingulate cortex. (B) In the subregions of OFG and INS, UCs had lower CT compared with HCs. (C) IBS subjects had lower CT in right aINS compared to HCs. Error bars reflect standard deviation. Asterisk indicates significant differences between groups ($q<0.05$) after controlling for sex, age, total gray matter volume and FDR correction.

correction (Table 2). As shown in Figure 1C, compared to HCs, IBS subjects showed significantly reduced CT in right aINS after FDR correction, a difference that was not affected by controlling for anxiety and depression.

Correlation of Cortical Thickness with Behavioral and Clinical Variables

In the UC group, symptom duration was *negatively* correlated with CT in left lateral OFG ($r = -.88$, $p = .0002$, $q = .0006$, Figure 2A) and left medial OFG ($r = -.78$, $p = .003$, $q = .003$, Figure 2B) and was *positively* correlated with CT in left postcentral gyrus ($r = .77$, $p = .003$, $q = .003$, Figure 2C). Adding anxiety and depression scores as covariates did not alter the results. No significant correlations with other clinical parameters (including the Mayo UCDAI) were observed.

Discussion

The primary goal of the current study was to assess regional CT differences between subjects with UC, and two comparison groups: a healthy control group and a disease control group without gut inflammation (IBS).The main findings of the study were: 1) Compared to both IBS and HCs, UC subjects showed *greater* CT in left cingulate cortical subregions, and in left primary somatosensory cortex (SI). 2) Compared with HCs, UC subjects showed *lower* CT in left OFG and in primary viscerosensory cortex (pINS). 3) Compared to HCs, IBS subjects showed *lower* CT in the interoceptive association cortex (aINS) in the right hemisphere. 4) There were large significant correlations of CT reductions in left OFG and CT increases in left SI with symptom duration in UC subjects, suggesting a role of chronic inflammation driven afferent input in these changes. The emerging pattern highlights significant differences in CT between patients with chronic gut inflammation, functional GI disorders and HCs, as well as some similarities.

Table 2. Significant cortical thickness differences in the ROIs between HCs, IBS and UC subjects with and without controlling for anxiety and depression scores.

ROI		Difference	F	P value	q value	F(A)	q(A)	F(D)	q(D)
lOFG	L	HC>UC	23.736	<.00001	.00023	15.898	.00411	23.592	.00020
lOFG	R	HC>UC	15.778	.00019	.00160	9.971	.01654	14.000	.00275
		HC>IBS	17.591	.00009	.00086	12.647	.00925	17.184	.00102
mOFG	L	HC>UC	23.124	.00001	.00023	13.904	.00715	26.905	.00009
mOFG	R	HC>IBS	9.052	.00383	.01686	8.744	.02156	9.802	.01304
Post	L	UC>HC	9.895	.00258	.01216	9.397	.01966	17.446	.00102
		UC>IBS	11.701	.00113	.00678	11.859	.01001	15.595	.00155
aINS	L	HC>UC	6.701	.01207	.04193	2.234	.26245	7.698	.02568
aINS	R	HC>IBS	18.098	.00007	.00082	12.384	.00925	16.893	.00102
mINS	L	HC>UC	10.304	.00213	.01173	3.859	.14306	12.453	.00489
pINS	L	HC>UC	30.701	<.00001	.00005	19.658	.00150	29.416	.00008
aMCC	L	UC>HC	18.231	.00007	.00008	11.277	.01137	18.651	.00080
		UC>IBS	19.862	.00004	.00006	19.387	.00150	21.006	.00040
pMCC	L	UC>HC	8.870	.00042	.01724	2.278	.26245	11.277	.00758
		UC>IBS	7.831	.00690	.02677	7.666	.03185	9.082	.01568
pgACC	L	UC>HC	11.713	.00112	.00678	8.839	.02156	8.901	.01607
		UC>IBS	10.127	.00232	.01175	10.014	.01654	9.690	.01304
sgACC	L	UC>HC	11.754	.00110	.00678	8.692	.02156	9.611	.01304
		UC>IBS	7.704	.00734	.02690	7.609	.03185	7.559	.02611

R: right; L: left; lOFG: lateral orbitofrontal gyrus; mOFG: medial orbitofrontal gyrus; Post: postcentral gyrus; aINS: aINSula; mINS: mid insula; pINS: posterior insula; aMCC: anterior mid cingulate cortex; pMCC: posterior mid cingulate cortex; pgACC: pregenual anterior cingulate cortex; sgACC: subgenual anterior cingulate cortex; q value: p value after FDR corrected at 5%, q value <.05 was considered significant; F(A): F score after controlling for anxiety; q(A): corrected p value after controlling for anxiety; F(D): F score after controlling for depression; q(D): corrected p value after controlling for depression.

Greater Regional CT in UC Patients

Somatosensory Cortex. In the current study, greater CT in primary somatosensory cortex (SI) was seen in the UC group. SI is part of the central pain processing network and its thickness is positively correlated with individual experimentally induced acute pain sensitivity in healthy subjects [44,45]. Chronic pain in human patient populations has been shown to be associated with cortical reorganization and changes in SI activity [38,46,47]. For example, SI cortical thickening has been reported in patients with migraine [48] and temporomandibular pain [43]. It has been suggested that the critical factor for S1 to undergo structural reorganization may be the presence of constant sensory input to this brain region [38,43,47]. Additionally, a voxel based morphometry study showed increased left pre- and postcentral gyri in chronic back pain patients [39]. In the current study, CT of left postcentral gyrus in UC groups showed a large positive correlation with symptom duration, consistent with a possible etiologic role of chronically enhanced viscerosensory input to the brain due to sensitization of visceral afferent pathways by chronic mucosal inflammation. However, the degree of somatosensory cortex changes did not correspond to the subjective pain reports, as UC subjects had greater CT in somatosensory cortex, but reported lower abdominal pain and discomfort compared to patients with IBS. Even though the reason(s) for these apparent discrepancies

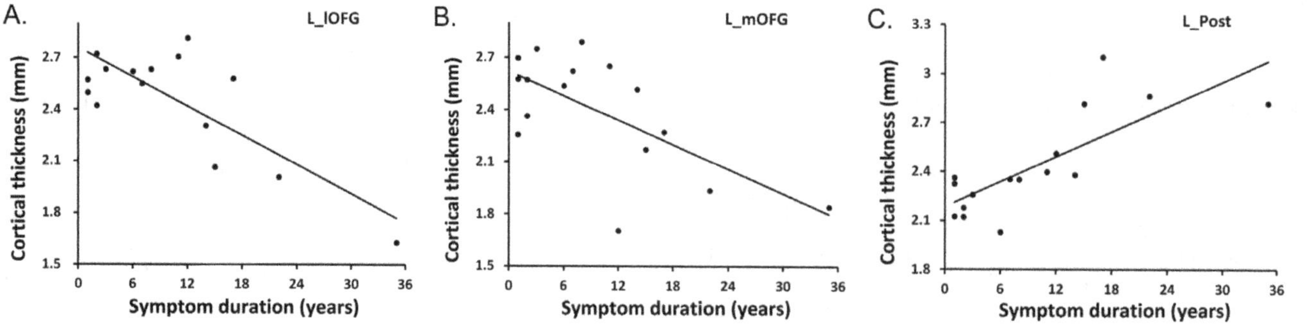

Figure 2. Correlation between cortical thickness and UC symptom duration. (A) Cortical thickness in left lateral orbitofrontal gyrus (L_lOFG) and (B) left medial orbitofrontal gyrus (L_mOFG) were negatively correlated with symptom duration in UC group. (C) Cortical thickness in left postcentral gyrus (L_Post) showed large positive correlation with UC symptom duration.

between CT differences in SI and subjective pain reports are not known, one may speculate that the subjective experience of chronic clinical visceral pain (as opposed to acute experimentally induced pain) is more related to activity and related structural changes in interoceptive association cortex (e.g. the aINS), rather than to primary sensory cortex [4,49].

Midcingulate Cortex. In the current study, compared to HCs and IBS subjects, the UC subjects had greater CT in subregions of the cingulate cortex, e.g. aMCC and pMCC. MCC is involved in emotion processing, skeletomotor regulation, chronic somatic and visceral pain, and along with the aINS (as part of the "salience network") integrating information to form conceptual pain [50–54]. Several studies have reported abnormal MCC activation by acute noxious visceral stimulation in IBS subjects [55–58]. Supporting a possible effect of repeated nociceptive stimuli on MCC structure, repeated application of thermal pain stimuli to healthy subjects over a period of 8 days resulted in gray matter increases in both MCC and SI [59]. Together with the observed greater CT in SI, the findings in UC patients are most consistent with the presence of a constant sensory input from the gut, due to sensitization of visceral afferent pathways by chronic mucosal inflammation. This interpretation is also consistent with the fact that in the current study, the IBS group (e.g. without chronically recurring mucosal inflammation) did not show significant CT change compared to HCs. Further support for differential brain mechanisms underlying chronic visceral pain comes from a recent PET ligand study which showed differences in neurokinin-1 receptor (NK-1R) binding potential (e.g. receptor availability) between patients with IBD (including Crohn's disease and UC) and IBS subjects [60]. Compared to HCs, IBD patients had low NK-1R availability in ACC and MCC, while IBS showed this deficit to a lesser extent. Animal studies have shown that the substance P/NK-1R signaling system is involved in cytogenesis, has neurotrophic and neuroprotective functions and inhibits apoptosis [61–63]. This implies a differential involvement of such neuroplastic mechanisms in the two visceral pain syndromes. Our findings differ from those reported in two other chronic inflammatory conditions, e.g. Crohn's disease [14] and osteoarthritis [64]. In both of these studies lower gray matter in the MCC was observed compared to HCs. Differences in patient populations and analysis methodology make it difficult to directly compare these studies with the current report [14,64].

Reduced Regional CT in IBS and UC Patients

INS Subregions. When compared to HCs, both disease groups showed lower CT in the INS, albeit in different subregions. Several studies in patients with chronic pain including IBS [7,9,12,13,64–68] compared to HCs, have found lower gray matter volumes and CT in the INS, even though subregions were often not specified. In the current study, UC compared to HCs had significantly reduced CT in the left pINS (observed differences in mINS were no longer seen after controlling for anxiety). It is likely that chronically enhanced afferent input from the gut due to recurrent mucosal inflammation is primarily associated with CT changes in the pINS, which represents the primary interoceptive cortex [37,69]. Even though there was no significant correlation between symptom duration or other behavioral measures with CT changes in the pINS, a chronic low back pain study showed that recovery of CT in pINS (and secondary somatosensory cortex) was correlated with reduction of pain intensity after treatment [12], implicating chronic nociceptive and inflammation related signaling as a factor in these CT changes.

In contrast to the UC group, IBS subjects had lower CT in a different subregion of the INS, e.g. the right aINS compared to HCs. The aINS functions as interoceptive association cortex integrates interoceptive input with emotional, salient and cognitive inputs, and provides output to autonomic and pain modulation systems [37,53,69–71]. The aINS also plays a central role in prediction, error processing, and self awareness of sensations [37,71]. Even though both patient groups had greater affective scores compared to HCs, IBS subjects reported more abdominal pain and discomfort compared to the UC group. However, there was no significant correlation of the observed changes with affective measures, symptom scores or duration of symptoms in IBS subjects.

Orbitofrontal Gyrus. UC subjects compared to HCs showed lower CT in the bilateral OFG, a brain region which plays an important role in interoception, emotion evaluation and regulation, and in cognitive reappraisal [43,72,73]. Decreased gray matter in OFG has also been found in other chronic pain disorders with inflammatory/nociceptive drive including hip osteoarthritis [64], low back pain [39] and migraine [74]. A negative correlation between left OFG thickness and symptom duration was observed in UC subjects, suggesting a role of chronic nociceptive input in the observed CT reductions. In contrast, no such correlation between IBS symptom duration and OFG structure were observed.

Limitations

Limitations of the study include the small sample size of the IBS and UC population, the group differences in level of anxiety and depression symptoms, and the heterogeneity of the groups in terms of sex. However, controlling for anxiety and depression, most of the observed results remained significant. In addition, our GLM and linear contrast were weighted to eliminate any bias caused by umbalanced representation of sexes. Furthermore, the fact that large correlations of some structural changes with disease duration were observed in the UC subjects, and the fact that some of the findings were similar to reports in subjects with other chronic inflammatory conditions [13,64], makes it unlikely that the findings are confounded by these limitations. Future, longitudinal studies in larger patient populations, including the correlation of plasma and mucosal inflammatory disease markers with structural brain changes both during disease flares and remissions are needed in order to better understand the role of colonic inflammation in remodeling of the brain. In such larger studies, presence of comorbidities in the IBS group, as well as differences in the impact of the IBS and UC on daily life activities and social interactions should be taken into account.

Conclusions

To our knowledge, this study represents the first comparison of brain structure between UC patients and both HCs and IBS subjects. The findings demonstrate significant differences in CT between UC and HC subjects, and differences between the two disease groups. Based on the correlation of structural changes with symptom duration in IBD, one may speculate that the observed gray matter reorganization of IBD subjects represents a consequence of chronic viscerosensory input to the brain due to sensitization of visceral afferent pathways by recurrent gut inflammation. The mechanisms by which such increased viscerosensory to the brain input can produce both increases and decreases of grey matter in different brain regions remains to be determined.

Acknowledgments

The authors would like to thank Ahmanson Lovelace Brain Mapping Center for expert technical assistance.

Author Contributions

Conceived and designed the experiments: JL EM. Performed the experiments: JYH ZJ CAM JS NH SS. Analyzed the data: JYH ZJ ID. Contributed reagents/materials/analysis tools: ZJ CAM ID YS KT. Wrote the paper: JYH JL AG EM.

References

1. Bielefeldt K, Davis B, Binion DG (2009) Pain and inflammatory bowel disease. Inflamm Bowel Dis 15: 778–788.
2. Berman SM, Naliboff BD, Suyenobu B, Labus JS, Stains J, et al. (2008) Reduced brainstem inhibition during anticipated pelvic visceral pain correlates with enhanced brain response to the visceral stimulus in women with irritable bowel syndrome. J Neurosci 28: 349–359.
3. Chang L, Munakata J, Mayer EA, Schmulson MJ, Johnson TD, et al. (2000) Perceptual responses in patients with inflammatory and functional bowel disease. Gut 47: 497–505.
4. Mayer EA, Berman S, Suyenobu B, Labus J, Mandelkern MA, et al. (2005) Differences in brain responses to visceral pain between patients with irritable bowel syndrome and ulcerative colitis. Pain 115: 398–409.
5. Schmidt-Wilcke T, Luerding R, Weigand T, Jurgens T, Schuierer G, et al. (2007) Striatal grey matter increase in patients suffering from fibromyalgia – a voxel-based morphometry study. Pain 132 Suppl 1: S109–116.
6. Seminowicz DA, Labus JS, Bueller JA, Tillisch K, Naliboff BD, et al. (2010) Regional gray matter density changes in brains of patients with irritable bowel syndrome. Gastroenterology 139: 48–57 e42.
7. Davis KD, Pope G, Chen J, Kwan CL, Crawley AP, et al. (2008) Cortical thinning in IBS: implications for homeostatic, attention, and pain processing. Neurology 70: 153–154.
8. Hsu MC, Harris RE, Sundgren PC, Welsh RC, Fernandes CR, et al. (2009) No consistent difference in gray matter volume between individuals with fibromyalgia and age-matched healthy subjects when controlling for affective disorder. Pain 143: 262–267.
9. Labus J, Dinov ID, Jiang Z, Ashe-McNalley C, Zamanyan A, et al. (2013) Irritable bowel syndrome in female patients is associated with alterations in structural brain networks. Pain.
10. Apkarian AV, Sosa Y, Sonty S, Levy RM, Harden RN, et al. (2004) Chronic back pain is associated with decreased prefrontal and thalamic gray matter density. J Neurosci 24: 10410–10415.
11. Schmidt-Wilcke T, Leinisch E, Ganssbauer S, Draganski B, Bogdahn U, et al. (2006) Affective components and intensity of pain correlate with structural differences in gray matter in chronic back pain patients. Pain 125: 89–97.
12. Seminowicz DA, Wideman TH, Naso L, Hatami-Khoroushahi Z, Fallatah S, et al. (2011) Effective treatment of chronic low back pain in humans reverses abnormal brain anatomy and function. J Neurosci 31: 7540–7550.
13. Frokjaer JB, Bouwense SA, Olesen SS, Lundager FH, Eskildsen SF, et al. (2012) Reduced cortical thickness of brain areas involved in pain processing in patients with chronic pancreatitis. Clin Gastroenterol Hepatol 10: 434–438 e431.
14. Agostini A, Benuzzi F, Filippini N, Bertani A, Scarcelli A, et al. (2013) New insights into the brain involvement in patients with Crohn's disease: a voxel-based morphometry study. Neurogastroenterol Motil.
15. Farmer MA, Chanda ML, Parks EL, Baliki MN, Apkarian AV, et al. (2011) Brain functional and anatomical changes in chronic prostatitis/chronic pelvic pain syndrome. J Urol 186: 117–124.
16. Wartolowska K, Hough MG, Jenkinson M, Andersson J, Wordsworth BP, et al. (2012) Structural changes of the brain in rheumatoid arthritis. Arthritis Rheum 64: 371–379.
17. Jones AK, Huneke NT, Lloyd DM, Brown CA, Watson A (2012) Role of functional brain imaging in understanding rheumatic pain. Curr Rheumatol Rep 14: 557–567.
18. Gwilym SE, Filippini N, Douaud G, Carr AJ, Tracey I (2010) Thalamic atrophy associated with painful osteoarthritis of the hip is reversible after arthroplasty: a longitudinal voxel-based morphometric study. Arthritis Rheum 62: 2930–2940.
19. Dinov ID, Torri F, Macciardi F, Petrosyan P, Liu Z, et al. (2011) Applications of the pipeline environment for visual informatics and genomics computations. BMC Bioinformatics 12: 304.
20. Dinov I, Lozev K, Petrosyan P, Liu Z, Eggert P, et al. (2010) Neuroimaging study designs, computational analyses and data provenance using the LONI pipeline. PLoS One 5.
21. Drossman DA (2000) Rome II: the functional gastrointestinal disorders: diagnosis, pathophysiology, and treatment: a multinational consensus. McLeanVA: Degnon Associates. xxvii, 764 p.
22. Drossman DA (2006) The functional gastrointestinal disorders and the Rome III process. Gastroenterology 130: 1377–1390.
23. Lewis JD, Chuai S, Nessel L, Lichtenstein GR, Aberra FN, et al. (2008) Use of the noninvasive components of the Mayo score to assess clinical response in ulcerative colitis. Inflamm Bowel Dis 14: 1660–1666.
24. Chang L, Lee OY, Naliboff B, Schmulson M, Mayer EA (2001) Sensation of bloating and visible abdominal distension in patients with irritable bowel syndrome. Am J Gastroenterol 96: 3341–3347.
25. Mykletun A, Stordal E, Dahl AA (2001) Hospital Anxiety and Depression (HAD) scale: factor structure, item analyses and internal consistency in a large population. Br J Psychiatry 179: 540–544.
26. Labus JS, Bolus R, Chang L, Wiklund I, Naesdal J, et al. (2004) The Visceral Sensitivity Index: development and validation of a gastrointestinal symptom-specific anxiety scale. Aliment Pharmacol Ther 20: 89–97.
27. Labus JS, Mayer EA, Chang L, Bolus R, Naliboff BD (2007) The central role of gastrointestinal-specific anxiety in irritable bowel syndrome: further validation of the visceral sensitivity index. Psychosom Med 69: 89–98.
28. Leung KTK (2011) Principal Ranking Meta-Algorithms: UNIVERSITY OF CALIFORNIA, LOS ANGELES.
29. Fischl B, Dale AM (2000) Measuring the thickness of the human cerebral cortex from magnetic resonance images. Proc Natl Acad Sci U S A 97: 11050–11055.
30. Mulder W, Osher S, Sethian JA (1992) Computing interface motion in compressible gas dynamics. Journal of Computational Physics 100: 209–228.
31. Osher S, Sethian JA (1988) Fronts propagating with curvature-dependent speed: algorithms based on Hamilton-Jacobi formulations. Journal of Computational Physics 79: 12–49.
32. Mazziotta J, Toga A, Evans A, Fox P, Lancaster J, et al. (2001) A probabilistic atlas and reference system for the human brain: International Consortium for Brain Mapping (ICBM). Philos Trans R Soc Lond B Biol Sci 356: 1293–1322.
33. Shi Y, Lai R, Gill R, Pelletier D, Mohr D, et al. (2011) Conformal metric optimization on surface (CMOS) for deformation and mapping in Laplace-Beltrami embedding space. Medical image computing and computer-assisted intervention: MICCAI International Conference on Medical Image Computing and Computer-Assisted Intervention 14: 327–334.
34. Tillisch K, Mayer EA, Labus JS (2011) Quantitative meta-analysis identifies brain regions activated during rectal distension in irritable bowel syndrome. Gastroenterology 140: 91–100.
35. Mayer EA, Bushnell MC, International Association for the Study of Pain. (2009) Functional pain syndromes: presentation and pathophysiology. Seattle: IASP Press. xviii, 580 p.
36. Agostini A, Benuzzi F, Filippini N, Bertani A, Scarcelli A, et al. (2012) New insights into the brain involvement in patients with Crohn's disease: a voxel-based morphometry study. Neurogastroenterol Motil.
37. Craig AD (2009) How do you feel – now? The anterior insula and human awareness. Nat Rev Neurosci 10: 59–70.
38. May A (2008) Chronic pain may change the structure of the brain. Pain 137: 7–15.
39. Ung H, Brown JE, Johnson KA, Younger J, Hush J, et al. (2012) Multivariate Classification of Structural MRI Data Detects Chronic Low Back Pain. Cereb Cortex.
40. Benjamini Y, Krieger AM, Yekutieli D (2006) Adaptive linear step-up procedures that control the false discovery rate. Biometrika 93: 491–507.
41. Benjamini Y, Hochberg Y (2000) On the Adaptive Control of the False Discovery Rate in Multiple Testing with Independent Statistics. Journal of Educational and Behavioral Statistics 25: 60–83.
42. Pike N (2011) Using false discovery rates for multiple comparisons in ecology and evolution. Methods in Ecology and Evolution 2: 278–282.
43. Moayedi M, Weissman-Fogel I, Crawley AP, Goldberg MB, Freeman BV, et al. (2011) Contribution of chronic pain and neuroticism to abnormal forebrain gray matter in patients with temporomandibular disorder. Neuroimage 55: 277–286.
44. Apkarian AV, Bushnell MC, Treede RD, Zubieta JK (2005) Human brain mechanisms of pain perception and regulation in health and disease. Eur J Pain 9: 463–484.
45. Erpelding N, Moayedi M, Davis KD (2012) Cortical thickness correlates of pain and temperature sensitivity. Pain 153: 1602–1609.
46. Moseley GL, Flor H (2012) Targeting cortical representations in the treatment of chronic pain: a review. Neurorehabil Neural Repair 26: 646–652.
47. Gustin SM, Peck CC, Cheney LB, Macey PM, Murray GM, et al. (2012) Pain and plasticity: is chronic pain always associated with somatosensory cortex activity and reorganization? J Neurosci 32: 14874–14884.
48. DaSilva AF, Granziera C, Snyder J, Hadjikhani N (2007) Thickening in the somatosensory cortex of patients with migraine. Neurology 69: 1990–1995.
49. Blankstein U, Chen J, Diamant NE, Davis KD (2010) Altered brain structure in irritable bowel syndrome: potential contributions of pre-existing and disease-driven factors. Gastroenterology 138: 1783–1789.
50. Taylor KS, Seminowicz DA, Davis KD (2009) Two systems of resting state connectivity between the insula and cingulate cortex. Hum Brain Mapp 30: 2731–2745.
51. Vogt BA, Berger GR, Derbyshire SW (2003) Structural and functional dichotomy of human midcingulate cortex. Eur J Neurosci 18: 3134–3144.

52. Vogt BA (2005) Pain and emotion interactions in subregions of the cingulate gyrus. Nat Rev Neurosci 6: 533–544.
53. Wiech K, Lin CS, Brodersen KH, Bingel U, Ploner M, et al. (2010) AINSula integrates information about salience into perceptual decisions about pain. J Neurosci 30: 16324–16331.
54. Meier ML, Brugger M, Ettlin DA, Luechinger R, Barlow A, et al. (2012) Brain activation induced by dentine hypersensitivity pain – an fMRI study. J Clin Periodontol 39: 441–447.
55. Labus JS, Naliboff BD, Berman SM, Suyenobu B, Vianna EP, et al. (2009) Brain networks underlying perceptual habituation to repeated aversive visceral stimuli in patients with irritable bowel syndrome. Neuroimage 47: 952–960.
56. Bernstein CN, Frankenstein UN, Rawsthorne P, Pitz M, Summers R, et al. (2002) Cortical mapping of visceral pain in patients with GI disorders using functional magnetic resonance imaging. Am J Gastroenterol 97: 319–327.
57. Verne GN, Himes NC, Robinson ME, Gopinath KS, Briggs RW, et al. (2003) Central representation of visceral and cutaneous hypersensitivity in the irritable bowel syndrome. Pain 103: 99–110.
58. Kwan CL, Diamant NE, Pope G, Mikula K, Mikulis DJ, et al. (2005) Abnormal forebrain activity in functional bowel disorder patients with chronic pain. Neurology 65: 1268–1277.
59. Teutsch S, Herken W, Bingel U, Schoell E, May A (2008) Changes in brain gray matter due to repetitive painful stimulation. Neuroimage 42: 845–849.
60. Jarcho JM, Feier NA, Bert A, Labus JA, Lee M, et al. (2013) Diminished neurokinin-1 receptor availability in patients with two forms of chronic visceral pain. Pain.
61. Lallemend F, Lefebvre PP, Hans G, Rigo JM, Van de Water TR, et al. (2003) Substance P protects spiral ganglion neurons from apoptosis via PKC-Ca2+-MAPK/ERK pathways. J Neurochem 87: 508–521.
62. Tulloch I, Ghazaryan N, Mexhitaj I, Ordonez D, Angulo JA (2011) Role of neurokinin-1 and dopamine receptors on the striatal methamphetamine-induced proliferation of new cells in mice. Brain Res 1399: 33–39.
63. Wang J, Angulo JA (2011) Synergism between methamphetamine and the neuropeptide substance P on the production of nitric oxide in the striatum of mice. Brain Res 1369: 131–139.
64. Rodriguez-Raecke R, Niemeier A, Ihle K, Ruether W, May A (2009) Brain gray matter decrease in chronic pain is the consequence and not the cause of pain. J Neurosci 29: 13746–13750.
65. Valfre W, Rainero I, Bergui M, Pinessi L (2008) Voxel-based morphometry reveals gray matter abnormalities in migraine. Headache 48: 109–117.
66. Kuchinad A, Schweinhardt P, Seminowicz DA, Wood PB, Chizh BA, et al. (2007) Accelerated brain gray matter loss in fibromyalgia patients: premature aging of the brain? J Neurosci 27: 4004–4007.
67. Schmidt-Wilcke T, Leinisch E, Straube A, Kampfe N, Draganski B, et al. (2005) Gray matter decrease in patients with chronic tension type headache. Neurology 65: 1483–1486.
68. Jiang Z, Dinov ID, Labus J, Shi Y, Zamanyan A, et al. (2013) Sex-related differences of cortical thickness in patients with chronic abdominal pain. PLoS One 8: e73932.
69. Farb NA, Segal ZV, Anderson AK (2012) Attentional modulation of primary interoceptive and exteroceptive cortices. Cereb Cortex 23: 114–126.
70. Lewis M, Haviland-Jones JM, Barrett LF (2008) Handbook of emotions. New York: Guilford Press. xvi, 848 p., [844] p. of plates p.
71. Paulus MP, Stein MB (2006) An insular view of anxiety. Biol Psychiatry 60: 383–387.
72. Rolls ET, Grabenhorst F, Parris BA (2008) Warm pleasant feelings in the brain. Neuroimage 41: 1504–1513.
73. Ray RD, Ochsner KN, Cooper JC, Robertson ER, Gabrieli JD, et al. (2005) Individual differences in trait rumination and the neural systems supporting cognitive reappraisal. Cogn Affect Behav Neurosci 5: 156–168.
74. Kim JH, Suh SI, Seol HY, Oh K, Seo WK, et al. (2008) Regional grey matter changes in patients with migraine: a voxel-based morphometry study. Cephalalgia 28: 598–604.

8

Small Intestine Inflammation in Roquin-Mutant and Roquin-Deficient Mice

Jeremy S. Schaefer, Dina Montufar-Solis, Niyati Nakra, Nadarajah Vigneswaran, John R. Klein*

Department of Diagnostic and Biomedical Sciences, University of Texas Health Science Center School of Dentistry, Houston, Texas, United States of America

Abstract

Roquin, an E3 ubiquitin ligase that localizes to cytosolic RNA granules, is involved in regulating mRNA stability and translation. Mice that have a M199R mutation in the Roquin protein (referred to as sanroque or *Roquin*$^{san/san}$ mice) develop autoimmune pathologies, although the extent to which these occur in the intestinal mucosa has not been determined. Here, we demonstrate that *Roquin*$^{san/san}$ mice reproducibly develop intestinal inflammation in the small intestine but not the colon. Similarly, mice generated in our laboratory in which the *Roquin* gene was disrupted by insertion of a gene trap cassette (*Roquin*$^{gt/gt}$ mice) had small intestinal inflammation that mimicked that of *Roquin*$^{san/san}$ mice. MLN cells in *Roquin*$^{san/san}$ mice consisted of activated proliferating T cells, and had increased numbers of CD44^{hi} CD62L^{lo} KLRG1^{+} short-lived effector cells. Proportionally more small intestinal intraepithelial lymphocytes in *Roquin*$^{san/san}$ mice expressed the ICOS T cell activation marker. Of particular interest, small intestinal lamina propria lymphocytes in *Roquin*$^{san/san}$ mice consisted of a high proportion of Gr-1^{+} T cells that included IL-17A^{+} cells and CD8^{+} IFN-γ^{+} cells. Extensive cytokine dysregulation resulting in both over-expression and under-expression of chemotactic cytokines occurred in the ileum of *Roquin*$^{san/san}$ mice, the region most prone to the development of inflammation. These findings demonstrate that chronic inflammation ensues in the intestine following Roquin alteration either as a consequence of protein mutation or gene disruption, and they have implications for understanding how small intestinal inflammation is perpetuated in Crohn's disease (CD). Due to the paucity of animal models of CD-like pathophysiology in the small intestine, and because the primary gene/protein defects of the Roquin animal systems used here are well-defined, it will be possible to further elucidate the underlying genetic and molecular mechanisms that drive the disease process.

Editor: Stefan Bereswill, Charité-University Medicine Berlin, Germany

Funding: Funding came from the United States National Institutes of Health (http://www.nih.gov/) (5R01DK035566). The funders had no role in study design, data collection and analysis, decision to publish, or preparation of the manuscript.

Competing Interests: The authors have declared that no competing interests exist.

* E-mail: john.r.klein@uth.tmc.edu

Introduction

Roquin, a RING finger E3 ubiquitin ligase that is characterized by a CCCH zinc finger found in RNA-binding proteins, localizes to cytosolic RNA granules that are involved in regulating mRNA stability and translation. As a member of the ubiquitin-mediated protein degradation pathway, E3 ligases determine the specificity of degradation by associating with a substrate [1]. E3 ligases are further defined by their catalytic domains: Homologous to E6-AP Carboxyl Terminus (HECT) domain proteins have intrinsic ligase activities, whereas Really Interesting New Gene (RING) domain proteins function as scaffolds in the degradation process [2]. Initial characterization of Roquin-defective mice (*Roquin*$^{san/san}$), which have an M199R mutation in the Roquin protein, revealed chronic inflammation consisting of lymphadenopathy, splenomegaly, thrombocytopenia, necrotizing hepatitis, and increased numbers of CD4^{+} follicular T cells and ICOS expression [3,4]. A recent study from our laboratory demonstrated that Roquin curtails IL-17 synthesis, and that the miR-223 microRNA is involved in regulating Roquin expression [5].

The extent to which Roquin is involved in driving autoimmunity has been brought into question, however, by a recent study using complete and conditional *Roquin* knockout mice [6]. Complete *Roquin* knockout resulted in a deformity of the caudal spine, and was generally lethal for most mice within 6 hours of birth, possibly due to a defect in lung development. Conditional knockouts in which the *Roquin* defect was targeted to T cells failed to exhibit a breach in self-tolerance or have changes in follicular T cell differentiation, although increased ICOS expression was noted [6]. Similar findings were observed for mice in which *Roquin* disruption was targeted to the entire hematopoietic system [6]. The reason for the discrepancy between findings from *Roquin*$^{san/san}$ and *Roquin*-deficient mice remains unclear; however, it is possible that a mutated form of the Roquin protein rather than total ablation of it is a contributing factor in promoting autoimmunity.

Based on the above observations, we were interested in determining the extent to which *Roquin*$^{san/san}$ mice, or mice in which the *Roquin* gene has been disrupted, develop intestinal inflammation. For the latter, we generated mice in which a gene trap was inserted into the *Roquin* gene (*Roquin*$^{gt/gt}$ mice). Here, we report that inflammation throughout the small intestine, but not in the colon, is a common feature of both *Roquin*$^{san/san}$ and *Roquin*$^{gt/gt}$ mice. Additionally, the ileum of *Roquin*$^{san/san}$ mice, the portion of the small intestine most prone to development of inflammation, had extensive cytokine dysregulation, activated T cells in mesenteric lymph nodes (MLN), small intestinal intraepithelial lymphocytes (siIELs) and small intestinal lamina propria lymphocytes (siLPLs), and pro-inflammatory cytokine production by siLPLs. These findings demonstrate alteration in the Roquin protein, either as a consequence of mutation or gene disruption, is a causal factor tied to the development of chronic inflammation in the small intestine.

Materials and Methods

Ethics Statement

All experiments were performed in accordance with the National Institutes of Health Guide for the Care and Use of Laboratory Animals using a protocol approved by the University of Texas Health Science Center Institutional Animal Welfare Committee (Permit Number: HSC-AWC-12-039).

Mice

Mating pairs of *Roquin*$^{san/+}$ mice were obtained from the Mutant Mouse Regional Resource Center (MMRRC) (University of California, Davis, CA) to establish a colony in the animal facility at The University of Texas Health Science Center at Houston. Heterozygous *Roquin*$^{san/+}$ mice were intercrossed to produce homozygous *Roquin*$^{san/san}$ mice. A mutagenically-separated PCR (MS-PCR) protocol [3] was used to determine zygosity. A PCR product of approximately 190 bp indicated the wild type allele while a product of approximately 215 bp denoted the presence of the *Roquin*^{san} mutation. Heterozygous mice displayed both products. Primers were: San forward, 5′-CAT-CAGGCTGGCCTCTAGTT-3′; San reverse M199, 5′- AA-GACCAGCTTCAGAGCTTCCTCCAGCA-3′; San revers-eR199, 5′-GAACCATCTTCTAAGGCCAGCGTGACCAG CTTCAGAGCTTCCTCCTACC-3′.

To generate *Roquin* gene trap mice, the SIGTR CC0753 ES cell line targeting the *Roquin* gene was purchased from the Mutant Mouse Regional Resource Center (MMRRC) (University of California, Davis, CA). Initial characterization of the ES cell line via Blasting of the sequence tag localized the gene trap within intron 1 of *Rc3h1*. In order to determine the precise location of the gene trap, we designed sequential PCR primers to amplify 2–4 kb regions between exon 1 and exon 2 in *Rc3h1*. PCR amplification using these *Rc3h1* specific primers coupled to the reverse β-geo specific primer revealed the location of the gene trap insertion to be between P5099 and P6546 of intron 1. The PCR product resulting from the amplification using the Rc3h1 P5099 and β-geo reverse primers was TOPO cloned and sequenced. Sequencing analysis identified the gene trap insertion point as following base pair 5809 within intron 1 of *Rc3h1* (Fig. S1).

The ES cell clones were expanded and microinjected into blastocysts to generate the gene trap chimeras at the Laboratory for Developmental Biology at The Brown Foundation Institute of Molecular Medicine (The University of Texas Health Science Center at Houston, Houston, TX). Chimeric mice were screened for the presence of the β-geo gene trap cassette using gene trap-specific primers. Gene trap-positive chimeras were backcrossed to the C57BL/6 background for more than eight generations. *Roquin*$^{gt/+}$ heterozygous mice were intercrossed to obtain homozygous *Roquin*$^{gt/gt}$ mice. PCR analysis using Roquin-specific primers that span the gene trap insertion point was performed to establish zygosity. The gene trap and Roquin-specific primers were: β-geo forward, 5′-CCCAACAGTTGCGCAGCCTGAAT-3′; β-geo reverse, 5′- CGCTGCACCATTCGCGTTAC-3′; Roquin P5634 forward, 5′-AGGCCAGCCTGGTGAAATAG-3′; Roquin P6120 reverse, 5′-AGGCCAGCCCAGTCTACAG-3′. *Roquin*$^{gt/gt}$ mice had a poor post-birth survival rate and most had a congenital caudal spine defect. Out of 29 litters obtained from heterozygous crosses, the ratio was 1.57 [wild type]: 4.3: [heterozygous]: 0.12 [homozygous gene trap] compared to the predicted simple Mendelian ratio of 1:2:1.

To measure Roquin and ICOS transcript levels, a Power SYBR Green PCR Master Mix kit (Applied Biosystems) was used according to the manufacturer's instructions. Total RNA was isolated using an miRNeasy Minikit (Qiagen, Valencia, CA) according to the manufacturer's instructions. cDNA was synthesized using a High-Capacity cDNA Reverse Transcription Kit (Applied Biosystems, Austin, TX). Samples were analyzed using the StepOnePlus real-time thermal cycler and software (Applied Biosystems). Relative gene expression was normalized to GAPDH. Roquin, IL-17A, and GAPDH gene-specific primers were designed and purchased from Integrated DNA Technologies (Coralville, IA). Primers were: Roquin forward, 5′-GGCTGCTCGATCTTTAGGTG-3′; Roquin reverse, 5′-TGTTCTCTCCTCAGAGCTTCG-3′; ICOS forward, 5′-TGACCCACCTCCTTTTCAAG-3′; ICOS reverse, 5′-TTAGGGTCATGCACACTGGA-3′; GAPDH forward, 5′-AGAACATCATCCCTGCATCC-3′; GAPDH reverse, 5′-AGCCGTATTCATTGTCATACC-3′.

Roquin western blotting was done using spleen tissues or cultured cells that had been lysed and homogenized in RIPA buffer (50 mM Tris-cl pH 7.4, 150 mM NaCl, 1% NP40, 1% SDS, 0.5% Na-deoxycholate, 1 mM PMSF, 50 mM NaF, aprotinin, leupeptin, pepstatin: 1 μg/ml each). 40 μg of cell lysates were electrophoresed through an 8% SDS polyacrylamide gel followed by overnight protein transfer to PVDF membranes. Membranes were blocked using 5% milk in TBS containing 0.1% Tween-20 (TBS-$T_{0.1}$). Membranes were probed with a Roquin antibody (Bethyl Laboratories, Montgomery, TX; A300-514A, [1:560]) overnight at 4°C with rocking, washed x3 with TBS-$T_{0.1}$, and incubated with an HRP-conjugated goat anti-rabbit antibody (Vector Laboratories, Burlingame, CA; [1:1500]). Enhanced chemiluminescent (SuperSignal West Pico Chemiluminescent Substrate [Thermo Fisher Scientific, Rockford, IL]) was used to detect the protein bands.

Adult female C57BL/6 mice, 8–10 weeks of age, were purchased from Harlan (Indianapolis, IN) and used for MLN, siIEL, and siLPL cell isolations, and for breeding with *Roquin*$^{gt/+}$ mice.

Histopathological and morphometric analysis

Mice were euthanized, intestinal tissues from the duodenum, jejunum, ileum, and cecum, and the ascending, transverse, and descending, colon, and the liver were harvested, fixed in 10% buffered formalin, processed for paraffin embedding, and 3 μM tissue sections were made and stained with hematoxylin and eosin (H&E). The degree of inflammation and related histologic changes were graded microscopically on cross-sections of intestinal tissues using a validated scoring system as described in our previously published paper [7]. Scoring for intestinal tissues consisted of score 0: no signs of inflammation; score 1: very low level of leukocytic infiltration in the lamina propria; score 2: low level of leukocytic infiltration in the lamina propria; score 3: moderate level of leukocytic infiltrate in the lamina propria with occasional crypt abscess; score 4: high levels of leukocytic in the lamina propria, crypt abscess, high vascular density, loss of goblet cells, and thickening of the intestinal wall; and score 5: transmural leukocytic infiltration, loss of goblet cells, high vascular density, and thickening of the intestinal wall. Scoring for the liver was done as described by others [8]. An experienced, board-certified pathologist performed histopathologic grading in a blinded manner.

Body weight of female *Roquin*$^{san/san}$ and C57BL/6 mice were recorded between 14 and 55 weeks of age. After euthanasia, spleen-to-body weight ratios were calculated from the body and spleen weights.

Leukocyte isolations and flow cytometric analyses

T cells were isolated from MLNs using a Mouse T-Cell Enrichment Kit (R&D, Minneapolis, MN) according to the manufacturer's protocol. siIELs were isolated using a protocol previously reported by our laboratory [9]. For isolation of siLPLs, the epithelial layer was first digested in DTT/EDTA [9], removed, and the remaining intestinal fragments were incubated in 50 ml of RPMI supplemented with 10% FBS, 0.36 mM $CaCl_2$, 100U/ml of Collagenase IV (Sigma, St. Louis, MO) for 1 h at 37°C with stirring. Cells were filtered through nylon wool, collected, and centrifuged at 400 g through a 40%/70% Percoll gradient. Viable cells were collected from the interface.

MLN cells, siIELs, and siLPLs were stained for identification of surface or intracellular markers as previously described [7] using combinations of the following antibodies: PE-anti-CD134 (OX40) (OX-86); PE-anti-CD278 (ICOS) (7E.17G9); PE-anti-FoxP3 (FJK-16 s); APC-anti-CD3ε (145-2C11); FITC-anti-CD44 (IM7); APC-anti-CD25 (PC61.5); AlexaFluor647-anti-Ki67 (SolA15); APC-anti-KLRG1 (2F1); APC- and PE-anti-IL-17A (17B7); FITC-anti-IFNγ (XMG1.2); PE-anti-CD8a (53–6.7); FITC rat IgG isotype control (eBRG1); biotin rat IgG isotype control; PE rat IgG2a isotype control (eBR2a); streptavidin APC (eBioscience, San Diego, CA, all reagents); FITC anti-mouse CD45R/B220 (RA3-6B2); PE-anti-CD3ε (145-2C11); FITC-anti-BrdU (3D4); PE-anti-CD62L (MEL-17) (Pharmingen, San Diego, CA, all reagents); biotin-anti Ly6C (HK1.4) (Southern biotechnology, Birmingham, AL). BrdU was administered by an i.p. injection of 1 mg BrdU at 72 and 48 hours prior to cell isolation.

Analyte arrays

Tissues from the ileum of normal and *Roquin*$^{san/san}$ mice were collected. Half was stored in RNAlater (Qiagen, Valencia, CA), half was used for histopathological analyses. RNA was isolated from tissues of three normal mice and three mice with pathology scores of 1.0. A RT^2 Profiler PCR Array Mouse Inflammatory Cytokines & Receptors kit (Qiagen) was used to measure the expression of 89 analytes consisting of genes for 28 chemokines, 13 chemokine receptors, 25 cytokines, 14 cytokine receptors, and 9 additional inflammation-related genes according to the manufacturer's protocols.

Statistical analysis

Determination of statistical significance was done using an unpaired two-sided Student's t-test.

Results

Roquin$^{san/san}$ and *Roquin*$^{gt/gt}$ mice develop inflammation in the small intestine and liver

We confirmed *Roquin*$^{san/san}$ mice to be homozygous mutant animals by MS-PCR [3]. As shown in Fig. 1A, normal mice had a single 190 bp PCR product. Homozygous *Roquin*$^{san/san}$ mutant mice had a single 215 bp PCR product. Heterozygous *Roquin*$^{san/+}$ mice had both PCR products. The average body weight of *Roquin*$^{san/san}$ mice from 14 to 55 weeks of age was significantly less than that of gender-matched normal animals (Fig. 1B), although with age the weight of *Roquin*$^{san/san}$ mice more closely approximated that of normal animals (Fig. 1C). Pathology scores did not show a significant positive or negative correlation with age (not shown). *Roquin*$^{san/san}$ mice had pronounced splenomegaly (Fig. 1D) that was characterized by florid follicular lymphoid hyperplasia (not shown). Histopathological analysis of intestinal tissues from *Roquin*$^{san/san}$ mice revealed inflammation throughout the small intestine and cecum with varying degrees of chronic inflammation spread along the entire length of the small intestine that was characterized by elongated crypts with flattened villi and increased siIELs. In focal areas, the intestinal inflammation was associated with ulceration of the villi, crypt abscess, and inflammatory cell infiltrates extending into the lamina propria. The pathology scores for the small intestine are shown in Fig. 1E. The distribution of pathology scores for the ileum of 23 *Roquin*$^{san/san}$ mice is displayed in Fig. 1F. Only 2 of 23 *Roquin*$^{san/san}$ mice had no pathology in the ileum. Tissue sections from the ileum of *Roquin*$^{san/san}$ mice with pathology scores of 2, 3, and 4 are shown in Fig. 1G–I, respectively. Inflammation in the colon of *Roquin*$^{san/san}$ mice was rare (not shown). Similar to other studies in which ICOS expression was elevated in splenic CD4$^+$ T cells of *Roquin*$^{san/san}$ mice [4], *Icos* gene expression was elevated in the ileum (Fig. 1J).

The liver of 26 *Roquin*$^{san/san}$ mice revealed moderate-to-severe hepatitis with an average pathology score of 3.96±0.29 (Fig. 2A). The degree of inflammation and liver cell death were graded with minor modification using a published scoring system for necroinflammatory activity [8]. Hematoxylin and eosin stained sections of *Roquin*$^{san/san}$ mice liver showed varying degrees of mononuclear cell infiltrate around central vein and periportal areas associated with lobular hepatocyte necrosis (Fig. 2C). Occasionally, chronic granulomatous inflammation consisting of lymphocytes, histiocytes and multinucleated giant cells were also noted around the central vein. The histopathological features of the liver from *Roquin*$^{san/san}$ mice with pathology scores of 5 are shown in Fig. 2B and C. A representative liver section from a normal animal without inflammation or hepatocyte death is shown (Fig. 2D).

To further understand the involvement of Roquin in modulating the inflammatory response, we generated Roquin-deficient mice using a Sanger Institute Gene Trap ES cell line (SIGTR CC0753) that targeted the *Roquin* gene (*Roquin*$^{gt/gt}$). Fig. 3A illustrates the location of the β-geo gene trap cassette and genotyping primers relative to the *Roquin* exons. Mice were bred onto the C57BL/6 background for more than eight generations. Mice homozygous for the gene trap had a single band of 800 bp; heterozygotes had two bands of 800 bp and 486 bp; wild type mice had a single 486 bp band (Fig. 3B). Roquin gene expression was reduced by 95% in the intestine compared to wild type or heterozygous animals (Fig. 3D). Importantly, however, the Roquin protein was undetectable in the spleen of *Roquin*$^{gt/gt}$ mice by western blotting (Fig. 3C). Tissue sections from the liver (grade 3), duodenum (grade 2), jejunum (grade 2), ileum (grade 2), and cecum (grade 3) of a *Roquin*$^{gt/gt}$ mouse are shown in Fig. 3E–I, respectively. Microscopic features of intestinal inflammation and chronic hepatitis in *Roquin*$^{gt/gt}$ mice were very similar to that of *Roquin*$^{san/san}$ mice. The average pathology score in the small intestine of three *Roquin*$^{gt/gt}$ mice was: 1.67±0.75 for the duodenum, 2.00±0.83 for the jejunum, 2.66±0.33 for the ileum, and 1.66±0.75 for the cecum. As with *Roquin*$^{san/san}$ mice, the most severe inflammation in *Roquin*$^{gt/gt}$ mice occurred in the ileum. All three *Roquin*$^{gt/gt}$ mice lacked colonic inflammation (not shown).

MLN cells in *Roquin*$^{san/san}$ mice have increased numbers of activated T cells, a higher proportion of proliferating T cells, and more short-lived effector cells (SLECs)

Compared to normal C57BL/6 mice (Fig. 4A), MLN T cells from *Roquin*$^{san/san}$ mice (Fig. 4B) had proportionally more CD3$^+$ OX40$^+$, CD3$^+$ ICOS$^+$, ICOS$^+$ CD44^{hi}, and CD3$^+$ B220$^+$ cells.

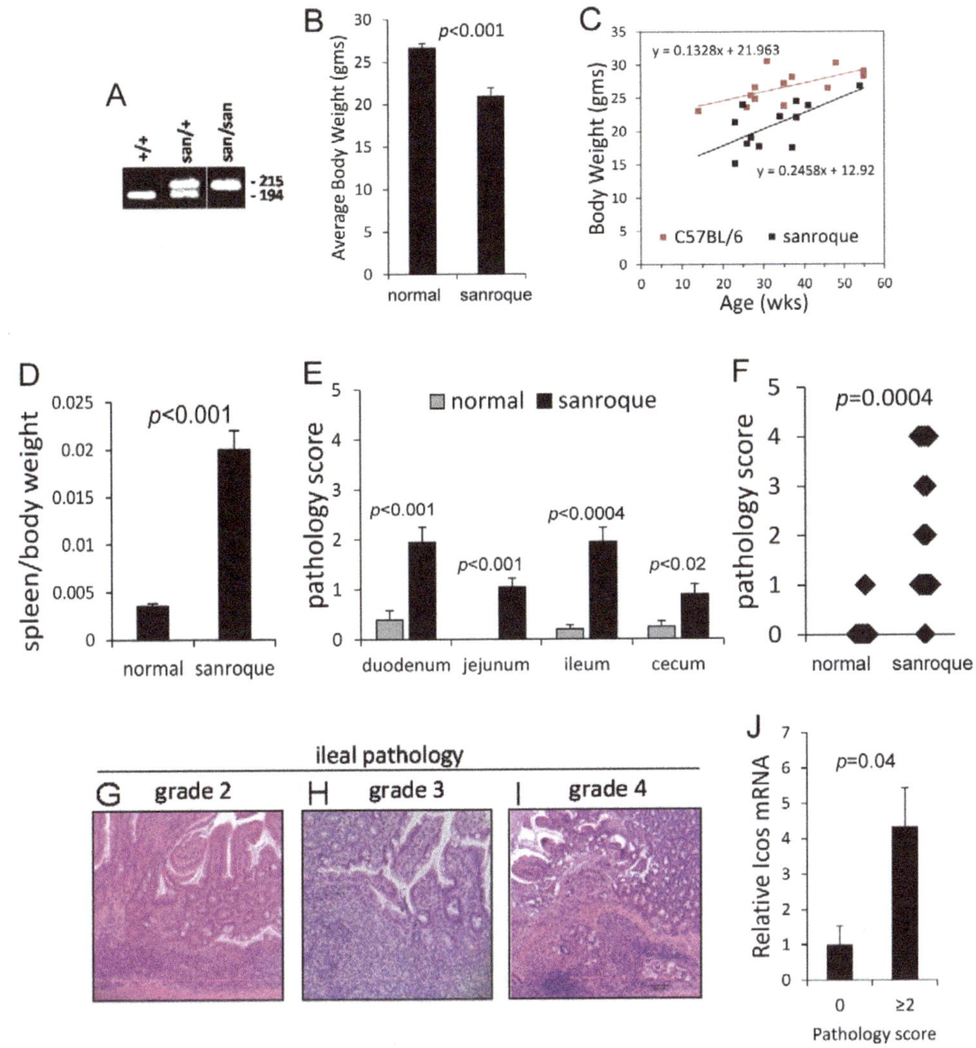

Figure 1. Morphometric and intestinal histopathological features of *Roquin*$^{san/san}$ mice. (**A**) MS-PCR was used to identify homozygous *Roquin*$^{san/san}$ mutant as demonstrated by the presence of a single 215 bp PCR product. Heterozygous *Roquin*$^{san/san}$ mice had two PCR products. *Roquin*$^{san/san}$ mice employed in the study were confirmed by MS-PCR. (**B, C**) Body weight of *Roquin*$^{san/san}$ mice 15–55 weeks of age was significantly less than that of gender-matched normal animals. Mean ± SEM of 13 normal and 12 *Roquin*$^{san/san}$ mice. (**D**) *Roquin*$^{san/san}$ mice also had pronounced splenomegaly with follicular lymphoid hyperplasia, a characteristic of this animal model. Mean ± SEM of 7 normal and 12 *Roquin*$^{san/san}$ mice ages 15–55 weeks. (**E**) Histopathological analysis of intestinal tissues revealed inflammation throughout the small intestine and cecum. Mean ± SEM of pathology scores of tissues from 23 *Roquin*$^{san/san}$ mice and 8–10 normal mice ages 15–55 weeks. (**F**) Distribution of pathology scores for the ileum of *Roquin*$^{san/san}$ mice as shown in panel E; note that only 2 of 23 *Roquin*$^{san/san}$ mice had no inflammation or mucosal injury in the ileum. (**G–I**) Representative H&E stained tissue sections from the ileum of *Roquin*$^{san/san}$ mice with pathology scores of 2, 3, and 4 that were characterized by villous atrophy and ulceration, crypt hyperplasia and increased intraepithelial mononuclear cell infiltrate. Original magnification, 200x. (**J**) *Icos* gene expression was elevated in the ileum of *Roquin*$^{san/san}$ mice. Mean ± SEM of three replicate samples ages 16, 17, and 26 weeks.

Additionally, ICOS was expressed at a higher MFI in *Roquin*$^{san/san}$ mice than normal mice (107 vs. 29, respectively). $CD25^+$ $FoxP3^+$ Tregs (gated onto $CD4^+$ cells) were more abundant in *Roquin*$^{san/san}$ mice, and $CD3^+$ T cells were more proliferative based on in vivo BrdU incorporation (Fig. 4). The elevated proliferative response of $OX40^+$ and $ICOS^+$ cells was further confirmed by ex vivo Ki67 staining (Fig. 5A and B). An additional important finding was the greater number of SLECs in the MLN of *Roquin*$^{san/san}$ mice (Fig. 5D) compared to normal mice (Fig. 5C) as defined by $CD44^{hi}$ $CD62L^{lo}$ $KLRG1^+$ expression.

Small intestine IELs and LPLs in *Roquin*$^{san/san}$ mice have unique phenotypic profiles linked to inflammation

We characterized siIELs and siLPLs from *Roquin*$^{san/san}$ mice according to expression of function-associated activation markers and pro-inflammatory cytokines. Findings from these studies revealed differences in the activation status of cells depending upon the mucosal lymphoid cell compartmentalization. Unlike MLN cells of *Roquin*$^{san/san}$ mice, few siIELs expressed OX40. ICOS was expressed on approximately one-quarter of all $CD3^+$ and $CD44^{hi}$ siIELs from *Roquin*$^{san/san}$ mice (Fig. 6B). IL-17A and IFN-γ were not produced to any appreciable level by either *Roquin*$^{san/san}$ or normal mice (Fig. 6A and B).

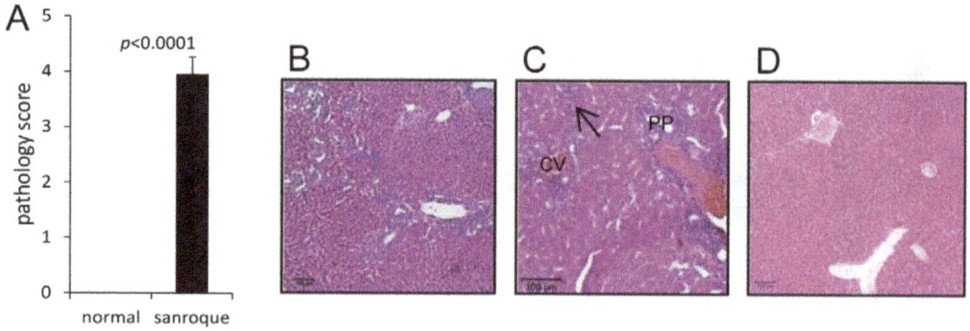

Figure 2. ***Roquin***$^{san/san}$ **mice have chronic hepatitis.** (**A**) Average pathology score of normal and *Roquin*$^{san/san}$ mice. Mean ± SEM of 6 normal and 26 *Roquin*$^{san/san}$ mice ages 15–55 weeks. (**B, C**) Representative H&E stained tissue sections of the liver from *Roquin*$^{san/san}$ mice with pathology scores of 5. (**C**) Mononuclear cell infiltrates are seen distributed in the periportal area (PP) and around the central veins (CV) of the hepatic lobules. Focal areas of hepatocyte necrosis (arrows) with mononuclear cell infiltration is found in the mid-zonal and pericentral areas of the hepatic lobules. (**D**) A representative H&E stained liver section from a normal C57BL/6 mouse devoid of inflammation. Original magnifications, B and D, 100×; C, 200×.

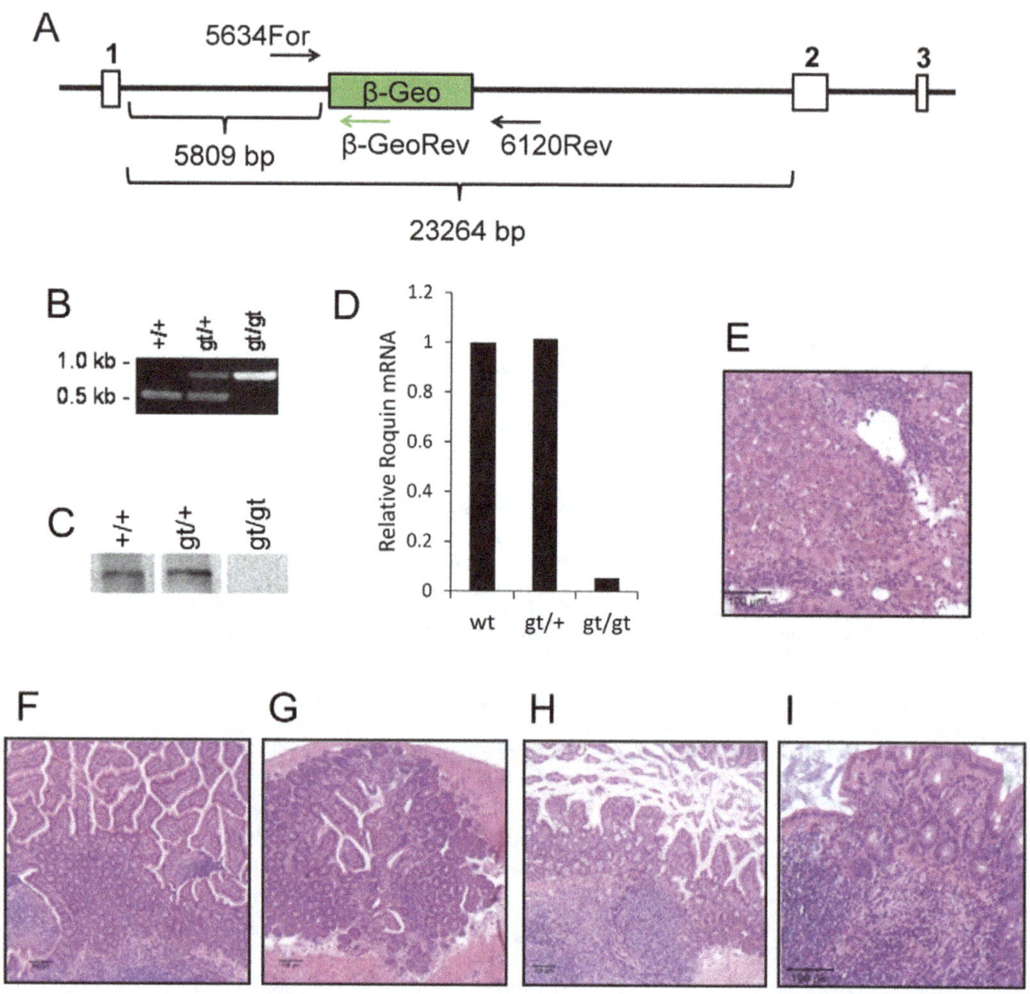

Figure 3. ***Roquin***$^{gt/gt}$ **gene trap mice develop extensive small intestine and liver inflammation.** (**A**) The location of the β-geo gene trap cassette and genotyping primers relative to the *Roquin* exons. (**B**) *Roquin*$^{gt/gt}$ mice were screened using gene trap-specific primers. Mice homozygous for the gene trap had a single band of 800 bp; heterozygotes had two bands of 800 bp and 486 bp; wild type mice had a single 486 bp band. Animal ages 16–22 weeks. (**C**) The Roquin protein was undetectable in the spleen of homozygous (gt/gt) mice by western blotting; 1animal each. Animal ages 16–22 weeks. (**D**) Roquin gene expression in the intestine of homozygous (gt/gt) mice was reduced by ~95%; 1animal each. Animal ages 16–22 weeks. Representative H&E stained tissue sections of the (**E**) liver, (**F**) duodenum, (**G**) jejunum, (**H**) ileum, and (**I**) cecum of a *Roquin*$^{gt/gt}$ mouse exhibited chronic hepatitis and intestinal inflammation. Pathology scores of sections are described in the text. E–I, original magnifications, 200×.

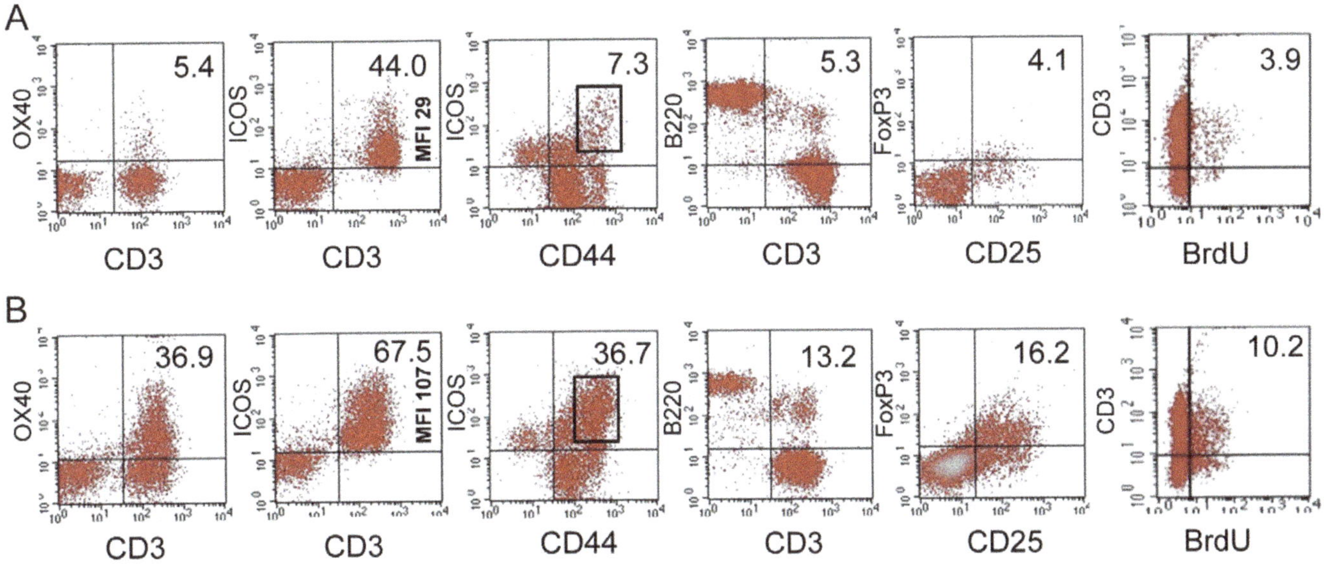

Figure 4. MLN cells in *Roquin*$^{san/san}$ mice have increased numbers of activated T cells, proliferating cells, and regulatory T cells. MLN lymphocytes from (**A**) normal and (**B**) *Roquin*$^{san/san}$ mice based on expression of OX40, ICOS, B220, FoxP3, and BrdU incorporation. FoxP3 CD25 expression was determined after gating onto CD4$^+$ cells. Representative data from 2-3 normal and 2-4 *Roquin*$^{san/san}$ mice.

The findings for siLPLs differed notably from that of siIELs in that only a small proportion of siLPLs were ICOS$^+$ in both normal and *Roquin*$^{san/san}$ mice. However, a high proportion of siLPLs from *Roquin*$^{san/san}$ mice expressed Gr-1, which included a subset of Gr-1$^+$ IL-17A$^+$ cells (Fig. 7B). Although Gr-1 is most frequently associated with myeloid cells, a population of Gr-1$^+$ CD8$^+$ cells, some of which express IFN-γ, has been identified [10]. Because Gr-1$^+$ siLPLs from *Roquin*$^{san/san}$ mice did not express F4/80 or CD11c antigens (not shown), and because the majority were CD3$^+$, they were not macrophages or dendritic cells. Additionally, there also were more CD3$^+$ siLPLs in *Roquin*$^{san/san}$ mice compared to normal mice (Fig. 7A and B), indicating that there had been an influx of T cells into the lamina propria of *Roquin*$^{san/san}$ mice.

We studied Gr-1$^+$ siLPLs from *Roquin*$^{san/san}$ mice and normal mice with regard to expression of IFN-γ in the CD8$^+$ population. These studies revealed significantly more IFN-γ synthesis by *Roquin*$^{san/san}$ mice compared to normal animals (Fig. 7B vs. A). Thus, siLPLs in *Roquin*$^{san/san}$ mice were a significant source of both IL-17A and IFN-γ, two potent pro-inflammatory cytokines.

Cytokine dysregulation in the ileum of *Roquin*$^{san/san}$ mice

To understand how Roquin regulates the inflammatory response, we analyzed tissue sections from the ileum of *Roquin*$^{san/san}$ and normal mice for expression of 89 inflammation-associated genes as described in the Materials and Methods. Shown in Table 1, eleven analytes were up-regulated and ten were down-regulated in the ileum of 3*Roquin*$^{san/san}$ mice relative to 4 normal controls. Interestingly, in both the up-regulated and down-regulated groups, there were several analytes having significant chemotactic activities. This suggested that the alteration in the Roquin protein had a major impact on cytokine synthesis in the small intestine, and it implied that this Roquin disruption likely contributed to the phenotypic manifestation of the intestinal inflammatory response. Analyte synthesis by non-intestinal tissues was not determined.

Discussion

CD is a form of inflammatory bowel disease (IBD) that can affect any region of the alimentary tract and may be associated with extra-intestinal inflammatory conditions such as iritis, arthritis, pulmonary inflammation, and skin disorders [8,11–13]. A number of mouse models exist for the study of IBD. These include cytokine knockouts such as IL-2$^{-/-}$ and IL-10$^{-/-}$ mice [14,15], as well as models involving the transfer of effector T cells into immunodeficient mice [16,17]. Inflammation in those models, however, is generally restricted to the colon. In contrast, there are few models of small intestinal inflammation that mimic CD. One of these is the SAMP1/yit mouse, which spontaneously develops ileitis by 20–30 weeks of age [18,19]. Although that model has been useful for understanding various aspects of the inflammatory response in the ileum, it is problematic for studies into the biomolecular basis of disease because the underlying genetic changes responsible for the inflammatory phenotype have not been fully characterized. Small intestine inflammation also develops in mice in which TNF has been over-expressed, such as in TNF$^{\Delta ARE}$ mice [20,21], and in certain mouse strains following infection with *Toxoplasma gondii* [22].

The present study demonstrates that *Roquin*$^{san/san}$ mice are susceptible to the development of chronic small intestine inflammation. Although some *Roquin*$^{san/san}$ mice had modest intestinal pathology (11 mice had pathology scores $\leq$1.0), 12 mice had pathology scores $\geq$2.0. Only 2 of 23 *Roquin*$^{san/san}$ mice lacked pathology in the ileum. These findings indicate that the *Roquin*$^{san/san}$ mouse is a reliable animal system to focus studies on small intestine inflammation. Additionally and importantly, because the basis for the genetic defect in *Roquin*$^{san/san}$ mice is known, i.e., it is due to a mutation or deletion in the expression of the Roquin protein, it will be possible to design studies aimed at understanding the regulatory mechanisms by which Roquin controls intestinal inflammation. We recently identified miR-223 as one of the regulatory elements involved in controlling Roquin protein expression, and demonstrated that altering miR-223 expression affects Roquin expression [5]. Studies are currently

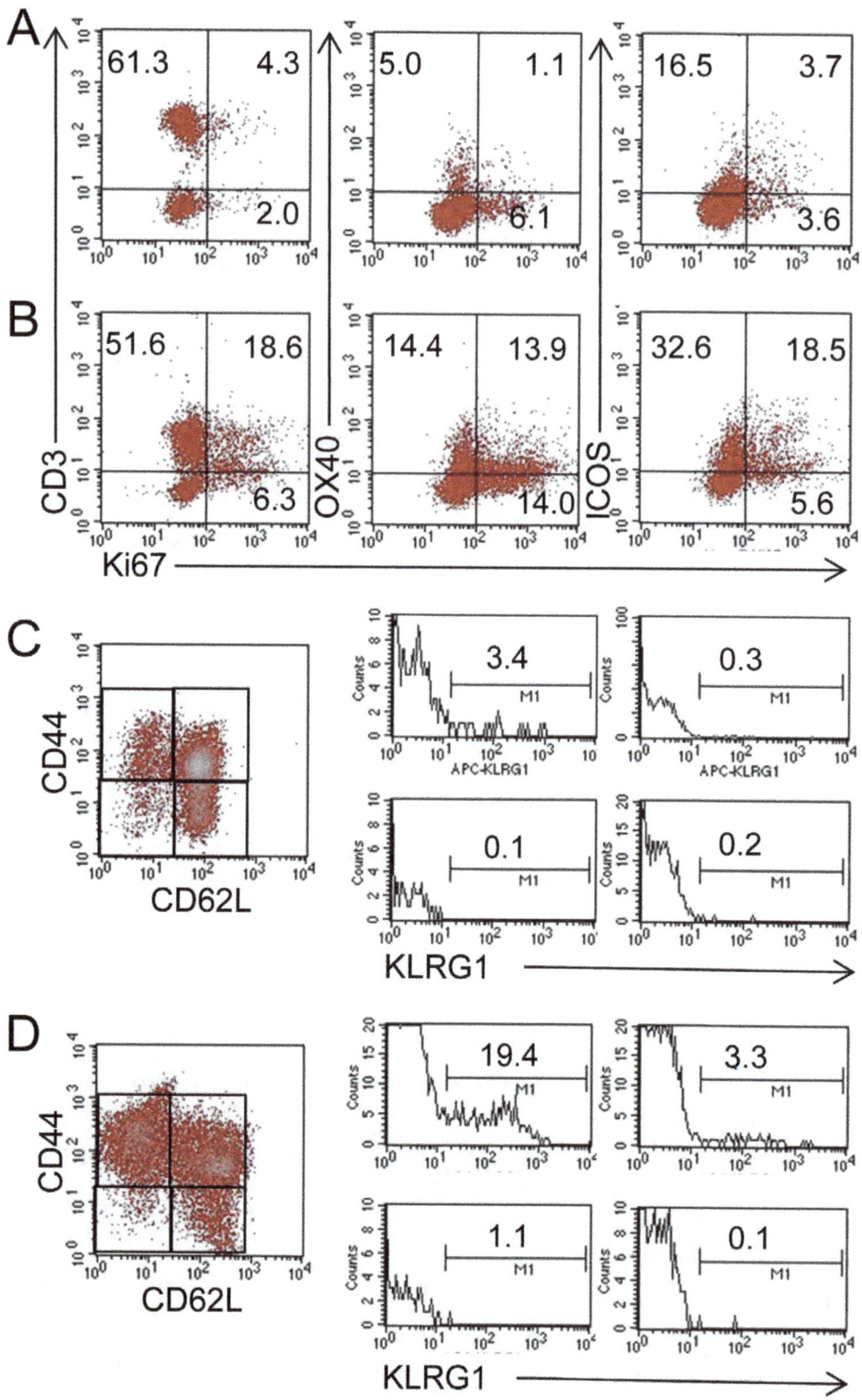

Figure 5. MLN cells from *Roquin*$^{san/san}$ mice are proliferative and have more SLECs. Based on Ki67 staining, (panel **B**) a greater proportion of OX40$^+$ cells and ICOS$^+$ MLN cells were proliferating T cells compared to MLN cells from (panel **A**) normal mice. Representative staining from 1 normal and 2 *Roquin*$^{san/san}$ mice. Similarly, there was a greater proportion of CD44^{hi} CD62L^{lo} KLRG1$^+$ SLECs present in MLN cells of (panel **D**) *Roquin*$^{san/san}$ mice compared to (panel **C**) normal mice. Representative data from 3 normal and 3 *Roquin*$^{san/san}$ mice.

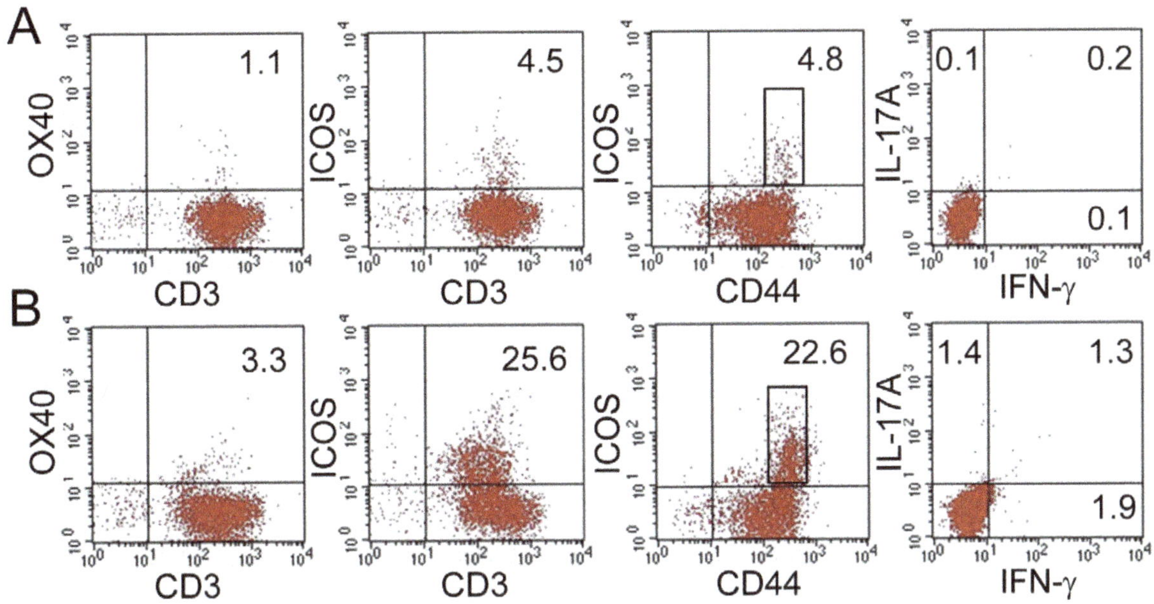

Figure 6. Characterization of siIELs in *Roquin*$^{san/san}$ mice. siIELs from *Roquin*$^{san/san}$ mice have more (panel **B**) ICOS^{+} T cells, including a subset of CD44^{hi} ICOS^{+} cells compared to (panel **A**) normal animals. Interestingly, neither IL-17A nor IFN-γ were produced to any appreciable levels in either type of mouse (panels A and B). Representative data from 2 normal and 2 *Roquin*$^{san/san}$ mice.

underway to identify transcriptional factors that regulate the expression of Roquin, miR-223, and other Roquin-associated miRNAs.

Roquin$^{gt/gt}$ mice generated in our laboratory and used here may prove to be useful for studies into the involvement of Roquin in controlling intestinal inflammation. However, studies with *Roquin*$^{gt/gt}$ mice were limited by the fact that most mice died at birth. Analysis of 29 litters from heterozygous crosses revealed a ratio of 1.57 [wild type]: 4.30: [heterozygous]: 0.12 [homozygous gene trap], which is starkly different from the predicted simple Mendelian ratio of 1:2:1, and therefore suggested a role for Roquin in embryonic development, possibly in the lung [6]. To overcome this, we are currently using *Roquin*$^{gt/gt}$ bone marrow to immunologically reconstitute irradiated normal animals, which will circumvent the deleterious effects of Roquin on non-hematopoietic tissues while retaining its effect within the immune system. It also will be of interest to explore the extent to which inflammation in *Roquin*$^{gt/gt}$ mice can be exacerbated following

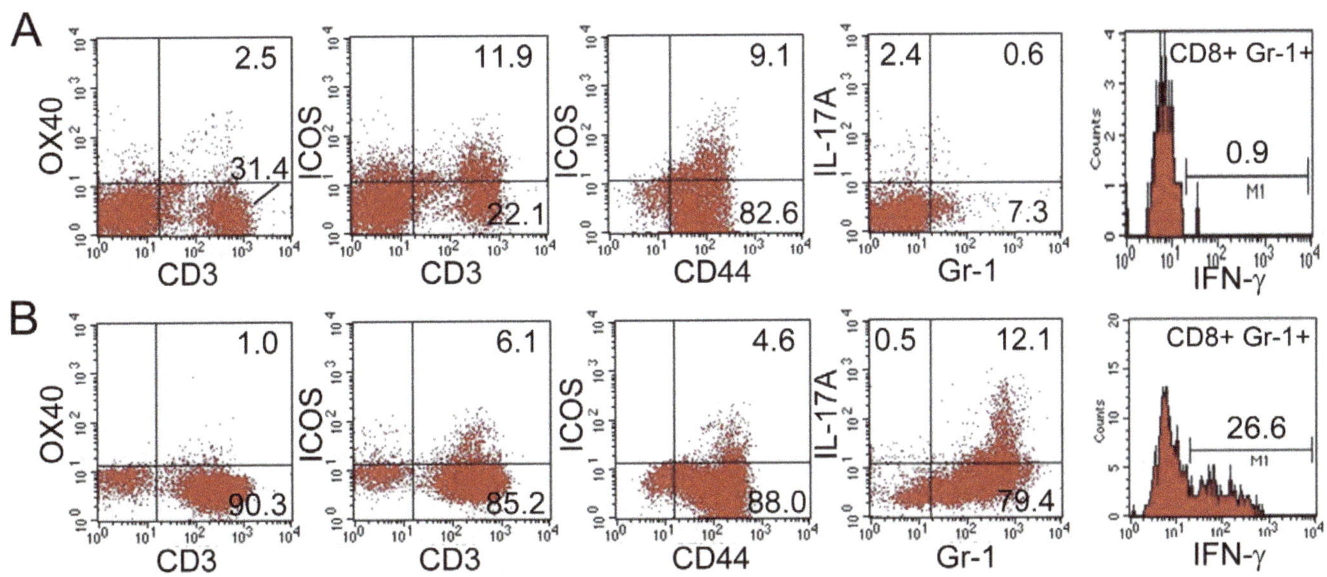

Figure 7. Unique phenotypic profile of siLPLs in *Roquin*$^{san/san}$ mice. siLPLs in *Roquin*$^{san/san}$ mice differed fundamentally from those in normal mice in that *Roquin*$^{san/san}$ mice had an unusually high proportion of GR-1^{+} T cells as determined by CD3 expression. The majority of those cells were CD44^{+} and they included a subset of IL-17A secreting cells. A subset of CD8^{+} Gr-1^{+} cells express IFN-γ (panel **B** compared to panel **A**). Representative data from 2–3 normal and *Roquin*$^{san/san}$ mice.

Table 1. Changes in analyte levels in the ileum of three *Roquin*$^{san/san}$ mice relative to four normal control mice.

Upregulated		**Down-regulated**	
Analyte	**Change**	**Analyte**	**Change**
IL5ra	6.962	Tnfrsf1b	−4.917
CCL1	5.961	Actb	−4.401
CCL24	5.622	CXCL5	−3.118
PPC	2.578	Spp1	−2.826
IL13	2.356	CCL5	−2.781
IL1α	2.317	CCL4	−2.201
CCL20	2.313	CCR7	−2.146
CXCL13	2.193	IL1β	−2.082
CXCL1	2.187	IL6st	−2.068
CCL25	2.156	IFNγ	−2.004
IL4	2.159		

exposure to pharmaceuticals such as piroxicam, a nonsteroidal anti-inflammatory drug that has been shown to accelerate the inflammatory response in IL-10$^{-/-}$ mice [23–25], and in mice exposed to dextran sulfate sodium.

We found both similarities and differences between our *Roquin*$^{gt/gt}$ mice and the *Rc3h1*$^{-/-}$ mice that were produced by others [6]. Similar to mice in that study, *Roquin*$^{gt/gt}$ mice generated in our laboratory had a poor post-birth survival rate and most had a congenital caudal spine defect. However, unlike *Rc3h1*$^{-/-}$ mice which generally lacked autoimmune disease [6], *Roquin*$^{gt/gt}$ animals that lived to adulthood had a disease phenotype associated with the small intestine and liver that resembled that of *Roquin*$^{san/san}$ mice. Whether these differences have to do with how Roquin-deficient animals were generated, or whether the intestine is more prone to autoimmune disease, is unclear. The *Roquin*$^{gt/gt}$ mice used in our studies were created via random insertion of a β-geo gene trap vector into the *Roquin* locus. Mapping of *Roquin*$^{gt/gt}$ mice by 5′RACE positioned the gene trap vector between exon 1 and 2. This procedure normally results in complete gene inactivation, as appeared to be the case based on the lack of detectable Roquin protein in western blots. Bertossi et al [6] targeted exons 4–6 of the *Roquin* locus by flanking the exons with loxP sites to create *Rc3h1*$^{-/-}$ mice. Although western blot data from *Rc3h1*$^{-/-}$ mouse embryonic fibroblasts indicated a true null mutation, it is possible that this knockout strategy may leave truncated versions of Roquin produced from the remaining exons. The presence of a secondary band of lower molecular weight in western blots of TCR-β^{+} splenocytes in CD4-directed conditional Roquin knock-out animals raises this possibility [6]. Regardless, our studies suggest that intestinal inflammation can develop in mice with either mutated Roquin or Roquin deletion.

The phenotypic profiles of MLN cells, siIELs, and siLPLs were revealing. MLN cells of *Roquin*$^{san/san}$ mice was characterized by an abundance of T cell activation markers, notably OX40, ICOS, and B220, as well as evidence for proliferating T cells, indicating replication of activated T cells. A second key feature of MLN T cells in *Roquin*$^{san/san}$ mice was the presence of CD44^{hi} CD62L^{lo} KLRG1^{+} SLECs. This is consistent with the finding of a population of SLECs in the spleen of *Rc3h1*$^{-/-}$ mice [6]. Similar findings linked to increased IFN-γ synthesis have been described for *Roquin*$^{san/san}$ mice [26]. Additional studies are planned in our laboratory using adoptive transfer experiments to trace the homing properties of the *Roquin*$^{san/san}$ SLECs to the gut, and using IL-7R expression to differentiate MLN SLECs from memory precursor effector cells (MPECs) [27]. Also of interest was the presence of increased numbers of FoxP3^{+} Tregs in the MLN of *Roquin*$^{san/san}$ mice. Although the significance of this is not yet clear, a recent study provided evidence for a functional role for ICOS^{+} FoxP3^{+} Tregs in the suppression of antigen-reactive T cells [28]. Additional analysis of that FoxP3^{+} T cell population in *Roquin*$^{san/san}$ mice may provide insight into how Roquin controls or fails to control autoimmunity.

siIELs from *Roquin*$^{san/san}$ mice were distinguished by the presence of ICOS^{+} CD44^{+} T cells; however, neither IL-17A nor IFN-γ were produced there to any appreciable degree. In contrast, ~80% of siLPLs from *Roquin*$^{san/san}$ mice were Gr-1^{+} T cells, a significant proportion of which produced IL-17A. Also among siLPLs was a subset of GR-1^{+} CD8^{+} IFN-γ-producing cells, which may be a CD8^{+} memory T cell population [10]. Taken together, these findings suggest that the siLPLs are the likely leukocyte population responsible for inflammatory destruction of the intestine in *Roquin*$^{san/san}$ mice.

The inflammatory response in the ileum of *Roquin*$^{san/san}$ mice was complex as seen from the analyte studies done using ileum tissues, which revealed dysregulation in the expression of twenty-one immunologically-related analytes, eleven of which were over-expressed and ten were down-regulated. Collectively, the cytokines that were over-expressed would have a significant effect on the recruitment of monocytes and macrophages (CCL1), T cells, NK cells, and B cells (CCL24, CCL25, CCL20), dendritic cells (CCL1, CCL20, CCL25), and eosinophils and neutrophils (CCL24, CCL20) into the small intestine. Additionally, the presence of IL-1a, IL-4, IL-5ra, IL-13, and CXCL1 would have a strong effect on driving and sustaining an inflammatory response. Conversely, several analytes with proinflammatory activities were down-regulated in *Roquin*$^{san/san}$ mice. These included IL6st, IL1β, and IFNγ. Likewise, gene expression for analytes with strong chemotactic activities for T cells, eosinophils and basophils (CCL4 and CCL5), and memory T cells (CCL7) were down-regulated. Suppressed levels of CCL5 in the ileum of *Roquin*$^{san/san}$ mice differs from what has been reported for *Roquin*$^{san/san}$ mice [3]; however, the latter study used splenocytes not intestinal cells for analysis. The findings reported here point to a dynamic host process that probably reflects an effort to maintain a normal homeostatic response in the small intestine of *Roquin*$^{san/san}$ mice. How that balance is shifted in one direction or the other may ultimately determine the extent to which inflammation is mild or severe in those animals. It also will be of interest to determine the extent to which intestinal antigenic challenge following virus, bacteria, or parasite infection alters the inflammatory response locally and the extent to which this reflects the pathology seen in Crohn's disease, as recently reported for collagen-induced arthritis [29].

The findings reported here demonstrate that mice having a mutated Roquin protein, or animals in which the *Roquin* gene has been disrupted, are prone to the development of intestinal inflammation that is principally localized in the small intestine. Because of the relatively few animal models of CD pathophysiology in the small intestine, and because the primary gene-protein defect of the animals used here is known, it will be possible to pursue the genetic and molecular mechanisms that drive this process. These and subsequent studies, including experimental intervention designed to force Roquin expression in vivo, could be of considerable value for expanding our knowledge of factors that are causative in initiating and maintaining chronic intestinal inflammatory responses.

Author Contributions

Conceived and designed the experiments: JSS DMS NV JRK. Performed the experiments: JSS DMS NN. Analyzed the data: JSS DMS NV JRK. Wrote the paper: JSS NV JRK.

References

1. Ciechanover A, Schwartz AL (1998) The ubiquitin-proteasome pathway: the complexity and myriad functions of proteins death. Proc Natl Acad Sci U S A 95: 2727–2730.
2. Lin AE, Mak TW (2007) The role of E3 ligases in autoimmunity and the regulation of autoreactive T cells. Curr Opin Immunol 19: 665–673.
3. Vinuesa CG, Cook MC, Angelucci C, Athanasopoulos V, Rui L, et al. (2005) A RING-type ubiquitin ligase family member required to repress follicular helper T cells and autoimmunity. Nature 435: 452–458.
4. Yu D, Tan AH, Hu X, Athanasopoulos V, Simpson N, et al. (2007) Roquin represses autoimmunity by limiting inducible T-cell co-stimulator messenger RNA. Nature 450: 299–303.
5. Schaefer JS, Montufar-Solis D, Vigneswaran N, Klein JR (2011) Selective upregulation of microRNA expression in peripheral blood leukocytes in IL-10−/− mice precedes expression in the colon. J Immunol 187: 5834–5841.
6. Bertossi A, Aichinger M, Sansonetti P, Lech M, Neff F, et al. (2011) Loss of Roquin induces early death and immune deregulation but not autoimmunity. J Exp Med 208: 1749–1756.
7. Schaefer JS, Montufar-Solis D, Vigneswaran N, Klein JR (2010) ICOS promotes IL-17 synthesis in colonic intraepithelial lymphocytes in IL-10−/− mice. J Leukoc Biol 87: 301–308.
8. Basseri B, Enayati P, Marchevsky A, Papadakis KA (2010) Pulmonary manifestations of inflammatory bowel disease: case presentations and review. J Crohns Colitis 4: 390–397.
9. Montufar-Solis D, Wang HC, Klein JR (2007) Stimulatory and costimulatory effects of IL-18 directed to different small intestinal CD43 T cell subsets. J Leukoc Biol 82: 1166–1173.
10. Matsuzaki J, Tsuji T, Chamoto K, Takeshima T, Sendo F, et al. (2003) Successful elimination of memory-type CD8+ T cell subsets by the administration of anti-Gr-1 monoclonal antibody in vivo. Cell Immunol 224: 98–105.
11. Manganelli C, Turco S, Balestrazzi E (2009) Ophthalmological aspects of IBD. Eur Rev Med Pharmacol Sci 13 Suppl 1: 11–13.
12. Reveille JD (2012) Genetics of spondyloarthritis – beyond the MHC. Nat Rev Rheumatol 8: 296–304.
13. Veloso FT (2011) Extraintestinal manifestations of inflammatory bowel disease: do they influence treatment and outcome? World J Gastroenterol 17: 2702–2707.
14. Sadlack B, Merz H, Schorle H, Schimpl A, Feller AC, et al. (1993) Ulcerative colitis-like disease in mice with a disrupted interleukin-2 gene. Cell 75: 253–261.
15. Kuhn R, Lohler J, Rennick D, Rajewsky K, Muller W (1993) Interleukin-10-deficient mice develop chronic enterocolitis. Cell 75: 263–274.
16. Claesson MH, Rudolphi A, Kofoed S, Poulsen SS, Reimann J (1996) CD4+ T lymphocytes injected into severe combined immunodeficient (SCID) mice lead to an inflammatory and lethal bowel disease. Clin Exp Immunol 104: 491–500.
17. Powrie F, Leach MW, Mauze S, Caddle LB, Coffman RL (1993) Phenotypically distinct subsets of CD4+ T cells induce or protect from chronic intestinal inflammation in C. B-17 scid mice. Int Immunol 5: 1461–1471.
18. Rivera-Nieves J, Bamias G, Vidrich A, Marini M, Pizarro TT, et al. (2003) Emergence of perianal fistulizing disease in the SAMP1/YitFc mouse, a spontaneous model of chronic ileitis. Gastroenterology 124: 972–982.
19. Matsumoto S, Okabe Y, Setoyama H, Takayama K, Ohtsuka J, et al. (1998) Inflammatory bowel disease-like enteritis and caecitis in a senescence accelerated mouse P1/Yit strain. Gut 43: 71–78.
20. Kontoyiannis D, Pasparakis M, Pizarro TT, Cominelli F, Kollias G (1999) Impaired on/off regulation of TNF biosynthesis in mice lacking TNF AU-rich elements: implications for joint and gut-associated immunopathologies. Immunity 10: 387–398.
21. Armaka M, Apostolaki M, Jacques P, Kontoyiannis DL, Elewaut D, et al. (2008) Mesenchymal cell targeting by TNF as a common pathogenic principle in chronic inflammatory joint and intestinal diseases. J Exp Med 205: 331–337.
22. Egan CE, Cohen SB, Denkers EY (2011) Insights into inflammatory bowel disease using Toxoplasma gondii as an infectious trigger. Immunol Cell Biol.
23. Srivastava AS, Feng Z, Mishra R, Malhotra R, Kim HS, et al. (2007) Embryonic stem cells ameliorate piroxicam-induced colitis in IL10−/− KO mice. Biochem Biophys Res Commun 361: 953–959.
24. Hale LP, Gottfried MR, Swidsinski A (2005) Piroxicam treatment of IL-10-deficient mice enhances colonic epithelial apoptosis and mucosal exposure to intestinal bacteria. Inflamm Bowel Dis 11: 1060–1069.
25. Berg DJ, Zhang J, Weinstock JV, Ismail HF, Earle KA, et al. (2002) Rapid development of colitis in NSAID-treated IL-10-deficient mice. Gastroenterology 123: 1527–1542.
26. Chang PP, Lee SK, Hu X, Davey G, Duan G, et al. (2012) Breakdown in repression of IFN-gamma mRNA leads to accumulation of self-reactive effector CD8+ T cells. J Immunol 189: 701–710.
27. Joshi NS, Cui W, Chandele A, Lee HK, Urso DR, et al. (2007) Inflammation directs memory precursor and short-lived effector CD8(+) T cell fates via the graded expression of T-bet transcription factor. Immunity 27: 281–295.
28. Vocanson M, Rozieres A, Hennino A, Poyet G, Gaillard V, et al. (2010) Inducible costimulator (ICOS) is a marker for highly suppressive antigen-specific T cells sharing features of TH17/TH1 and regulatory T cells. J Allergy Clin Immunol 126: 280–289, 289 e281–287.
29. Ji YR, Kim HJ, Yu DH, Bae KB, Park SJ, et al. (2012) Enforced expression of roquin protein in T cells exacerbates the incidence and severity of experimental arthritis. J Biol Chem 287: 42269–42277.

9

Macrophages and Dendritic Cells Emerge in the Liver during Intestinal Inflammation and Predispose the Liver to Inflammation

Yohei Mikami[1,2], Shinta Mizuno[1], Nobuhiro Nakamoto[1], Atsushi Hayashi[1,3], Tomohisa Sujino[1], Toshiro Sato[1], Nobuhiko Kamada[4], Katsuyoshi Matsuoka[1], Tadakazu Hisamatsu[1], Hiroshi Ebinuma[1], Toshifumi Hibi[1], Akihiko Yoshimura[2]*, Takanori Kanai[1]*

1 Division of Gastroenterology and Hepatology, Department of Internal Medicine, Keio University School of Medicine, Tokyo, Japan, **2** Department of Microbiology and Immunology, Keio University School of Medicine, Tokyo, Japan, **3** Research Laboratory, Miyarisan Pharmaceutical, Tokyo, Japan, **4** Department of Pathology and Comprehensive Cancer Center, University of Michigan Medical School, Ann Arbor, Michigan, United States of America

Abstract

The liver is a physiological site of immune tolerance, the breakdown of which induces immunity. Liver antigen-presenting cells may be involved in both immune tolerance and activation. Although inflammatory diseases of the liver are frequently associated with inflammatory bowel diseases, the underlying immunological mechanisms remain to be elucidated. Here we report two murine models of inflammatory bowel disease: RAG-$2^{-/-}$ mice adoptively transferred with $CD4^+CD45RB^{high}$ T cells; and IL-$10^{-/-}$ mice, accompanied by the infiltration of mononuclear cells in the liver. Notably, $CD11b^-CD11c^{low}$PDCA-1^+ plasmacytoid dendritic cells (DCs) abundantly residing in the liver of normal wild-type mice disappeared in colitic $CD4^+CD45RB^{high}$ T cell-transferred RAG-$2^{-/-}$ mice and IL-$10^{-/-}$ mice in parallel with the emergence of macrophages (Mφs) and conventional DCs (cDCs). Furthermore, liver Mφ/cDCs emerging during intestinal inflammation not only promote the proliferation of naïve $CD4^+$ T cells, but also instruct them to differentiate into IFN-γ-producing Th1 cells *in vitro*. The emergence of pathological Mφ/cDCs in the liver also occurred in a model of acute dextran sulfate sodium (DSS)-induced colitis under specific pathogen-free conditions, but was canceled in germ-free conditions. Last, the Mφ/cDCs that emerged in acute DSS colitis significantly exacerbated Fas-mediated hepatitis. Collectively, intestinal inflammation skews the composition of antigen-presenting cells in the liver through signaling from commensal bacteria and predisposes the liver to inflammation.

Editor: David L. Boone, University of Chicago, United States of America

Funding: This study was supported in part by Grants-in-Aid for Scientific Research [21390233], Scientific Research on Priority Areas [22021038] from the Japanese Ministry of Education, Culture, Sports, Science and Technology; a Grant-in-Aid for Young Scientists [22790667] from the Japanese Ministry of Health, Labour and Welfare; Health and Labour Sciences Research Grants for research on intractable diseases from the Japanese MIKAMI ET AL Ministry of Health, Labour and Welfare; a Keio University Grant-in-Aid for Encouragement of Young Medical Scientists. The funders had no role in study design, data collection and analysis, decision to publish, or preparation of the manuscript.

Competing Interests: AH is employed by a commercial company, Miyarisan Pharmaceutical.

* E-mail: takagast@z2.keio.jp (TK); yoshimura@a6.keio.jp (AY)

Introduction

Patients with inflammatory bowel diseases (IBD) are susceptible to developing extraintestinal disorders in the joints, eyes, skin, or liver [1]. For example, primary sclerosing cholangitis (PSC) has been diagnosed in 3.7% of patients with ulcerative colitis [2] and in 3.4% of those with Crohn's disease [3]. The liver and the biliary system are the usual sites for extraintestinal lesions, despite being located between systemic and portal circulations. The portal vein contains a large amount of gut-derived products, such as short-chain fatty acids and microbe-associated molecular patterns (MAMPs) [4]. Although MAMPs, such as LPS from gram-negative commensal bacteria, act as a strong stimulants for antigen-presenting cells (APCs) [5], the liver has been shown to be an immunologically tolerant organ [6,7]. The portal venous tolerance system is regulated by various immune compartments which contain natural killer (NK) cell, natural killer T (NKT) cell, and regulatory T cells, macrophages (Mφ) such as Kupffer cells, and dendritic cells (DCs) [8]. Recent studies have shown that plasmacytoid DCs (pDCs), a subgroup of resident DCs, induce anergy or rapid depletion of antigen-specific T cells in the liver via a $CD4^+$ T cell-independent mechanism [9,10]. These findings suggest that regulation and dysregulation of APCs in the liver contribute to liver tolerance and inflammation, respectively. However, the mechanisms of immune regulation and dysregulation in human IBD and experimental colitis models are not yet fully understood. A few studies have focused on the role of gut microbiota and MAMPs in promoting high-fat induced steatohepatitis [11], however, mechanism of immunological dysregulation in the liver during colitis still remains to be elucidated.

Our group has previously reported that increased numbers of Mφs and conventional DCs (cDCs) in experimental colitis models [12] and human IBD [13] have pro-inflammatory characteristics through excess production of IL-12 and IL-23 in response to

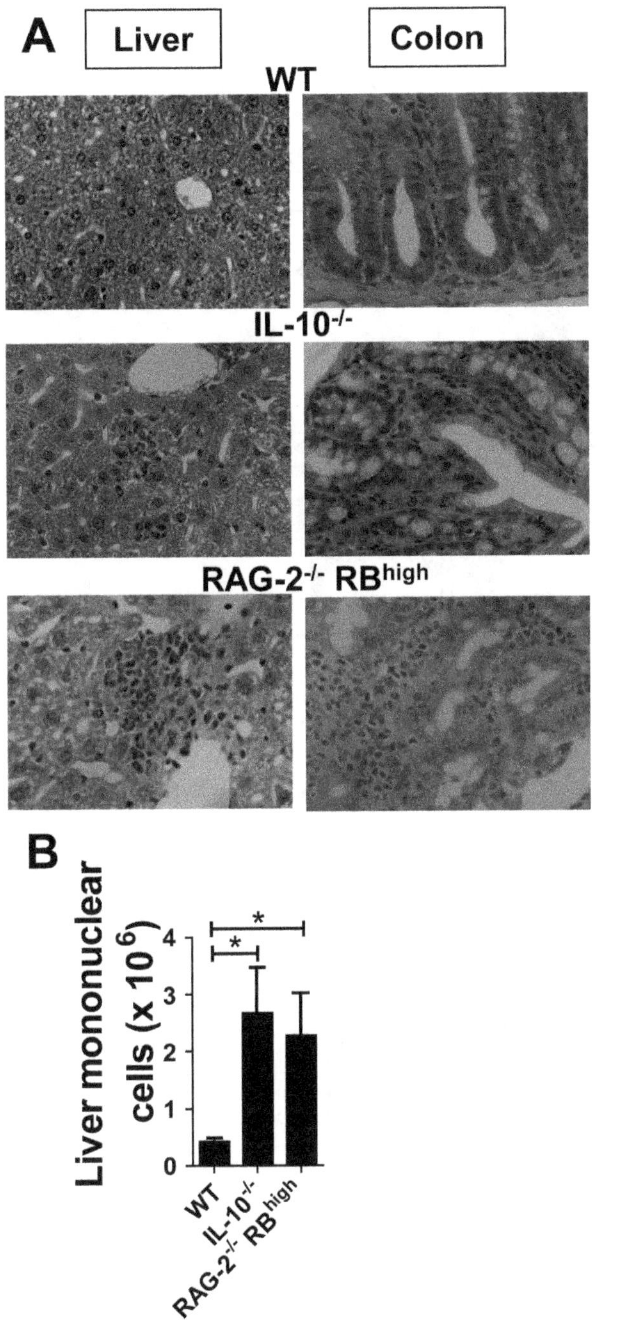

Figure 1. Accumulation of mononuclear cells in the liver develops in chronic colitis models. (**A**) H&E specimens of the liver (left) and colon (right) derived from WT, IL-10$^{-/-}$ mice, and RAG-2$^{-/-}$ RB^{high} mice. Magnification: ×100 (left) and ×400 (right). (**B**) Absolute number of hepatic mononuclear cells. FACS data are representative of three independent experiments. Values are expressed as means ± SEM for each group. WT (*n* = 5), IL-10$^{-/-}$ mice (*n* = 7) and RAG-2$^{-/-}$ RB^{high} mice (*n* = 4). **P*<0.05.

bacteria. This leads to the development of Th1 immunity in inflamed intestinal mucosa. More recently, we demonstrated that migrating macrophages contribute to the induction of acute liver inflammation in murine hepatitis models [14].

To clarify hepatic immunological regulation under colitic conditions, we used three murine IBD models: (1) RAG-2$^{-/-}$ mice adoptively transferred with splenic CD4$^+$CD45RB^{high} T cells from wild-type (WT) mice [15]; (2) an acute dextran sulfate sodium (DSS)-induced colitis model [16]; and (3) IL-10$^{-/-}$ mice [17] that spontaneously develop chronic IBD-like colitis.

Materials and Methods

Mice

WT C57BL/6J mice (8–12 weeks old) were purchased from Japan Clea (Tokyo, Japan). C57BL/6-Ly5.1 mice and RAG-2$^{-/-}$ mice were obtained from Taconic Laboratory (Hudson, NY, USA) and the Central Laboratories for Experimental Animals (Kawasaki, Japan), respectively. IL-10$^{-/-}$ mice were purchased from Jackson Laboratories (Bar Harbor, Maine, USA). Recipient RAG-2$^{-/-}$ mice were used when they were 6 or 14 weeks old. Colitic IL-10$^{-/-}$ mice were used when they were 20 weeks old. Germ-free (GF) C57BL/6-Ly5.2 mice (8 weeks old) were purchased from Sankyo Laboratories (Tokyo, Japan). GF mice were maintained in vinyl isolators within the gnotobiotic facility of the Miyarisan pharmaceutical company (Tokyo, Japan).

All experiments were approved by the Committee on the Ethics of Animal Experiments of Keio University School of Medicine, and conducted in accordance with institutional guidelines and Home Office regulations. [No. 24-026-1].

Adoptive Transfer Studies

For adoptive transfer, CD4$^+$ T cells were isolated from spleen cells of C57BL/6-Ly5.1 mice using the anti-CD4 (L3T4)-MACS system (Miltenyi Biotec, Auburn, CA, USA) according to the manufacturer's instructions. Enriched CD4$^+$ T cells (96–97% pure) were labeled with PE-conjugated anti-mouse CD4 (RM4-5; BD bioscience, San Diego, CA, USA) and FITC-conjugated anti-CD45RB (16A; BD bioscience). CD4$^+$CD45RB^{high} cells were purified (>98.0%) using a FACS Aria (Becton Dickinson Co.). RAG-2$^{-/-}$ mice (6 weeks old) were injected i.p. with 3×10^5 CD4$^+$CD45RB^{high} T cells. At 6 weeks post-transfer, these mice developed a wasting disease and colitis as previously reported [15].

For adoptive retransfer, lamina propria (LP) CD4$^+$ T cells were isolated from colon LP mononuclear cells of RAG-2$^{-/-}$ RB^{high} mice using the anti-CD4 (L3T4)-MACS system. Isolated LP CD4$^+$ T cells were injected i.p. into RAG-2$^{-/-}$ mice (RAG-2$^{-/-}$ LP CD4$^+$ mice). Mice were maintained under specific pathogen-free (SPF) conditions in the Animal Care Facility of Keio University.

DSS-induced Colitis Model

Mice were treated under SPF conditions with 2% DSS (MW 50 kDa; Ensuiko Sugar Refining Co., Yokohama, Japan) in drinking water for 7 days (>4 mice per group). Mice were treated under GF conditions with 1% DSS in drinking water for 7 days followed with regular drinking water for 3 days (>4 mice per group).

Animal Models of Liver Injury

Concanavalin A (Con A, type IV) was purchased from Sigma-Aldrich (St. Louis, MO, USA). Intravenous injections of Con A (20 mg/kg) were administered into the tail vein of animals 10 h before examination. The Fas-activating antibody Jo2 (0.3 mg/kg of body weight; BD bioscience) was injected i.p. and mice were sacrificed 6 h later [18,19].

Preparation of Liver Mononuclear Cells

Liver mononuclear cells were separated from the liver as previously described [20]. Livers were perfused through the portal vein with PBS, then minced and passed through a 100 μm nylon mesh. The filtrate was centrifuged at 50×*g* for 1 min, and the

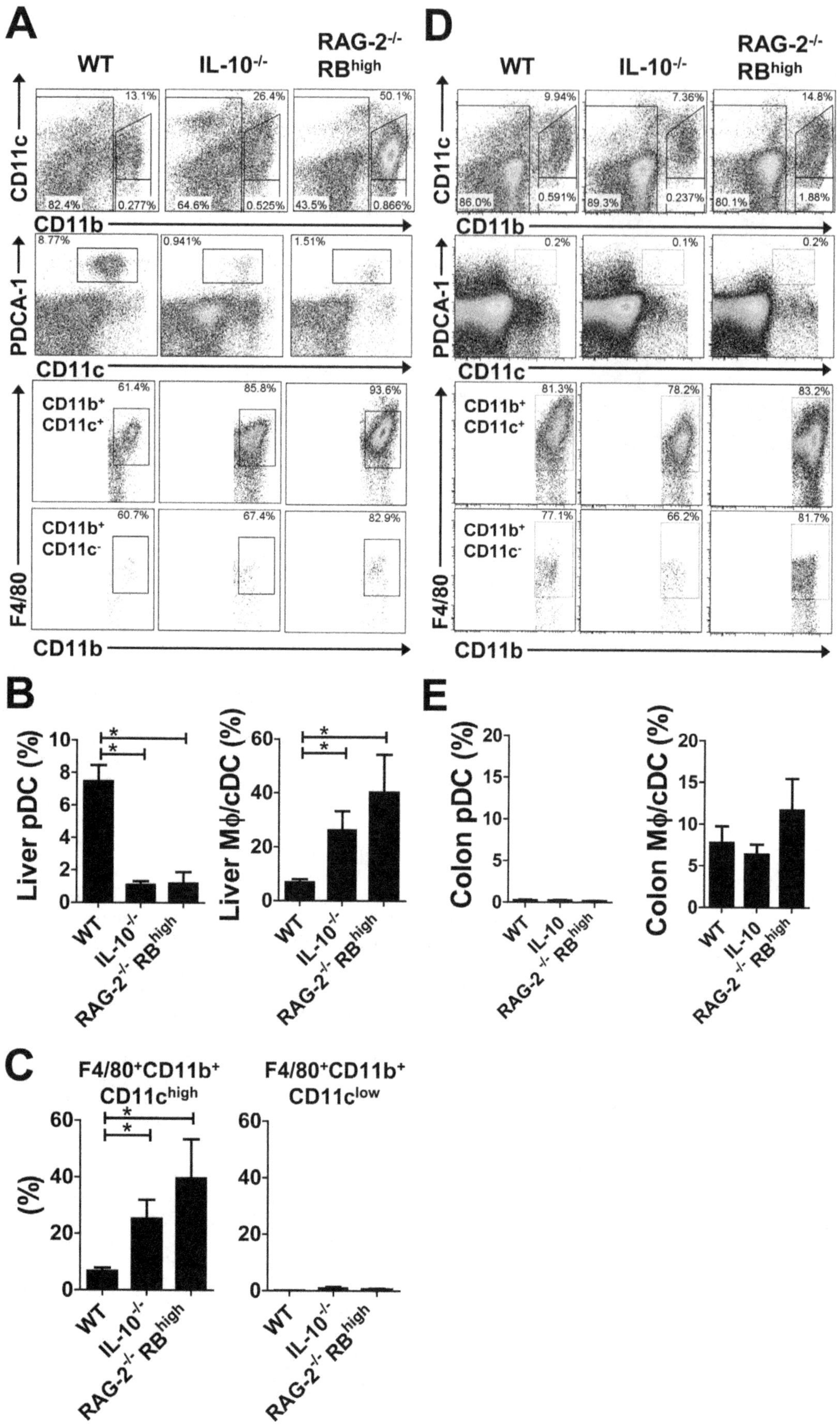
A
WT
IL-10-/-
RAG-2-/- RBhigh
CD11c
CD11b
PDCA-1
F4/80
CD11b+ CD11c+
CD11b+ CD11c-
D
B
Liver pDC (%)
Liver Mϕ/cDC (%)
C
F4/80+CD11b+ CD11chigh
F4/80+CD11b+ CD11clow
(%)
E
Colon pDC (%)
Colon Mϕ/cDC (%)

Figure 2. Chronic intestinal inflammation was associated with reciprocal changes in the balance of APCs. (**A**) Flow cytometry results related to mononuclear cells isolated from the livers of WT (left column), IL-10$^{-/-}$ (middle), and RAG-2$^{-/-}$ RB^{high} (right) mice. Dead cells were excluded with 7AAD staining, followed by proper use of a FSC/SSC gate. CD11b^{-}, CD11b^{+}CD11c^{high}, and CD11b^{+}CD11c^{low} cells were gated from the cells shown in the first row. CD11b^{-} cells are shown in the second row and PDCA-1^{+}CD11b^{-}CD11c^{int} cells were analyzed. The expression of F4/80 in CD11b^{+}CD11c^{high} cells and CD11b^{+}CD11c^{low} cells are analyzed in the third row and the fourth row. (**B**) Proportion of PDCA-1^{+}CD11b^{-}CD11c^{int} pDCs and F4/80^{+}CD11b^{+} Mφ/cDCs among whole mononuclear cells. (**C**) Proportion of F4/80^{+} CD11b^{+}CD11c^{high} Mφ/cDCs and F4/80^{+} CD11b^{+}CD11c^{low} Mφ/cDCs among whole mononuclear cells. (**D**) Flow cytometry analysis of mononuclear cells isolated from the colons of WT (left column), IL-10$^{-/-}$ (middle), and RAG-2$^{-/-}$ RB^{high} (right) mice. (**E**) Proportion of PDCA-1^{+}CD11b^{-}CD11c^{+} pDCs and F4/80^{+}CD11b^{+}CD11c^{-} Mφ/cDCs among whole mononuclear cells. FACS data are representative of three independent experiments expressed as means ± SEM for each group. WT ($n=4$), IL-10$^{-/-}$ ($n=4$) and RAG-2$^{-/-}$ RB^{high} ($n=3$) mice. *$P<0.05$.

supernatant washed once. Cells were suspended in Histopaque solution (Sigma-Aldrich) and overlaid on HBSS. After centrifugation (780×*g* for 20 min), cells were collected from the upper phase.

Preparation of LP Mononuclear Cells

Cell isolation was performed as previously described [21]. Dissected colon mucosa was incubated with Ca^{2+}, Mg^{2+}-free HBSS containing 1 mM DTT (Sigma-Aldrich) and 5 μM EDTA (Gibco) for 30 min, then treated with 3 mg/ml collagenase (Roche Diagnostics GmbH, Germany) and 0.01% DNase (Worthington Biomedical Co., Freehold, NJ, USA) for 1 h. Cells were pelleted twice through a 40% isotonic Percoll solution and then subjected to Ficoll-Hypaque density gradient centrifugation (40%/75%).

Histological Examination

Liver and colon were fixed in 10% formalin and embedded in paraffin. Sections were stained with H&E and then examined. Histological examination of acute colitis was performed as described previously [22]. Briefly, histological activity score was assessed as the sum of three parameters as follows: extent, 0–3 (0, none; 1, mucosa; 2, mucosa and submucosa; 3, transmural); inflammation, 0–3 (0, none; 1, slight; 2, moderate; 3, severe); crypt damage, 0–4 (0, none; 1, basal 1/3 lost; 2, basal 2/3 lost; 3, only surface epithelium intake; 4, entire crypt and epithelium lost). The score of each parameter was multiplied by a factor of 1–4 (1, 0–25%; 2, 26–50%; 3, 51–75%; 4, 76–100%) according to the percentage of epithelial involvement.

Flow Cytometry

After blocking with anti-FcR (CD16/32, BD bioscience) for 20 min, cells were incubated with specific mAbs at 4°C for 30 min. The following mAbs were used: anti-mouse CD3e-APC-Cy7; anti-CD4-PE-Cy7; anti-NK1.1-APC; anti-CD11b-PE-Cy7; anti-CD11cFITC; 7-AAD; anti-PDCA-1-APC; anti-CCR9-PE; anti-IFN-γ-FITC; and anti-IL-17-APC (eBioscience, BD bioscience). Background fluorescence was assessed by staining with irrelevant anti-rat isotypes (BD bioscience). Stained cells were analyzed by flow cytometry (FACS Canto II, Becton Dickinson Co.) and data analyzed using FlowJo software (Tree Star Inc.) [12].

Quantitative RT-PCR (qPCR)

All qPCR assays were performed as described previously [14]. RNA was extracted from LP mononuclear cells using TRIzol reagent (Invitrogen, Carlsbad, CA, USA) and cDNA was synthesized from 100 ng of total RNA using TaqMan® Reverse Transcription Reagents (Applied Biosystems, Foster City, CA, USA). Reverse transcription was performed at 25°C for 10 min, 48°C for 30 min, and then 95°C for 5 min. cDNA was analyzed by qPCR using TaqMan® Universal PCR Master Mix (Applied Biosystems) in an Applied Biosystems StepOne™/StepOnePlus™ Real-Time PCR System. Cycling conditions for PCR amplification were 50°C for 2 min and 95°C for 10 min, followed by 40 cycles of 95°C for 10 s, then 60°C for 1 min. Relative quantification was achieved by normalizing to the β-actin gene (Applied Biosystems). The following probes were purchased from Applied Biosystems: *Ifng* (99999071_m1), *Tnf* (99999068_m1) and *Actb* (01205647_g1).

In vitro Proliferation Assays

APCs, PDCA-1^{+} pDCs from the livers of C57BL/6 mice, CD11b^{+} Mφs from the inflamed livers of Con A-injected C57BL/6 mice (Con A Mφs), IL-10$^{-/-}$ mouse Mφs, and DSS-treated C57BL/6 mouse Mφs (DSS Mφs) were isolated using a FACS Aria (Becton Dickinson Co.). Enriched naïve CD4^{+} splenocytes obtained from OT-II mice were sorted using a CD4^{+} CD62L^{+} T Cell Isolation Kit II (Miltenyi Biotech, Auburn, CA, USA) and labeled with 1 mM CFSE (Molecular Probes, Eugene, OR, USA) for 10 min at 37°C, followed by the addition of 1.0 ml of FCS for 2 min and washed three times in PBS. CFSE-labeled CD4+ naïve cells (1×10^{5} cells/well) were co-cultured with pDCs or Mφs (2×10^{4} cells/well) in 96-well round-bottom plates for 72 h in the presence of OVA peptides (1 μM). After incubation, cells were collected, incubated with anti-CD4-PE-Cy7 and anti-CD3e-APC-Cy7 and analyzed by FACS; 7-AAD was added to exclude dead cells. Proliferation analysis is based on division times of CFSE^{+}CD4^{+} T cells.

Unlabeled CD4^{+} naïve T cells (1×10^{5} cells/well) were also co-cultured with pDCs or Mφs (2×10^{4} cells/well) for 120 h in the presence of OVA peptides followed by incubation with anti-IFN-γ and/or anti-IL-17 mAbs, and then treated with a Cytofix/Cytoperm kit (BD bioscience). Culture supernatant was collected and analyzed with the BD™ Cytometric Beads Array Mouse Th1/Th2/Th17 Cytokine Kit (Becton Dickinson Co.).

Statistical Analysis

Results are expressed as mean ± SEM. Data groups were analyzed with GraphPad Prism using Tukey-Kramer test and Student's *t*-tests. A *P*-value less than 0.05 was considered statistically significant.

Results

Accumulation of Mononuclear Cells was Induced in the Liver of Mice with Chronic Colitis

To investigate hepatic immunological regulation in the colitic condition, we first used two murine IBD models, RAG-2$^{-/-}$ mice adoptively transferred with splenic CD4^{+}CD45RB^{high} T cells from WT mice (RAG-2$^{-/-}$ RB^{high} mice) and IL-10$^{-/-}$ mice. Consistent with previous reports [15], RAG-2$^{-/-}$ RB^{high} mice showed severe colitis, and infiltration of mononuclear cells in the portal vein area of the liver (Fig. 1A). This was not observed in WT mice. IL-10$^{-/-}$ mice spontaneously developed colitis, characterized by prominent epithelial hyperplasia with leukocyte infiltration into the liver (Fig. 1A). Consistently, the absolute number of liver

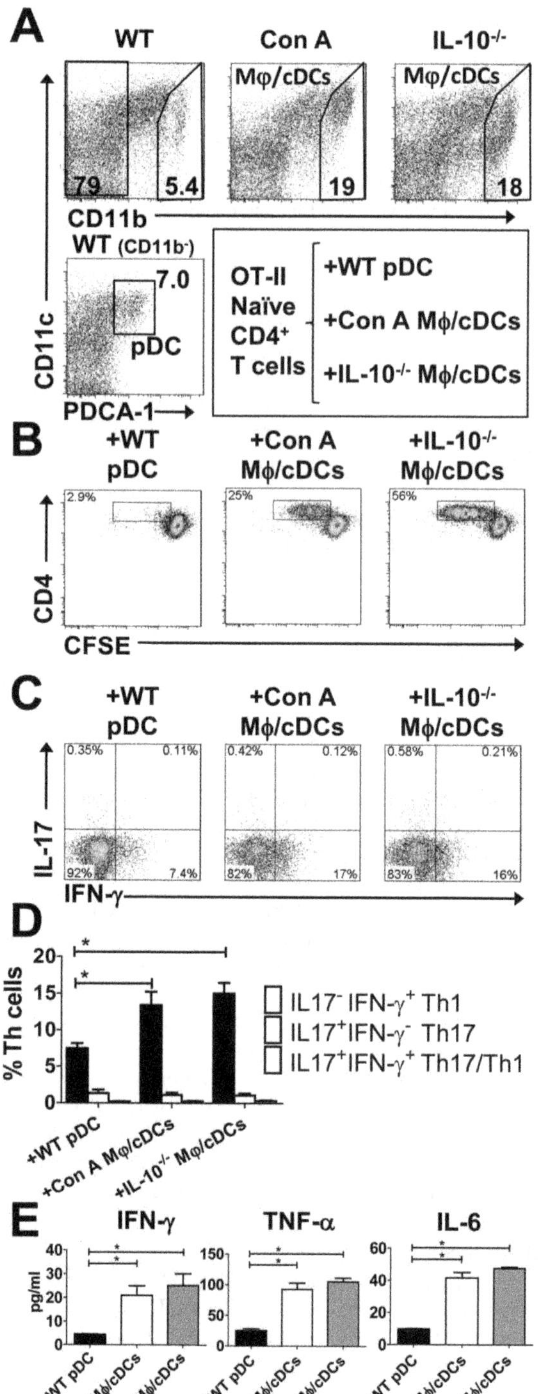

Figure 3. Hepatic Mφ/cDCs cells under colitic conditions induce a Th1 inflammatory response. (**A**) FACS analysis of PDCA-1^+CD11b^-CD11c^{int} pDCs from the livers of WT (left column) mice. We also analyzed CD11b^+CD11c^- Mφs from the livers of ConA-treated (middle) and IL-$10^{-/-}$ (right) mice, respectively. Dead cells were excluded with 7AAD staining. (**B**) Proliferation of naïve CFSE-labeled splenic $CD4^+$ T cells from OT-II mice, and co-cultured WT pDCs, ConA Mφs, or IL-$10^{-/-}$ Mφs in the presence of OVA. Dead cells were excluded with 7AAD staining and $CD4^+$ T cells gated on $CD3^+$ $CD4^+$ cells are shown (B and C). Data are representative of three independent experiments. (**C**) Intracellular IFN-γ and IL-17A expression in $CD4^+$ T cells co-cultured with WT pDCs, ConA Mφs, or IL-$10^{-/-}$ Mφs in the presence of OVA. Data are representative of three independent experiments. (**D**) Proportion of IFN-γ^+IL-$17A^-$, IFN-γ^-IL-$17A^+$, and IFN-γ^+IL-$17A^+$ cells among the Th cell population. (**E**) Cytokine concentrations in the culture supernatant of OT-II $CD4^+$ T cells that were co-cultured with WT pDCs or ConA Mφs. Data are representative of three independent experiments. Each experiment was performed using duplicate samples. $^*P<0.05$.

mononuclear cells in both colitis models was significantly increased when compared with age-matched C57BL/6 mice (Fig. 1B). Liver enzymes (aspartate aminotransferase and alanine aminotransferase) demonstrated no significant changes between WT mice and the two colitis groups (data not shown).

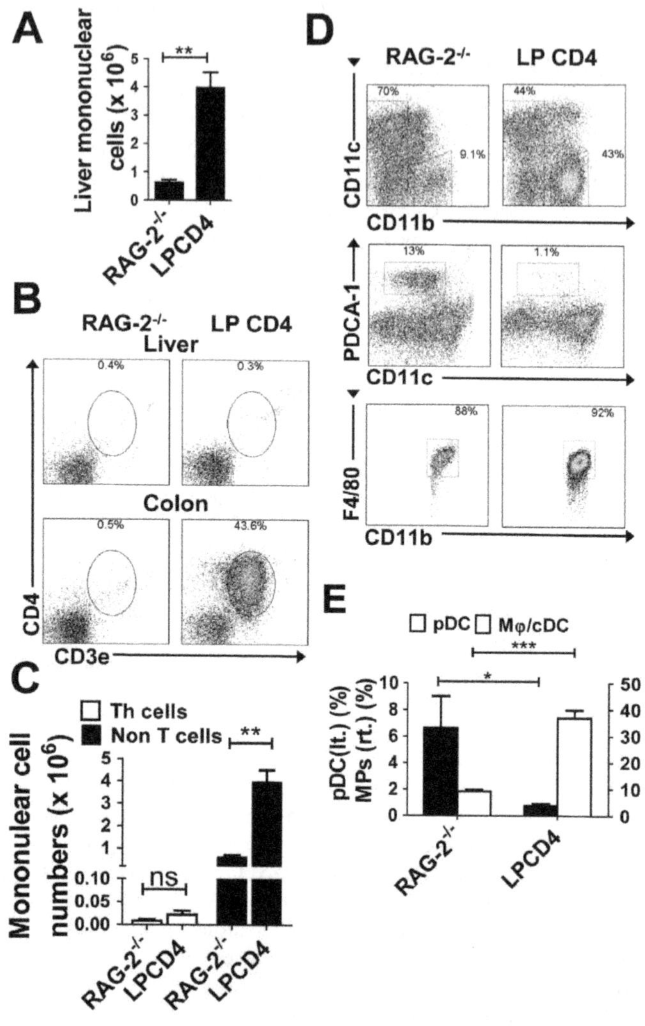

Figure 4. Immune dysregulation in the liver independent of T cell accumulation in the liver. (**A**) Numbers of hepatic mononuclear cells. Data are presented as the mean ± SEM for each group. RAG-$2^{-/-}$ mice ($n=4$) and RAG-$2^{-/-}$ LP $CD4^+$ mice ($n=4$). (**B**) Representative data from flow cytometry analysis of Th cells in each organ. Dead cells were excluded by 7AAD staining. (**C**) Numbers of hepatic $CD3^+$ $CD4^+$ Th cells and non-T cells. (**D**) Representative data from flow cytometry analysis of pDCs and Mφs in the liver of each experimental group. Dead cells were excluded using 7AAD staining. Scatter plots for CD11b^-CD11c^{int} and CD11b^+CD11c^- cells are shown in the middle and bottom rows, respectively. (**E**) Proportion of PDCA-1^+CD11b^-CD11c^{int} pDCs and F4/80^+CD11b^+CD11c^- Mφs among whole mononuclear cells. Data are representative of three independent experiments. Values are presented as the mean ± SEM from seven mice in each group. $^*P<0.05$, $^{**}P<0.01$, $^{***}P<0.005$.

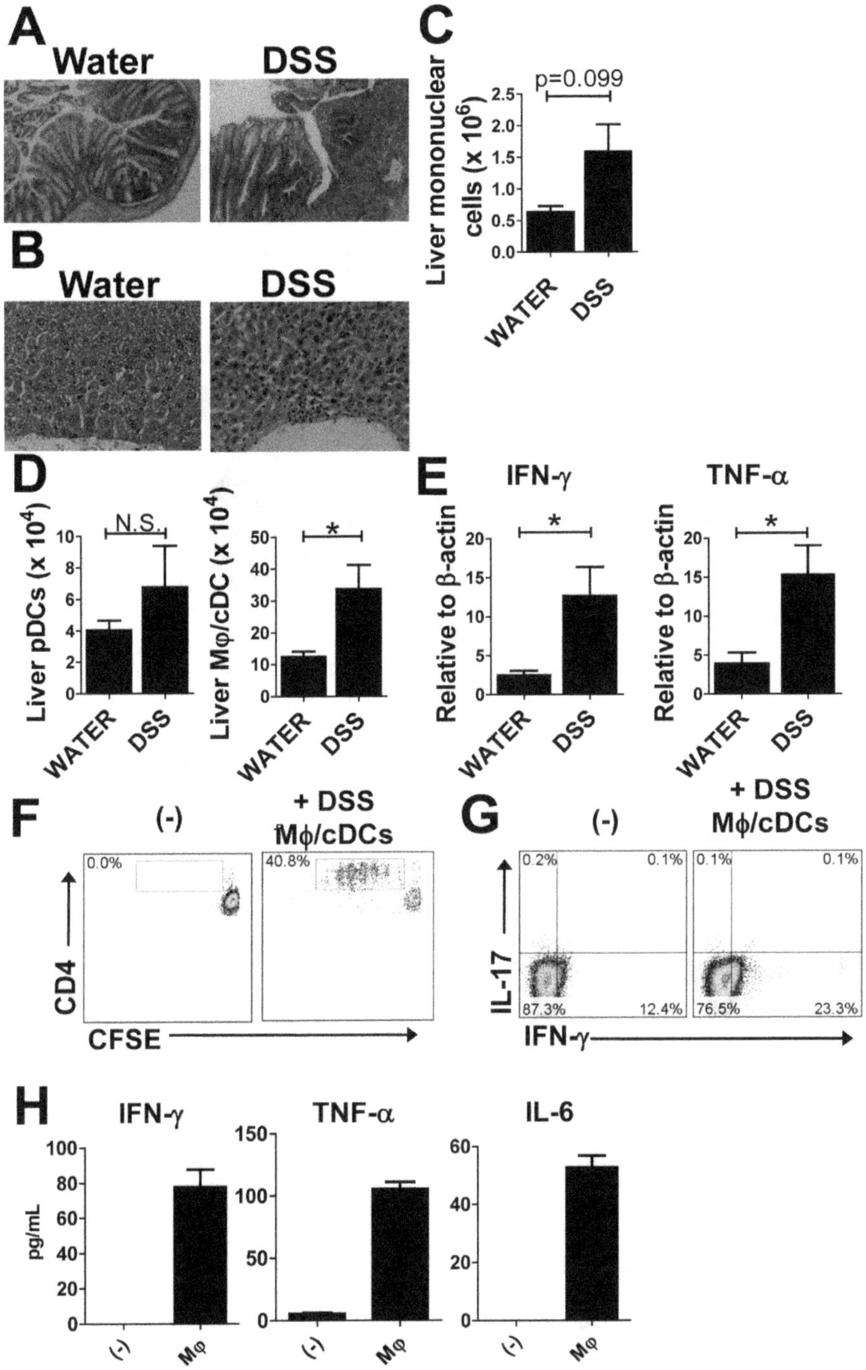

Figure 5. Accumulation of liver macrophages in acute colitis models. (**A**) H&E specimens of the colon taken from mice treated with water (left) or 2% DSS (right). Magnification, ×40 (**B**) H&E specimens of livers from mice treated with water (left) and DSS (right). Magnification, ×100 (**C**) The number of liver mononuclear cells from water- and DSS-treated mice. (**D**) The absolute number of PDCA-1^{+}CD11b^{-}CD11c^{int} pDCs and CD11b^{+}CD11c^{-} Mφs among whole mononuclear cells. Data are representative of three independent experiments. (**E**) Levels of mRNA transcripts for IFN-γ, TNF, and IL-6 in the liver. Values are presented as the mean ± SEM for each group ($n=4$, water-treated group; $n=5$, DSS-treated group). *$P<0.05$. N.S., no significant difference. (**F–H**) Hepatic DSS Mφs induce a Th1 inflammatory response. (**F**) Proliferation of naïve CFSE-labeled splenic $CD4^{+}$ T cells. (**G**) Intracellular IFN-γ and IL-17A expression in naïve CFSE-unlabeled splenic $CD4^{+}$ T cells from OT-II mice that were co-cultured with or without hepatic Mφs from DSS-treated WT mice in the presence of OVA. Dead cells were excluded with 7AAD staining, and $CD4^{+}$ T cells gated on $CD3^{+}$ $CD4^{+}$ cells are shown. Data are representative of two independent experiments. (**H**) Representative cytokine concentrations in culture supernatants from two independent experiments. Each experiment was performed using duplicate samples.

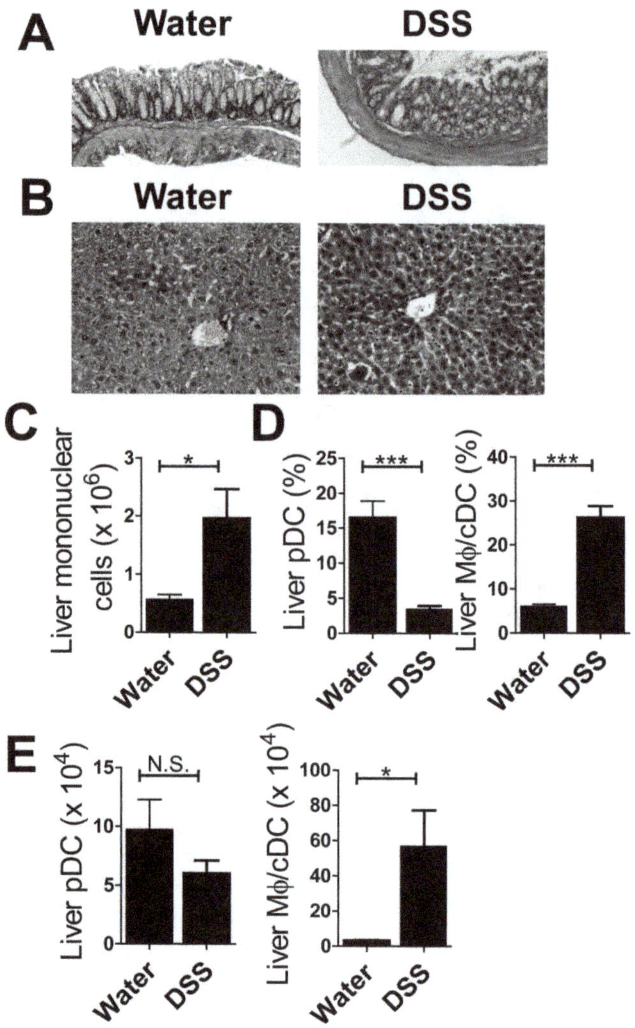

Figure 6. Hepatic infiltration of Macrophages are obserbed in DSS-treated RAG-2$^{-/-}$ mice. (**A**) H&E specimens of colon from mice treated with water (left) or 4% DSS (right). Magnification, ×100 (**B**) H&E specimens of liver from water- (left) and DSS-treated (right) mice. Magnification, ×200 (**C**) The number of liver mononuclear cells for each group of mice. (**D**) Proportion and (**E**) absolute number of PDCA-1^{+}CD11b^{-}CD11c^{int} pDCs and CD11b^{+}CD11c^{-} macrophages among whole mononuclear cells. Data are representative of two independent experiments. Values are presented as the mean ± SEM for each group (*n* = 4, water-treated group; *n* = 4, DSS-treated group). *$P<0.05$. N.S., no significant difference.

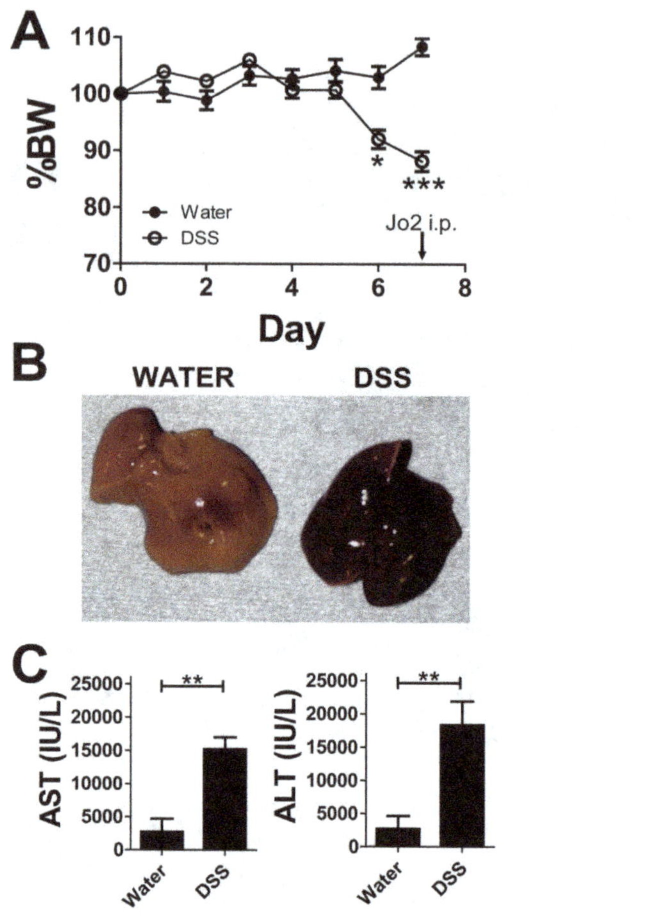

Figure 7. Newly recruited macrophages in the liver during colitis predispose it to inflammation. WT mice were treated under SPF conditions with 2% DSS for 5 days and subsequently with water for 2 days (*n* = 5 mice per group). The Fas-activating antibody, Jo2, was injected i.p. into mice. (**A**) Changes in body weight are expressed as a percentage of original weight. Values are presented as the mean ± SEM for each group. Data are representative of two independent experiments. (**B**) Macroscopic view of livers from water- (left) and DSS-treated mice. (**C**) Levels of aspartate aminotransferase (left) and alanine aminotransferase (right) in water- and DSS-treated mice 6 h after Jo2 injection.

Chronic Colitis is Associated with APC Balance in the Liver

Since it has been reported that Mφ/cDCs and pDCs represent subgroups of APCs differentiated from Mφ/DC precursors [23], we further investigated the composition of APCs in the liver. Analysis of flow cytometry data revealed that the proportion of CD11b^{+}CD11c$^{high/low}$ Mφ/cDCs in the livers (Fig. 2A, first row) of RAG-2$^{-/-}$ RB^{high} and IL-10$^{-/-}$ mice was significantly increased when compared with WT mice. Almost all CD11b^{+}CD11c$^{high/low}$ Mφ/cDCs expressed F4/80 (Fig. 2A, third and fourth rows), therefore we classified them as mononuclear phagocyte system cells. In contrast, the proportion of CD11b^{-}CD11c^{low}PDCA-1^{+} pDCs in the livers of WT mice was significantly higher than those in RAG-2$^{-/-}$ RB^{high} and IL-10$^{-/-}$ mice (Fig. 2A, second row). Statistical analysis confirmed reciprocal changes, where a decrease in the proportion (and absolute number) of pDCs corresponded to an increase in Mφ/cDCs in the liver of colitic mice (Fig. 2B). F4/80^{+} CD11b^{+}CD11c^{high} cells, but not F4/80^{+}CD11b^{+}CD11c^{low} cells, were predominant in hepatic Mφ/cDCs (Fig. 2C). Only a small number of pDCs were found in the LP of the colon under both healthy and colitic conditions (Fig. 2D and E).

Hepatic Mφ/cDCs Under Colitic Conditions Induce a Th1 Inflammatory Response

Owing to finding drastic compositional changes of liver APCs in colitic conditions, we assessed the function of hepatic CD11b^{-}CD11c^{low}PDCA-1^{+} pDCs isolated from the livers of WT mice (WT pDCs), and CD11b^{+}CD11c$^{-/+}$ Mφ/cDCs isolated from the livers of colitic IL-10$^{-/-}$ mice (IL-10$^{-/-}$ Mφ/cDCs) (Fig. 3A). The positive controls were Mφ/cDCs isolated from ConA-treated livers (ConA Mφ/cDCs) (Fig. 3A). We co-cultured pDCs or Mφ/cDCs with naïve CFSE-labeled CD4^{+} T cells in the

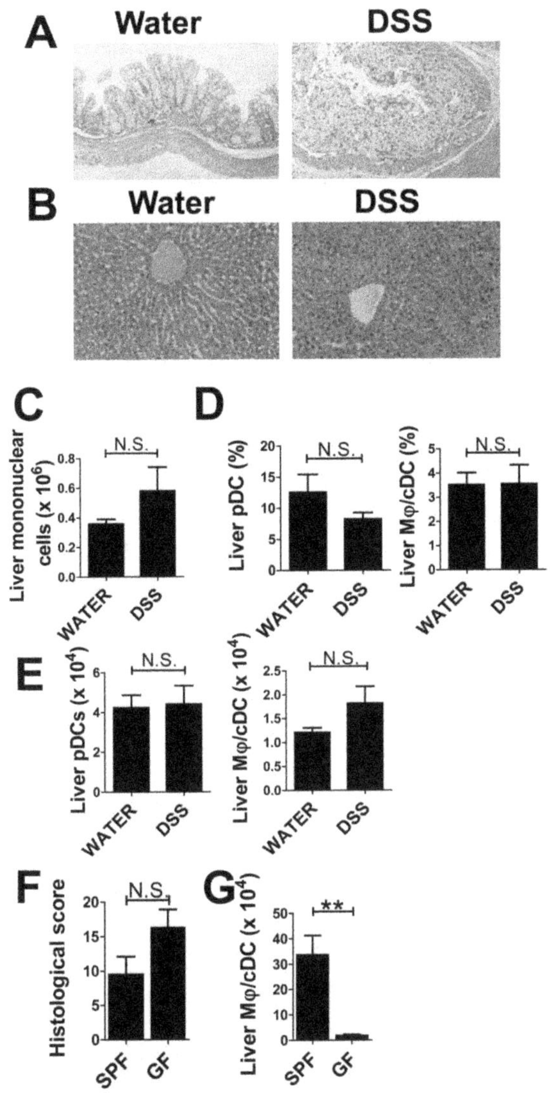

Figure 8. GF condition abrogates the compositional changes of hepatic APCs in acute colitis models. (**A**) H&E staining of colon sections taken from mice treated with water (left) or DSS (right). Magnification, ×100. (**B**) H&E staining of liver sections from water- (left) and DSS-treated (right) mice. Magnification, ×100. (**C**) Number of liver mononuclear cells. (**D**) Proportion and (**E**) absolute number of PDCA-$1^+CD11b^-CD11c^{int}$ pDCs and $CD11b^+CD11c^-$ Mφs among whole mononuclear cells. (**F, G**) Comparisons between SPF and GF in the histology (F) and the numbers of Mφs (G) in DSS-treated mice. Data are representative of two independent experiments. Values are presented as the mean ± SEM for each group ($n = 5$, water-treated GF group; $n = 4$, DSS-treated GF group; $n = 5$, DSS-treated SPF group). N.S., no significant difference.

presence of OVA peptides. After 72 h in culture, $CD4^+$ T cells had extensively divided in the presence of Mφ/cDCs from not only Con A-treated mice but also colitic IL-$10^{-/-}$ mice, but divided little in the presence of WT pDCs (Fig. 3B). To further assess pro-inflammatory responses of Mφ/cDCs, we examined cytokine production from cultured $CD4^+$ T cells. Flow cytometry showed a significant increase in the proportion of IFN-γ-expressing $CD4^+$ T cells following co-culture with IL-$10^{-/-}$ Mφ/cDCs. A similar result was seen with ConA Mφ/cDCs; however, there was no significant increase in IL-17-producing $CD4^+$ T cells (Fig. 3C and D). Consistent with these data, culture supernatants from $CD4^+$ T cells following co-culture with IL-$10^{-/-}$ Mφ/cDCs or ConA Mφ/cDCs exhibited a significant increase in IFN-γ and other pro-inflammatory cytokines such as IL-6 and TNF-α (Fig. 3E).

Immune Dysregulation in the Liver

Given the evidence that activated Mφ/cDCs in the liver instruct naïve $CD4^+$ T cells to differentiate into Th1 cells (Fig. 3C), we then examined whether the primary recruitment of colitogenic Th1 cells to the liver or other mechanisms induced a dysregulation in the balance of Mφ/cDCs and pDCs in the liver under colitic conditions, as mononuclear cells expanded in the liver in colitic RAG-$2^{-/-}$ RB^{high} mice and IL-$10^{-/-}$ mice (Fig. 1). As an alternative mechanism, the breakdown of the colonic barrier and sequential uptake of MAMPs or other gut-derived antigens during the colitis state may play an important role in drastic changes of APCs in the liver. To minimize the effects of liver-infiltrating T cells, we used an adoptive retransfer system: colitogenic LP $CD4^+$ T cells obtained from established RAG-$2^{-/-}$ RB^{high} mice were transferred into RAG-$2^{-/-}$ mice to generate RAG-$2^{-/-}$ LP $CD4^+$ mice, as colitogenic $CD4^+$ T cells residing in the intestine express gut-specific homing receptors and have an ability to preferentially migrate to the intestine but not to liver [24,25]. These mice developed severe colitis (data not shown) and also showed significant increases in the number of liver-infiltrating mononuclear cells (Fig. 4A). The RAG-$2^{-/-}$ LP $CD4^+$ mice showed almost no $CD3^+CD4^+$ T cell infiltration in the liver, but did exhibit severe colitis with marked infiltrations of $CD3^+CD4^+$ T cells in the colon (Fig. 4B). We confirmed statistically that the significant increases in liver mononuclear cells in RAG-$2^{-/-}$ LP $CD4^+$ mice was due to the emergence of non-T cells (possibly APCs) (Fig. 4C). We further investigated compartments of APCs in the liver of RAG-$2^{-/-}$ LP $CD4^+$ mice. Consistent with the data from colitic RAG-$2^{-/-}$ RB^{high} or IL-$10^{-/-}$ mice (Fig. 2), RAG-$2^{-/-}$ LP $CD4^+$ mice also showed reciprocal changes; a significant decrease in pDCs corresponded with an increase in Mφ/cDCs (Fig. 4D and E). RAG-$2^{-/-}$ LP $CD4^+$ mice exhibited severe colitis without infiltration of T cells in the liver (Fig. 4B and 4C). These data suggest that intestinal inflammation induce changes in the compartments of APCs.

Accumulation of Mφ/cDCs in the Livers of Mice with DSS-induced Colitis

To further determine whether hepatic immune dysregulation is caused by barrier disruption of the intestinal wall, we looked at livers from immune-sufficient WT mice subjected to DSS-induced colitis under SPF conditions. Seven days after the start of DSS administration, mice exhibited severe colitis and infiltration of mononuclear cells in the liver (Fig. 5A and B). Consistent with histological data, liver mononuclear cells were upregulated in DSS-treated mice when compared with water-treated mice (Fig. 5C). Flow cytometry revealed that the number of Mφ/cDCs was significantly increased in the livers of DSS-treated mice; however, there were no significant changes in the numbers of pDCs (Fig. 5D). Expression levels of IFN-γ and TNF-α in the liver were significantly increased in DSS-treated mice (Fig. 5E). Furthermore, hepatic Mφ/cDCs in the DSS-treated mice promoted proliferation of $CD4^+$ T cells (Fig. 5F), and increased the proportion of IFN-γ-expressing $CD4^+$ T cells (Fig. 5G). We detected a significant increase in pro-inflammtory cytokines in co-culture supernatants (Fig. 5H).

We also confirmed the reciprocal changes for pDCs and Mφ/cDCs in DSS-treated RAG-$2^{-/-}$ mice, which had severe colitis and infiltration of mononuclear cells in the liver (Fig. 6A, B and C). The proportion of pDCs was decreased in DSS-treated RAG-$2^{-/}$

− mice (Fig. 6D). Furthermore, the proportion and number of Mφ/cDCs was increased, even in mice lacking $CD4^+$ T cells (Fig. 6D and E). These data suggest that colon inflammation induces the recruitment of Mφ/cDCs and these newly recruited Mφ/cDCs stimulate Th1 cells or promote differentiation of Th1 cells.

We also assessed whether these Mφ/cDCs that emerged under colitic conditions contributed to acute liver inflammation, which had been initially induced by Fas-activating antibody (Jo2) [18,19]. As shown in Fig. 7A, DSS-treated mice with significant body weight loss underwent Jo2 treatment. The livers of DSS-induced colitic mice in which Jo2 was administered showed significant blood accumulation (Fig. 7B). Consistently, the levels of aspartate aminotransferase and alanine aminotransferase were significantly increased in DSS mice after Jo2 treatment compared with non-DSS mice (Fig. 7C).

Leukocyte Infiltration was not Detected in Acute Colitis Models Under GF Conditions

We investigated whether MAMPs or other bacterial degradation products induce hepatic immune dysregulation and analyzed the livers of mice treated with DSS under GF conditions. Bacteria do not reside in the intestines of GF mice, meaning there is no inflow of bacterial components into the liver. Mice treated with DSS under GF conditions showed severe colitis; however, there was no evidence of leukocyte infiltration (Fig. 8A and B). Consistent with histological data, we observed no significant changes in the number of liver mononuclear cells for controls and DSS-treated mice (Fig. 8C). Flow cytometry data showed that there were no significant changes in the ratios of pDCs to Mφ/cDCs (Fig. 8D); or in the absolute numbers of these cells in the livers of DSS-treated mice (Fig. 8E). DSS-treated GF mice also exhibited severe colitis compared with SPF mice (Fig. 8F), but Mφ/cDCs were not increased (Fig. 8G). These findings indicate that bacterial products play a crucial role in inducing infiltration of Mφ/cDCs into the liver.

Discussion

In this study we demonstrated: (1) hepatic pDCs are decreased and Mφ/cDCs are increased in mice with chronic intestinal inflammation; (2) newly emerged Mφ/cDCs during the development of colitis possess pro-inflammatory characteristics that drive differentiation of naïve T cells toward Th1 cells; (3) Mφ/cDCs that emerge during colitis possibly result in the exacerbation of hepatitis symptoms; and (4) the reciprocal changes we observed in the compartments of the liver's innate immune system during intestinal inflammation were mainly caused by MAMPs, other bacterial degradation products, or bacteria themselves subsequent to the disruption of the intestinal wall. Changes in APC compartments were seen not only in RAG-$2^{-/-}$ RB^{high} mice and DSS-administered mice but also in RAG-$2^{-/-}$ mice retransferred with gut-tropic colitogenic LP $CD4^+$ T cells in SPF conditions; but were not seen in mice of the DSS colitis model in the GF condition that lack commensal bacteria in the gut.

Previous studies have suggested a relationship between intestinal and liver inflammation [2,3,11,26]. These previous reports support our hypothesis that intestinal inflammation skews the balance of immune cells in the liver. However, no expansive research has been conducted to clarify the inflammatory relationship between the liver and the intestine. In this study, we are the first to demonstrate distinctive changes in compartments (pDCs vs. Mφ/cDCs) of hepatic immune cells due to chronic intestinal inflammation. Increased hepatic Mφ/cDCs appeared irrespective of whether the colitis model was acute or chronic. Immunological changes were not only observed in the liver during colitis, but also in ConA-induced liver injury (Fig. 3A) [14], suggesting that these changes are universal phenomena during liver stress.

We hoped to elucidate how these crucial changes of hepatic APCs occur during intestinal inflammation. The liver is between the portal and systemic circulatory systems. The liver receives continuous blood supplements from the intestine via the portal vein and is presumably exposed to MAMPs or other degradation products from viable or non-viable commensal bacteria [8]. We used a GF system to demonstrate the importance of bacterial components in causing immunological dysregulation in the liver. Most models of experimental colitis fail to develop under GF conditions [27,28]; however, we used a DSS model, which is known to result in the development of severe colitis [29,30]. DSS-treated mice under SPF conditions exhibited Mφ/cDC infiltration into the liver (Fig. 5 and 8). This was not observed for DSS-treated mice under GF conditions despite the existence of severe colitis. This means that the accumulation of Mφ/cDCs is not just a consequence of nonspecific inflammation related with colitis. Mice under GF conditions lack the protective effects against colitis from microbiota [31], but also lack the stimulant transferred from the intestine to the liver. These data suggest that stimulation from degradation products from intestinal commensal bacteria play an important role in recruitment of Mφ/cDCs.

Various commensal bacteria that usually reside in the intestine (such as *C. coccoides*, *C. leptum* and *Enterococcus)* were found in ConA-treated and untreated livers [20]. Such a finding lends support to the hypothesis that intestinal bacterial products or bacteria themselves are transferred from the intestine to the liver. The rate (and amount) of uptake of bacteria-derived products, such as microbial DNA and LPS, is thought to increase during colitis because of the fragility of the colon wall [11,32]. Further study is required to estimate the amount and type of bacterial products that stimulate the liver during colitis.

Despite our finding that recruitment of Mφ/cDCs is stimulated by bacterial degradation products or bacteria themselves, several scenarios may be considered as additional mechanisms underlying the accumulation of Mφ/cDCs. First, activated Mφ/cDCs themselves migrate from the intestine to the liver. Alternatively, circulating monocytes accumulate in the liver stimulated by pro-inflammatory cytokines transferred via the portal vein, such as TNF-α produced by LP $CD4^+$ T cells or APCs in the intestine [30]. However, pro-inflammatory cytokines are produced in the colon of GF mice, so this possibility may only have a partial effect. Whether increased Mφ/cDCs originate from monocytes or resident macrophages in the liver should be explored in future studies. Third, activated T cells migrate from the intestine to the liver and stimulate the liver to recruit and activate circulating or resident Mφ/cDCs. RAG-$2^{-/-}$ LP $CD4^+$ mice (Fig. 3) and DSS-treated RAG-$2^{-/-}$ (Fig. 6) mice show increased Mφ/cDCs without infiltration of T, B, and NKT cells in the liver, which suggests that Mφ/cDCs are recruited to the liver independently of T, B, and NKT cells. However, there still remains involvement of cytokines, DSS itself and other types of the cells such as NK cells and liver sinusoidal endothelial. Macrophages accumulated during both acute and chronic colitis models in the liver produced inflammatory cytokines and promoted differentiation of Th1 cells or activation of NK cells. Thus, it is likely that systemic IFN-γ production leads subsequent upregulation of the sensitivity of FAS-mediated signal in the liver.

The current study suggests that hepatic APC compartments alter in parallel with the progression of colitis, and increased Mφ/

cDCs have pro-inflammatory characteristics. Two major hepatic diseases presenting as extraintestinal manifestations in IBD patients are PSC and autoimmune hepatitis. The prevalence of these liver diseases is reported, both in Crohn's disease and ulcerative colitis, to correlate with the severity and expansion of the intestinal disease [3,26,33]. The active disease is associated with ongoing extraintestinal manifestations in patients with Crohn's disease [26]. The prevalence of PSC was 5.5% in patients with substantial colitis and 0.5% in patients with distal colitis [2]. Therefore, Mφ/cDCs infiltrating into the liver in the colitis models may be involved in the pathogenesis of IBD-related liver diseases. However, liver enzymes demonstrated no significant changes during colitis unlike autoimmune hepatitis or PSC. Thus, we hypothesized that accumulated Mφ/cDCs may increase the susceptibility of hepatitis. We combined the Fas-mediated model of hepatitis with the DSS colitis models to show the clinical importance of our study. Fas-mediated hepatitis models are widely used as a model of hepatitis [18,19]. TNF-α released by activated hepatic macrophages is one of the very important factors that damage hepatocytes, which are highly sensitive to cell-extrinsic stimulation in Fas-mediated hepatitis [19]. We also suggest the importance of the infiltration of macrophages in fulminant hepatitis models [10]. Mφ/cDCs recruited to the liver during colitis in a T cell-independent manner produce pro-inflammatory cytokines and promote Th1 reaction. $CD11b^{+}CD11c^{low/+}$ Mφ/cDCs are already detectable in healthy WT mice (Fig. 2B), but previous studies suggest that these resident macrophages including Kupffer cells have a immunoregulatory character, such as producing IL-10 [6,34]. Taken together with the previous studies and our findings, Mφ/cDCs infiltrating into the liver during colitis may contribute to making the hepatitis worse. Some additional stimulation would be needed for breaking down liver tolerance and causing hepatitis or cholangitis which mimics liver diseases associated with IBD.

An additional finding of our study is that pDCs are significantly decreased in the late phase of colitis in the chronic models. Hepatic pDCs plays an important role in maintaining liver homeostasis [9,10,14], so not only increased Mφ/cDCs but decreased pDCs may have effects on the infiltration of mononuclear cells in the liver during chronic colitis. This is known as sustained negative regulation of LPS signaling in response to a second LPS stimulus. pDCs express certain toll-like receptors (TLR) [14], with the number of spleen pDCs decreasing following TLR treatment [35]. These previous reports suggest that pDCs are one of the initial sensors of MAMPs or other degradation products, and possibly decrease when the endotoxin tolerance is broken down. Further studies will be needed to address this issue.

In conclusion, the findings from our study suggest that dysregulation in the balance of liver APCs, especially in the recruitment of pro-inflammatory Mφ/cDCs, during colitis occurs in a T-cell-independent manner for chronic and acute murine colitis models. This report may provide the basis for a novel strategy to treat intractable immune diseases in the liver. We have also highlighted the relevance of the relationship between liver and intestine immunology during intestinal inflammation.

Acknowledgments

We thank A. Matsumoto, T. Handa, Y. Ono, N. Taniki, K. Takeshita, K. Saigusa and K. Kimura for their help with some of the experiments. We are grateful to M. K. Tokutake and M. Takabe for their assistance with the care of experimental animals.

Author Contributions

Conceived and designed the experiments: YM AY TK. Performed the experiments: YM SM NN AH. Analyzed the data: YM T. Sujino T. Sato KM T. Hisamatsu HE T. Hibi NK. Wrote the paper: YM AY TK.

References

1. Baumgart DC, Sandborn WJ (2007) Inflammatory bowel disease: clinical aspects and established and evolving therapies. Lancet 369: 1641–1657.
2. Olsson R, Danielsson A, Jarnerot G, Lindstrom E, Loof L, et al. (1991) Prevalence of primary sclerosing cholangitis in patients with ulcerative colitis. Gastroenterology 100: 1319–1323.
3. Rasmussen HH, Fallingborg JF, Mortensen PB, Vyberg M, Tage-Jensen U, et al. (1997) Hepatobiliary dysfunction and primary sclerosing cholangitis in patients with Crohn's disease. Scand J Gastroenterol 32: 604–610.
4. Tremaroli V, Backhed F (2012) Functional interactions between the gut microbiota and host metabolism. Nature 489: 242–249.
5. Kaisho T, Takeuchi O, Kawai T, Hoshino K, Akira S (2001) Endotoxin-induced maturation of MyD88-deficient dendritic cells. J Immunol 166: 5688–5694.
6. Crispe IN (2009) The liver as a lymphoid organ. Annu Rev Immunol 27: 147–163.
7. Crispe IN (2003) Hepatic T cells and liver tolerance. Nat Rev Immunol 3: 51–62.
8. Thomson AW, Knolle PA (2010) Antigen-presenting cell function in the tolerogenic liver environment. Nat Rev Immunol 10: 753–766.
9. Goubier A, Dubois B, Gheit H, Joubert G, Villard-Truc F, et al. (2008) Plasmacytoid dendritic cells mediate oral tolerance. Immunity 29: 464–475.
10. Tokita D, Sumpter TL, Raimondi G, Zahorchak AF, Wang Z, et al. (2008) Poor allostimulatory function of liver plasmacytoid DC is associated with pro-apoptotic activity, dependent on regulatory T cells. J Hepatol 49: 1008–1018.
11. Gabele E, Dostert K, Hofmann C, Wiest R, Scholmerich J, et al. (2011) DSS induced colitis increases portal LPS levels and enhances hepatic inflammation and fibrogenesis in experimental NASH. J Hepatol 55: 1391–1399.
12. Kamada N, Hisamatsu T, Okamoto S, Sato T, Matsuoka K, et al. (2005) Abnormally differentiated subsets of intestinal macrophage play a key role in Th1-dominant chronic colitis through excess production of IL-12 and IL-23 in response to bacteria. J Immunol 175: 6900–6908.
13. Kamada N, Hisamatsu T, Okamoto S, Chinen H, Kobayashi T, et al. (2008) Unique CD14 intestinal macrophages contribute to the pathogenesis of Crohn disease via IL-23/IFN-gamma axis. J Clin Invest 118: 2269–2280.
14. Nakamoto N, Ebinuma H, Kanai T, Chu PS, Ono Y, et al. (2012) CCR9(+) Macrophages Are Required for Acute Liver Inflammation in Mouse Models of Hepatitis. Gastroenterology 142: 366–376.
15. Powrie F, Leach MW, Mauze S, Caddle LB, Coffman RL (1993) Phenotypically distinct subsets of CD4+ T cells induce or protect from chronic intestinal inflammation in C. B-17 scid mice. Int Immunol 5: 1461–1471.
16. Ishii K, Kanai T, Totsuka T, Uraushihara K, Ishikura T, et al. (2004) Hyperexpression of inducible costimulator on lamina propria mononuclear cells in rat dextran sulfate sodium colitis. J Gastroenterol Hepatol 19: 174–181.
17. Kuhn R, Lohler J, Rennick D, Rajewsky K, Muller W (1993) Interleukin-10-deficient mice develop chronic enterocolitis. Cell 75: 263–274.
18. Murthy A, Defamie V, Smookler DS, Di Grappa MA, Horiuchi K, et al. (2010) Ectodomain shedding of EGFR ligands and TNFR1 dictates hepatocyte apoptosis during fulminant hepatitis in mice. J Clin Invest 120: 2731–2744.
19. Ogasawara J, Watanabe-Fukunaga R, Adachi M, Matsuzawa A, Kasugai T, et al. (1993) Lethal effect of the anti-Fas antibody in mice. Nature 364: 806–809.
20. Ojiro K, Ebinuma H, Nakamoto N, Wakabayashi K, Mikami Y, et al. (2010) MyD88-dependent pathway accelerates the liver damage of Concanavalin A-induced hepatitis. Biochem Biophys Res Commun 399: 744–749.
21. Mikami Y, Kanai T, Sujino T, Ono Y, Hayashi A, et al. (2010) Competition between colitogenic Th1 and Th17 cells contributes to the amelioration of colitis. Eur J Immunol 40: 2409–2422.
22. Kimura K, Kanai T, Hayashi A, Mikami Y, Sujino T, et al. (2012) Dysregulated balance of retinoid-related orphan receptor gammat-dependent innate lymphoid cells is involved in the pathogenesis of chronic DSS-induced colitis. Biochem Biophys Res Commun 427: 694–700.
23. Geissmann F, Manz MG, Jung S, Sieweke MH, Merad M, et al. (2010) Development of monocytes, macrophages, and dendritic cells. Science 327: 656–661.
24. Mora JR, Bono MR, Manjunath N, Weninger W, Cavanagh LL, et al. (2003) Selective imprinting of gut-homing T cells by Peyer's patch dendritic cells. Nature 424: 88–93.
25. Nemoto Y, Kanai T, Kameyama K, Shinohara T, Sakamoto N, et al. (2009) Long-lived colitogenic CD4+ memory T cells residing outside the intestine participate in the perpetuation of chronic colitis. J Immunol 183: 5059–5068.

26. Vavricka SR, Brun L, Ballabeni P, Pittet V, Prinz Vavricka BM, et al. (2011) Frequency and risk factors for extraintestinal manifestations in the Swiss inflammatory bowel disease cohort. Am J Gastroenterol 106: 110–119.
27. Podolsky DK (2002) Inflammatory bowel disease. N Engl J Med 347: 417–429.
28. Sartor RB (2006) Mechanisms of disease: pathogenesis of Crohn's disease and ulcerative colitis. Nat Clin Pract Gastroenterol Hepatol 3: 390–407.
29. Hayashi A, Sato T, Kamada N, Mikami Y, Matsuoka K, et al. (2013) A Single Strain of Clostridium butyricum Induces Intestinal IL-10-Producing Macrophages to Suppress Acute Experimental Colitis in Mice. Cell Host Microbe 13: 711–722.
30. Maslowski KM, Vieira AT, Ng A, Kranich J, Sierro F, et al. (2009) Regulation of inflammatory responses by gut microbiota and chemoattractant receptor GPR43. Nature 461: 1282–1286.
31. Rakoff-Nahoum S, Paglino J, Eslami-Varzaneh F, Edberg S, Medzhitov R (2004) Recognition of commensal microflora by toll-like receptors is required for intestinal homeostasis. Cell 118: 229–241.
32. Henao-Mejia J, Elinav E, Jin C, Hao L, Mehal WZ, et al. (2012) Inflammasome-mediated dysbiosis regulates progression of NAFLD and obesity. Nature 482: 179–185.
33. Bjornsson E, Olsson R, Bergquist A, Lindgren S, Braden B, et al. (2008) The natural history of small-duct primary sclerosing cholangitis. Gastroenterology 134: 975–980.
34. Knolle P, Schlaak J, Uhrig A, Kempf P, Meyer zum Buschenfelde KH, et al. (1995) Human Kupffer cells secrete IL-10 in response to lipopolysaccharide (LPS) challenge. J Hepatol 22: 226–229.
35. Swiecki M, Wang Y, Vermi W, Gilfillan S, Schreiber RD, et al. (2011) Type I interferon negatively controls plasmacytoid dendritic cell numbers in vivo. J Exp Med 208: 2367–2374.

10

Temporal Colonic Gene Expression Profiling in the Recurrent Colitis Model Identifies Early and Chronic Inflammatory Processes

Bas Kremer[1,3]*, Rob Mariman[1,2], Marjan van Erk[3], Tonny Lagerweij[1], Lex Nagelkerken[1]

1 Department of Metabolic Health Research, TNO, Leiden, The Netherlands, **2** Department of Immunohematology and Bloodtransfusion, Leiden University Medical Centrum, Leiden, The Netherlands, **3** Department of Microbiology and Systems Biology, TNO, Zeist, The Netherlands

Abstract

The recurrent TNBS-colitis model in BALB/c mice has been proposed as a model of Inflammatory Bowel Disease with a shifting pattern of local cytokines with the expression of Th1 cytokines during the early phase, Th17 cytokines during the intermediate phase and Th2 cytokines during late fibrotic stages. In this study, we evaluated the development of pathology in time–in conjunction with genome-wide gene expression in the colons–in response to three weekly intrarectal instillations of TNBS. During this time-frame mice develop colitis with extensive cellular infiltration of (sub)mucosa and mildly to moderately affected crypt architecture. These pathological processes were sensitive to local treatment with budesonide. Gene expression profiling confirmed an acute phase response after each intrarectal TNBS-challenge. In addition, a chronic inflammatory process developed over time particularly evident from a gradual increase in expression of mast cell related genes. The changes in pathological hallmarks were consistent with a temporal expression of mRNA encoding a selection of chemokines. In conclusion, the early stages of the recurrent TNBS-colitis model reflect several aspects of inflammatory bowel disease which are sensitive to immunomodulation.

Editor: Benoit Foligne, Institut Pasteur de Lille, France

Funding: No current external funding sources for this study.

Competing Interests: BK, LN and MvE are employed by TNO, a not-for-profit organization regulated by public law. TNO is an independent research organization dealing with health-related research, not part of any government, university or company. There are no patents, products in development, or marketed products to declare. The organization may benefit from its knowledge, by supporting companies in their product development by consultancy and research. In these cases, the authors will not receive additional salary, additional personal income, or any form of financial support.

* E-mail: bas.kremer@tno.nl

Introduction

Inflammatory Bowel Diseases (IBD), with Ulcerative Colitis (UC) and Crohn's Disease (CD) as major entities, are chronic inflammatory disorders of the gastrointestinal tract, affecting an estimated 3.6 million people in Europe and the US [1]. IBD may be chronic or relapsing in nature, possibly due to a process of inflammation following an exaggerated immune response against enteric microorganisms. These processes affect intestinal function leading to diarrhea, cramping, and abdominal pain. Although considerable progress has been achieved with regard to the multifactorial nature of IBD [2], current therapies show limited efficacy [3].

Although there is a clear medical need to develop novel anti-inflammatory therapy for IBD, the evaluation of novel therapeutic strategies is hampered by the availability of suitable preclinical efficacy models. Most frequently, acute colitis models such as dextrane sodium sulphate (DSS) and the 2,4,6-trinitrobenzene sulfonic acid (TNBS) induced colitis are used [4,5]. These models are characterized by severe acute inflammation of the colon representing histopathological aspects that reflect human IBD. Whereas the DSS-colitis model involves activation of the innate immune system in particular, the TNBS model was shown to depend on a local Th-1 biased response [6]. The acute chemically induced IBD models have been shown of great value for a better understanding of acute inflammatory disease processes in IBD. In addition, efficacies of a limited number of relevant treatments have been reported in these models [7–9].

As an alternative to chemically induced colitis, several models helped to gain valuable insight into the underlying pathology of IBD, such as the model based on transfer of $CD45RB^{Hi}$ $CD4^{+}$ T cell to immunodeficient recipients or the development of colitis in IL-10 deficient mice [10,11]. These models put emphasis on the role of the intestinal microbiota eliciting a chronic inflammatory response in the gut. However, because these models are performed in an immunodeficient environment with disturbed immunoregulatory circuits they are not always suitable for the evaluation of novel therapeutic strategies.

In recent years, several groups have demonstrated that repeated intrarectal administrations of low-dose TNBS to mice and rats result in chronic colitis [12,13]. This colitis model has primarily been used to study fibrotic processes as a consequence of chronic intestinal inflammation [14,15]. Recently, we have implemented a modified protocol of the chronic TNBS colitis model with reduced duration, in which treatment with probiotics was shown to prevent the onset of chronic colitis and associated clinical symptoms, suggesting sensitivity to immunomodulation [16].

In this report, we characterize the processes underlying the development of pathology in this model by temporal gene expression profiling in the colon with the aim to further substantiate the value of this model for both mechanistic and pre-clinical efficacy studies. We show that the recurrent TNBS-induced colitis model combines histopathological features with aspects of active inflammation and chronic processes of cellular infiltration, angiogenesis and tissue remodeling, which are all relevant to human IBD.

Results

Recurrent TNBS-colitis: a Model with Low Mortality Sensitive to Intrarectal Budesonide

In this study, we evaluated early stages of the recurrent TNBS colitis model and confined ourselves to 4 weeks of follow-up after skin sensitization and three weekly intrarectal challenges with increasing dosages of TNBS, thereby combining two previously published protocols [5,15]. This adapted protocol consistently resulted in mild to moderate colitis, reflected by significant growth

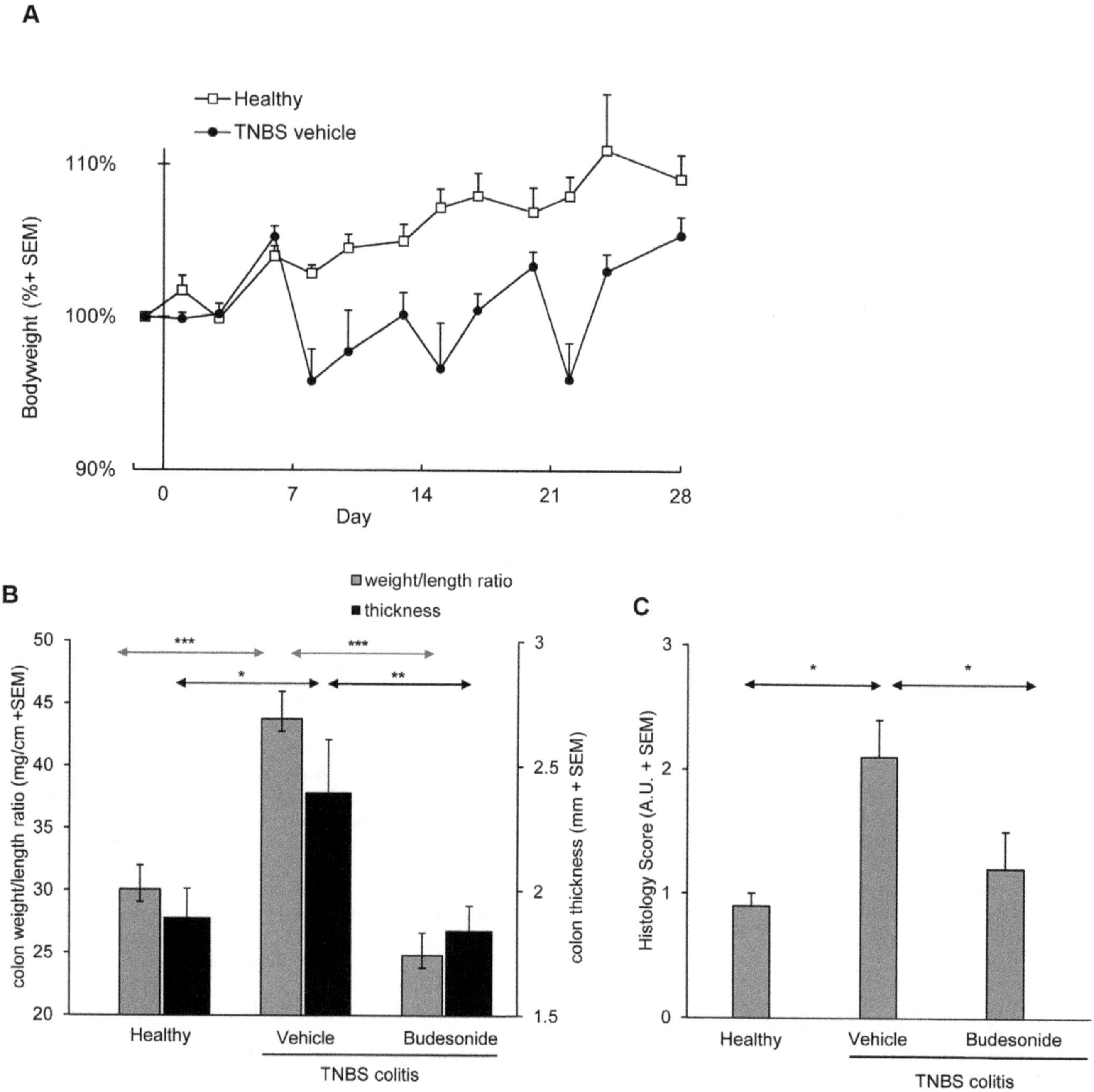

Figure 1. Disease characteristics of the recurrent TNBS model and efficacy of budesonide treatment. The development of colitis induction is evident from periods of loss of body weight following each rectal instillation of TNBS (Figure 1A; AUC $p<0.005$). At end-point, inflamed colons show significantly increased weight/length ratios and colon thickness (Figure 1B); both aspects are suppressed by budesonide. TNBS colitis induction is associated with a significantly increased histological score (Figure 1C); this score is significantly lower in budesonide treated animals. Bars represent group mean values of 10–12 mice/group, error bars represent SEM. Mann-Whitney U-test; *$p<0.05$, **$p<0.01$, ***$p<0.001$.

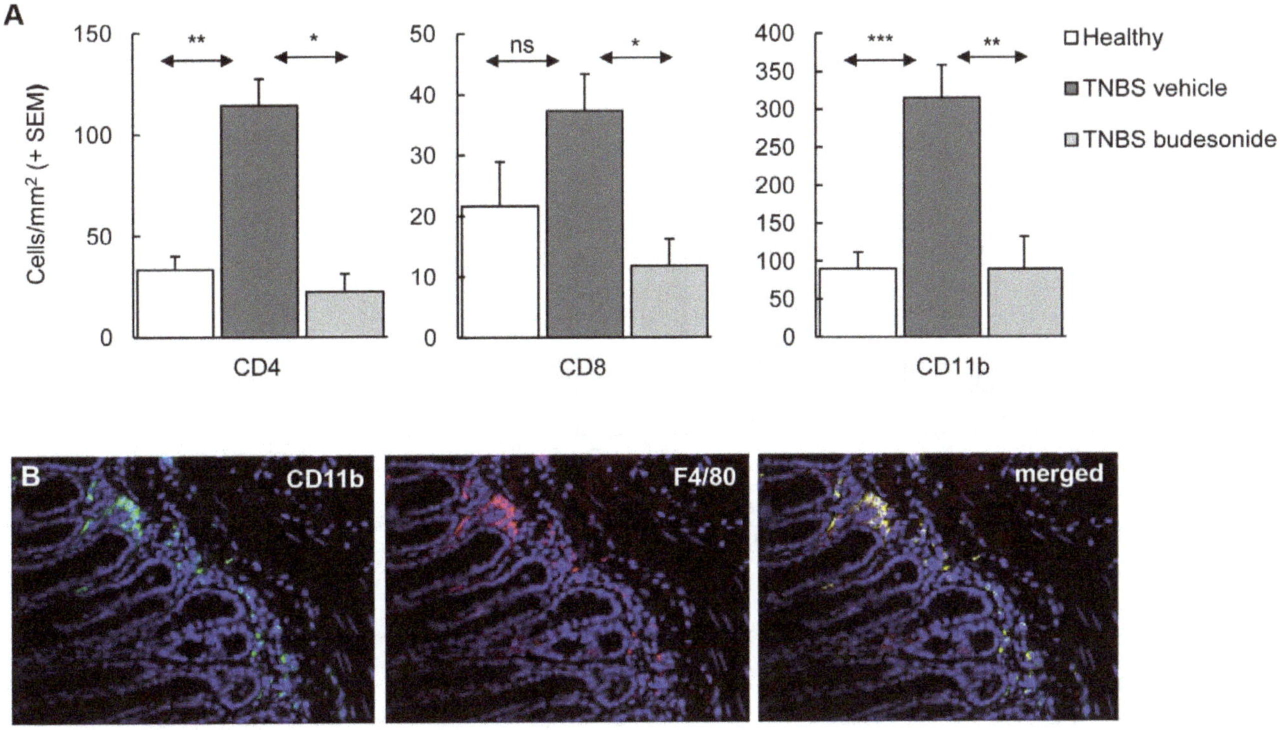

Figure 2. Colitis induction is associated with increased numbers of innate and adaptive immune cells. The composition of the cellular infiltrate and the effect of budesonide treatment were analyzed by immunohistochemistry. (**A**) Enumeration of the cells showed significantly increased cell numbers per mm^2 tissue due to TNBS colitis induction. Budesonide treatment significantly reduced the number of these infiltrating cells. Bars represent group mean values of 10–12 mice/group, error bars represent SEM. Mann-Whitney U-test; *$p<0.05$, **$p<0.01$, ***$p<0.001$. (**B**) Double staining of CD11b+ and F480+ cells using fluorescence microscopy confirmed co-expression of these two cell surface markers.

retardation ($p<0.005$) (Figure 1A). Each rectal TNBS instillation induced transient loss of body weight of 5 to 15%. Average mortality was less than 15% and in particular associated with the first rectal challenge. At endpoint, colitis was evident from an increased colon weight/length ratio and increased thickening of the colon (Figure 1B). These macroscopic changes were associated with increased histology scores in the distal part of the colon (Figure 1C). Infiltration of mucosa and submucosa by CD4$^+$ and CD8$^+$ T cells, CD11b$^+$ cells (Figure 2A), confirmed as macrophages by F4/80 staining (Figure 2B) was associated with mild to moderate damage of the mucosal architecture.

All of these aspects were suppressed in mice treated by intrarectal administration of budesonide. Besides, budesonide treatment was associated with weight loss, typical for chronic exposure to corticosteroids in mice.

Multiplex analysis of 23 different cytokines and chemokines in serum collected at endpoint revealed significantly increased levels of IFN-γ, IL-1β, IL-17, MCP-1 and MIP-1β in mice with colitis, but not in mice treated with budesonide. Furthermore, budesonide suppressed IL-12p40 levels even compared to the serum concentrations in healthy control mice (Table 1).

Altogether, several inflammatory characteristics relevant to IBD are represented in this model and shown to be sensitive to corticosteroid treatment.

Alterations in Gene Expression during the Development of Recurrent TNBS Colitis

Because the adapted recurrent TNBS colitis model showed involvement of relevant pathological processes and sensitivity to treatment, we sought to gain more insight into processes involved in the early development of colitis in this model. Therefore, we evaluated gene expression in colons of mice sacrificed at different time-points, i.e. before the first and 2 or 7 days after each rectal TNBS instillation. Evaluation of colon macroscopy at each of these time-points showed that TNBS administration was associated with transient shortening of the colons, whereas colon weight increased gradually in time (Figure 3). Histological evaluation of the colons revealed marked areas of hemorrhages and complete destruction of crypt architecture two days after each TNBS instillation; this mucosal damage had partially recovered seven days after each instillation (data not shown).

Genome wide expression profiling was performed on RNA isolated from distal colon tissue of five TNBS-treated mice at each selected time-point. Based on False Discovery Rate (FDR) correction, a total of 2074 genes of the 14285 transcripts that passed the filtering procedure, showed significantly different levels of mRNA at one or more time-points in comparison to mRNA from healthy mice. Differentially expressed genes that showed similar expression profiles are clustered in a heatmap (Figure 4A). The first TNBS challenge was associated with enhanced expression of a limited number of genes, whereas enhanced expression of a large number of genes occurred shortly after the second challenge on day 16 (Figure 4B). These patterns were largely normalized on day 21. Importantly, the third challenge resulted in extensive changes in gene expression on days 23 and 28. Forty-two % of the genes that showed increased expression on day 28 were also enhanced on day 23 and therefore not normalized. Furthermore, 27% of the genes differentially expressed on day 28, were not different from healthy on any of the earlier time-

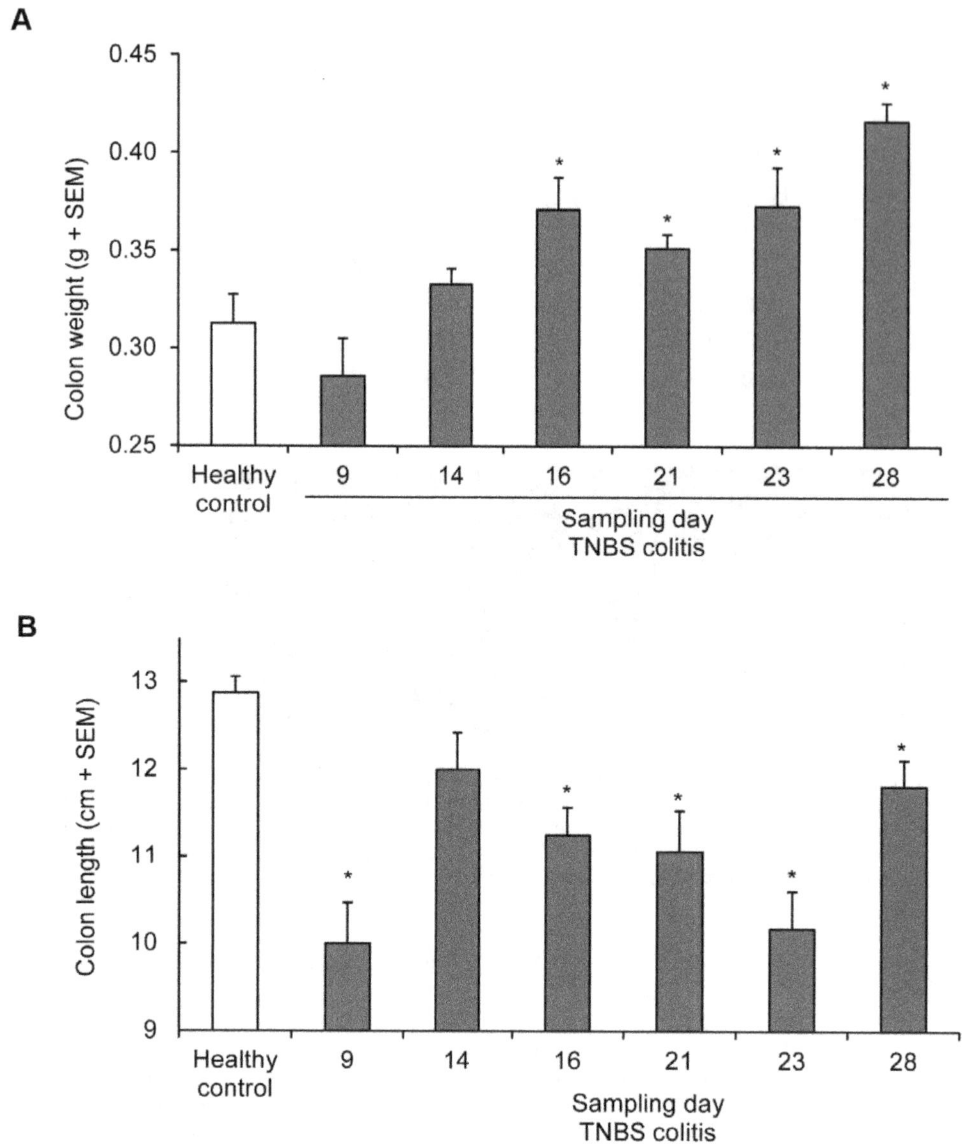

Figure 3. Disease characteristics of the recurrent TNBS model in time. Results of the time-course study in the recurrent TNBS colitis model. At each time-point indicated in Figure 8, 8 animals were sacrificed and colon length (**A**) and weight (**B**) was determined. Colitis is associated with a gradual increase in colon weight whereas the colon length is severely affected by each TNBS administration followed by a gradual relaxation.

points, suggesting developing pathology upon multiple TNBS instillations.

To further elucidate the cellular processes associated with the induction of colitis by repeated TNBS instillations, we performed gene ontology analysis on the FDR filtered gene data set using MetaCore^{TM} software. Enriched processes with more than 15 genes and p-values below $10-^{5}$ were considered to be significant (Table S1), which include general terms like "inflammation", but also detailed underlying subcategories. Five major processes important for human pathogenesis of IBD were identified in this model, i.e. I) tissue morphogenesis, II) the response to wounding, III) immune/inflammatory responses, IV) cell adhesion and V) angiogenesis. Gene expression associated with immune/inflammatory responses was particularly evident 2 days after each TNBS challenge. Furthermore, several processes gradually developed in time, in particular processes associated with epithelial cell growth and tissue repair/wound healing (Table S1). Altogether, several processes found in human IBD are reflected in this recurrent TNBS model and these will be discussed more detailed in the next paragraphs. The key transcription factors involved in the processes underlying the development of colitis in this model were identified by MetaCore^{TM} analysis. As shown in Table 2, Nuclear factor kappa-light-chain-enhancer of activated B cells (*NF-κB*), activator protein 1 (*AP-1*), CAMP responsive element binding protein 1 (*CREB1*), were central to the process at most time-points, in accordance with an inflammatory process. Networks involving Hepatocyte-Nuclear Factor-4α (*hnf4α*) were only observed on day 16 and 23, consistent with its role in the acute phase response.

Chemokines, Cytokines and Cell-adhesion Molecules in Recurrent TNBS-colitis

Each of the repeated challenges with TNBS was followed by increased expression of genes encoding mediators of acute inflammation such TNF-α, IL-1β, CHI3L1, as well as calprotectin

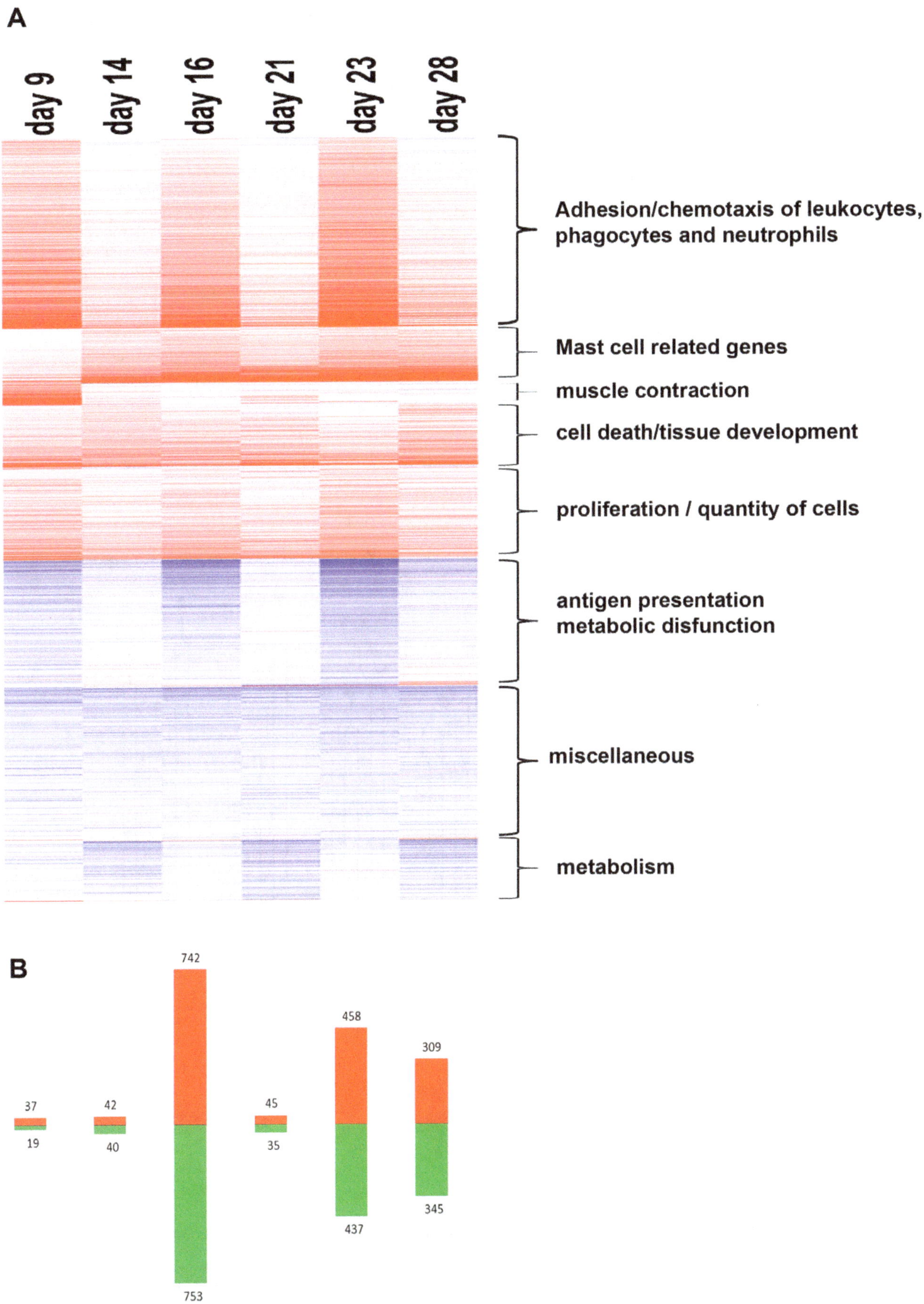
A
day 9
day 14
day 16
day 21
day 23
day 28
Adhesion/chemotaxis of leukocytes, phagocytes and neutrophils
Mast cell related genes
muscle contraction
cell death/tissue development
proliferation / quantity of cells
antigen presentation
metabolic disfunction
miscellaneous
metabolism
B
37
19
42
40
742
753
45
35
458
437
309
345

Figure 4. Transcriptome analysis in the recurrent TNBS-induced colitis model. To determine temporal patterns of gene expression levels that were affected by the repeated TNBS instillations, microarray analysis was performed on RNA isolated from colon tissue of colitic mice at day 9, 14, 16, 21, 23, and 28 (n = 5/group) (**A**) A heat-map of the genes with significantly modified gene expression revealed multiple clusters with different temporal expression patterns. (**B**) Bar graph indicates the number of up regulated (red) and down-regulated genes during colitis development at each time point. Genes were considered significant with a False discovery rate (FDR) p value <0.05. FDR was used to correct for multiple comparisons.

or calgranulin C (S100a8 -a9). These S100-proteins are relevant to the pathogenesis, disease activity, diagnosis, and therapeutic management of IBD [17]. Apart from this acute response towards TNBS instillations, the adaptive arm of the immune system appeared to be of importance from day 23 onwards as shown by gene ontology analysis in Metacore^{TM}. This analysis also revealed a role for cell adhesion molecules and chemokines. The KEGG list of 69 cell adhesion molecules (CAMs), chemokines and chemokine receptors, that was previously applied to illustrate an important role of these molecules in mucosal biopsies of UC and CD patients [18], was used to evaluate their expression during the development of recurrent TNBS-colitis. A heat-map of the molecules on this list that showed significantly altered expression at one or more time points is presented in Figure 5A. Several endothelial and leukocyte CAMs that were increased in patients with colonic IBD were also enhanced in the mouse model, e.g. CD62L, ICAM1, MAD-CAM1, SELE, THY1, JAM3, and PECAM1. Moreover, several chemokines involved in the recruitment of leukocytes, i.e., CCL2 (MCP-1), CCL3 (MIP-1α), CCL4 (MIP-1β), CCL7 (MCP-3), CCL9 (MIP-1γ), CCL24 (eotaxin-2), CXCL-1 (KC), and CXCL-2 (MIP-2α) were induced as well. Not all transcripts related to immune responses were up-regulated. Several genes encoding

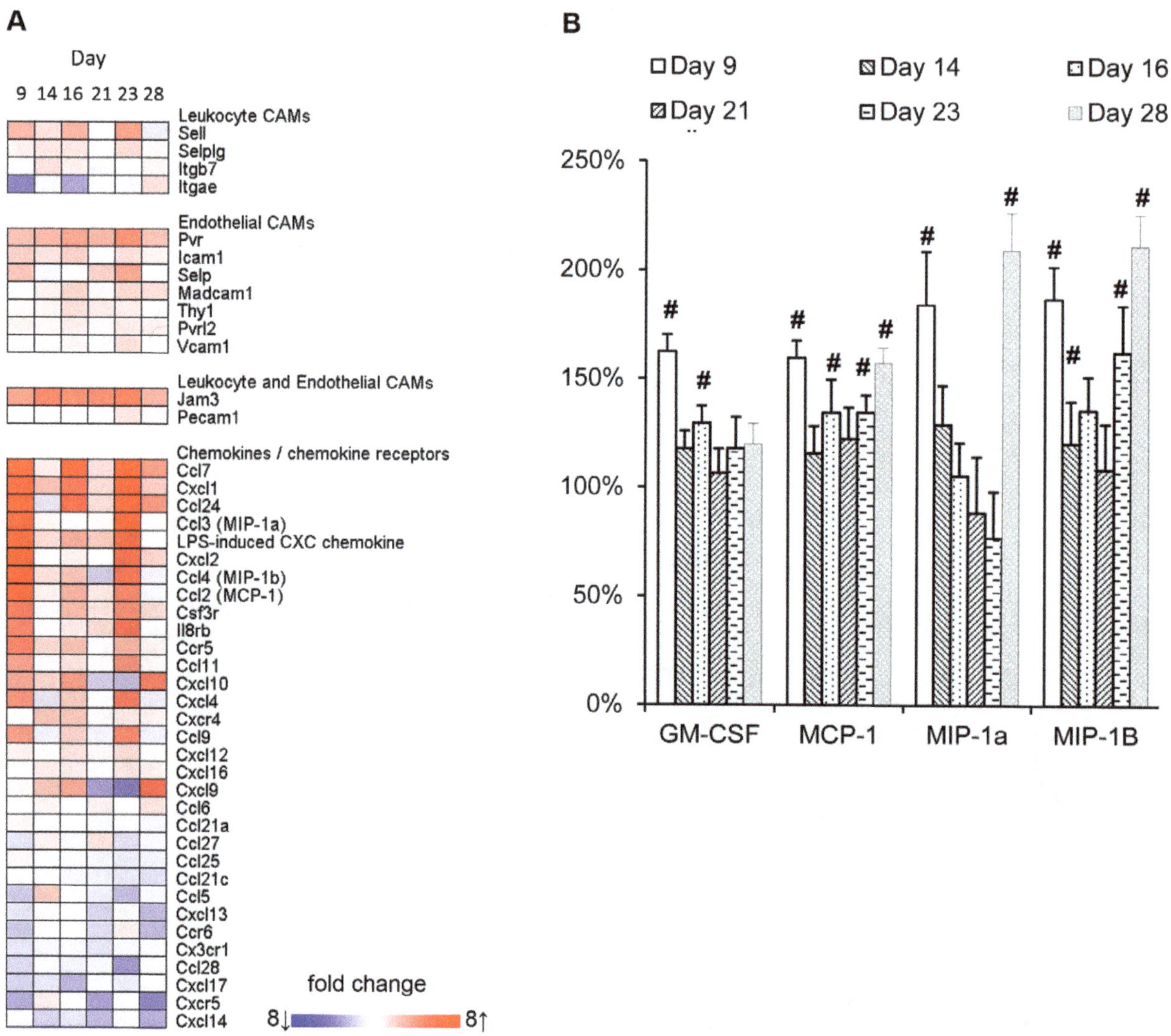

Figure 5. Effect of recurrent TNBS administrations on cell adhesion molecules and chemokines. (**A**) Local mRNA expression of cell adhesion molecules and chemokines was determined within the time-course microarray experiment. The size of the effect of TNBS-induced colitis on gene expression in comparison to healthy colons is indicated in a heatmap. These differences are based on mean expression levels of 5 individual animals per time-point. (**B**) Circulating serum chemokines were analyzed by multiplex technology. Relative serum concentrations of concentrations of GM-CSF, MCP-1 (CCL2), MIP-1α (CCL3), and MIP-1β (CCL4) are graphically depicted; significant differences are indicated by #.

Table 1. Relative circulating cytokine concentrations in TNBS-induced colitis[a].

	Group								
Cytokine	**Healthy (n = 14)**			**Vehicle (n = 19)**			**Budesonide(n = 15)**		
Eotaxin	100%	±	5%	102%	±	9%	89%	±	10%
G-CSF	100%	±	10%	114%	±	9%	83%	±	8%[c]
GM-CSF	100%	±	4%	108%	±	5%	98%	±	7%
IFNγ	100%	±	10%	137%	±	12%[b]	93%	±	14%[c]
IL-10	100%	±	25%	194%	±	37%	54%	±	16%
IL-12p40	100%	±	8%	87%	±	7%	28%	±	4%[c]
IL-12p70	100%	±	15%	117%	±	19%	89%	±	11%
IL-13	100%	±	9%	133%	±	12%	82%	±	10%[c]
IL-17	100%	±	13%	153%	±	17%[b]	94%	±	12%[c]
IL-1α	100%	±	19%	93%	±	12%	87%	±	17%
IL-1β	100%	±	8%	135%	±	12%[b]	82%	±	9%[c]
IL-2	100%	±	11%	118%	±	12%	84%	±	12%
IL-3	100%	±	13%	137%	±	14%	104%	±	13%
IL-4	100%	±	15%	111%	±	12%	85%	±	14%
IL-5	100%	±	6%	111%	±	12%	72%	±	8%[c]
IL-6	100%	±	15%	122%	±	9%	82%	±	9%[c]
IL-9	100%	±	9%	118%	±	8%	84%	±	8%[c]
KC	100%	±	7%	107%	±	7%	81%	±	4%[c]
MCP-1	100%	±	9%	131%	±	9%[b]	86%	±	16%[c]
MIP-1α	100%	±	8%	95%	±	7%	96%	±	10%
MIP-1β	100%	±	6%	121%	±	6%[b]	100%	±	10%
Rantes	100%	±	6%	91%	±	5%	80%	±	7%
TNFα	100%	±	10%	106%	±	9%	116%	±	20%

[a]In two independent studies, serum concentrations of 23 cytokines were determined by multiplex technology on day 28. In Table S2 concentrations are presented as pg/ml ± SEM. In each study, values were normalized and expressed as a percentage of the mean concentration of the corresponding healthy control mice. Relative concentrations and shown as % ±SEM.
[b]significantly ($p<0.05$) different relative serum concentration from that in healthy mice.
[c]significantly ($p<0.05$) different relative serum concentration from that in vehicle treated mice.

chemokines, including CCL21, and 25, and CXCL12, 14, and 15, showed gradually decreased expression during the development of colitis, indicative of a changing chemotactic profile during the progression of colon inflammation. Multiplex analysis on serum samples revealed that concentrations of GM-CSF, MCP-1, MIP-1α, and MIP-1β were significantly increased at one or more time-points during the experiment, although they did not reflect colon tissue gene expression profiles for these chemokines (Figure 5B).

As reported previously, repeated challenges with TNBS are associated with a changing cytokine profile in colon, suggesting for a shift from Th1 to a Th17 profile, and eventually Th2 cells with fibrosis [15]. In line with this study, IFN-γ gene expression was increased in our study, with a maximum on day 16, whereas IL-4 gene expression remained unchanged until the third TNBS challenge, after which a significant increase was observed (Figure 6A). However, mRNA expression profiles of cytokines considered significant for IBD or colitis, such IL-12p40, IL-23p19, IL-12p35, IL-17 did not differ from those in healthy tissue (data not shown).

To establish whether these IBD-related cytokines were reflected in the periphery, serum samples were subjected to cytokine analysis employing multiplex technology. A shown in Figure 6B, we did not obtain evidence for a biased cytokine profile at any time-point.

Involvement of Mast Cells and α-defensins in TNBS-colitis

A small subset of genes showed gradually increasing expression levels in time. This cluster mainly comprised mast cell specific genes (Figure 7A), including mast cell protease 1, 4, and 6 (*mcpt1, 4, 6*), mast cell chymase (*cma2,*), carboxypeptidase A3 (*cpa3*), tryptase α/β1 (*tpsab*), and high-affinity IgE Fc receptor (*fcer1a*). Gene expression was induced up to 233-fold (*mcpt1,* day 28). The highest expression levels of these genes were observed during the later stages of this model, i.e. on days 23 and 28. Immunohistochemical staining of FcεRI+ confirmed the presence of large numbers of mast cells in the lamina propria of affected colon tissue (data not shown). This was in line with increased numbers of mast cells stained by toluidine blue in affected colon tissue (Figure 7B). These results suggest a gradual increase of mast cells associated with the development of chronic colitis in this model.

Another set of genes that showed strongly affected expression levels encoded for antimicrobial peptides. Expression of many members of the α-defensin family was transiently increased on day 9, immediately following the first intrarectal TNBS instillation (Figure 7C). A subset of these defensins, including α-defensin 1 (*defa1*) and four α-defensin-related cryptdins (*defcr5, 6, 20* and *21* and *defcr-rs1*) also showed increased expression on day 28. These genes were induced up to 132-fold (*defcr-rs1,* day 28). This

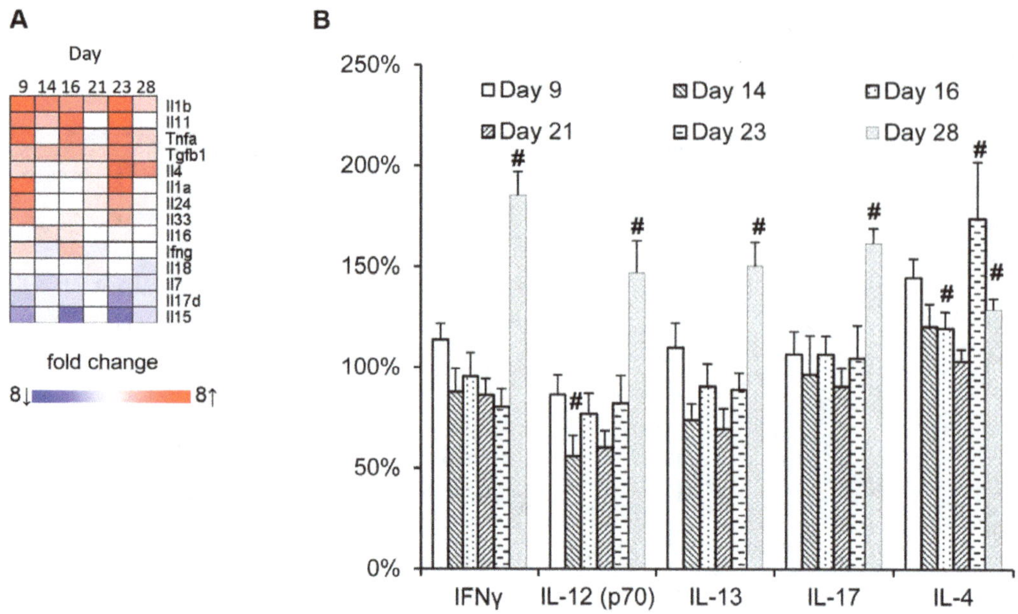

Figure 6. Effect of recurrent TNBS administrations on local and circulating cytokine profiles. (**A**) Local mRNA expression of cytokines was determined within the time-course microarray experiment. The size of the effect of TNBS-induced colitis on gene expression in comparison to healthy colons is indicated in a heatmap. These differences are based on mean expression levels of 5 individual animals per time-point. (**B**) Relative serum concentrations of Th1/Th2/Th17 hallmark cytokines at different time-points during the development of colitis. Concentrations of IFN-γ and IL-12p70, IL-4 and IL-13, and IL-17 are graphically depicted; significant differences are indicated by #.

modulation was restricted to α-defensins, as the level β-defensin gene expression remained unchanged.

Discussion

To gain insight into the pathogenesis of IBD, a variety of animal models reflecting different aspects of the disease are used [10,11,19]. Most IBD models result from exogenous manipulation; they can be categorized based on induction by chemicals, immune cell transfer, or gene targeting [19]. Models based on immune cell transfer, such as the $CD45RB^{Hi}$ T-cell transfer model, and models based on gene targeting, such as the IL-10 knockout mouse model, present excellent models to study mechanisms involved in the pathogenesis IBD [20]. Nonetheless, these models have the disadvantage of lacking a fully functional immune system. These limitations do not apply for models of colitis induced by DSS or TNBS. However, these models usually have the disadvantage of being mediated by damage and being relatively insensitive to anti-inflammatory drugs. In this respect the recurrent TNBS colitis model is more promising. This model has been proposed because the induced pathology reflects the chronic and relapsing immune activation processes underlying human IBD resulting in late onset of fibrosis [13,15]. In this report, we show results obtained in a modified version of this model, limiting the duration to first three weeks of colitis development. We show its sensitivity to immunosuppression by local corticosteroid treatment with budesonide which is a relevant compound in clinical treatment of patients with CD. Moreover, we recently showed that the model is sensitive to pretreatment with probiotic bacteria [16].

Our initial work to develop a model for colitis was largely inspired by the work of Neurath et al. who showed that TNBS-induced colitis is mediated by Th1 cells [21]. However, in our hands this model showed in SJL mice substantial mortality and variation, which was partly explained by the source of the animals and the type of chow diet (data not shown). Modifications to the protocol, as indicated by Wirtz et al [5], i.e. skin sensitization with TNBS prior to intrarectal challenges with TNBS, decreased the mortality rate in this model. Nevertheless, the limited therapeutic window of 2 days in the acute model prompted us to evaluate the characteristics of a recurrent TNBS-colitis model described by Fichtner-Feigl et al [15], allowing for prolonged treatment during a period of several weeks.

Our study further characterizes the processes underlying or associated with the early stage development of colitis in this model, i.e. a time frame of 3 weeks, by performing genome wide transcriptome analysis on colon tissue. This approach revealed that each intrarectal TNBS challenge induced a complex set of genes encoding molecules that are generally associated with an acute phase inflammatory response, such as TNFα, IL-6, calgranulins S100a8 and 9, and reg3γ. In addition, each intrarectal TNBS challenge was associated with an enhanced expression of genes encoding a set of chemokines; MCP-1 (CCL-2), MIP-1α (CCL3) and MIP-1β (CCL4), CCL7, CCL9, CCL11, CCL24, CXCL2 and CXCL4, showed a similar acute phase expression pattern, consistent with the influx of inflammatory cells. Moreover, serum concentrations of GM-CSF, MCP-1, MIP-1α, and MIP-1β were significantly increased in particular two days after each TNBS challenge. These data suggest that each TNBS challenge induces transient chemokine production in the colon, which likely drives the attraction of innate and adaptive immune cells to the site of TNBS-induced tissue damage. The involvement of these chemokines is relevant for human IBD since the majority is also elevated in tissues of UC and CD patients [22–24].

In addition, CXCL1 and CXCL2, which are chemokines with strong angiogenic effects, were strongly induced by the first intrarectal TNBS challenge and this was followed by the enrichment of a large cluster of genes encoding factors that are involved in angiogenesis, including FGF, endothelin-1, and VEGF-D. These data are suggestive for a link between the process of inflammation and angiogenesis in this model. Impor-

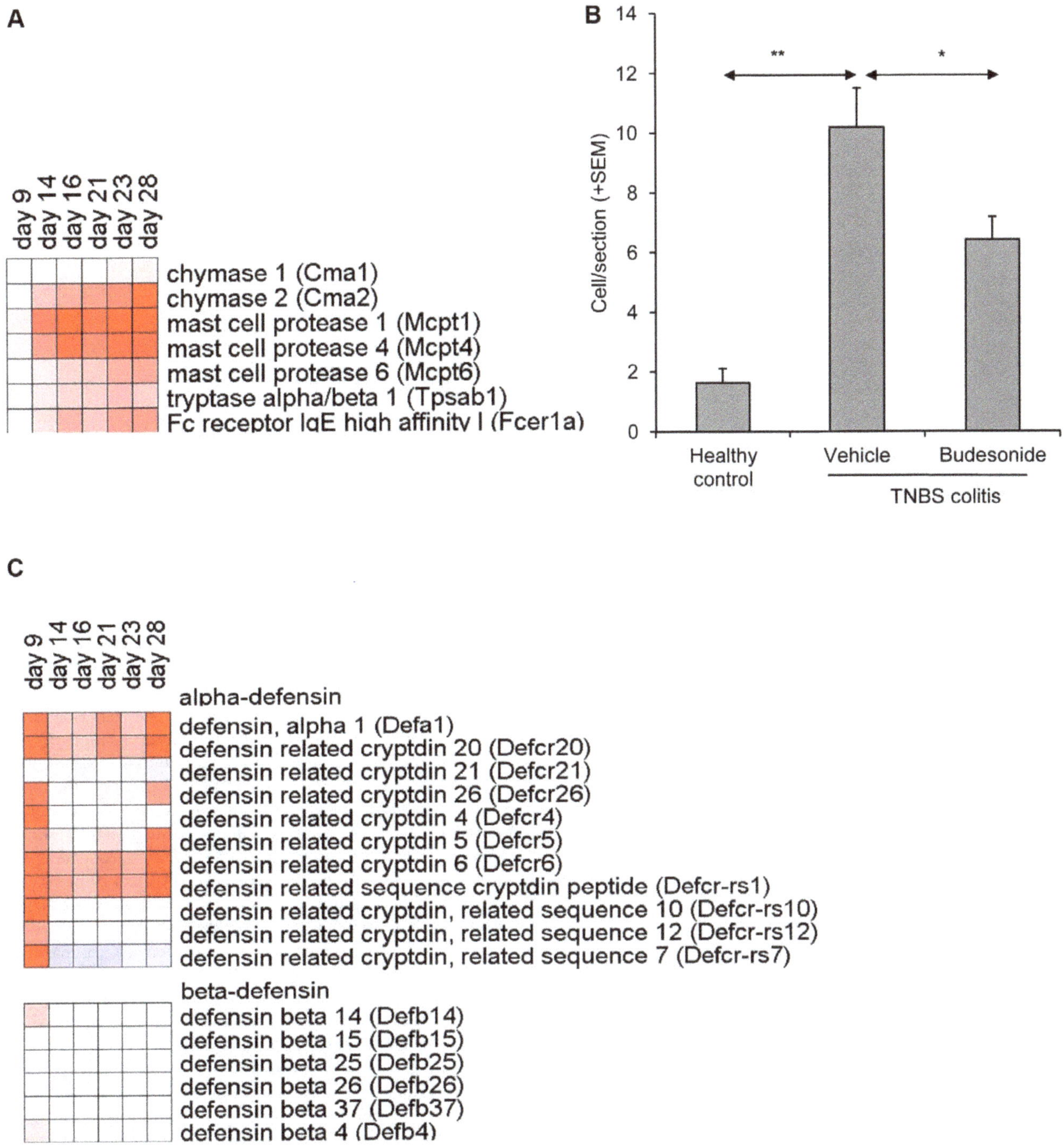

Figure 7. TNBS -induced colitis is associated with increased numbers of mast cells and α-defensins. (**A**) mRNA expression of selected mast cell specific genes in affected colon tissue (n = 5/group). Heatmap represents fold changes in TNBS colitis mice as compared to healthy control mice. (**B**) Quantification of toluidine blue positive cells confirmed TNBS induced up-regulation of mast cells. (**C**) mRNA expression of α- and β-defensin genes in affected colon tissue.

tantly, angiogenesis has been described as an important component in the pathogenesis and potential target for treatment of IBD [25].

Interestingly, the expression of a set of genes encoding chemokines involved in homeostatic processes, including CCL21, CCL25, CCL27 and CCL28, was gradually down-regulated in our TNBS colitis model. As these chemokines are involved in mucosal lymphoid structure development [26], our findings suggest that normal lymphatic tissue regeneration is affected in the model. This was substantiated by the observation that colitic tissue contained lower levels of transcripts associated with B cells (Cd19, Cxcr5, Tnfrsf13c, and Pou2af1) and intraepithelial lymphocytes [27] (IL-15, IL-7, and CD3γ).

Many genes that showed reduced expression upon TNBS colitis induction were related to metabolic processes. These main affected metabolic functions based on gene expression shifts comprise of

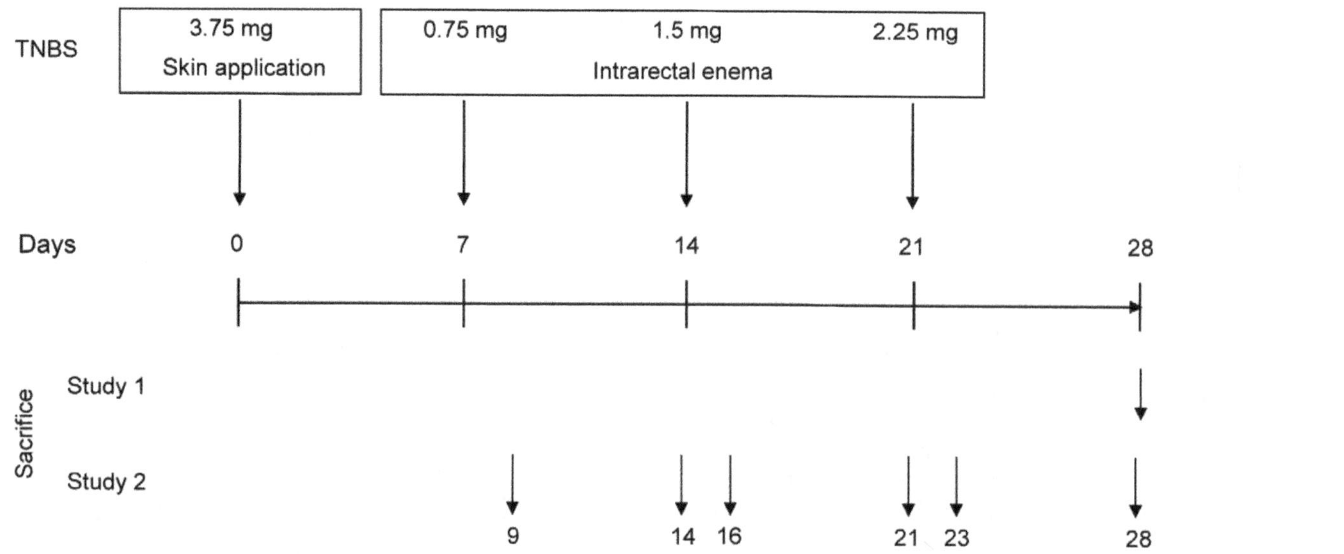

Figure 8. Schematic representation of the colitis induction protocol. Induction of colitis is achieved by dorsal skin application of TNBS in ethanol on day 0, followed by rectal TNBS/ethanol instillations on day 7, 14, and 21. The necropsy time-points for study 1, i.e. TNBS disease induction and corticosteroid treatment, and study 2, i.e. the time-course experiment, are presented in the upper part of the schematic. Severity of colitis induction was assessed by measurement of colon weight, length and thickness and by histopathological evaluation of the distal part of the colon. At each necropsy, serum was collected for cytokine profiling and colon tissue was sampled for RNA isolation.

changes in oxidative stress response processes, methylation, lipid biosynthesis, and small molecule metabolism. These observations reflect the strong connection between immune and metabolic response systems in the gut, as described Shulzhenko et al [28].

Mast cell influx is one of the key features of the model presented in this paper, as observed by microarray and histological examination. The transcriptomics data revealed progressively elevated mRNA levels of genes encoding mast cell specific products such as proteases 1, 4 and 6 (mcpt-1, -4, -6), carboxypeptidase 3 (cpa3), and high affinity Fc receptor for IgE (FcεRI). Mast cell infiltration was confirmed by increased numbers of toluidine blue positive mast cells as well as increases in FcεRI+ cells in the affected lamina propria. The attraction of mast cell progenitors from the blood depends on several factors, in particular local chemokine expression. These include, CCL2, CCXL4, CCL3, CCL24, and CCL11 [26,29]. These chemokines were up- regulated during acute inflammation phases of the model and may therefore contribute to the temporal migration/ recruitment of these cells to the inflamed mucosa. Interestingly, protective effects of probiotics in this model were associated with reduced expression of these chemokines [16]. Also in biopsies of CD and UC patients mucosal accumulation of mast cells has been observed [30–33]; however, the causative relationship between the development of IBD and numbers or activation state of mast cells has not been established. As mast cells are known to produce and release a plethora of mediators involved in pro-inflammatory as well as regulatory and active tissue repair processes [32,34,35], we hypothesize that they may exert differential effects depending on the stage of the inflammation processes.

The induction of colitis was associated with an increased expression of a cluster α-defensins together with the expression of other antimicrobial peptides, such as angiogenin 4 (ang4), regenerating islet derived antimicrobial peptides RegIIIγ and RegIV (reg3g and reg4, respectively), and secretory phospholipase A2 type IIA (pla2a2a/pla2g2a). Although all of these anti-microbial peptides have been described as products of Paneth cells in the small intestine, we have not been able to demonstrate the origin of these transcripts in the colon. Staining with Lendrum's phloxine-tartrazine or immunohistochemical staining for lysozyme P did not confirm the presence of Paneth cells in the affected colon tissue (data not shown). It is tempting to speculate that these genes are indicative of the presence of metaplastic Paneth cells, which have been reported in both colonic CD and UC biopsies [36–38], whereas they are not found in healthy colon tissue [39,40]. In patients these cells showed increased expression of human α-defensins DEFA5 and DEFA6 in the colon [22,38,41,42]. Additional studies are needed to establish the

Table 2. Master regulators in colitis development.

Transcription factor[a]	Central regulator of	Time-point[b]					
		9	14	16	21	23	28
SP1	Lipid metabolism, inflammation		++	++		++	++
HNF4α	Endodermal development			++		++	
c-myc	cell proliferation	+	+	+		+	+
CREB1	Inflammation			+		+	+
p53	Apoptosis, cell cycle	+	+	+		+	+
NF-κB	Inflammation	+	+	+	+	+	
AP1	Inflammation			+		+	+
C/EBP-β	Lipid metabolism, inflammation			+			+
ESR1	Metabolism, inflammation					+	+

[a]Transcription factors were identified in biological networks generated using MetaCore™ software. Transcription factors represented in this table were identified in significant networks containing a minimal of 8 nodes.
[b]Level of significance of the transcription factor network is classified based on z-scores: +, z-score between 50 and 100; ++, z-score above 100. No score means that the networks for these transcription factors were not identified at the time-point or had a z-score below 50.

origin of the antimicrobial peptide gene expression in affected colon tissue.

In conclusion, this recurrent TNBS-colitis model, adapted to comprise both transient acute inflammatory processes and gradually developing chronic inflammation, reflects several clinical and histopathological features of human IBD. The temporal gene expression profiles generated in this study revealed distinct processes involved in the onset and progression of disease in this model, and this knowledge may help to identify novel targets and therapeutic approaches for IBD.

Materials and Methods

Mouse Colitis Model

All experiments were performed with female BALB/c mice (8 wk old, 18–22 g) obtained from Janvier (St. Berthevin, France). Mice were conventionally housed under controlled temperature (22–24°C) and photoperiod (12 h light-dark cycle), and had free access to standard mouse chow (SSNIFF R/M-H, BioServices B.V., Uden, The Netherlands) and acidified tap water. Animal experiments were approved by the Institutional Animal Care and Use Committee of The Netherlands Organization for Applied Scientific Research (TNO), approval number DEC2982 and were in compliance with European Community specifications regarding the use of laboratory animals.

To induce colitis, mice were exposed to intracolonic administration of step-wise increasing doses of TNBS (Figure 8). Seven days prior to the first intracolonic TNBS administration, mice were sensitized by a single application of 3.75 mg of TNBS (Sigma-Aldrich, Zwijndrecht, The Netherlands) in 48% (v/v) ethanol on the shaved dorsal skin. On days 7, 14 and 21, mice were lightly anaesthesized with isoflurane and subsequently 0.75, 1.5 and 2.25 mg TNBS in 40% (v/v) ethanol was administered per rectum via a 2.0 mm tube (Unomedical A/S, Birkerød, Denmark) connected with a 1.0 ml syringe, which was advanced into the rectum for approximately 3 cm. Upon administration of 150 µl of TNBS solution, mice were held in a vertical position for 30 seconds to allow for equal distribution.

Study Design

In this report, the results of 2 experiments (Figure 8) are discussed in detail. In study 1, induction of colitis was performed as described above and at day 28 all animals were sacrificed for assessment of all relevant parameters. In this study, local budesonide (3 mg/kg) treatment was included as a positive treatment control. Budesonide was administered 3× per week starting one day prior to the first rectal TNBS administration, i.e. day 6. Budesonide (Sigma-Aldrich, Zwijndrecht, The Netherlands) was prepared in PBS containing 2.5% (v/v) Tween-80 and 2.5% (v/v) ethanol. In study 2, we performed a time-course study to evaluate the development of colitis by macroscopy, cytokine profiling and gene expression profiling. In this study, one group of animals ($n = 8$) was included for each time-point in the study. The selected time-points 2 and 7 days after each TNBS administration, 8 mice were sacrificed, as indicated in Figure 8.

Colon Macroscopy

Severity of colitis was assessed by macroscopical analysis directly upon sacrifice. After colon length was measured, feces were removed by gentle pressure with forceps. Subsequently, colon weight was measured. Finally, colon thickness was measured with a digital caliper at 1, 2, and 3 cm from the anus.

Histological Assessment of Colitis

Following measurement of macroscopy parameters, colons were dissected and fragments were fixed in 4% buffered formalin and embedded in paraffin. Sections of 5 µm were stained by hematoxylin-eosin-saffron. Inflammation was scored in a blinded manner for 3 non-sequential sections per colon fragment at a 400× magnification, according to a semi quantitative (0–4) scoring system, based on number of infiltrating cells and mucosal damage. Mast cells were evaluated after staining with toluidine blue [43] at a 400× magnification.

Immunohistochemical Analysis of Cellular Infiltrates

Dissected colon fragments were immediately immersed in Tissue Tek OCT compound (Sakura Finetel, Torrance, CA, USA) and cryopreserved in liquid nitrogen. Immunohistochemistry was performed on 6 µm sections with primary antibodies specific for CD4 (L3T4.), CD8 (53–6.7), CD11b (M1/70), and F4/80 (CI-A3-1all obtained from BD Biosciences (San Diego, CA, USA). After incubation, biotinylated antibodies were detected by incubation with streptavidin-HRP (Vector Laboratories, Burlingame, CA, USA) using 3-amino-9-ethylcarbozole (Sigma) as a substrate. Immunopositive cells were counted at a 400× magnification and normalized against the colon tissue surface area. For immunofluorescence, primary antibodies and according Texas red and fluorescein labeled secondary antibodies were applied. Slides were covered with Vectashield (H1000) mounting medium with DAPI Vector).

Cytokine and Chemokine Quantification in Serum

Cytokine concentrations in serum obtained at each sacrifice were determined by Multiplex analyses. For this purpose, serum was diluted and assayed with the Bio-Plex Pro 23-Plex Panel, for IL-1α, -1β, -2, -3, -4, -5, -6, -9, -10, -12(p40), -12(p70), -13, -17, IFN-γ, TNF-α, RANTES, MIP-1α and -1β, MCP-1, KC, G-CSF, GM-CSF, and eotaxin protein (Bio-Rad Laboratories, Hercules, CA, USA). The beads were read on a LiquiChip 200, (Qiagen, Hombrechtikon, Switzerland), and data were analyzed by the five parameter curve fitting in Luminex100 IS Software. Cytokine concentrations were corrected for the dilution factor and presented in pg/ml or as relative concentrations to the average concentration in healthy mice.

Transcriptome Analysis

Total RNA from frozen intestinal tissue was isolated using TRIzol reagent (Invitrogen, Breda, The Netherlands) according to the manufacturer's instructions. RNA was treated with DNAse and purified using Nucleospin RNAII Total RNA Isolation kit (Macherey-Nagel, Düren, Germany), according to manufacturer's protocol.

The quality control of RNA samples, RNA labeling and hybridization were performed at ServiceXS (Leiden, The Netherlands). RNA concentration was assessed using a Nanodrop ND-1000 spectrophotometer (Nanodrop Technologies, Wilmington, DE, U.S.A). The RNA quality and integrity was determined using Lab-on-Chip analysis on an Agilent 2100 Bioanalyzer (Agilent Technologies, Inc., Santa Clara, CA, U.S.A.). The RNA integrity numbers (RIN) of all RNA samples had values above 7.3. Biotinylated cRNA was prepared using the Illumina TotalPrep RNA Amplification Kit (Ambion, Inc., Austin, TX, U.S.A.) according to the manufacturer's specifications starting with 500 ng total RNA. Per sample, 750 ng of cRNA was used to hybridize to the Sentrix MouseRef-8 BeadChips (Illumina, Inc., San Diego, CA, U.S.A.). Each BeadChip contains eight arrays and each of the arrays harbors 25697 probes. Hybridization and washing were performed according to the Illumina standard assay procedure. Scanning was performed on the Illumina iScanner (Illumina, Inc., San Diego, CA, U.S.A.). Image analysis and extraction of raw and background subtracted expression data were performed with Illumina Beadstudio v3 Gene Expression software using default settings. The data discussed in this publication have been deposited in NCBI's Gene Expression Omnibus [44] and are accessible through GEO Series accession number GSE35609 (http://www.ncbi.nlm.nih.gov/geo/query/acc.cgi?acc = GSE35609). GeneSpring GX 11.0 was used for quantile normalization of the probe-level, background subtracted expression values. After the normalization, unexpressed probes were removed from the further analyses. All expression values below 5 (2.322 on log2 scale) were floored to 5. Differentially expressed probes were identified using the limma package of the R/Bioconductor project, applying linear models and moderated t-statistics that implement empirical Bayes regularization of standard errors [45]. The statistical analyses were performed through The Remote Analysis Computation for gene Expression data (RACE) suite at http://race.unil.ch [46]. False Discovery Rate (FDR) corrected p-values of 0.05 was used as threshold for significance of the differential expression. Fold changes relative to healthy control mice are presented. GEO Processes were identified using Metacore Software V6.11.

RT-qPCR for a set of genes (CCL2, CCL11, CCL24, cldn-1, cldn-4, cldn-11) showed a high correlation with data obtained by microarrays, and thereby confirmed the relative gene expression presented in the figures (data not shown).

Author Contributions

Conceived and designed the experiments: BK RM LN. Performed the experiments: TL RM. Analyzed the data: BK RM MvE. Wrote the paper: BM RM LN.

References

1. Engel MA, Neurath MF (2010) New pathophysiological insights and modern treatment of IBD. Journal of Gastroenterology 45: 571–583.
2. Xavier RJ, Podolsky DK (2007) Unravelling the pathogenesis of inflammatory bowel disease. Nature 448: 427–434.
3. Kozuch PL, Hanauer SB (2008) Treatment of inflammatory bowel disease: A review of medical therapy. World Journal of Gastroenterology : WJG 14: 354–377.
4. Kawada M, Arihiro A, Mizoguchi E (2007) Insights from advances in research of chemically induced experimental models of human inflammatory bowel disease. World Journal of Gastroenterology : WJG 13: 5581–5593.
5. Wirtz S, Neufert C, Weigmann B, Neurath MF (2007) Chemically induced mouse models of intestinal inflammation. Nature Protocols 2: 541–546.
6. Neurath M, Fuss I, Strober W (2000) TNBS-colitis. International Reviews of Immunology 19: 51–62.
7. Paiotti AP, Miszputen SJ, Oshima CT, Artigiani Neto R, Ribeiro DA, et al. (2011) Etanercept attenuates TNBS-induced experimental colitis: Role of TNF-alpha expression. Journal of Molecular Histology 42: 443–450.
8. Shen C, de Hertogh G, Bullens DM, Van Assche G, Geboes K, et al. (2007) Remission-inducing effect of anti-TNF monoclonal antibody in TNBS colitis: Mechanisms beyond neutralization? Inflammatory Bowel Diseases 13: 308–316.
9. Mencarelli A, Renga B, Palladino G, Distrutti E, Fiorucci S (2009) The plant sterol guggulsterone attenuates inflammation and immune dysfunction in murine models of inflammatory bowel disease. Biochemical Pharmacology 78: 1214–1223.
10. Elson CO, Cong Y, Lorenz R, Weaver CT (2004) New developments in experimental models of inflammatory bowel disease. Current Opinion in Gastroenterology 20: 360–367.
11. Strober W, Fuss IJ (2006) Experimental models of mucosal inflammation. Advances in Experimental Medicine and Biology 579: 55–97.
12. Fichtner-Feigl S, Fuss IJ, Preiss JC, Strober W, Kitani A (2005) Treatment of murine Th1- and Th2-mediated inflammatory bowel disease with NF-kappa B decoy oligonucleotides. The Journal of Clinical Investigation 115: 3057–3071.
13. Lawrance IC, Wu F, Leite AZ, Willis J, West GA, et al. (2003) A murine model of chronic inflammation-induced intestinal fibrosis down-regulated by antisense NF-kappa B. Gastroenterology 125: 1750–1761.
14. Fichtner-Feigl S, Strober W, Geissler EK, Schlitt HJ (2008) Cytokines mediating the induction of chronic colitis and colitis-associated fibrosis. Mucosal Immunology 1 Suppl 1: S24–7.
15. Fichtner-Feigl S, Fuss IJ, Young CA, Watanabe T, Geissler EK, et al. (2007) Induction of IL-13 triggers TGF-beta1-dependent tissue fibrosis in chronic 2,4,6-trinitrobenzene sulfonic acid colitis. Journal of Immunology (Baltimore, Md.: 1950) 178: 5859–5870.
16. Mariman R, Kremer B, van Erk M, Lagerweij T, Koning F, et al. (2012) Gene expression profiling identifies mechanisms of protection to recurrent trinitrobenzene sulfonic acid colitis mediated by probiotics. Inflammatory Bowel Diseases 18: 1424–1433.
17. Manolakis AC, Kapsoritakis AN, Tiaka EK, Potamianos SP (2011) Calprotectin, calgranulin C, and other members of the s100 protein family in inflammatory bowel disease. Digestive Diseases and Sciences 56: 1601–1611.
18. Arijs I, De Hertogh G, Machiels K, Van Steen K, Lemaire K, et al. (2011) Mucosal gene expression of cell adhesion molecules, chemokines, and chemokine receptors in patients with inflammatory bowel disease before and after infliximab treatment. The American Journal of Gastroenterology 106: 748–761.
19. Wirtz S, Neurath MF (2007) Mouse models of inflammatory bowel disease. Advanced Drug Delivery Reviews 59: 1073–1083.
20. Strober W (2008) Why study animal models of IBD? Inflammatory Bowel Diseases 14 Suppl 2: S129–31.
21. Neurath MF, Fuss I, Kelsall BL, Stuber E, Strober W (1995) Antibodies to interleukin 12 abrogate established experimental colitis in mice. The Journal of Experimental Medicine 182: 1281–1290.
22. Noble CL, Abbas AR, Cornelius J, Lees CW, Ho GT, et al. (2008) Regional variation in gene expression in the healthy colon is dysregulated in ulcerative colitis. Gut 57: 1398–1405.
23. Noble CL, Abbas AR, Lees CW, Cornelius J, Toy K, et al. (2010) Characterization of intestinal gene expression profiles in crohn's disease by genome-wide microarray analysis. Inflammatory Bowel Diseases 16: 1717–1728.
24. Gijsbers K, Geboes K, Van Damme J (2006) Chemokines in gastrointestinal disorders. Current Drug Targets 7: 47–64.
25. Danese S, Sans M, de la Motte C, Graziani C, West G, et al. (2006) Angiogenesis as a novel component of inflammatory bowel disease pathogenesis. Gastroenterology 130: 2060–2073.
26. Zimmerman NP, Vongsa RA, Wendt MK, Dwinell MB (2008) Chemokines and chemokine receptors in mucosal homeostasis at the intestinal epithelial barrier in inflammatory bowel disease. Inflammatory Bowel Diseases 14: 1000–1011.
27. Porter BO, Malek TR (2000) Thymic and intestinal intraepithelial T lymphocyte development are each regulated by the gammac-dependent cytokines IL-2, IL-7, and IL-15. Seminars in Immunology 12: 465–474.
28. Shulzhenko N, Morgun A, Hsiao W, Battle M, Yao M, et al. (2011) Crosstalk between B lymphocytes, microbiota and the intestinal epithelium governs immunity versus metabolism in the gut. Nature Medicine 17: 1585–1593.
29. Hallgren J, Gurish MF (2011) Mast cell progenitor trafficking and maturation. Advances in Experimental Medicine and Biology 716: 14–28.
30. Stenton GR, Vliagoftis H, Befus AD (1998) Role of intestinal mast cells in modulating gastrointestinal pathophysiology. Annals of Allergy, Asthma & Immunology : Official Publication of the American College of Allergy, Asthma, & Immunology 81: 1–11; quiz 12–5.
31. Raithel M, Matek M, Baenkler HW, Jorde W, Hahn EG (1995) Mucosal histamine content and histamine secretion in crohn's disease, ulcerative colitis and allergic enteropathy. International Archives of Allergy and Immunology 108: 127–133.
32. He SH (2004) Key role of mast cells and their major secretory products in inflammatory bowel disease. World Journal of Gastroenterology : WJG 10: 309–318.
33. Andoh A, Deguchi Y, Inatomi O, Yagi Y, Bamba S, et al. (2006) Immunohistochemical study of chymase-positive mast cells in inflammatory bowel disease. Oncology Reports 16: 103–107.
34. Rijnierse A, Nijkamp FP, Kraneveld AD (2007) Mast cells and nerves tickle in the tummy: Implications for inflammatory bowel disease and irritable bowel syndrome. Pharmacology & Therapeutics 116: 207–235.
35. Theoharides TC, Alysandratos KD, Angelidou A, Delivanis DA, Sismanopoulos N, et al. (2012) Mast cells and inflammation. Biochimica Et Biophysica Acta 1822: 21–33.

36. Cunliffe RN, Rose FR, Keyte J, Abberley L, Chan WC, et al. (2001) Human defensin 5 is stored in precursor form in normal paneth cells and is expressed by some villous epithelial cells and by metaplastic paneth cells in the colon in inflammatory bowel disease. Gut 48: 176–185.
37. Fahlgren A, Hammarstrom S, Danielsson A, Hammarstrom ML (2003) Increased expression of antimicrobial peptides and lysozyme in colonic epithelial cells of patients with ulcerative colitis. Clinical and Experimental Immunology 131: 90–101.
38. Perminow G, Beisner J, Koslowski M, Lyckander LG, Stange E, et al. (2010) Defective paneth cell-mediated host defense in pediatric ileal crohn's disease. The American Journal of Gastroenterology 105: 452–459.
39. Sommers SC (1966) Mast cells and paneth cells in ulcerative colitis. Gastroenterology 51: 841–850.
40. Boulton RA, Usselmann B, Mohammed I, Jankowski J (2003) Barrett's esophagus: Environmental influences in the progression of dysplasia. World Journal of Surgery 27: 1014–1017.
41. Wehkamp J, Stange EF (2006) Paneth cells and the innate immune response. Current Opinion in Gastroenterology 22: 644–650.
42. Zilbauer M, Jenke A, Wenzel G, Goedde D, Postberg J, et al. (2011) Intestinal alpha-defensin expression in pediatric inflammatory bowel disease. Inflammatory Bowel Diseases 17: 2076–2086.
43. Strobel S, Miller HR, Ferguson A (1981) Human intestinal mucosal mast cells: Evaluation of fixation and staining techniques. Journal of Clinical Pathology 34: 851–858.
44. Edgar R, Domrachev M, Lash AE (2002) Gene expression omnibus: NCBI gene expression and hybridization array data repository. Nucleic Acids Research 30: 207–210.
45. Smyth GK (2004) Linear models and empirical bayes methods for assessing differential expression in microarray experiments. Statistical Applications in Genetics and Molecular Biology 3: Article3.
46. Psarros M, Heber S, Sick M, Thoppae G, Harshman K, et al. (2005) RACE: Remote analysis computation for gene expression data. Nucleic Acids Research 33: W638–43.

11

Anti-Inflammatory Effects of Resveratrol, Curcumin and Simvastatin in Acute Small Intestinal Inflammation

Stefan Bereswill[1], Melba Muñoz[1], André Fischer[1], Rita Plickert[1], Lea-Maxie Haag[1], Bettina Otto[1], Anja A. Kühl[2], Christoph Loddenkemper[2], Ulf B. Göbel[1], Markus M. Heimesaat[1]*

1 Institut für Mikrobiologie und Hygiene, Charité – Universitätsmedizin Berlin, Berlin, Germany, 2 Institut für Pathologie, Charité - Universitätsmedizin Berlin, Berlin, Germany

Abstract

Background: The health beneficial effects of Resveratrol, Curcumin and Simvastatin have been demonstrated in various experimental models of inflammation. We investigated the potential anti-inflammatory and immunomodulatory mechanisms of the above mentioned compounds in a murine model of hyper-acute Th1-type ileitis following peroral infection with *Toxoplasma gondii*.

Methodology/Principal Findings: Here we show that after peroral administration of Resveratrol, Curcumin or Simvastatin, mice were protected from ileitis development and survived the acute phase of inflammation whereas all Placebo treated controls died. In particular, Resveratrol treatment resulted in longer-term survival. Resveratrol, Curcumin or Simvastatin treated animals displayed significantly increased numbers of regulatory T cells and augmented intestinal epithelial cell proliferation/regeneration in the ileum mucosa compared to placebo control animals. In contrast, mucosal T lymphocyte and neutrophilic granulocyte numbers in treated mice were reduced. In addition, levels of the anti-inflammatory cytokine IL-10 in ileum, mesenteric lymph nodes and spleen were increased whereas pro-inflammatory cytokine expression (IL-23p19, IFN-γ, TNF-α, IL-6, MCP-1) was found to be significantly lower in the ileum of treated animals as compared to Placebo controls. Furthermore, treated animals displayed not only fewer pro-inflammatory enterobacteria and enterococci but also higher anti-inflammatory lactobacilli and bifidobacteria loads. Most importantly, treatment with all three compounds preserved intestinal barrier functions as indicated by reduced bacterial translocation rates into spleen, liver, kidney and blood.

Conclusion/Significance: Oral treatment with Resveratrol, Curcumin or Simvastatin ameliorates acute small intestinal inflammation by down-regulating Th1-type immune responses and prevents bacterial translocation by maintaining gut barrier function. These findings provide novel and potential prophylaxis and treatment options of patients with inflammatory bowel diseases.

Editor: Niyaz Ahmed, University of Hyderabad, India

Funding: This work was supported by grants from the German Research Foundation (DFG, SFB633) to MMH and MM (TP B6), AF, SB, and UBG (TP A7), AAK and CL (TP Z1), BO and L-MH (GRACO). The funders had no role in study design, data collection and analysis, decision to publish, or preparation of the manuscript.

Competing Interests: The authors have declared that no competing interests exist.

* E-mail: markus.heimesaat@charite.de

Introduction

Several nutritional compounds are the focus of public attention because of their potential beneficial health effects. Some compounds derived from plants and herbs (e.g. Resveratrol, Curcumin) have been proven effective in traditional medicine as herbal remedies for inflammatory disorders such as hepatitis, arthritis, and colitis [1]. Both, Resveratrol and Curcumin also exert pharmacological effects in various experimental models of acute and chronic inflammation [1]. In addition, some pharmaceutical compounds (e.g. statins) have shown to possess anti-inflammatory, immuno-modulatory properties apart from their original indication for disease treatment [2].

Resveratrol (3,5,4′-trihydoxy-*trans*-stilbene) is a polyphenol found in grape skins and red wine. Resveratrol has been reported to exert multiple health-promoting benefits such as anti-inflammatory, anti-oxidant, anti-tumor, anti-platelet aggregation, anti-aging and anti-atherogenic effects [3]. Anti-inflammatory properties of Resveratrol have been described in several diseases such as arthritis [4], pancreatitis [5], and experimental colitis [6].

Curcumin is a polyphenol derived from the root of the turmeric plant *Curcuma longa* and responsible for the yellow-orange color and the spicy taste of curries [7]. Curcumin exerts anti-infectious, anti-tumor, and anti-inflammatory properties [8]. Preventive as well as therapeutic anti-inflammatory effects of Curcumin treatment have been observed in various animal models [9].

Simvastatin belongs to the class of cholesterol-lowering statins that are widely used to reduce cardiovascular morbidity and mortality in patients with or without coronary artery disease [10]. Statins have been also proposed to exert anti-inflammatory effects that are not directly related to their cholesterol-lowering activity [2] by interfering with endothelial adhesion and leukocyte migration to sites of inflammation [11].

Within eight to ten days following peroral infection with the parasite *Toxoplasma (T.) gondii*, susceptible mice develop severe small intestinal necrosis (pan-ileitis), induced by IL-23 [12] and mediated by a strong Th1-type immune response with a subsequent storm of pro-inflammatory cytokines including IL-12, IFN-γ, TNF-α, and nitric oxide (NO) [13]. Furthermore, inflammation triggers characteristic quantitative as well as qualitative ileum flora shifts [14,15]. We demonstrated earlier that luminal concentrations of commensal Gram-negative bacteria such as *E. coli* increase and aggravate ileitis development through TLR4-dependent signaling pathways [15]. Moreover, commensal gut bacteria translocate through the leaky epithelial barrier into the intestinal submucosa and spread to adjacent organs through blood or lymphatic vessels leading to sepsis and multi-organ failure [12]. Taken together, the Th1-type immunopathology in the *T. gondii*-mediated ileitis model is triggered by the commensal microbiota and thus resembles the immunological key features of acute episodes in inflammatory bowel disease (IBD) such as Crohn's disease (ileitis terminalis) in humans. However, experimental models of small intestinal inflammation are scarce and most of the experimental IBD models assess the large intestine. Given that Resveratrol, Curcumin or Simvastatin have been shown to suppress immune responses, we investigated the immuno-modulatory effects of these compounds in this well characterized model of ileitis. Our results showed the anti-inflammatory and immuno-modulating properties of all three compounds. Amelioration of ileitis was accompanied by reduced immunopathology and an integral gut barrier function that prevented bacterial translocation. These findings provide novel potential therapeutic options for patients during the acute episodes of Crohn's disease.

Results

Resveratrol treatment prolongs survival in an acute ileitis model

To investigate the beneficial effects of Resveratrol, Curcumin, and Simvastatin on small intestinal inflammation, we infected C57BL/10 mice with *T. gondii* and compared survival rates between treated and Placebo control mice. Whereas all untreated control mice had died at day 11 p.i., 20% of Curcumin- and 40% of Simvastatin- or Resveratrol-treated animals survived the acute phase of inflammation (**Fig. 1**). Furthermore, Resveratrol treated mice displayed significantly higher survival rates until the end of the experiment as compared to Placebo controls (40% survival, 19 days post infection; $p<0.005$, Kaplan Meier analysis; **Fig. 1**). Thus, Resveratrol treatment prolongs survival in our hyper-acute ileitis model.

Simvastatin, Curcumin, and Resveratrol ameliorate acute small intestinal inflammation

Mice orally treated with Simvastatin, Resveratrol or Curcumin displayed significantly less macroscopic signs of intestinal inflammation. Within 8 days p.i., Placebo control mice had lost approximately 15% of their initial body weight whereas mice treated with either compound displayed significant less weight loss (between 9 and 11%; $p<0.005$) (**Fig. 2 A**). Given that ileal inflammation is accompanied by a significant shortening of the upper intestinal tract, we determined the lengths of the small intestine between treated and control animals. *T. gondii* infection resulted in less significant shortening of the small intestinal length

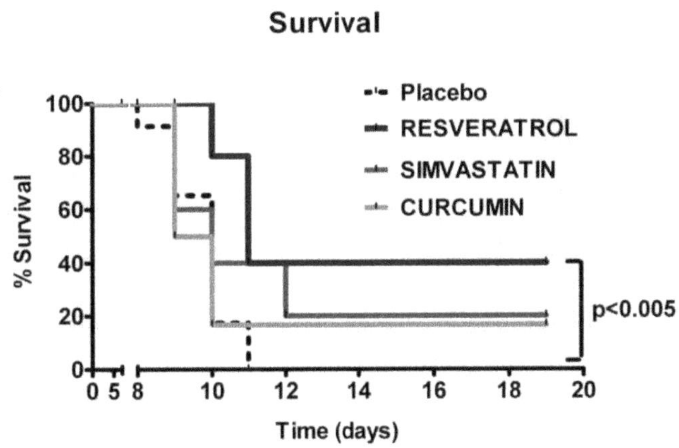

Figure 1. Survival rates of mice treated with Placebo (n = 23), Simvastain (n = 5), Resveratrol (n = 5) or Curcumin (n = 6) from d-2 until d8 p.i.. Mortality of animals was monitored daily until d19 p.i.. Significance levels (as compared with Placebo controls) were determined by Kaplan-Meier analysis.

in treated mice compared with the Placebo group (16–18% vs. 22% respectively; $p<0.05$) (**Fig. 2 B**). Moreover, animals treated with Simvastatin, Resveratrol or Curcumin displayed only mild signs of inflammation in their ileal mucosa including edema and cell-free exudate into the lumen but maintained an intact epithelium. In contrast, severe ileal inflammation including initial necrosis was observed in the control group ($p<0.0001$) (**Fig. 2 C**). Thus, oral treatment of Simvastatin, Resveratrol or Curcumin ameliorates acute small intestinal *T. gondii*-induced inflammation.

To examine whether differences in *T. gondii* loads within the ileum might have contributed to the beneficial effects observed after peroral treatment with Simvastatin, Resveratrol or Curcumin, we assessed *T. gondii* DNA concentrations in treated and untreated mice. Neither the amount of *T. gondii* DNA nor the number of parasitophorous vacuoles containing *T. gondii* tachyzoites in the ileum differed significantly between treated and Placebo groups at the same time point (data not shown).

Immuno-modulatory effects of Simvastatin, Resveratrol or Curcumin treatment in the mucosa *in situ* during acute ileitis

To further elucidate potential immuno-modulatory mechanisms by which the compounds under investigation exerted their beneficial effects, we assessed the number of several immune cell subsets in the ileal mucosa and submucosa of treated vs control mice with ileitis (**Fig. 3 A–D**). Because acute inflammation in *T. gondii* ileitis is T-cell driven and Th1 dominated [13], and there is strong evidence that regulatory T cells accumulate at inflamed tissue sites in IBD patients [16], we quantified $CD3^+$ and $FOXP3^+$ T cells in the ileum *in situ* by immunohistochemistry. Ileitis resulted in a significant accumulation of $CD3^+$ cells within the ileum mucosa and submucosa ($p<0.000001$ vs naïve mice) (**Fig. 3 A**). This increase of T lymphocytes, however, was significantly less pronounced in mice treated either with Resveratrol or Curcumin ($p<0.05$ vs. Placebo) (**Fig. 3 A**). Furthermore acute ileitis was accompanied by a 50% reduction of $FOXP3^+$ T lymphocytes in the ileum on d8 p.i. ($p<0.00001$ as compared to non-infected, naïve animals, **Fig. 3 B**). Most importantly, mice from either the Simvastain, Resveratrol or Curcumin treatment group displayed 20–30% higher $FOXP3^+$ cell numbers as compared to Placebo controls with ileitis on d8 p.i. ($p<0.05$-0.00001) (**Fig. 3 B**).

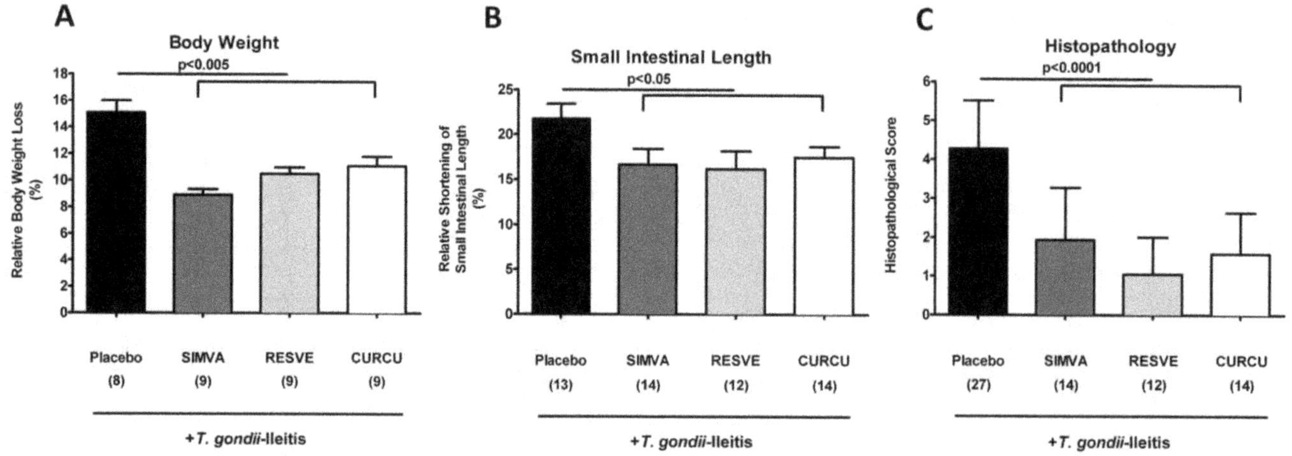

Figure 2. Less small intestinal immunopathology after treatment with Simvastain, Resveratrol or Curcumin (8 days after *T. gondii* infection). (**A**) Relative body weight loss of mice after treatment with Placebo (n = 8), Simvastain (SIMVA; n = 9), Resveratrol (RESVE; n = 9) or Curcumin (CURCU; n = 9) from d-2 until d8 p.i. (**B**) Relative small intestinal shortening of mice after treatment with Placebo (n = 13), Simvastain (SIMVA; n = 14), Resveratrol (RESVE; n = 12) or Curcumin (CURCU; n = 14) from d-2 until d8 p.i. (**C**) Histopathology of the terminal ileum of mice treated with Placebo (n = 27), Simvastain (SIMVA; n = 14), Resveratrol (RESVE; n = 12) or Curcumin (CURCU; n = 14) from d-2 until d8 p.i.. Mean values, standard deviations, and significance levels as indicated were determined by the Student's t test. Data are pooled from at least three independent experiments.

Given that neutrophilic granulocytes are important effector innate immune cells during acute ileitis development, we investigated the recruitment of myeloperoxidase-7$^+$ (MPO-7$^+$) cells in the small intestinal lamina propria of both treated and control mice in the acute phase of disease (**Fig. 3 C**). On d8 p.i., a more than 5-fold increase in MPO-7$^+$ cells was observed within the ileum of Placebo control animals compared to naïve mice, which were non-infected and untreated ($p<0.005$). However, Simvastatin, Resveratrol or Curcumin treated mice displayed 25–50% fewer MPO-7$^+$ cells as compared to Placebo controls ($p<0.05$) (**Fig. 3 C**).

In addition, we evaluated cell proliferation and regeneration in ileal sections on d8 p.i. using Ki-67, an antibody that recognizes a nuclear cell proliferation-associated antigen expressed in all active stages of the cell cycle [17]. After *T. gondii* infection, Ki-67$^+$ cell numbers increased significantly as compared to naïve mice ($p<0.00001$) (**Fig. 3 D**). Mice treated with either Resveratrol or Curcumin, however, displayed 50% more Ki-67$^+$ cells than Simvastatin- or Placebo treated animals on d8 p.i. ($p<0.005$).

Taken together, treatment with Simvastatin, Resveratrol or Curcumin modulates small intestinal immune cell responses during acute ileitis by decreasing CD3$^+$ and MPO7$^+$ cell accumulation but increasing FOXP3$^+$ and Ki-67$^+$ cell numbers.

Pro- and anti-inflammatory cytokine responses after peroral treatment of mice with acute ileitis

Given that treated mice were resistant to the development of *T. gondii*-induced ileitis compared to untreated mice but *T. gondii* DNA concentration in the ileum did not differ significantly between these groups, we hypothesized that differential pro-inflammatory cytokine expression profiles within the ilea, mesenteric lymph nodes (MLNs) or spleens might explain the reduced immunopathology observed after treatment with the compounds mentioned above at d8 p.i..

The analysis of mRNA in the ileum *in situ* revealed that IL-23p19 ($p<0.001$), IFN-γ ($p<0.05$), and TNF-α ($p<0.01$) expressions were significantly down-regulated in Curcumin-treated mice at d8 p.i. as compared to untreated controls (**Fig. 4 A**), whereas Resveratrol treated animals exhibited lower IL-6 ileal mRNA expression (**Fig. 4 B**). In addition, IFN-γ ($p<0.05$) and MCP-1 ($p<0.05$) secretion into *ex vivo* ileum cultures were significantly lower after Resveratrol, Curcumin or Simvastatin treatment compared to Placebo (**Fig. 5 A–B**). Furthermore, significantly higher amounts of the anti-inflammatory cytokine IL-10 were found in the ilea ($p<0.01$-0.001), MLNs ($p<0.01$-0.005) and spleens ($p<0.05$-0.01) after either treatment regimen compared to Placebo controls with ileitis (**Fig. 6 A–C**).

Taken together, our results show that treatment with either Simvastain, Resveratrol or Curcumin modulates the cytokine profile within the small intestine which agrees with changes of immune cell subsets (fewer T cells and neutrophils, more Tregs) observed in treated mice pointing towards less pro- and more anti-inflammatory responses.

Reduced pro-inflammatory gut bacterial species in the small intestine of mice treated with Simvastatin, Curcumin or Resveratrol

Because we have shown that *E. coli* overgrowth in the terminal ileum aggravates *T. gondii* induced inflammation [14,15], we compared the composition of the ileum microflora of mice after treatment with Simvastatin, Curcumin or Resveratrol at d8 p.i.. Cultural analysis demonstrated that the total bacterial load increased during ileitis, but was significantly reduced by 1 to 2 orders of magnitude in treated mice as compared to Placebo controls (**Fig. 7 A**) ($p<0.05$-0.0005). A more detailed cultural analysis revealed that following treatment concentrations of pro-inflammatory bacterial species such as *E. coli* (**Fig. 7 B**) and enterococci (**Fig. 7 C**) were significantly reduced by 3.0 – 3.5 ($p<0.000001$) and 1.0 – 1.5 ($p<0.0005$) orders of magnitude, respectively, whereas the potentially anti-inflammatory lactobacilli and bifidobacteria populations were slightly increased by up to 1.0 log orders (**Fig. 7 D**) ($p<0.05$-0.0005). Counts of *Clostridium* and *Eubacterium* spp. were unaffected after treatment (data not shown). Interestingly, changes in the ileal flora

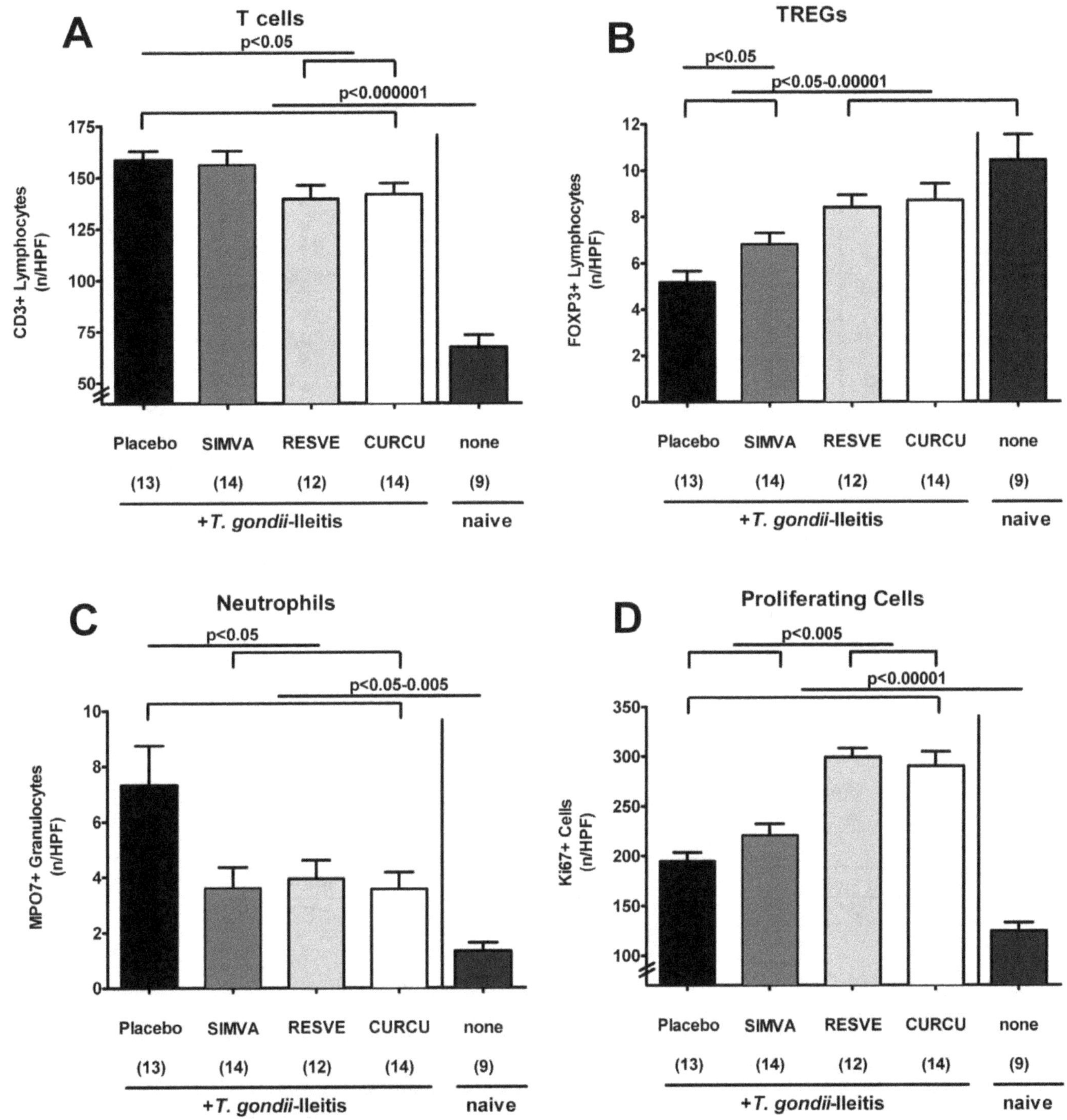

Figure 3. Quantification of defined cell population in the ileum of mice *in situ* after treatment with Simvastain, Resveratrol or Curcumin (8 days after *T. gondii* infection). The average number of cells positive for (**A**) CD3, (**B**) FOXP3, (**C**) MPO7 (Myeloperoxidase), and (**D**) Ki-67 from at least six high power fields (HPF, 400× magnification) per animal were determined microscopically in immunostained ileum sections at d8 p.i. after treatment of mice with Placebo, Simvastain (SIMVA), Resveratrol (RESVE), or Curcumin (CURCU) from d-2 until d8 p.i. and naïve, uninfected animals. Numbers of analyzed animals are given in parentheses. Mean values, standard errors of the mean, and significance levels as indicated were determined by the Student's t test. Data are pooled from at least three independent experiments.

composition were comparable in the respective treatment groups. Furthermore, a direct antimicrobial effect of Simvastatin, Resveratrol or Curcumin was ruled out by specific *in vitro* testing of the substances in the presence of the highly susceptible laboratory strain *Bacillus subtilis* (data not shown). Thus, shifts in bacterial ileal flora concentrations (lower bacterial loads and less *E. coli* overgrowth) in treated mice during ileitis were not due to direct antimicrobial effects but rather agrees with the observed macroscopic and microscopic anti-inflammatory effects of the respective substances.

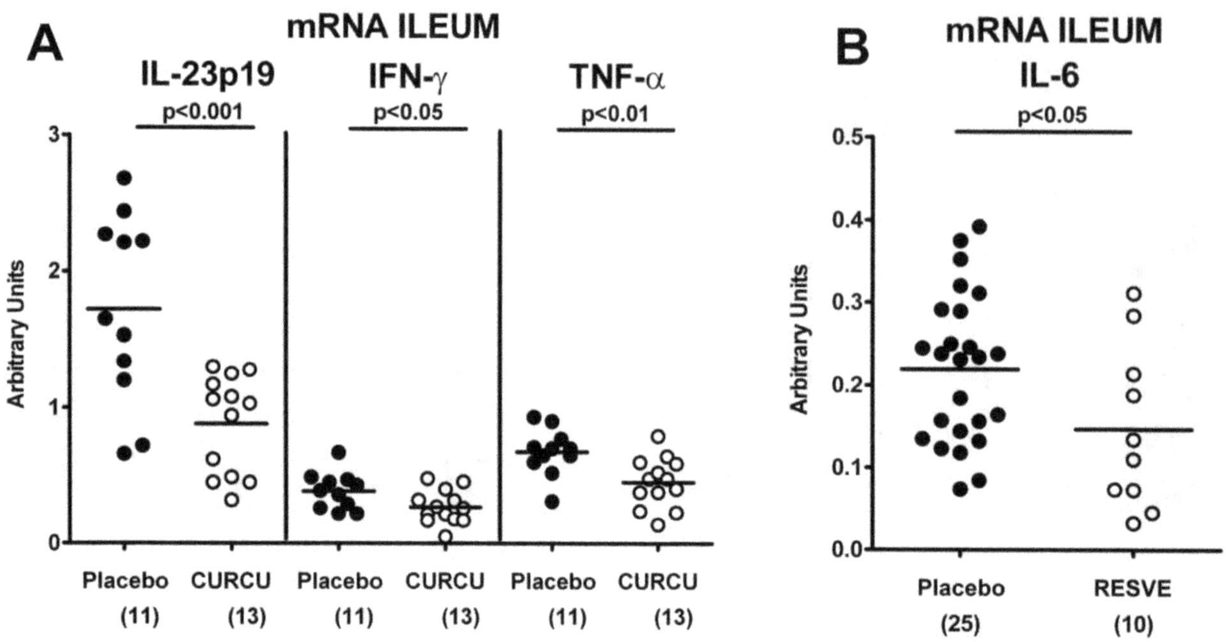

Figure 4. m-RNA Expression of pro-inflammatory cytokines in ilea of mice 8 days after *T. gondii* infection and treatment with (A) Curcumin or (B) Resveratrol from d-2 until d8 p.i. compared to Placebo controls. RT-PCR results of IL-23p19, IFN-γ and TNF-α (**A**) and IL-6 (**B**) expression from individual mice are expressed as fold changes relative to HPRT mRNA expression (arbitrary units). Numbers of analyzed animals are given in parentheses. Mean values and significance levels as indicated were determined by the Student's t test. Data are pooled from at least three independent experiments.

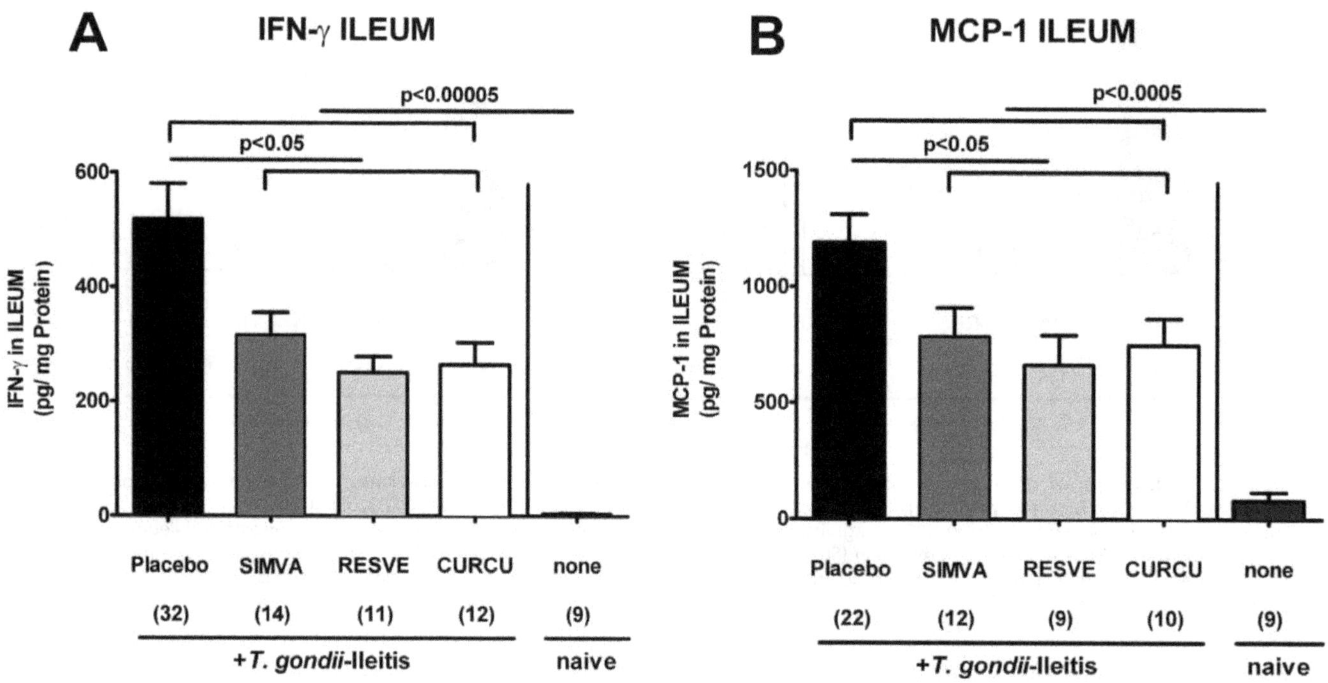

Figure 5. (A) IFN-γ and (B) MCP-1 concentrations (CBA-ELISA) in supernatants of ileum cultures from naïve, uninfected animals and mice treated with Simvastatin (SIMVA), Resveratrol (RESVE) or Curcumin (CURCU) from d-2 until d8 p.i. as compared to Placebo controls (8 days after *T. gondii* infection). Numbers of analyzed animals are given in parentheses. Mean values, standard errors of the mean, and significance levels as indicated were determined by the Student's t test. Data are pooled from at least two independent experiments.

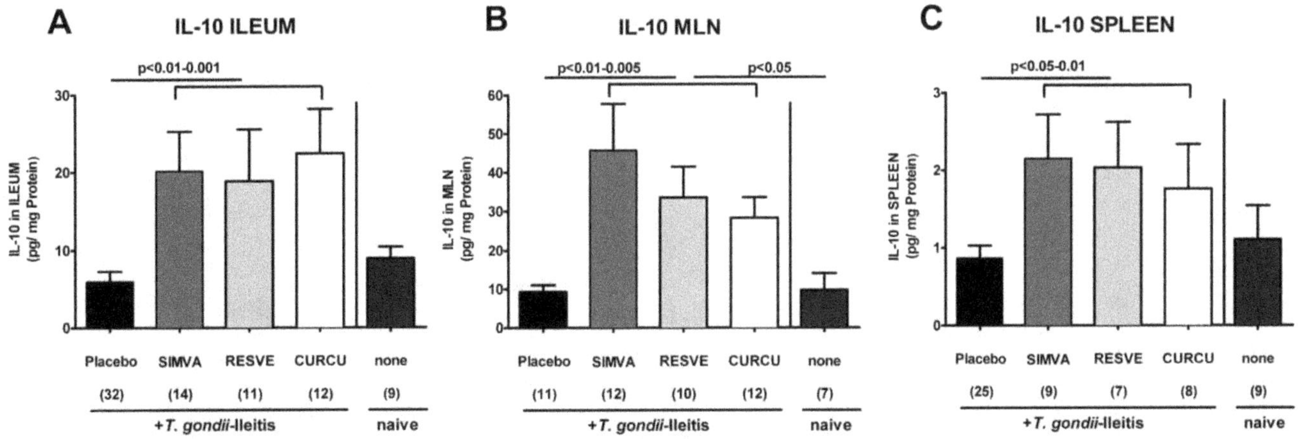

Figure 6. IL-10 concentrations (CBA-ELISA) in supernatants of Ileum (A), MLN (B) and spleen (C) cultures from naïve, uninfected animals and mice treated with Simvastatin (SIMVA), Resveratrol (RESVE) or Curcumin (CURCU) from d-2 until d8 p.i. as compared to Placebo controls (8 days after *T. gondii* infection). Numbers of analyzed animals are given in parentheses. Mean values, standard errors of the mean, and significance levels as indicated were determined by the Student's t test. Data are pooled from at least two independent experiments.

Simvastatin, Curcumin or Resveratrol treatment prevents bacterial translocation during *T. gondii*-induced ileitis

Since we have recently demonstrated that acute ileitis is accompanied by translocation of living bacteria from the commensal gut flora into adjacent organs [15] we lastly investigated translocation rates following Resveratrol, Simvastatin, or Curcumin treatment. Bacterial translocation into MLNs was detected in all animals at day 8 p.i.. (**Fig. 8 A**). Living bacteria translocated into the spleen in 78.1%, 57.1%, 55.6%, or 33.3% of cases after treatment with Placebo, Resveratrol, Simvastatin, or Curcumin, respectively (**Fig. 8 B**). The translocation rates into liver (**Fig. 8 C**) and kidney (**Fig. 8 D**) were much lower in Resveratrol- (57.1% and 42.9%, respectively) and Curcumin- (55.6% and 22.2%, respectively) treated animals as compared to the Placebo (77.8% and 66.7%, respectively) and Simvastatin (77.8% and 66.7%, respectively) groups. Oral treatment with Simvastatin (22.2%) or Curcumin (11.1%) resulted in less frequent bacteremia (and thus subsequently less frequent potential lethal sepsis) as compared to Placebo controls (29.6%) at d8 p.i. (**Fig. 8 E**). Surprisingly, all blood samples taken from Resveratrol treated mice bacteria remained sterile. The translocating bacterial species that could be cultured from the organs were predominantly *E. coli* and enterococci, the bacterial groups that were overgrowing the ileum lumen during ileitis as described above. No living bacteria could be cultured from the respective organs of naïve (non-infected, untreated) mice with intact small intestinal barrier function.

Thus, Simvastatin, Curcumin and Resveratrol treatment remarkably reduced bacterial translocation into subepithelial tissues thereby minimizing bacteria/TLR ligation and preventing immune cell activation and subsequent inflammatory response initiation.

Discussion

Inflammatory bowel diseases (IBD) such as Crohn's disease (also termed ileitis terminalis) and ulcerative colitis are characterized by chronic intestinal inflammation with acute episodes of multi-factorial etiology [18,19]. The vast majority of experimental studies concerning intestinal inflammation have been performed in murine models affecting the colon. Thus, we used our well-established, hyper-acute model of *small* intestinal inflammation following *T. gondii* infection to investigate anti-inflammatory and immuno-modulatory effects of Resveratrol, Curcumin, and Simvastatin in ileal inflammation. The immunopathology observed after *T. gondii* infection is driven by Th1 cells and by the bacterial gut flora. This situation resembles immunopathology during acute episodes of Crohn's disease [20]. Furthermore, the underlying immunopathology is characterized by an overproduction of pro-inflammatory cytokines such as IL-12, IFN-γ, TNF-α, and IL-23, a key regulator of the immune response cascade [12,13,21].

Here, we demonstrate that hyper-acute inflammation in the *small* intestine is ameliorated by either Resveratrol, Curcumin or Simvastatin treatment. In addition, the anti-inflammatory effects of the compounds under investigation during the acute phase of ileitis (on day 8 after ileitis induction by peroral infection with *T. gondii*) were comparable: animals from all three treatment groups were protected from immunopathology development and exhibited better clinical conditions, less body weight loss and shortening of the small intestinal length. Untreated mice also displayed severe pan-ileitis whereas treated animals (irrespective of the compound used) only showed minor mucosal changes with an intact epithelial lining. Furthermore, reduced ileal inflammation in Resveratrol and Curcumin treated mice might result from compensatory higher proliferation rates of intestinal epithelial cells found in the ileal mucosa as shown by higher $Ki67^+$ cell numbers after respective treatment.

Moreover, the amelioration of immunopathology was accompanied by a reduced accumulation of $CD3^+$ T lymphocytes as well as lower expression of the key regulator IL-23 and pro-inflammatory cytokines IFN-γ and TNF-α in the small intestinal lamina propria after Resveratrol or Curcumin treatment. Furthermore, ileal secretion of IFN-γ and the monocyte chemotactic protein MCP-1 was significantly decreased after treatment with Simvastatin, Resveratrol, or Curcumin. In parallel, myeloperoxidase-7^+ neutrophilic granulocytes recruitment was diminished thereby limiting oxidative stress in the ileum and maintaining an integral epithelial cell barrier function. In addition, numbers of $FOXP3^+$ cells were diminished in untreated mice, but significantly increased (comparable to the observed numbers in naïve mice) in treated animals after ileitis induction which correlates with increased concentrations of the anti-inflammatory cytokine IL-10 observed in ileum, MLNs, and spleen at d8 p.i..

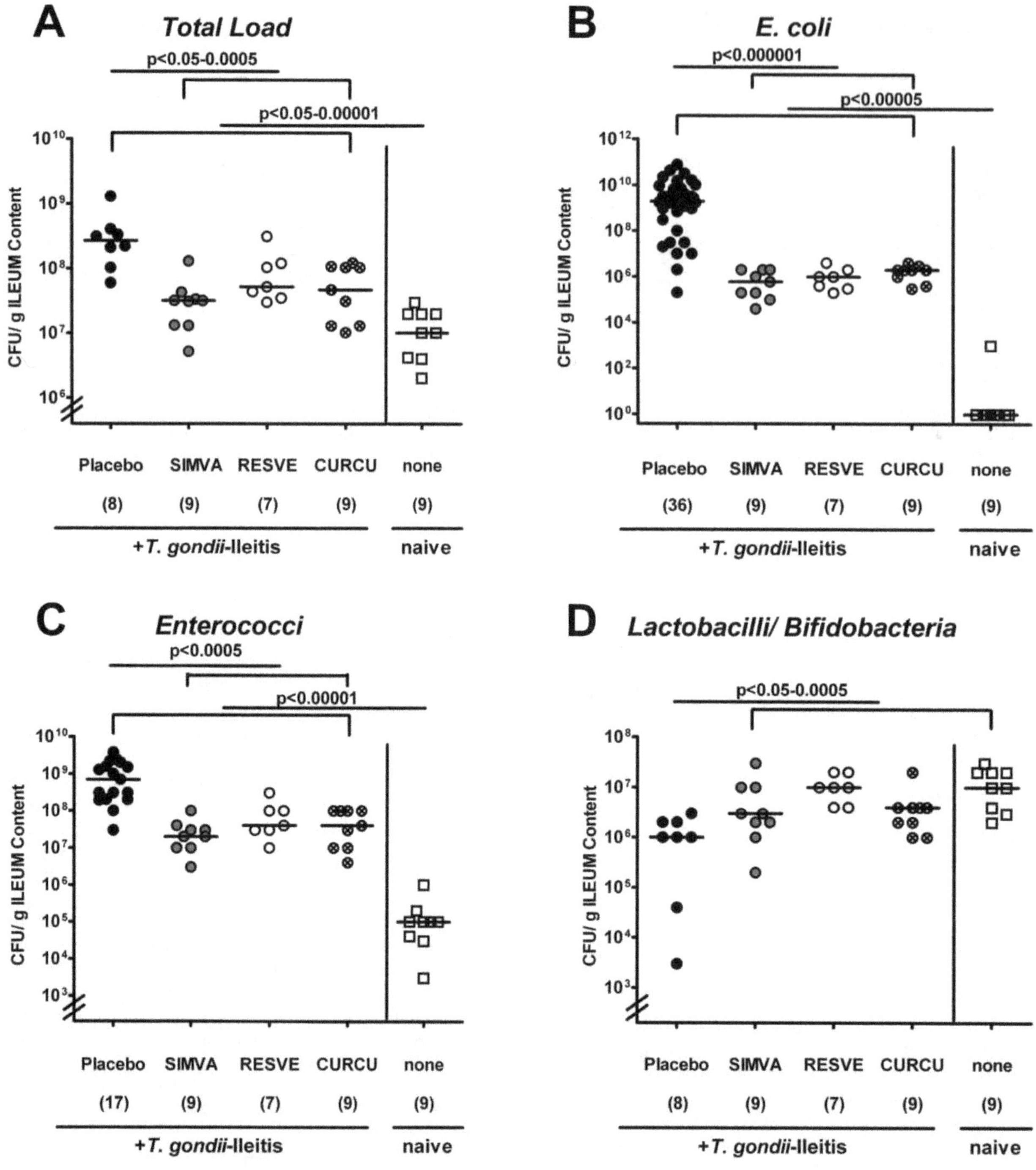

Figure 7. Changes in the composition of the luminal ileum flora obtained from uninfected animals (none) and *T. gondii*-infected mice treated with Simvastain (SIMVA), Resveratrol (RESVE) or Curcumin (CURCU) from d-2 until d8 p.i. as compared to Placebo controls (8 days after *T. gondii* infection). Detailed cultural analysis was performed on appropriate selective media, bacterial species identified by biochemical analysis and reconfirmed by comparative sequence analysis (see Methods). Individual bacterial counts (CFU, colony forming units) of (**A**) Total bacterial load, (**B**) *E. coli*, (**C**) enterococci, (**D**) lactobacilli/bifidobacteria obtained from respectively treated mice (numbers of animals are given in parentheses), medians and levels of significance determined by Mann-Whitney-U test are indicated. Data are pooled from two representative experiments.

Simvastatin has been shown to inhibit acute as well as chronic inflammatory responses in a cholesterol-independent manner by interfering with endothelial adhesion and leukocyte migration to sites of inflammation [11,22]. In rats with normal blood cholesterol levels, simvastatin was found to ameliorate immunopathology in an acute TNBS colitis model by blocking neutrophil accumulation in the small intestine and lowering serum TNF-α levels [23].

Curcumin exerts its anti-inflammatory effects in murine colitis models by inhibiting COX2- and pro-inflammatory cytokine expression such as nitric oxide [9,24,25] and suppressing NF-κB activation [26,27].

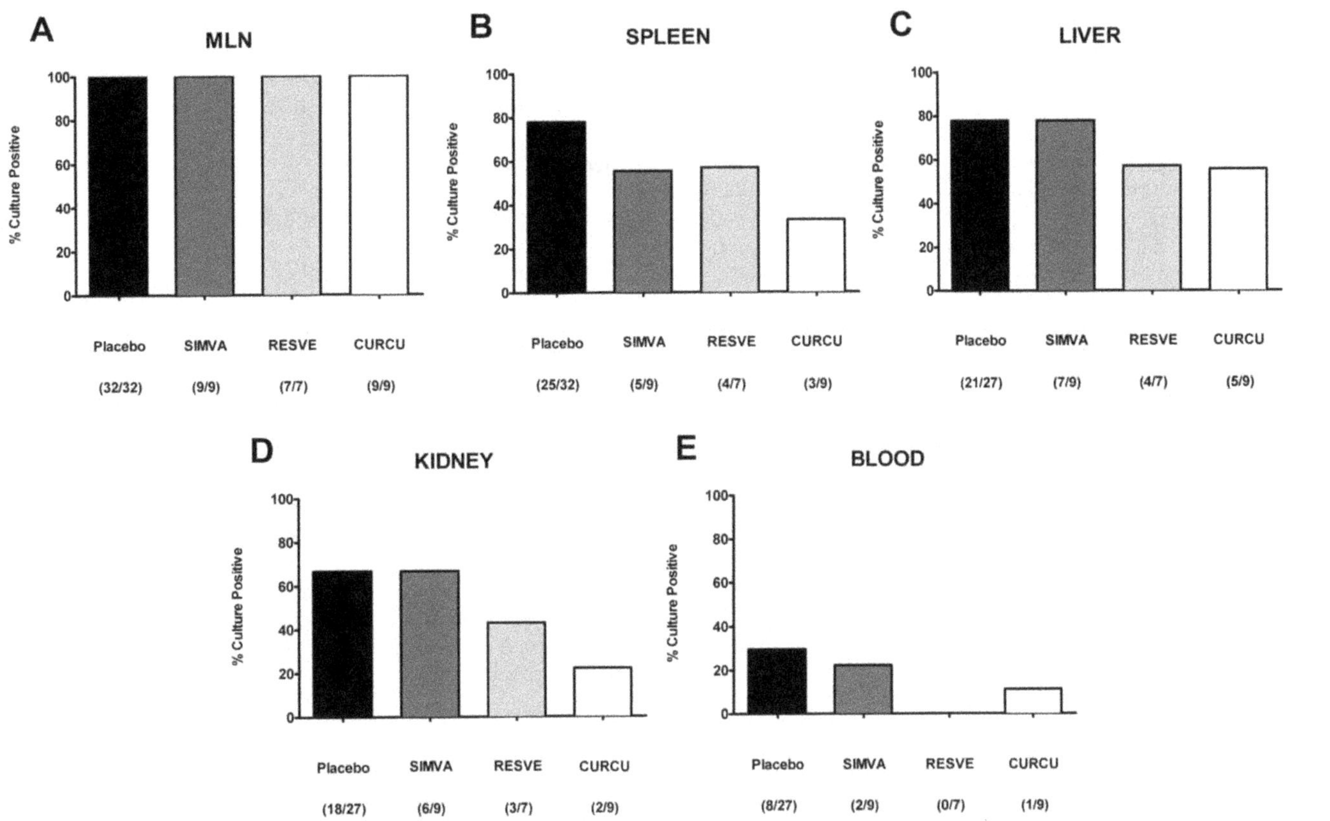

Figure 8. Bacterial translocation into (A) MLN, (B) Spleen, (C) Liver, (D) Kidney, and (E) Blood of mice treated with Simvastain (SIMVA), Resveratrol (RESVE) or Curcumin (CURCU) from d-2 until d8 p.i. as compared to Placebo controls (8 days after *T. gondii* infection). Organs or blood were cultivated in thioglycolate broth for maximum 7 days. Turbid broths were sub-cultivated on solid media (refer to Materials). Indicated are relative rates of positive samples (in %) and absolute numbers of positive samples out of total number analyzed in parentheses.

In acute TNBS rat colitis model, a decreased neutrophil influx and IL-1β production as well as an enhanced apoptosis of colonic mucosa was observed following Resveratrol treatment [28]. In chronic DSS-induced colitis, both decreased expression of pro-inflammatory cytokines (TNF-α, NO, and IL-1β) and increased anti-inflammatory mediators (IL-10) in the colonic mucosa contributed to attenuate inflammation after Resveratrol treatment [29]. In addition, even low dose Resveratrol treatment exerted anti-inflammatory effects in an acute DSS-induced colitis model by reducing expression levels of prostaglandin-E2, COX2, and NO [6].

Changes in commensal gut flora composition observed in acute *T. gondii*-induced ileitis resemble the gut flora changes found in humans with IBD [14,15]. Shifts in the ileal flora composition become overt around d5 p.i., the time point when first significant defects of the epithelial barrier are histologically detectable. Ileitis development is accompanied by decreased species diversity, decreased loads of potentially anti-inflammatory species such as lactobacilli and bifidobacteria and a marked increase in commensal, potentially pro-inflammatory *E. coli* in the ileum lumen by 6–8 orders of magnitude. Furthermore, overgrowing *E. coli* within the gut aggravates Toll-like receptor- (TLR-) 4 driven immune responses during *T. gondii*-induced ileitis [15]. In addition, overgrowing bacteria easily translocate through a disrupted epithelial cell barrier into the intestinal lamina propria, lymphoid tissues (e.g. the ileum draining MLNs) and subsequently come in contact with immune cells thereby exacerbating intestinal inflammation. Lastly, when translocating bacteria reach the systemic blood stream, peritonitis, sepsis and subsequent multiple organ failure occurs with fatal consequences [14,15]. Therefore, we investigated whether Simvastatin, Resveratrol or Curcumin could prevent gut flora composition changes and bacterial translocation after *T. gondii* infection. Interestingly, treatment with either compound significantly diminished total bacterial ileal burdens as compared to untreated animals. Strikingly, lower *E. coli* and enterococci counts were found in treated mice whereas lactobacilli and bifidobacteria populations were slightly but significantly increased. In addition, ileitis development is accompanied by a marked decrease in the lactobacilli and bifidobacteria populations [14] and strikingly, after either treatment these lactobacilli and bifidobacteria populations remained at comparable levels with naïve, uninfected mice. Remarkably, none of the compounds had a direct anti-microbial effect *in vitro*.

Larrosa and co-workers reported in 2009 similar flora shifts in an acute DSS-induced colitis model, however, to a much lesser extent: After low-dose Resveratrol treatment, rats exhibited increases in lactobacilli and bifidobacteria populations within the colonic lumen and blocked the increase in enterobacteria (mainly *E. coli*) [6]. In several studies, a protective effect of lactobacilli and bifidobacteria in DSS-colitis could be demonstrated [30], as well as modulatory effects upon pro-inflammatory responses in intestinal epithelial cells that have been challenged with pathogenic enterobacteria [31]. Thus, abundance of anti-inflammatory lactobacilli and bifidobacteria together with scarcity of pro-inflammatory *E. coli* markedly limit inflammation during *T. gondii* ileitis.

Resveratrol, Simvastatin, or Curcumin treatment might have an anti-inflammatory effect by directly interfering with the TLR/MyD88 signaling pathway. Recent findings in acute TNBS-induced colitis model in rats demonstrate that Curcumin-induced inhibition of intestinal inflammation involves TLR-4 and MyD88 [32].

Furthermore, an effect of Curcumin on matrixmetalloproteinases (MMPs; important in the pathogenesis of human IBD [33]) was recently described [34]: Curcumin down-regulated MMP-9 (gelatinase-B) activity on inflammation-induced intestinal epithelial cells *in vitro*. We have recently shown that non-selective MMP- as well as selective gelatinase blockage by a synthetic compound ameliorated *T. gondii* ileitis [12]. However, MMP-2, but not MMP-9 played a crucial role in mediating small intestinal pathology. MMP-9 is proposed to play an important role in experimental colitis [35]. Interestingly, neutrophils have been proposed as an important source for MMPs. Thus, inhibition of neutrophil migration by the investigated compounds might also down-modulated MMP secretion thereby diminishing epithelial cell inflammation.

In a recent study, Curcumin has been shown to inhibit oxidative stress [36] that in turn has been associated with tight junction opening, thereby modifying intestinal permeability [37]. In the present study, bacterial translocation rates (due to compromised epithelial barrier function) into spleen and cardiac blood after treatment with either compound were lower as compared to the Placebo group. Therefore, Resveratrol, Simvastatin, and Curcumin might modulate tight junction protein expression and function.

Most strikingly, 20 to 40% of the animals treated with Resveratrol, Simvastatin, or Curcumin survived the acute phase of inflammation whereas all untreated mice had died at d11 p.i.. In addition, 40% of Resveratrol treated mice displayed a long-term survival (until the end of the observation period until d19 p.i.; $p<0.005$ vs. Placebo). The long-term survival effect of Resveratrol is remarkable for three reasons: First, in our study, the duration of treatment (before and during course of acute inflammation) was rather short: Resveratrol treatment was initiated two days prior to ileitis induction and lasted 10 days in total; at d8 p.i. treatment was withdrawn. Second, given that the bioavailibility of the compound is low, short-term and local rather than systemic effects are observed within the gut lumen (effective until d8/d9 p.i.). Because *T. gondii*-induced ileitis compromises the intestinal absorption capacity, Resveratrol absorption after oral application is also reduced. Third, Resveratrol treatment improves survival in a hyper-acute small intestinal inflammation model where all Placebo control mice died. Thus far, Resveratrol treatment has only been shown to reduce mortality in a chronic colitis model [29]. We might hypothesize that Resveratrol treatment prevents bacterial translocation into the systemic circulation because in our study, we did not observe bacterial growth in any of blood cultures drawn from Resveratrol treated mice. Therefore, mice are protected from a bacteremia-induced sepsis that leads to death. Furthermore, fewer bacteria translocation rates into sub-epithelial tissues might be due to a less compromised epithelial barrier function. Fewer translocation rates are mirrored by an IL-6 decrease in the ileum of Resveratrol treated animals. Our findings agree with those in the literature suggesting that genes belonging to the IL-6 pathway are down-regulated in Resveratrol treated mice in experimental colitis [6] and other inflammation models [38].

In conclusion, here we show for the first time that Resveratrol, Curcumin, and Simvastatin exert potent anti-inflammatory effects in a hyper-acute Th1-type driven small intestinal inflammation model. In addition, Resveratrol, Curcumin, and Simvastatin represent novel and promising intervention strategies for prophylaxis and therapy of small intestinal inflammation in IBD.

Materials and Methods

Ethics Statement

All animal experiments were conducted according to the German animal protection laws (LaGeSo Berlin, TVV G0145/10 and G0146/10) with approval from the Charité – Universitätsmedizin ethical committee. Animal welfare was monitored twice daily by assessment of clinical conditions and weight loss of mice.

Mice, parasites and ileitis induction

C57BL/10ScSn (wildtype) mice used for experiments were 3 months old and bred under specific pathogen-free (SPF) conditions in the Forschungsinstitut für Experimentelle Medizin (Charité, Berlin, Germany). For induction of ileitis, mice were infected orally with 100 *T. gondii* cysts (ME49 strain) from homogenized brains of intraperitoneally infected NMRI mice in a volume of 0.3 ml phosphate-buffered saline (PBS, pH 7.4) by gavage, as described previously [14].

Compounds

Resveratrol, Curcumin, and Simvastatin were dissolved in 2% Carboxy-Methyl-Cellulose (in PBS; all purchased from Sigma-Aldrich, München, Germany) and administered to mice with a daily dose of 20 mg, 100 mg, and 20 mg per kg body weight, respectively. Mice received the respective verum compound or the carrier solution (serving as Placebo control) perorally by gavage (in a 0.3 ml volume) once daily starting 2 days before *T. gondii* infection until the end of the experiment at day (d) 8 post infection (p.i.).

Sampling procedures and determination of small intestinal shortening

Mice were sacrificed by isoflurane 8 days after infection (Abbott, Wiesbaden, Germany). Cardiac blood and tissue samples from liver, spleen, kidneys, mesenteric lymph nodes and terminal ileum were removed under sterile conditions. Intestinal samples from each mouse were collected in parallel for histological, microbiological, immunological and molecular analyses. The relative shortening of the small intestine was calculated by dividing the difference of the mean length of small intestine from age- and sex-matched naïve control mice minus the length of infected mice at day 8 p.i. and then multiplied by 100 over the mean length of naïve control mice small intestines (relative shortening in length = (mean d0 – d8 p.i.)×100/mean d0). Results were expressed as % shortage.

Histologic scores and determination of parasite load

Histologic scores of ileitis and parasite loads were determined in tissue samples from terminal ileum immediately fixed in 5% formalin and embedded in paraffin as described earlier [14,15]. Sections (5 μm) were stained with hematoxylin and eosin and examined by light microscopy. Our standardized histological inflammation score ranging from 0 to 6 (0, normal; 1, edematous blubbing; 2, cell-free exudate into the lumen, but intact epithelium; 3, cellular shedding into the lumen; 4, beginning epithelial disintegration; 5, mucosal destruction <50% of small intestine length; 6, complete destruction >50% of small intestine length, severe necroses) was used for blinded duplicate evaluation (by M.M.H. and M.M.). Numbers of parasitophorous vacuoles containing tachyzoites or tachyzoite antigens were determined by immunohistology using a rabbit anti-*T. gondii*- IgG antiserum and counted in the terminal ileum, as previously described [21]. In addition, *T. gondii* DNA in ileal biospies was quantified as described earlier [12].

Immunohistochemistry

In situ immunohistochemical analysis of ileum paraffin sections were performed as described previously [39]. Primary antibodies against CD3 (# N1580, Dako, Glostrup, Denmark, dilution 1:10), FOXP3 (FJK-16s, eBioscience, San Diego, USA, 1:100), myeloperoxidase-7 (MPO7, # A0398, Dako, 1:500), and Ki-67 (TEC3, Dako, 1:100) were used. For each animal, the average number of positive stained cells within at least six independent high power fields (HPF, high power visual field in 400× magnification) were determined microscopically by two independent investigators (M.M.H. and C.L.) and subjected to statistical analysis as indicated.

Real-time PCR

RNA was isolated from organs, reverse transcribed and analyzed as described previously [12]. Mouse IL-23p19, IFN-γ and TNF-α mRNA expressions were detected and analyzed using Light Cycler Data Analysis Software, Roche. Expression levels were calculated relative to the HPRT expression (and indicated as "Arbitrary Units").

Cytokine detection in ileum, MLN, and spleen culture supernatants

Ileum biopsies were cut longitudinally, washed with PBS and strips of 1 cm^2, MLNs or spleen placed in 24-flat-bottom well culture plates (Nunc, Wiesbaden, Germany) containing 500 µl serum-free RPMI 1640 medium supplemented with penicillin (100 U/ml) and streptomycin (100 µg/ml; PAA Laboratories). After 18 h at 37°C, culture supernatants were tested for IFN-γ, MCP-1, and IL-10 concentrations by the Mouse Inflammation Cytometric Bead Array (CBA; BD Biosciences).

Cultural analysis of the ileum microflora and bacterial translocation

Culture-based analysis of the ileum flora was performed as described earlier [14]. For qualitative detection of bacterial translocation, cardiac blood (approx. 0.5 ml) or the respective organ (liver, spleen, MLN, kidney) was immediately transferred into thioglycolate broth under sterile conditions and incubated for maximum 7 days at 37°C. Bacterial growth was monitored daily by turbidity assessment. Aliquots from turbid broths were cultivated on solid media under aerobic, microaerophilic and obligate anaerobic conditions and the bacterial species identified microbiologically and biochemically as described earlier [14].

Antimicrobial effects of Simvastatin, Curcumin and Resveratrol were assessed *in vitro* by inoculating a blank susceptibility disk (Oxoid, Basingstoke, UK) with 10 µl of either compound. Before, the blank disc was placed onto an Müller-Hinton agar plate (Oxoid) that was inoculated with a highly susceptible *Bacillus subtilis* ATCC 6633 strain. After overnight incubation (37°C), lack of growth inhibition around the disk was indicating a negative antimicrobial result [40].

Statistical analysis

Mean values, medians, standard deviations, standard errors of the mean, and levels of significance were determined using appropriate tests as indicated (Student's t-Test, Mann-Whitney U-Test or the log-rank test for Kaplan-Meier analysis of survival). Two-sided probability (p) values ≤ 0.05 were considered significant. All experiments were repeated at least twice.

Acknowledgments

The authors thank Michaela Wattrodt, Ursula Rüschendorf, Ines Puschendorf, Simone Spieckermann, Gernot Reifenberger, Uwe Lohmann and the staff of the animal research facility for excellent technical assistance and Günther Heimesaat for critical discussions.

Author Contributions

Conceived and designed the experiments: MMH AF SB. Performed the experiments: MMH MM AF RP BO L-MH SB. Analyzed the data: MMH MM AF RP BO L-MH AAK CL. Contributed reagents/materials/ analysis tools: CL AAK. Wrote the paper: MMH MM AF RP L-MH BO AAK SB UBG.

References

1. Jain SK (1994) Ethnobotany and research on medicinal plants in India. Ciba Found Symp 185: 153–164; discussion 164-158.
2. Kobashigawa JA, Katznelson S, Laks H, Johnson JA, Yeatman L, et al. (1995) Effect of pravastatin on outcomes after cardiac transplantation. N Engl J Med 333: 621–627.
3. Baur JA, Pearson KJ, Price NL, Jamieson HA, Lerin C, et al. (2006) Resveratrol improves health and survival of mice on a high-calorie diet. Nature 444: 337–342.
4. Elmali N, Baysal O, Harma A, Esenkaya I, Mizrak B (2007) Effects of resveratrol in inflammatory arthritis. Inflammation 30: 1–6.
5. Ma ZH, Ma QY, Wang LC, Sha HC, Wu SL, et al. (2005) Effect of resveratrol on peritoneal macrophages in rats with severe acute pancreatitis. Inflamm Res 54: 522–527.
6. Larrosa M, Yanez-Gascon MJ, Selma MV, Gonzalez-Sarrias A, Toti S, et al. (2009) Effect of a low dose of dietary resveratrol on colon microbiota, inflammation and tissue damage in a DSS-induced colitis rat model. J Agric Food Chem 57: 2211–2220.
7. Calabrese V, Butterfield DA, Stella AM (2003) Nutritional antioxidants and the heme oxygenase pathway of stress tolerance: novel targets for neuroprotection in Alzheimer's disease. Ital J Biochem 52: 177–181.
8. Huang TS, Lee SC, Lin JK (1991) Suppression of c-Jun/AP-1 activation by an inhibitor of tumor promotion in mouse fibroblast cells. Proc Natl Acad Sci U S A 88: 5292–5296.
9. Sugimoto K, Hanai H, Tozawa K, Aoshi T, Uchijima M, et al. (2002) Curcumin prevents and ameliorates trinitrobenzene sulfonic acid-induced colitis in mice. Gastroenterology 123: 1912–1922.
10. Simes J, Furberg CD, Braunwald E, Davis BR, Ford I, et al. (2002) Effects of pravastatin on mortality in patients with and without coronary heart disease across a broad range of cholesterol levels. The Prospective Pravastatin Pooling project. Eur Heart J 23: 207–215.
11. Diomede L, Albani D, Sottocorno M, Donati MB, Bianchi M, et al. (2001) In vivo anti-inflammatory effect of statins is mediated by nonsterol mevalonate products. Arterioscler Thromb Vasc Biol 21: 1327–1332.
12. Munoz M, Heimesaat MM, Danker K, Struck D, Lohmann U, et al. (2009) Interleukin (IL)-23 mediates Toxoplasma gondii-induced immunopathology in the gut via matrixmetalloproteinase-2 and IL-22 but independent of IL-17. J Exp Med 206: 3047–3059.
13. Liesenfeld O, Kosek J, Remington JS, Suzuki Y (1996) Association of CD4+ T cell-dependent, interferon-gamma-mediated necrosis of the small intestine with genetic susceptibility of mice to peroral infection with Toxoplasma gondii. J Exp Med 184: 597–607.
14. Heimesaat MM, Bereswill S, Fischer A, Fuchs D, Struck D, et al. (2006) Gram-negative bacteria aggravate murine small intestinal Th1-type immunopathology following oral infection with Toxoplasma gondii. J Immunol 177: 8785–8795.
15. Heimesaat MM, Fischer A, Jahn HK, Niebergall J, Freudenberg M, et al. (2007) Exacerbation of murine ileitis by Toll-like receptor 4 mediated sensing of lipopolysaccharide from commensal Escherichia coli. Gut 56: 941–948.
16. Maul J, Loddenkemper C, Mundt P, Berg E, Giese T, et al. (2005) Peripheral and intestinal regulatory CD4+ CD25(high) T cells in inflammatory bowel disease. Gastroenterology 128: 1868–1878.
17. Gerdes J, Li L, Schlueter C, Duchrow M, Wohlenberg C, et al. (1991) Immunobiochemical and molecular biologic characterization of the cell

proliferation-associated nuclear antigen that is defined by monoclonal antibody Ki-67. Am J Pathol 138: 867–873.
18. Podolsky DK (2002) Inflammatory bowel disease. N Engl J Med 347: 417–429.
19. Basset C, Holton J (2002) Inflammatory bowel disease: is the intestine a Trojan horse? Sci Prog 85: 33–56.
20. Liesenfeld O (2002) Oral infection of C57BL/6 mice with Toxoplasma gondii: a new model of inflammatory bowel disease? J Infect Dis 185 Suppl 1: S96–101.
21. Vossenkamper A, Struck D, Alvarado-Esquivel C, Went T, Takeda K, et al. (2004) Both IL-12 and IL-18 contribute to small intestinal Th1-type immunopathology following oral infection with Toxoplasma gondii, but IL-12 is dominant over IL-18 in parasite control. Eur J Immunol 34: 3197–3207.
22. Maher BM, Dhonnchu TN, Burke JP, Soo A, Wood AE, et al. (2009) Statins alter neutrophil migration by modulating cellular Rho activity–a potential mechanism for statins-mediated pleotropic effects? J Leukoc Biol 85: 186–193.
23. Jahovic N, Gedik N, Ercan F, Sirvanci S, Yuksel M, et al. (2006) Effects of statins on experimental colitis in normocholesterolemic rats. Scand J Gastroenterol 41: 954–962.
24. Camacho-Barquero L, Villegas I, Sanchez-Calvo JM, Talero E, Sanchez-Fidalgo S, et al. (2007) Curcumin, a Curcuma longa constituent, acts on MAPK p38 pathway modulating COX-2 and iNOS expression in chronic experimental colitis. Int Immunopharmacol 7: 333–342.
25. Ung VY, Foshaug RR, MacFarlane SM, Churchill TA, Doyle JS, et al. Oral administration of curcumin emulsified in carboxymethyl cellulose has a potent anti-inflammatory effect in the IL-10 gene-deficient mouse model of IBD. Dig Dis Sci 55: 1272–1277.
26. Jobin C, Bradham CA, Russo MP, Juma B, Narula AS, et al. (1999) Curcumin blocks cytokine-mediated NF-kappa B activation and proinflammatory gene expression by inhibiting inhibitory factor I-kappa B kinase activity. J Immunol 163: 3474–3483.
27. Jian YT, Mai GF, Wang JD, Zhang YL, Luo RC, et al. (2005) Preventive and therapeutic effects of NF-kappaB inhibitor curcumin in rats colitis induced by trinitrobenzene sulfonic acid. World J Gastroenterol 11: 1747–1752.
28. Martin AR, Villegas I, La Casa C, de la Lastra CA (2004) Resveratrol, a polyphenol found in grapes, suppresses oxidative damage and stimulates apoptosis during early colonic inflammation in rats. Biochem Pharmacol 67: 1399–1410.
29. Sanchez-Fidalgo S, Cardeno A, Villegas I, Talero E, de la Lastra CA () Dietary supplementation of resveratrol attenuates chronic colonic inflammation in mice. Eur J Pharmacol 633: 78–84.
30. Fooks LJ, Gibson GR (2002) Probiotics as modulators of the gut flora. Br J Nutr 88 Suppl 1: S39–49.
31. Candela M, Perna F, Carnevali P, Vitali B, Ciati R, et al. (2008) Interaction of probiotic Lactobacillus and Bifidobacterium strains with human intestinal epithelial cells: adhesion properties, competition against enteropathogens and modulation of IL-8 production. Int J Food Microbiol 125: 286–292.
32. Lubbad A, Oriowo MA, Khan I (2009) Curcumin attenuates inflammation through inhibition of TLR-4 receptor in experimental colitis. Mol Cell Biochem 322: 127–135.
33. Baugh MD, Perry MJ, Hollander AP, Davies DR, Cross SS, et al. (1999) Matrix metalloproteinase levels are elevated in inflammatory bowel disease. Gastroenterology 117: 814–822.
34. Claramunt RM, Bouissane L, Cabildo MP, Cornago MP, Elguero J, et al. (2009) Synthesis and biological evaluation of curcuminoid pyrazoles as new therapeutic agents in inflammatory bowel disease: effect on matrix metalloproteinases. Bioorg Med Chem 17: 1290–1296.
35. Medina C, Santana A, Paz MC, Diaz-Gonzalez F, Farre E, et al. (2006) Matrix metalloproteinase-9 modulates intestinal injury in rats with transmural colitis. J Leukoc Biol 79: 954–962.
36. Aggarwal BB, Sung B (2009) Pharmacological basis for the role of curcumin in chronic diseases: an age-old spice with modern targets. Trends Pharmacol Sci 30: 85–94.
37. Rapin JR, Wiernsperger N (2010) Possible links between intestinal permeablity and food processing: A potential therapeutic niche for glutamine. Clinics (Sao Paulo) 65: 635–643.
38. Ahn J, Lee H, Kim S, Ha T (2007) Resveratrol inhibits TNF-alpha-induced changes of adipokines in 3T3-L1 adipocytes. Biochem Biophys Res Commun 364: 972–977.
39. Heimesaat MM, Fischer A, Siegmund B, Kupz A, Niebergall J, et al. (2007) Shift towards pro-inflammatory intestinal bacteria aggravates acute murine colitis via Toll-like receptors 2 and 4. PLoS One 2: e662.
40. Kouri TT, Gant VA, Fogazzi GB, Hofmann W, Hallander HO, et al. (2000) Towards European urinalysis guidelines. Introduction of a project under European Confederation of Laboratory Medicine. Clin Chim Acta 297: 305–311.

12

Administration of Reconstituted Polyphenol Oil Bodies Efficiently Suppresses Dendritic Cell Inflammatory Pathways and Acute Intestinal Inflammation

Elisabetta Cavalcanti[1], Elisa Vadrucci[1,2], Francesca Romana Delvecchio[2,3], Francesco Addabbo[1], Simona Bettini[4], Rachel Liou[5], Vladia Monsurrò[6], Alex Yee-Chen Huang[5], Theresa Torres Pizarro[7], Angelo Santino[8,9], Marcello Chieppa[1,2,3*,9]

1 Laboratory of Experimental Immunopathology, IRCCS "de Bellis," Castellana Grotte (BA), Italy, **2** Laboratory of Mucosal Immunology, Mario Negri South, Santa Maria Imbaro (CH), Italy, **3** Laboratory of Translational Medicine, ARCHES, Castellana Grotte (BA), Italy, **4** Department of Engineering for Innovation, University of Salento, Lecce, Italy, **5** Department of Pediatrics, Case Western Reserve University School of Medicine, Cleveland, Ohio, United States of America, **6** Department of Pathology and Diagnostic, University of Verona Medical School, Verona, Italy, **7** Department of Pathology, Case Western Reserve University School of Medicine, Cleveland, Ohio, United States of America, **8** Institute of Science of Food Production, CNR, Lecce, Italy

Abstract

Polyphenols are natural compounds capable of interfering with the inflammatory pathways of several *in vitro* model systems. In this study, we developed a stable and effective strategy to administer polyphenols to treat *in vivo* models of acute intestinal inflammation. The *in vitro* suppressive properties of several polyphenols were first tested and compared for dendritic cells (DCs) production of inflammatory cytokines. A combination of the polyphenols, quercetin and piperine, were then encapsulated into reconstituted oil bodies (OBs) in order to increase their stability. Our results showed that administration of low dose reconstituted polyphenol OBs inhibited LPS-mediated inflammatory cytokine secretion, including IL-6, IL-23, and IL-12, while increasing IL-10 and IL-1Rα production. Mice treated with the polyphenol-containing reconstituted OBs (ROBs) were partially protected from dextran sodium sulfate (DSS)-induced colitis and associated weight loss, while mortality and inflammatory scores revealed an overall anti-inflammatory effect that was likely mediated by impaired DC immune responses. Our study indicates that the administration of reconstituted quercetin and piperine-containing OBs may represent an effective and potent anti-inflammatory strategy to treat acute intestinal inflammation.

Editor: Andreas Zirlik, University Heart Center Freiburg, Germany

Funding: This work was supported by "My First AIRC Grant (MFAG 10684) Italian Cancer Association" Via Corridoni, 7 20122 Milano Italy; the Italian Ministry of Health, "GR2009" the Fondazione Cassa di Risparmio di Puglia, PON02_00186_2937475 "Pro.Ali.Fun" and 5 per mille 2010 (ARCHES, Castellana Grotte, Bari); A.Y.H. is supported by NIH R01 CA154656 and the St. Baldrick's Foundation; T.T.P is supported by NIH P01 DK091222. The funders had no role in study design, data collection and analysis, decision to publish, or preparation of the manuscript.

Competing Interests: The authors have declared that no competing interests exist.

* E-mail: transmed@irccsdebellis.it

9 These authors contributed equally to this work.

Introduction

Intestinal inflammatory disorders, including inflammatory bowel diseases (IBD)s, are common multifactorial clinical pathologies resulting from uncontrolled and deregulated gut mucosal immune responses[1]. In fact, the intestinal immune system is characterized by unique features that are specific for surveying the largest exposed surface of the body that is in direct contact with the external environment, and for balancing physiological inflammation while maintaining normal gut homeostasis[2]. Several different cells serve important roles in this complex immune surveillance. Dendritic cells (DCs), for example, play a pivotal role in switching the adaptive immune response from a tolerogenic to an inflammatory state[3]. It has been postulated that triggering oral tolerance in patients with IBD is due, in part, to defective inflammatory cytokine production by intestinal resident DCs[4].

Intestinal DC cytokine production is unique and imprinted by exposure to epithelial factors, including TSLP and TGFβ[5] [6] [7]. Disruption of the epithelial barrier changes the gut milieu towards an inflammatory phenotype that facilitates intestinal DC accumulation to the site of inflammation[8] [9] [10] and promotes the secretion of inflammatory mediators, including TNFα, IL-12, and IL-18[11] [12]. Taken together, various therapeutic approaches that target inflammatory DCs by dampening proinflammatory cytokine production have been evaluated[13]. Clinical therapies currently available include, for example, the systemic administration of antibodies against TNFα. Treatment with anti-TNF, in fact, is proven to be effective even in cases of chronic disease; however, a significant percentage of patients do not respond or become resistant to anti-TNF therapy[14].

Several studies have described the beneficial effects of plant-derived polyphenols as natural ligands that are able to reduce inflammation, with some inhibiting production of TNFα from cell lines of different origins in both *in vitro* and *in vivo* models[15]. Little is known, however, regarding the immunomodulatory effects of polyphenols on DCs, likely due to their chemical characteristics that impart instability, particularly in an *in vivo* setting, and limit their translational potential[16] [17]. Quercetin, similarly to many other phytochemicals, is a hydrophobic compound characterized by low solubility in water and consequent low bioavailability. These major limitations can be bypassed by developing efficient delivery systems that have the ability to protect, as well as release, polyphenols at the appropriate site of action. A wide variety of new delivery systems has been proposed, including liposomes, nanoparticles, and nanoemulsions[18]. Among these, plant OBs represent a convenient and feasible option to achieve the aforementioned goals. OBs are lipid storage vesicles that are naturally found in plant seeds. Isolated OBs are remarkably stable due to the steric hindrance and electro-negative repulsion provided by surface proteins of the organelles[19] [20]. According to the relative proportions of triacylglycerols (TAGs), PLs, and proteins, stable OBs can be technically reconstituted with these three essential constituents[21]. Reconstituted oil bodies (ROBs), as well as native OBs, have been previously reported as useful vehicles for the stabilization of curcumin, another polyphenol[22].

In the present study, we pre-selected the most effective combination of polyphenols to suppress *in vitro* LPS-induced inflammatory cytokine secretion from DCs. We then encapsulated the selected polyphenols into ROBs that efficiently decreased polyphenol degradation. The combined administration of ROBs containing quercetin and piperine (ROBs-QP) improved the efficacy of suppression of LPS-induced inflammatory cytokine production from DCs, even at a low dose. The two ROBs efficiently synergized to induce significant TNFα suppression. Inhibition of DC inflammatory pathways was confirmed by a decrease in phospho-p38 and COX-2 that was particularly evident when the two nanocapsules were administered together. Finally, we addressed the *in vivo* efficiency by evaluating the ability to protect C57Bl/6 mice from acute colitis induced by 2% DSS administration [23]. In this animal model, administration of ROBs-QP was able to delay weight loss, reduce the inflammatory score, and improve survival. These findings suggest that administration of ROBs-QP suppresses the DC inflammatory program *in vitro* and *in vivo*, thus ameliorating acute colitis and possibly other chronic intestinal inflammatory disorders, and provide the rationale for further *in vivo* usage of the proposed compounds.

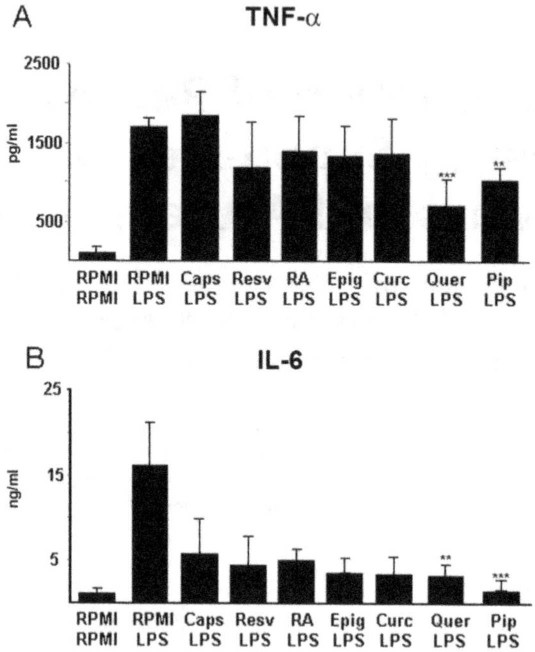

Figure 1. Polyphenol administration to BMDCs interferes with LPS-mediated TNFα and IL-6 production. 25 μM of each polyphenol was administered on day 5 and 7; LPS [1 μg/ml] was administered on day 8. SNs were collected 24 h later, and TNFα and IL-6 protein levels were assessed by ELISA. Both cytokine concentrations were significantly inhibited when cells were exposed to Quercetin (Querc) and Piperine (Pip) when compared to control (RPMI+LPS). Data are shown as mean ± S.D. of five independent experiments. Differences where considered between control (RPMI-LPS) and LPS-Quer- or LPS-Pip-treated cells $^{**}P<0.01$, $^{***}P<0.001$. Capsaicin (Caps), Resveratrol (Resv), Rosmarinic Acid (RA), Epigallocatechin (Epig) and Curcumin (Curc).

Results

Quercetin administration during DC maturation inhibits LPS-mediated TNFα and IL-6 production

We first compared a battery of synthetic and commercially available polyphenols for their ability to inhibit LPS-induced inflammatory cytokine production from DCs. Bone marrow-derived DCs (BMDCs) received 25 μM of a single polyphenol on the third and fifth day of *in vitro* culture. On day 7, DCs were exposed to LPS [1 μg/ml], and 24 hours later, supernatants (SNs) were collected, and IL-6 and TNFα protein levels were determined by ELISA (Fig. 1). Quercetin was consistently the most efficient inhibitor of both TNFα and IL-6 protein production compared to other polyphenols, while piperine appeared to have specificity for IL-6 inhibition. Surprisingly, *trans*-resveratrol, one of the most studied polyphenols, proved to be one of the least efficient inhibitors (Fig. 1).

ROB encapsulation efficiently stabilizes quercetin

Plant OBs share a common structure comprised of a hydrophobic core of triacylglycerols (TAGs) and sterols surrounded by a monolayer of polar phospholipids (PLs) embedded with associated proteins (Fig. 2a). Figure 2F clearly shows rapid polyphenol degradation once dissolved in 0.1 M phosphate buffer of pH 7 at 37°C to a final concentration of 12.5 μM. Free quercetin was almost completely degraded in 4 hours, with approximately 50% degradation at 30 min (Fig. 2F). Furthermore, 4 hours following quercetin incubation in phosphate buffer, the presence of an additional peak, eluting with a retention time of around 20 min (Fig. 2G, H, I), was observed by chromatograms of RP-HPLC analysis. After 48 hours in phosphate buffer, both of these compounds were almost completely degraded (Fig. 2I). These data were further supported by the formation of degradation product upon analysis of UV-Vis absorption spectra obtained at different time points (data not shown). This analysis showed a gradual blue shift from the maximum absorbance at around 370 nm to about 330 nm, confirming the loss of conjugation of the chromophore. These results were in agreement with those already reported by others[24].

Quercetin was then encapsulated into ROBs (ROBs-Q) to improve its stability and bioavailability. ROBs-Q were imaged by confocal laser scanning microscopy (CLSM) and images showed the presence of micro/nanocapsules of expected size and shape (Fig. 2E). Quercetin encapsulated into ROBs showed 100% stability up to three days. After six (144 h) and 10 days (240 h), 50% and 20%, respectively, of the initial active compound were detected (Fig. 2F and L–N). Furthermore, the RP-HPLC elution profiles showed that for ROBs-Q, the degradation product was always a minor peak up to 20 days of incubation (data not shown).

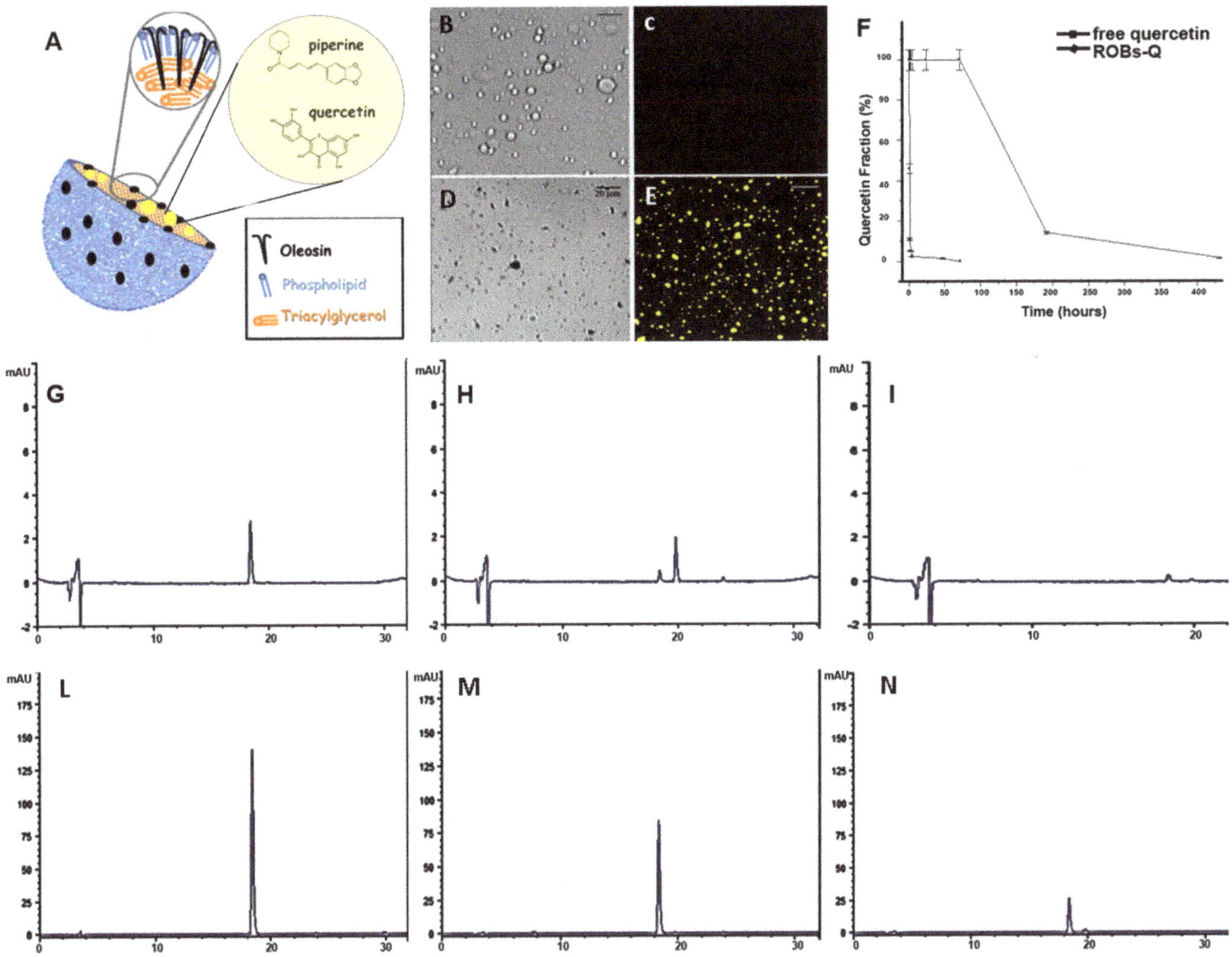

Figure 2. Characterization of polyphenol-embedded ROBs. A) model structure of a natural oil body: external PL monolayer, embedded proteins (*i.e.* oleosin) and TAGs; Piperine and quercetin were encapsulated in the core. B and D) CLSM micrograph of empty ROBs and quercetin encapsulated ROBs imaged by transmitted light. C and E) LSM micrograph of empty ROBs and ROBs quercetin imaged by fluorescence light using an excitation wavelength of 488 nm and emission recorded with a 505–530 nm filter set. F) Degradation profiles of free (squares) and NE (circles) quercetin incubated in 0.1 M phosphate buffer pH 7 at 37°C in the dark for different times; HPLC chromatograms of free quercetin (12.5 μM) incubated with 0.1 M phosphate buffer pH 7 in the dark at 37°C after 0 h (G), 4 h (H) and 48 h (I) compared to HPLC chromatograms of quercetin encapsulated ROBs (12.5 μM) treated in the same experimental conditions at 48 h (2 days, L), 144 h (6 days, M) and 432 h (18 days, N).

Polyphenol embedded ROBs potently inhibit inflammatory cytokine secretion from DCs

BMDCs were exposed to several ROBs-QP concentrations to address potential toxicity of the treatment. We observed a significant increase in apoptosis when DCs were treated with 100 μM of ROBs-QP. The percentage of apoptotic DCs obtained from 25 μM ROBs-QP treated wells was always below 18% and never significantly higher than the percentage of apoptotic cells observed in the untreated wells (data not shown). BMDCs were exposed to 25 μM of ROBs-embedded quercetin or piperine (ROBs-Q or ROBs-P, respectively), or ROBs containing the combination of the two polyphenols (ROBs-QP) at the same concentrations. Our results showed that ROBs-QP efficiently inhibited TNFα and IL-6 production (Fig. 3). Of note, ROBs-QP did not affect production of cytokines since cytokine production was comparable to untreated DCs in the absence of TLR4 engagement by LPS. Empty ROBs failed to decrease TNFα and IL-6 protein levels, revealing that the polyphenol content, and not the protective shell, was responsible for inhibition of inflammatory cytokine production (Fig. 3). To exclude eventual induction of cells proliferation, we collected and counted the cells following the supernatant collection. DCs proliferation was never observed (data not shown).

LPS- and PG-associated ph-p38 is decreased following ROBs-QP administration

As shown in Figure 4A and B, BMDCs exposed to either LPS or PG acutely activated the MAPK p38 signaling pathway. Treated cells significantly increased levels of p38 MAPK phosphorylation as compared to basal levels. Time course experiments (Baseline, 10′, 30′, 120′) indicated both TLR4- and TLR2-dependent activation of p38 MAPK peaks during the first 10 min and remained sustained for 2 h. Quantitative analysis of phosphorylation levels also revealed a different order of magnitude for LPS- and PG-mediated phosphorylation of p38 MAPK (Fig. 4A and B).

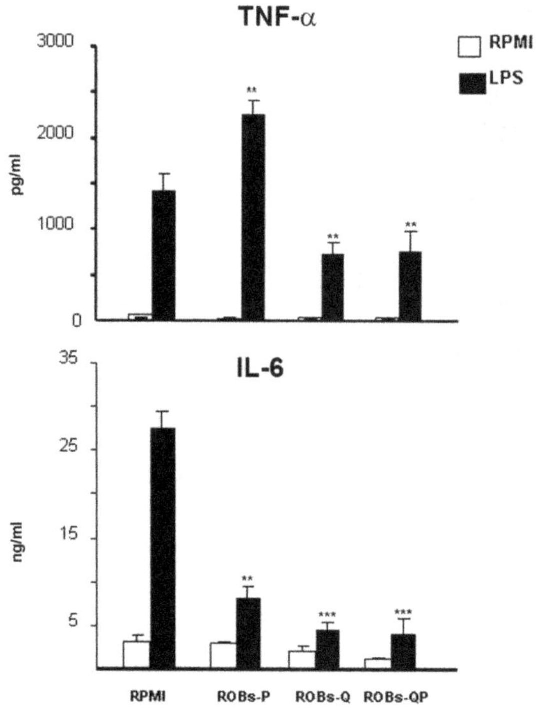

Figure 3. ROB-embedded polyphenol mix interferes with production of LPS-mediated cytokines from DCs. ROB-embedded piperine (ROBs-P), quercetin (ROBs-Q) or a mix of the two (ROBs-QP) were administered on day 5 and 7 [25 μM] to DC cultures. LPS [1 μg/ml] was administered on day 8. SNs were collected 24 h later and TNFα and IL-6 content evaluated by ELISA. Data are shown as mean ± S.D. of five independent experiments; $^{**}P<0.01$, $^{***}P<0.001$.

Administration of low dose ROBs-QP promotes a unique pattern of cytokine production

Most of the *in vivo* studies following polyphenol administration failed translation into clinical practice due to rapid polyphenol degradation in water and the high dosage required to obtain significant results. DCs were treated as previously described using different doses of ROBs–QP, and production of several DC-derived cytokines was evaluated. Figure 5 shows that ROBs-QP effectively inhibits the production of acute phase inflammatory cytokines, including TNFα, IL-6, IL-23 and IL-12. Administration of 100 μM of ROBs-QP reduced DC activity, as demonstrated by decreased cytokine production, and 50 μM ROBs-QP revealed low toxicity as viability was comparable among treated and untreated DCs. Administration of 50 μM ROBs-QP decreased TNFα, IL-12 IL-23, IL-6, CCL3, CXCL1 and even IL-10 production. IL-1Rα, IL-1β, CCL5 and TGFβ secretion was not affected. Administration of 25–12.5 μM ROBs-QP still had the ability to inhibit the acute inflammatory pathway and to induce increased levels of anti-inflammatory cytokines. Efficacy of ROBs-QP was lost at 6.25 μM, with the exception of IL-6 production that was still potently inhibited.

Intraperitoneal delivery of ROBs-QP ameliorates acute intestinal inflammation induced by administration of 2% DSS

The efficiency of polyphenol stabilization following encapsulation of ROBs, combined with an effective dose needed to obtain suppression of acute inflammatory cytokine production, allowed us to design appropriate *in vivo* treatment strategies. Two groups of C57Bl/6 mice received 2% DSS in their drinking water to induce acute colitis[23]. Mice were carefully observed and weight, general health conditions, and fecal blood were monitored daily. Starting from day 3 of DSS colitis, the mice received ROBs-QP by intraperitoneal injection [0.5 μM/g] three times per week. Administration of ROBs-QP effectively delayed the presence of fecal blood and prevented weight loss. In vehicle treated mice, diarrhea and weight loss were detected at day 5, followed shortly after by the presence of fecal blood. In these mice, weight loss at day 6 and day 8 was 5% and 18%, respectively. Administration of ROBs-QP significantly delayed weight loss that was 2% at day 6 and 8, and reached 13% at day 10 (Fig. 6A). Mice in which disease reached maximal severity, defined by the ethical approval protocol for animal research (see methods), were euthanized. ROBs-QP treatment prolonged mice survival (Fig. 6B) and reduced the overall disease activity index (Fig. 6C). At day 9, equal numbers of mice per group were sacrificed, and colon tissues and MLNs were harvested. Colons from ROBs-QP treated mice appeared less inflamed as shown by quantitative parameters, including colonic length and weight (Fig. 6D). From these mice, we evaluated MLNs for the number of $CD4^{+}Foxp3^{+}$ cells. ROBs-QP treatment induced a 15% increase in the $CD4^{+}Foxp3^{+}$ population. In addition, reduced colon length, increased diarrhea and rectal bleeding occurred in DSS-treated mice; however, all of these symptoms were reduced by ROBs-QP administration. Profound differences between vehicle- and ROBs-QP-treated mice were observed at day 9, and revealed that vehicle-treated mice showed furry hair, while ROBs-QP-treated mice showed normal hair. In addition, the severity of fecal bleeding was vastly reduced in ROBs-QP-treated mice (Fig. 6F). Representative histology obtained from the colon of vehicle- and ROBs-QP-treated mice was observed at day 9 (Fig. 7A). Signs of inflammation and infiltrating granulocytes can be detected in both samples. It is possible to observe a lower grade of inflammation in the samples obtained from ROBs-QP treated mice. We further analyzed COX2 in colon lysates from these same donors. Figure 7B shows reduced expression of the inflammatory mediator COX2 in colon lysates. Consistently with other studies levels of COX-2 was remarkably increased in colon obtained from 2%DSS treated mice. ROBs-QP administration remarkably reduced COX-2 induction, likely via the reduced P38 activation. The constitutive isoform COX1 showed no detectable differences between vehicle- and ROBs-QP-treated colons. Furthermore, we mechanically stripped the epithelial cells layer to investigate the ROBs-QP mediated COX2 reduction in the non-epithelial compartment. As shown in figure 7B, COX2 reduction was still detected in ROBs-QP-treated cells, thus suggesting that the non-epithelial colon compartment is also affected by ROBs-QP administration.

Discussion

In this study, we evaluated an effective method to obtain alternatively activated DCs by administration of a polyphenol mix, embedded in ROBs. DCs are critical players of the inflammatory response, with the ability to capture, process, and present antigens to direct the adaptive immune response. Upon TLR engagement, immature DCs profoundly change and become mature cells[25] [26]. These cells are commonly characterized by low endocytosis, altered surface marker expression (*e.g.*, costimulatory proteins, such as CD80 and CD86), switching of chemokine receptor expression, and cytokine production[27] [28]. As previously discussed, alternatively activated DCs, even upon TLR engagement, do not promote inflammation and are involved in promoting tolerance[29]. In the intestine, a single monolayer of

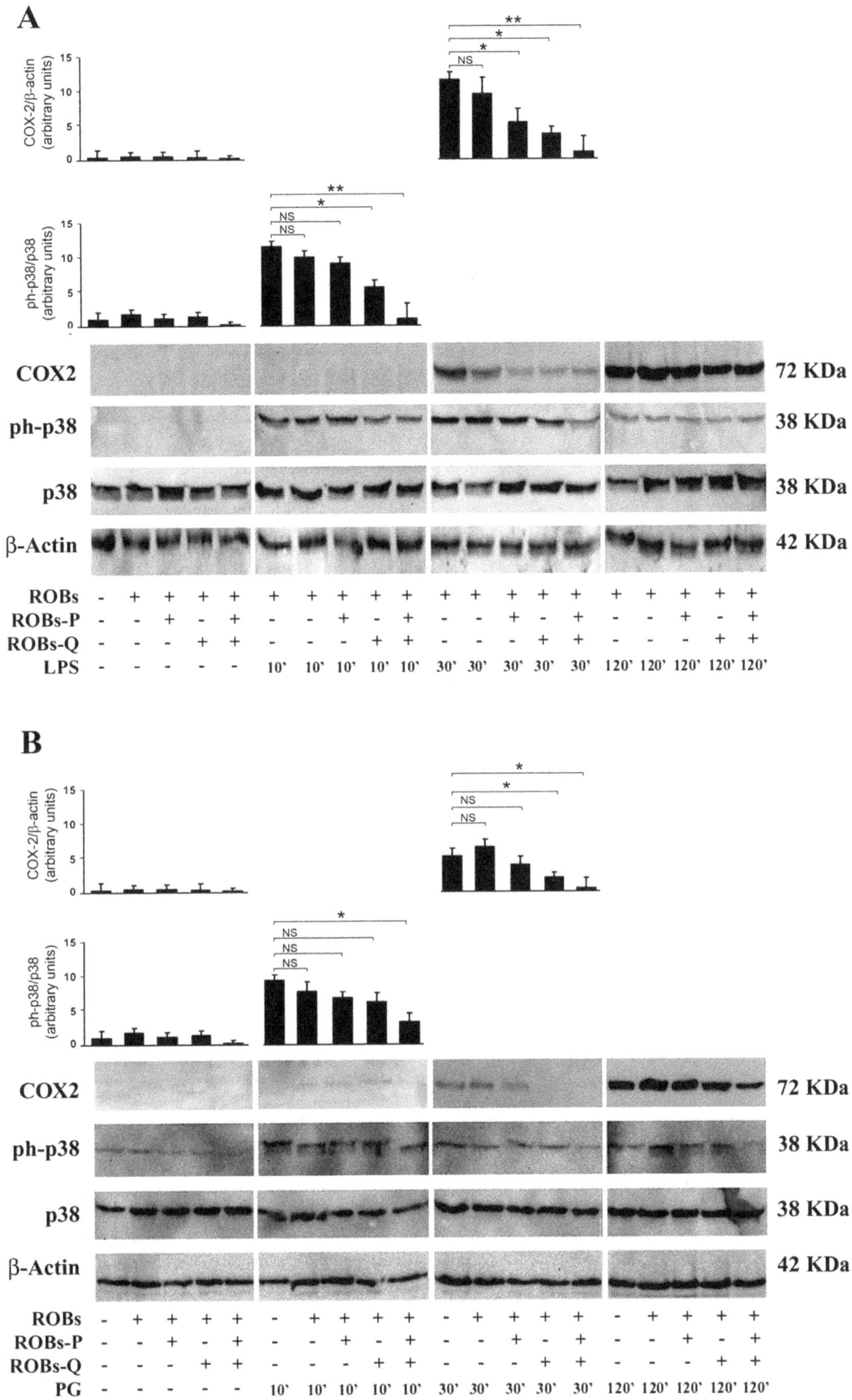
A
COX-2/β-actin (arbitrary units)
ph-p38/p38 (arbitrary units)
NS
COX2
ph-p38
p38
β-Actin
72 KDa
38 KDa
38 KDa
42 KDa
ROBs
ROBs-P
ROBs-Q
LPS
10' 10' 10' 10' 10' 30' 30' 30' 30' 30' 120' 120' 120' 120' 120'
B
COX-2/β-actin (arbitrary units)
ph-p38/p38 (arbitrary units)
NS
COX2
ph-p38
p38
β-Actin
72 KDa
38 KDa
38 KDa
42 KDa
ROBs
ROBs-P
ROBs-Q
PG
10' 10' 10' 10' 10' 30' 30' 30' 30' 30' 120' 120' 120' 120' 120'

Figure 4. Modulated activation of pro-inflammatory MAPK p38 signaling and inducible COX-2 on ROBs-QP treated DCs. DCs were cultured in the presence of either ROBs-P, ROBs-Q or ROBs-QP as mentioned previously; empty ROBs were used as control. LPS (A) or PG (B) was administered at indicated time points. DC lysates were subjected to immunoblotting with antibodies to detect total and phosphorylated forms of p38 MAPK and COX-2. Representative immunoblots from at least three independent experiments are shown for each condition. Each bar represents the mean ± SEM of densitometric analyses for phosphorylated proteins normalized to their respective total forms; *P<0.05, **P<0.01 vs. basal conditions.

epithelial cells separates billions of bacteria from the largest concentrated population of immune cells [2]. Normal intestinal homeostasis is preserved through dynamic mechanisms[8] [9] [10]. The intestinal milieu is able to educate resident DCs to develop into alternatively activated DCs that will not produce inflammatory mediators, even following TLR engagement[30] [5] [6] [7]. Chronic intestinal inflammation is often characterized by loss of alternatively activated DCs and the presence of pro-inflammatory DCs. The present study was undertaken to explore the possibility of promoting alternatively activated DCs by administration of nutritionally-derived compounds, commonly found in the diet. Several studies have reported that polyphenol intake is associated with reduced risks of cardiovascular and neurodegenerative diseases, as well as cancer development [31] [32] [33] [34]. This action appears to be related to the modulation of NF-kB and MAPK activation[35] [36]. Numerous studies have evaluated the possibility of polyphenols to serve as a potential therapy for patients with IBD [37]. Results from these studies were somewhat inconsistent, and required a high polyphenol concentration in order to obtain significant results *in vivo*.

We first evaluated the effects of different polyphenols using an *in vitro* DC culture system. Our goal was to obtain inflammatory-impaired DCs that would significantly reduce proinflammatory cytokine production upon TLR engagement. Despite the low chemical stability in aqueous buffer, we compared the anti-inflammatory effects of several polyphenols, including capsaicin, resveratrol, retinoic acid, epigallocatechin, curcumin, quercetin and piperine, in *in vitro* cultured DCs. LPS-induced TNFα production was evaluated in treated vs. untreated cells. Quercetin appeared to be consistently the most efficient suppressor of TNFα; these results are consistent with previous reports demonstrating the anti-inflammatory effects of quercetin metabolites[38]. Despite the poor inhibitory properties of TNFα, most of the polyphenols tested were able to suppress IL-6 production. We performed an *in vitro* time course study to evaluate the effects of quercetin. Concomitant administration of LPS and polyphenols appeared ineffective. Administration of polyphenols from the first day of culture induced similar effects to treating twice, on days 3 and 5. TNFα and IL-6 levels detected in the SN of DCs receiving a single dose of polyphenols, either on day 3 or 5, were higher compared to those receiving doses on both day 3 and 5 (data not shown). Since previous reports suggested that piperine acts as a potent bioenhancer for the activity of other polyphenols[39], we evaluated the concomitant administration of both quercetin and piperine. Our results showed that inhibition of both TNFα and IL-6 can be further enhanced when DCs are treated with both quercetin and piperine. Piperine's ability to improve polyphenol inhibition may be due to upregulation of either cytochrome P450, family 4, subfamily f, polypeptide 18 (Cyp4f18) and cytochrome P450, family 4, subfamily a, and/or polypeptide 12a (Cyp4a12a) (data not shown).

Clinical use of polyphenols has been negatively influenced by the chemical characteristics that make them unstable. Indeed, free quercetin is almost completely degraded in 4 hours, and only 30 minutes are needed to observe approximately 50% degradation (Fig. 2F). The mechanism of quercetin degradation in the dark has been proposed to involve the addition of a water molecule to the 2,3 double bond (see structure in fig. 2A) and a further oxidation step, as reported by Dall'Acqua *et al.* (2012)[40]. On the basis of these results, we decided to encapsulate quercetin into ROBs-Q with the intent to improve its stability and bioavailability. As expected, encapsulation of ROBs greatly stabilized quercetin, which showed 100% stability up to three days. These results emphasized the improved efficacy of lipid-based micro/nano particles for quercetin stabilization. We administered ROBs-QP to BMDCs and demonstrated robust suppression of TLR4- and TLR2-mediated inflammatory pathways. The signal cascade involving the P38 pathway was also reduced upon ROBs-QP administration; thus, encouraging further investigation as IBD patients are characterized by macrophages with increased P38α expression. Consistent with other studies demonstrating the ability of LPS and PG to induce COX-2 expression, protein levels of inducible COX-2 were significantly increased in treated cells as early as 30′ with treatment, and remained elevated after 2 hours of stimulation. Interestingly, ROBs-Mix exposed BMDCs, treated with either LPS or PG, significantly reduced p38 MAPK phosphorylation at 10′ and 30′. Single polyphenol ROB administration failed to prevent p38 MAPK phosphorylation. Consequently, in ROBs-Mix exposed BMDCs, COX-2 was significantly reduced 30′ following LPS or PG administration. This effect was lost at 2 h, most likely due to other pathways activated at the same time. We propose that co-treatment with ROBs-P and ROBs-Q might result in a functional synergistic pharmacological effect that goes undetected when only one polyphenol is given, and these effects are at least in part due to the activation of intracellular p38 MAPK.

Following inhibition of the signaling cascade involving the P38 pathway, the release of inflammatory cytokines appeared to be suppressed. Results from dose response studies reveal the pattern of inflammatory cytokine inhibition by ROBs-QP administration. IL-6 is consistently reduced even at a very low dosage (up to 6.25 μM), similarly to other NF-kB-dependent cytokines, such as IL-1α, IL-1β, IL-12, and IL-23. Secretion of anti-inflammatory cytokines, including IL-10 and IL-1Ra, was increased, most efficiently by 25 μM ROBs administration. Nevertheless, it is important to note that the ratio between inflammatory and anti-inflammatory cytokines favors the latter, even at low dosages of ROBs. Production of TGFβ is decreased, as the detectable concentrations of SNs from ROBs-QP treated DCs are similar to untreated DCs. This cytokine secretion path reveals the ROBs-QP DCs become inflammatory impaired. The chemokine profile induced by 25 μM ROBs administration reveals an inhibition of the macrophage inflammatory protein (CCL3), at the same time no significant difference was detected in the production of CCL5 and CXCL1. All together, these data encouraged us to investigate the efficiency of ROBs in an *in vivo* model of acute intestinal inflammation. We evaluated intraperitoneal ROBs-QP treatment starting from day 3 following DSS administration. We decided to start ROB administration when intestinal inflammation is initiated, as our goal was to evaluate a treatment, rather than a prevention, strategy. We evaluated QP presence in the blood and bile of treated mice at 1, 3, 5 and 24 h following ROBs-QP

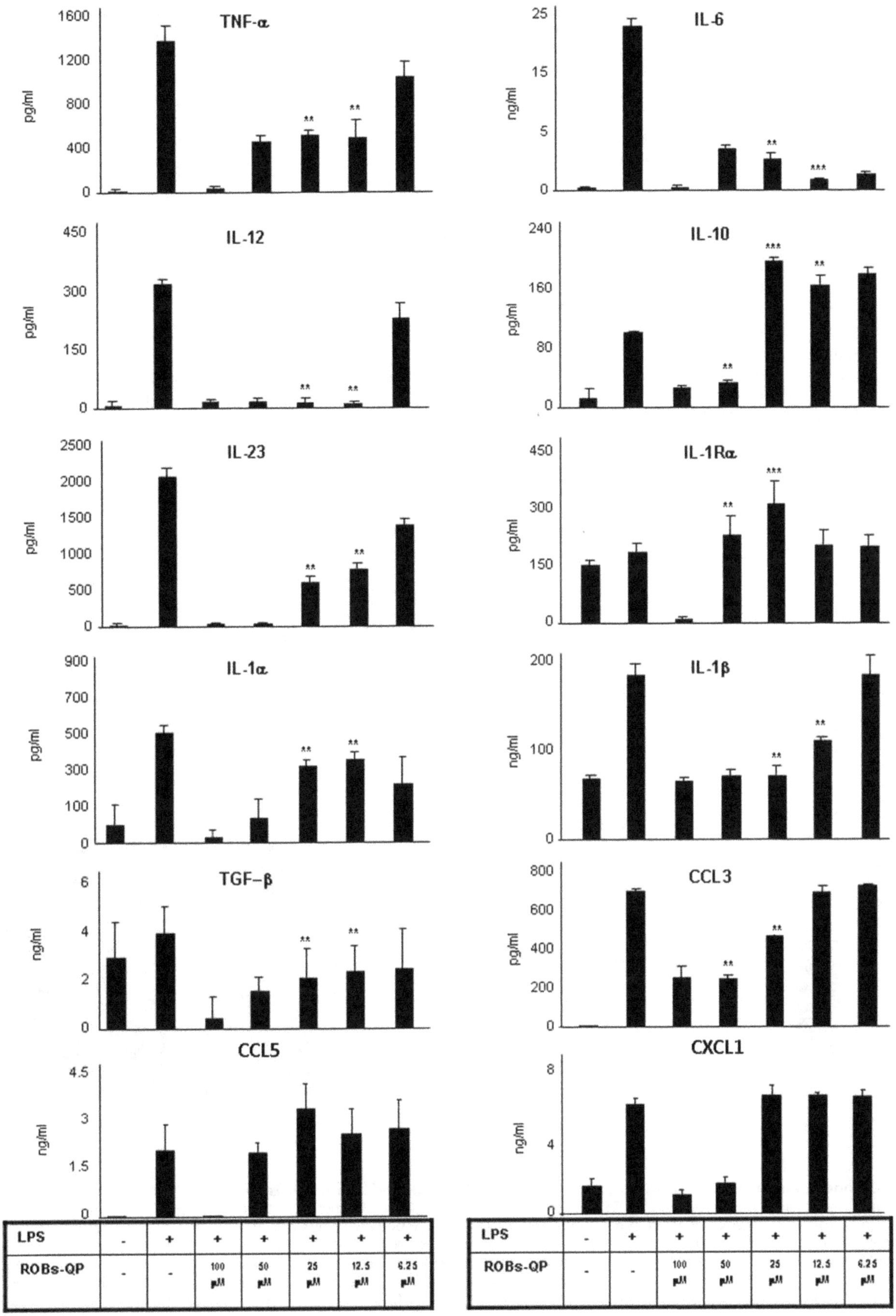
TNF-α
pg/ml
IL-6
ng/ml
IL-12
pg/ml
IL-10
pg/ml
IL-23
pg/ml
IL-1Rα
pg/ml
IL-1α
pg/ml
IL-1β
ng/ml
TGF-β
ng/ml
CCL3
pg/ml
CCL5
ng/ml
CXCL1
ng/ml
LPS - + + + + + +
ROBs-QP - - 100 μM 50 μM 25 μM 12.5 μM 6.25 μM

Figure 5. ROBs-QP administration promotes a unique cytokine profile in LPS-treated DCs. BMDCs were exposed to different ROBs-QP concentrations on day 5 and 7. LPS [1 µg/ml] was administered on day 8, and 24 h later SNs were collected. Cytokine protein levels were measured by ELISA. Data are shown as mean ± S.D. of five independent experiments. Statistically significant differences were considered when $^{**}P<0.01$; $^{***}P<0.001$ between control (LPS, no polyphenols) and LPS-ROBS-QP-treated cells.

administration. We were able to detect quercetin in the bile of treated mice at 1 and 3 h following ROBs-QP administration although the detected amount was close to the detection limit of the instrument (1 ng). In our experimental conditions, we were never able to detect quercetin in the serum of treated mice. Our results clearly demonstrate that ROBs-QP administration results in a potent reduction of DSS-induced colitis. The small increase in the percentages of MLN $CD4^{+}Foxp3^{+}$ T cells may explain the results obtained. Histology from ROBs-QP treated mice indicates a delay in the DSS-induced inflammatory cascade. Furthermore, mice appeared healthy for a longer period, fecal blood was reduced, and survival was prolonged. Colitis is present in both treated and untreated mice exposed to 2% DSS for 9 days, although the histology of ROBs-QP treated mice reveals lower areas of inflammation. Granulocytes infiltrate is comparable in the two groups, consistently with the *in vitro* data showing CXCL1 production unaffected by ROBs-QP administration. The reduced expression of the inflammatory mediator COX2 in the colon lysates with or without epithelial cells indicates that ROBs-QP administration *in vivo* is efficiently affecting lamina propria resident cells including DCs, monocytes and macrophages. Taken together, these results demonstrate that the administration of ROBs containing a polyphenol mix of quercetin and piperine efficiently inhibits LPS-mediated inflammatory responses from DCs. ROB encapsulation protects polyphenols from degradation and improves the efficiency of polyphenol administration. *In vivo*, significant results can be observed in models of acute intestinal

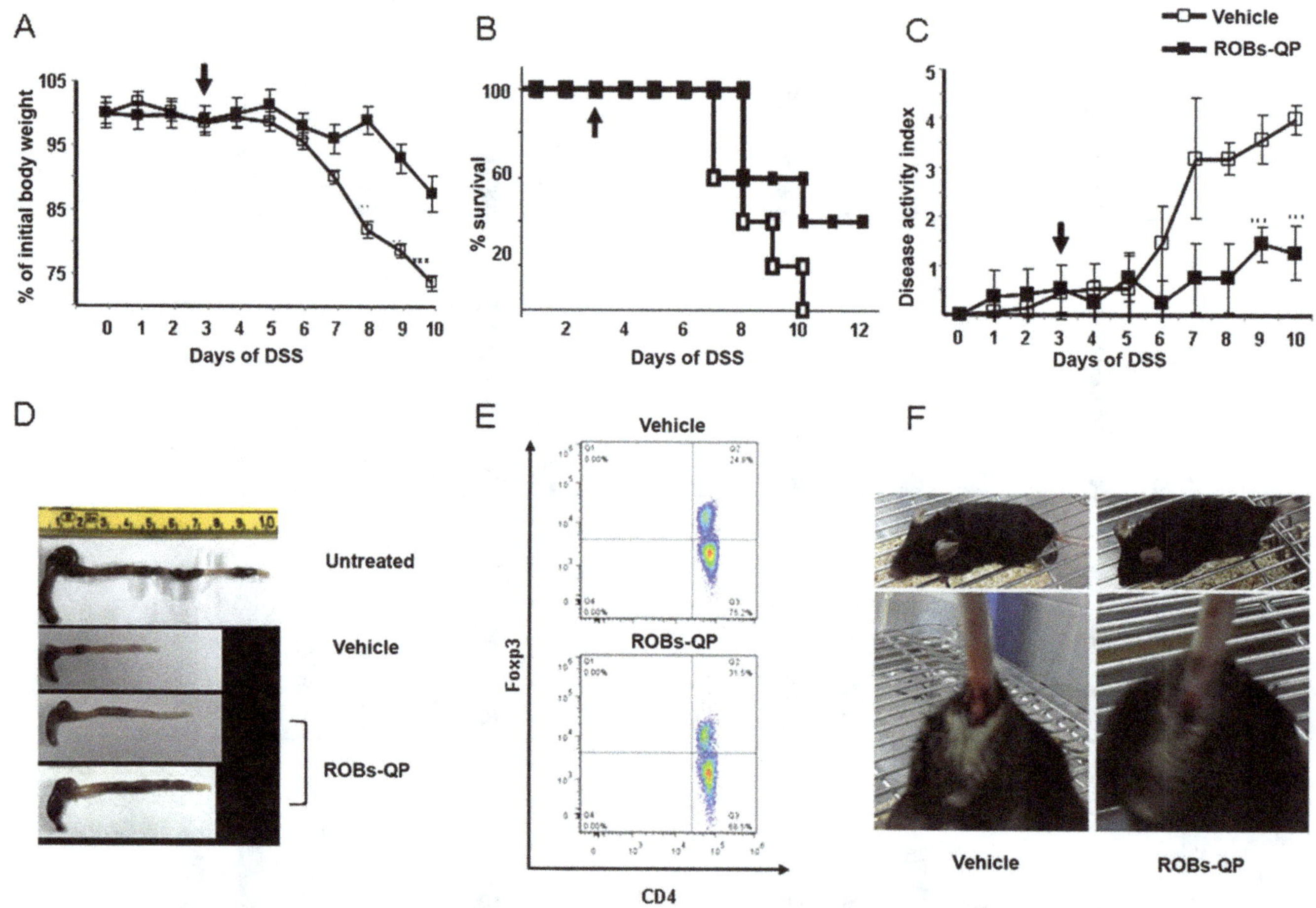

Figure 6. Intraperitoneal administration of ROBs ameliorates 2% DSS-mediated acute colitis. Sex- and weight-matched mice were divided in 2 groups (10 mice each). Mice received 2% DSS in drinking water from day 0, and either ROBs-QP or vehicle starting from day 3. Body weight and presence of diarrhea and rectal bleeding were monitored daily. (A) Average body weight is shown as mean ± SEM. Arrow indicates the beginning of ROBs-QP administration; $^{*}P<0.05$, $^{**}P<0.01$. (B) Survival rate is shown as percentage of initial number of either untreated or ROBs-QP-treated mice; N = 10/group, $P\leq0.01$ vs. all treated groups. (C) Disease Activity Index (DAI) was calculated daily. The values represent the mean of 6 mice (3 females and 3 males) ± SEM; $^{*}P<0.05$, $^{**}P<0.01$. (D) Macroscopic changes at day 9 of representative colons isolated from mice treated with 2% DSS. (E) At day 9, mice were sacrificed and MLNs explanted, and percentages of $CD4^{+}Foxp3^{+}$ cells were assessed by FACS; figure shows a representative dot plot. (F) Fur and perianal beading of representative untreated vs. ROBs-QP-treated mice 9 days after the beginning of 2% DSS administration.

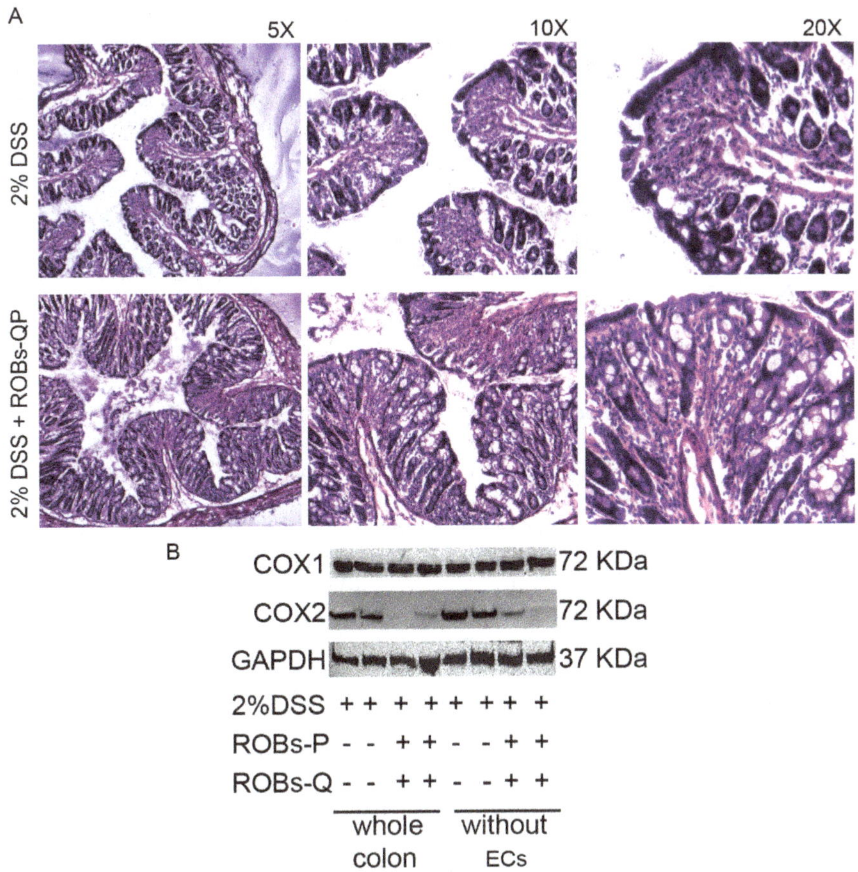

Figure 7. ROBs-QP *in vivo* administration reduced expression of COX2 in colon lysates even in absence of the epithelial cells layer. (A) Histology from ROBs-QP treated mice indicates signs of inflammation and infiltrating granulocytes in the colon of vehicle- and ROBs-QP-treated mice. (B) Western blot staining of colon lysates obtained from mice treated as previously described. Reduced expression of COX2 can be observed with or without epithelial cells from colon lysates of ROBs-QP-treated colons. The constitutive isoform COX1 showed no detectable differences.

inflammation, thus opening new possibilities for novel therapeutic approaches for the treatment of chronic inflammatory diseases.

Methods

Ethics statement

C57BL/6 mice were purchased from Charles River Breeding Laboratories. All animal experiments were carried out in accordance with Directive 86/609 EEC enforced by Italian D.L.n 116 1992 and approved by the official RBM veterinarian. When required, euthanasia was performed by cervical dislocation. The protocol was approved by the Committee on the Ethics of Animal Experiments of Ministero della Salute - Direzione Generale Sanità Animale (Prot. 2012/00000923 A00:Eo_GINRC).

Generation and culture of DCs

DCs were harvested from murine bone marrow (BM). Briefly, BM from the tibiae and femurs of 6- to 8-week-old male C57BL/6 mice were flushed with RPMI and depleted of red blood cells with ACK cell lysing buffer (GIBCO). Cells were plated in 6-well culture plates (1×10^6 cells/ml; 3 ml/well) in RPMI supplemented with 10% heat-inactivated FBS, 100 U/ml penicillin, 100 mg/ml streptomycin, 25 µg/ml rmGM-CSF, and 25 µg/ml rmIL-4 at 37°C in a humidified 5% CO_2 atmosphere. On day 3, BMDCs were harvested and plated at 1×10^6/ml in 24-well culture plates. On day 5 and day 7, BMDCs were administered polyphenols (25 µM). LPS was administered [1 µg/ml] at day 8 for 24 h.

Enzyme-linked immunosorbent assay (ELISA)

Cell culture SNs were analyzed for TNFα, IL-6, IL-10, IL-12 p70, IL-23, IL-1Rα, IL-1α IL-1β, CCL3 and TGFβ proteins in triplicate, using an ELISA kit, as described by the manufacturer (R&D Systems, Minneapolis, MN).

Cell cultures and Western blot analysis

BMDCs in primary culture were grown in RPMI 10% FBS in 12 multiwell plates. At day 5 and 7, BMDCs were stimulated with encapsulated polyphenols followed by co-administration of either LPS or peptidoglycan (PG) at various time intervals (10, 30, 120 min) to better evaluate the modulation of intracellular pathway activation downstream of TLR4 or TLR2 agonism. Activation of p42/44 MAPK, p38 MAPK, and NF-κB pathways was assessed. Phosphorylation at Thr^{202}/Tyr^{204} and at Thr^{180}/Tyr^{182} was considered an indicator of activation for p42/44 and p38 MAPK, respectively. Phosphorylation of IκBα at $Ser^{32}/^{36}$, as well as phosphorylation of p65 subunit at Ser^{536}, was assumed to be an indicator for NF-κB activation. Cell lysates were prepared using 100 µl of lysis buffer (100 mM NaCl, 40 mM HEPES, pH 7.5, 1% Triton X-100, 1 mM Na_3VO_4, 4 mM $Na_4P_2O_7$, 10 mM EDTA, 1 mM PMSF, 10 mM NaF, 2 µg/ml aprotinin, and 2 µg/ml leupeptin). Equal amounts of protein (25 µg) were separated by

10% SDS-PAGE and subjected to immunoblotting with the following primary antibodies (dilution 1:1,000): COX-2, p65, ph-p65, (Santa Cruz Biotecnology, Santa Cruz, CA); IκBα, ph-IkBα, ERK1/2, ph-ERK1/2, p38 MAPK, and ph-p38 MAPK, (Cell Signaling Technology). The β-actin antibody was from Sigma. Incubation with horseradish peroxidase-linked anti-mouse, anti-rabbit, and anti-goat secondary antibodies (Santa Cruz Biotecnology) (1:3,000) was performed for 1 h at room temperature. Immunoblotting results were visualized by Molecular Imager ChemiDoc XRS System (Bio-Rad Laboratories). Images were captured with QuantityOne Software (Bio-Rad Laboratories) and blots quantified by scanning densitometry (Image J; National Institutes of Health, Bethesda, MD).

Histological examination

Tissue section from the distal colon were fixed in 10% buffered formalin and embedded in paraffin. Sections of 6 μm were stained with hematoxylin and eosin (H&E). Images were acquired using Leica LMD 6500.

Purification of OBs

OBs were extracted from almond seeds. OB purification was carried out by a two-layer flotation procedure as previously reported [22], and a further purification step was performed consisting of two sequential washings with 2.0 M NaCl. OBs were finally resuspended in 150 mM Tris–HCl, pH 7.5, containing 0.6 M sucrose.

Quercetin and piperine encapsulation into ROBs

Quercetin and piperine were encapsulated into the ROBs using the above reported protocol [22] with few modifications. Natural OBs were resuspended in 150 mM TRIS-HCl pH 7.5, containing 0.5 M sucrose, 1 mM EDTA, 10 mM KCl, 1 mM $MgCl_2$, 5 mM ascorbic acid (buffer A) and twice extracted with chloroform: methanol (2:1), in order to separate PLs and proteins from TAGs. After centrifugation at 1000 *g* for 5 minutes, the upper phase was extracted with five volumes of diethyl ether anhydrous (to recover TAGs). All the recovered fractions were dried by a rotavapor.

ROB reconstitution mixture consisted of the whole chloroform-methanol phase (PLs) with a quercetin (or piperine)/TAGs ratio of 1/250 starting from 2 mg of each phytochemical. The final volume was adjusted to 3 ml by the addition of buffer A. Samples were sonicated by a Brandson digital Sonifier 250-D at an amplitude of 40% and a cycle of 30 seconds pulse on and 30 seconds off for three times. After sonication, samples were centrifuged at 2000 *g* for 10 minutes and ROBs containing quercetin or piperine were recovered from the top of the centrifuge-tubes.

HPLC analysis was carried out extracting the encapsulated phytochemicals using 2 volumes of ultrapure water, 2 volumes of methyl-butyl-ether, and 1 volume of methanol. After centrifugation at 1000 *g* for 5 minutes, the methyl-butyl-ether phase was recovered, dried (rotavapor), and resuspended into 50% ethanol. Quercetin was quantified by reverse phase-HPLC using the method described above [41] onto a 1100 Agilent work chromatographic station equipped with a photodiodes array UV-Vis detection system. The elution profile was monitored at 370 nm. Quercetin, purchased from Sigma-Aldrich, was used as standard.

Quercetin-loaded ROBs were imaged by confocal microscopy using an excitation wavelength of 488 nm; emission was recorded with a 505–530 nm filter set. Empty ROBs were imaged by transmitted light microscopy. Confocal micrographs were taken with a Leica confocal scanning system mounted to a Leica TCS SP5 (Leica Microsystem GmbH, Mannheim, Germany).

In vivo treatment with nanocapsules

Acute colitis was induced by administration of 2% DSS in drinking water. Sex- and weight-matched mice were divided in 2 groups (10 mice each). 2% DSS in drinking water was administered starting from day 0. Starting at day 3, mice were either injected intraperitoneally with ROBs-QP [0.5 μM/g] or vehicle three times per week. Mice were monitored on a daily basis for the following 10 days. Body weight, stool consistency, and rectal bleeding were recorded. Mice were sacrificed at day 10, and colon and MLN tissues were explanted to evaluate clinical severity of colitis. Colon length was measured as an indicator of colonic inflammation. Colons were placed onto a non-absorbent surface and measured with a ruler, taking care not to stretch the tissue. The colon/body weight index was calculated as the ratio of the colon wet weight and the total body weight (BW) of each mouse. Body weight, occult and rectal bleeding, and stool consistency were monitored daily after DSS administration. Disease activity index (DAI) was determined by scoring change in body weight, occult blood and gross bleeding as described in the literature[42] [43]. Single cell preparations obtained from the MLNs were used to evaluate $CD4^{+}Foxp3^{+}$ cells according to the flow cytometry FOXP3 staining kit (eBioscience). Epithelial cells layer was mechanically stripped from the colon. The colon was cut in half, longitudinally opened and cleaned. The colon sections were washed 3 times with 2.5 mM EDTA at 4°C, the epithelial cells containing supernatant removed and the colon lysated.

Acknowledgments

For the scientific discussion, we thank all members of LAB-81, Dr. Anna Bagorda and "The Italian Translations Company", LLC ?http:// italiantranslationscompany.weebly.com/.

Author Contributions

Conceived and designed the experiments: MC AS AH TP. Performed the experiments: EC EV FRD FA SB RL VM. Analyzed the data: MC VM EC. Contributed reagents/materials/analysis tools: MC AS. Wrote the paper: MC EC TP.

References

1. Strober W, Fuss I, Mannon P (2007) The fundamental basis of inflammatory bowel disease. The Journal of clinical investigation 117: 514–521.
2. Maynard CL, Elson CO, Hatton RD, Weaver CT (2012) Reciprocal interactions of the intestinal microbiota and immune system. Nature 489: 231–241.
3. Sun CM, Hall JA, Blank RB, Bouladoux N, Oukka M, et al. (2007) Small intestine lamina propria dendritic cells promote de novo generation of Foxp3 T reg cells via retinoic acid. J Exp Med 204: 1775–1785.
4. Kraus TA, Toy L, Chan L, Childs J, Mayer L (2004) Failure to induce oral tolerance to a soluble protein in patients with inflammatory bowel disease. Gastroenterology 126: 1771–1778.
5. Iliev ID, Mileti E, Matteoli G, Chieppa M, Rescigno M (2009) Intestinal epithelial cells promote colitis-protective regulatory T-cell differentiation through dendritic cell conditioning. Mucosal immunology 2: 340–350.
6. Hanabuchi S, Ito T, Park WR, Watanabe N, Shaw JL, et al.(2010)Thymic stromal lymphopoietin-activated plasmacytoid dendritic cells induce the generation of FOXP3+ regulatory T cells in human thymus. Journal of immunology 184: 2999–3007.
7. Rimoldi M, Chieppa M, Larghi P, Vulcano M, Allavena P, et al. (2005) Monocyte-derived dendritic cells activated by bacteria or by bacteria-stimulated epithelial cells are functionally different. Blood 106: 2818–2826.
8. Rescigno M, Chieppa M (2005) Gut-level decisions in peace and war. Nature medicine 11: 254–255.

9. Hart AL, Al-Hassi HO, Rigby RJ, Bell SJ, Emmanuel AV, et al. (2005) Characteristics of intestinal dendritic cells in inflammatory bowel diseases. Gastroenterology 129: 50–65.
10. Rivollier A, He J, Kole A, Valatas V, Kelsall BL (2012) Inflammation switches the differentiation program of Ly6Chi monocytes from antiinflammatory macrophages to inflammatory dendritic cells in the colon. J Exp Med 209: 139–155.
11. de Baey A, Mende I, Baretton G, Greiner A, Hartl WH, et al. (2003) A subset of human dendritic cells in the T cell area of mucosa-associated lymphoid tissue with a high potential to produce TNF-alpha. Journal of immunology 170: 5089–5094.
12. Middel P, Raddatz D, Gunawan B, Haller F, Radzun HJ (2006) Increased number of mature dendritic cells in Crohn's disease: evidence for a chemokine mediated retention mechanism. Gut 55: 220–227.
13. Ng SC, Kamm MA, Stagg AJ, Knight SC (2010) Intestinal dendritic cells: their role in bacterial recognition, lymphocyte homing, and intestinal inflammation. Inflamm Bowel Dis 16: 1787–1807.
14. Perrier C, Rutgeerts P (2011) Cytokine blockade in inflammatory bowel diseases. Immunotherapy 3: 1341–1352.
15. Romier B, Schneider YJ, Larondelle Y, During A (2009) Dietary polyphenols can modulate the intestinal inflammatory response. Nutrition reviews 67: 363–378.
16. Chen X, Yang L, Howard OM, Oppenheim JJ (2006) Dendritic cells as a pharmacological target of traditional Chinese medicine. Cellular & molecular immunology 3: 401–410.
17. Manjeet KR, Ghosh B (1999) Quercetin inhibits LPS-induced nitric oxide and tumor necrosis factor-alpha production in murine macrophages. International journal of immunopharmacology 21: 435–443.
18. Cai X, Dou J, Yu A, Zhai G (2013) Bioavailability of Quercetin: Problems and Promises. Current medicinal chemistry 20: 2572–82.
19. Chen MC, Chyan CL, Lee TT, Huang SH, Tzen JT (2004) Constitution of stable artificial oil bodies with triacylglycerol, phospholipid, and caleosin. J Agric Food Chem 52: 3982–3987.
20. Peng CC, Lin IP, Lin CK, Tzen JT (2003) Size and stability of reconstituted sesame oil bodies. Biotechnol Prog 19: 1623–1626.
21. Tzen JT, Chuang RL, Chen JC, Wu LS (1998) Coexistence of both oleosin isoforms on the surface of seed oil bodies and their individual stabilization to the organelles. J Biochem 123: 318–323.
22. Bettini S, Vergara D, Bonsegna S, Giotta L, Toto C, et al. (2013) Efficient stabilization of natural curcuminoids mediated by oil body encapsulation. Rsc Advances 3: 5422–5429.
23. Kim JJ, Shajib MS, Manocha MM, Khan WI (2012) Investigating intestinal inflammation in DSS-induced model of IBD. J Vis Exp. 1;(60). pii: 3678. doi: 10.3791/3678
24. Burn PL, Holmes AB, Kraft A, Bradley DDC, Brown AR, et al. (1992) Synthesis of a Segmented Conjugated Polymer-Chain Giving a Blue-Shifted Electroluminescence and Improved Efficiency. Journal of the Chemical Society-Chemical Communications: 32–34.
25. Nish S, Medzhitov R (2011) Host defense pathways: role of redundancy and compensation in infectious disease phenotypes. Immunity 34: 629-636.
26. Macagno A, Napolitani G, Lanzavecchia A, Sallusto F (2007) Duration, combination and timing: the signal integration model of dendritic cell activation. Trends Immunol 28: 227–233.
27. Inaba K, Turley S, Yamaide F, Iyoda T, Mahnke K, et al. (1998) Efficient presentation of phagocytosed cellular fragments on the major histocompatibility complex class II products of dendritic cells. J Exp Med 188: 2163–2173.
28. Parlato S, Santini SM, Lapenta C, Di Pucchio T, Logozzi M, et al. (2001) Expression of CCR-7, MIP-3beta, and Th-1 chemokines in type I IFN-induced monocyte-derived dendritic cells: importance for the rapid acquisition of potent migratory and functional activities. Blood 98: 3022–3029.
29. Chieppa M, Bianchi G, Doni A, Del Prete A, Sironi M, et al. (2003) Cross-linking of the mannose receptor on monocyte-derived dendritic cells activates an anti-inflammatory immunosuppressive program. J Immunol 171: 4552–4560.
30. Bernardo D, Sanchez B, Al-Hassi HO, Mann ER, Urdaci MC, et al. (2012) Microbiota/host crosstalk biomarkers: regulatory response of human intestinal dendritic cells exposed to Lactobacillus extracellular encrypted peptide. PLoS One 7: e36262.
31. Kasimsetty SG, Bialonska D, Reddy MK, Thornton C, Willett KL, et al. (2009) Effects of pomegranate chemical constituents/intestinal microbial metabolites on CYP1B1 in 22Rv1 prostate cancer cells. J Agric Food Chem 57: 10636–10644.
32. Kawai Y, Nishikawa T, Shiba Y, Saito S, Murota K, et al. (2008) Macrophage as a target of quercetin glucuronides in human atherosclerotic arteries: implication in the anti-atherosclerotic mechanism of dietary flavonoids. J Biol Chem 283: 9424–9434.
33. Shirai M, Moon JH, Tsushida T, Terao J (2001) Inhibitory effect of a quercetin metabolite, quercetin 3-O-beta-D-glucuronide, on lipid peroxidation in liposomal membranes. J Agric Food Chem 49: 5602–5608.
34. Yang JH, Hsia TC, Kuo HM, Chao PD, Chou CC, et al. (2006) Inhibition of lung cancer cell growth by quercetin glucuronides via G2/M arrest and induction of apoptosis. Drug Metab Dispos 34: 296–304.
35. Ruiz PA, Braune A, Holzlwimmer G, Quintanilla-Fend L, Haller D (2007) Quercetin inhibits TNF-induced NF-kappaB transcription factor recruitment to proinflammatory gene promoters in murine intestinal epithelial cells. J Nutr 137: 1208–1215.
36. Romier B, Van De Walle J, During A, Larondelle Y, Schneider YJ (2008) Modulation of signalling nuclear factor-kappaB activation pathway by polyphenols in human intestinal Caco-2 cells. Br J Nutr 100: 542–551.
37. Sanchez de Medina F, Vera B, Galvez J, Zarzuelo A (2002) Effect of quercitrin on the early stages of hapten induced colonic inflammation in the rat. Life Sci 70: 3097–3108.
38. Comalada M, Camuesco D, Sierra S, Ballester I, Xaus J, et al. (2005) In vivo quercitrin anti-inflammatory effect involves release of quercetin, which inhibits inflammation through down-regulation of the NF-kappaB pathway. Eur J Immunol 35: 584–592.
39. Kesarwani K, Gupta R, Mukerjee A (2013) Bioavailability enhancers of herbal origin: An overview. Asian Pac J Trop Biomed 3: 253–266.
40. Dall'Acqua S, Miolo G, Innocenti G, Caffieri S (2012) The photodegradation of quercetin: relation to oxidation. Molecules 17: 8898–8907.
41. D'Introno A, Paradiso A, Scoditti E, D'Amico L, De Paolis A, et al. (2009) Antioxidant and anti-inflammatory properties of tomato fruits synthesizing different amounts of stilbenes. Plant Biotechnol J 7: 422–429.
42. Cooper HS, Murthy SN, Shah RS, Sedergran DJ (1993) Clinicopathologic study of dextran sulfate sodium experimental murine colitis. Lab Invest 69: 238–249.
43. Naito Y, Takagi T, Kuroda M, Katada K, Ichikawa H, et al. (2004) An orally active matrix metalloproteinase inhibitor, ONO-4817, reduces dextran sulfate sodium-induced colitis in mice. Inflamm Res 53: 462–468.

13

CD98 Positive Eosinophils Contribute to T Helper 1 Pattern Inflammation

Fu-Min Xue[1], Huan-Ping Zhang[2], Hui-Jie Hao[1], Zhao-Yang Shi[1], Chuan Zhou[1], Baisui Feng[1], Ping-Chang Yang[2]*

1 Department of Gastroenterology, The First Affiliated Hospital of Zhengzhou University, Zhengzhou, China, 2 Department of Pathology & Molecular Medicine, McMaster University, Hamilton, Ontario, Canada

Abstract

Background and Aims: The pathogenesis of inflammatory bowel disease (IBD) has not been fully understood yet. Eosinophils (Eo) are one type of the major proinflammatory cells of the chronic inflammation in the intestine. CD98 is involved in the pathogenesis of a number of inflammations. This study aims to elucidate the role of CD98$^+$ Eos in the initiation of intestinal inflammation.

Methods: The colon biopsies were collected from 60 patients with IBD. The expression of CD98 in the biopsies was examined by immunohistochemistry. The serum levels of the flagellin (FGN) antibody and Eo-derived mediators in the culture supernatants were assessed by enzyme-linked immunosorbent assay. The role of FGN on Eo activation was examined in a cell culture model. The role of FGN in the induction of colitis was observed in a mouse model.

Results: Compared to normal controls, the frequency of CD98$^+$ Eos was markedly increased in the IBD colon mucosa. FGN were detected in the colon biopsies and in the sera of IBD patients. Exposure to FGN induced the expression of galectin 3 (the ligand of CD98) in dendritic cells. The exposure to galectin 3 activated the CD98$^+$ Eos. After treatment with FGN intrarectally, mice with eosinophilia showed severe inflammation in the colon.

Conclusions: The interaction of galectin 3 and CD98 can induce Eos to release chemical mediators that contributes to the initiation of the intestinal inflammation.

Editor: Jörn Karhausen, Duke University Medical Center, United States of America

Funding: This study was supported by grants from the Natural Science Foundation of China (#81070288), the Canadian Institutes of Health Research (#191063, #220058 and #177843), Natural Sciences, Engineering Research Council of Canada (NSERC, #371268). The funders had no role in study design, data collection and analysis, decision to publish, or preparation of the manuscript.

Competing Interests: The authors have declared that no competing interests exist.

* E-mail: yangp@mcmaster.ca

These authors contributed equally to this work.

Introduction

Inflammatory bowel disease (IBD) is a chronic inflammatory disorder of the intestine. The precise etiology of IBD is unclear. IBD includes two subtypes, ulcerative colitis (UC) and Crohn's disease (CD). The inflammation in UC is limited to the mucosa of the colon, while CD may occur anywhere in the gastrointestinal tract that is characterized as transmural inflammation accompanying with or without granuloma in the intestinal tissue. The treatment of IBD is unsatisfactory currently [1].

Eosiniophils (Eos) contain a number of chemical mediators, such as Eo cationic protein (ECP), Eo peroxidase (EPO), Eo-derived neurotoxic protein (ENP) and major basic protein (MBP). Eos release chemical mediators upon activation [2]. The mediators are involved in the pathogenesis of allergic diseases such as asthma [3]. Besides, Eos are also involved in the pathogenesis of a number of other disorders, such as rheumatoid arthritis [4], infectious diseases [5] and idiopathic [6] inflammatory disorders. Eos normally distribute in the intestine with a plausible function to expel the parasitic infection [7]. The chemical mediators of Eos are involved in the intestinal inflammation. Yet, the mechanism by which Eos induce inflammation in the intestine remains to be further understood.

CD98 is a glycoprotein [8] that is encoded by two genes, the *SLC3A2* and *SLC7A5*. CD98 forms the large neutral amino acid transporter that is a heterodimeric membrane transport protein to transport branched-chain (valine, leucine, isoleucine) and aromatic (tryptophan, tyrosine) amino acids [9]. Intestinal epithelial cells express CD98 under the physiological conditions. Recent reports indicate that CD98 is involved in the intestinal inflammation, which can be upregulated by interferon (IFN)-γ in the intestine [8]. Others also indicate that CD98 is involved in the pathogenesis of colitis and cancer [9,10]; the underlying mechanism is not fully elucidated yet.

Galectin-3 (Gal-3) is a member of the lectin family; it is encoded by a single gene, *LGALS3*, located on chromosome 14, locus q21–q22 [11]. Gal-3 is expressed by a number of cells. Published data indicate that Gal-3 is involved in the pathogeneses of cancer, inflammation, fibrosis, heart disease, and stroke. Gal-3 is the ligand of CD98 [12]. Dendritic cell (DC) express Gal-3 in response to appropriate stimulation [13]. Whether the interaction of DC-derived Gal-3 and CD98$^+$ Eos plays any roles in the initiation of intestinal inflammation, such as IBD, is unclear. In the present study, we collected the colon biopsies from a group of IBD patients and found that Eos highly expressed CD98 in the IBD colon mucosa. DC-derived Gal-3 interacted with CD98 to activate Eos that contributed to the initiation of intestinal inflammation.

Materials and Methods

Reagents

Flagellin was purchased from Austral Biologicals (San Ramon, CA). Antibody of flagellin was purchased from Biodesign (Saco, Maine). Antibodies (S-17, C-terminus; N-20, N-terminus) and shRNA kits of CD98, TLR5 (B-24) and Gal-3 (H-5) were purchased from Santa Cruz Biotech (Santa Cruz, CA). Enzyme-linked immunosorbent assay (ELISA) kit for flagellin and rhGal-3 were purchased from R&D Systems (Shanghai, China). Anti-TLR5 antibody was purchased from Abcam (Cambridge, MA). Magnetic cell sorting reagents were purchased from Miltenyi Biotec (Auburn, CA). ELISA kits of EPO, EDN, MBP and ECP, neutralizing polyclonal antibodies of CD98 and Gal-3 were purchased from Uscn Life Science Inc. (Wuhan, China).

Mice

BALB/c mice (6–8 weeks old) were purchased from the Beijing Experimental Animal Institute (Beijing, China). Mice were maintained in a pathogen-free environment. The experimental procedures were approved by the Animal Care Committee at Zhengzhou University.

Human Subjects and Colon Biopsy

Sixty IBD patients (at remission stage) were recruited from the Department of Gastroenterology, Zhengzhou University and the China PLA General Hospital. The diagnosis of IBD was followed our routine procedures that were also published elsewhere [14,15]. The colon biopsies were taken from the inflamed area of the intestine. The normal control tissue was obtained from the colon (non-polyp tissue) of 10 patients with colon polyposis. The demographic information of the IBD patients was listed in Table 1. The collection of colon biopsies was followed the established procedures in our departments. Informed, written consent was obtained from each patient. The study using human specimens in this study was approved by the Human Study Ethic Committees at Zhengzhou University and the China PLA General Hospital.

Serum Collection

Ten milliliter blood was collected from each IBD patient and 30 healthy subjects. The sera were isolated and stored at −80°C until use.

Immunohistochemistry

The colon biopsies were frozen with liquid nitrogen. The cryosections were prepared and stained with antibodies of MBP (dilution: 1:200) and CD98 (dilution: 1:100) at 4°C overnight. The sections were then incubated with the horseradish peroxidase- or the alkaline phosphate-labeled secondary antibodies for 1 h at room temperature. The sections were finally stained with haematoxylin and observed with a light microscope. All the sections were coded; the observers were not aware of the code to avoid bias. The positively stained cells were counted in twenty fields (×400) per sample.

Table 1. Demographic and disease features of patients.

Group	Crohn's disease	Ulcerative colitis	Colon polyp
Sex	M: 15; F: 15	M: 15; F: 15	M: 5; F:5
Age	33.6 (28–66)	36.3 (23–74)	41.2 (18–61)
Weight (kg)	56.4 (51–75)	62 (54–77)	59 (55–71)
Duration of (months)	42 (26–65)	45 (34–86)	33 (12–45)
Prednisolone (mg/day)	15 (5–20)	15 (5–20)	0
Race	Asian	Asian	Asian
Outpatient	30	30	10
Previous hospitalizations	18	19	0
Localization			
Colon	30 (100%)	30 (100%)	10
Terminal ileum	6 (20%)		
Upper gastrointestinal	1 (3%)		
Left-sided Ulcerative colitis	0	4 (13.3%)	
Extensive Ulcerative colitis	0	3 (10.0%)	
Behavior			
Inflammatory	30 (100%)	30 (100%)	0
Stricturing	3 (10.0%)		
Penetrating	0		
Perianal disease	4 (13.3%),	4 (13.3%)	0
Treatment			
Steroids	30 (100%),	30 (100%)	0
Infliximab	5 (16.6%),	0	
Antibiotics	11 (36.7%),	14 (46.7%)	0
Mesalamine	3 (10.0%),	7 (23.3%)	0

Data are shown as medians (interquartile ranges).

ELISA

The serum levels of flagellin antibody, EPO, EDN, MBP and ECP were determined by ELISA with commercial reagent kits following the manufacturer's instructions.

Generation of Human DCs

Twenty healthy volunteers were selected as blood donors. Peripheral blood mononuclear cells (PBMCs) were separated using the Histopaque (SG-1.077; Sigma) density gradients. The CD11c$^+$ DCs were separated from the PBMCs by magnetic cell sorting (MACS). As checked by flow cytometry (FACS), the purity of the separated DCs was over 90%. The cells were cultured in RPMI 1640 medium containing 10% fetal calf serum, 2 mM l-glutamine, 100 U/ml penicillin, 100 μg/ml streptomycin, 25 mM HEPES (4-(2-hydroxyethyl)-1-piperazineethanesulfonic acid) and Granulocyte-macrophage colony-stimulating factor (20 ng/ml) under 37°C in 5% CO_2 environment. Three days later, the cells were collected and used for further experiments.

Quantitative Real-time RT-PCR (qRT-PCR)

The expression of Gal-3 in DCs was determined by qRT-PCR. Twenty-five ng cDNA were amplified in 50 μl 1 × SYBR-Green I PCR master mix, containing 200 nM primers for Gal-3. The experiments were performed in triplicate using a qRT-PCR thermal cycler (Bio-Rad). The negative controls (master mix containing untranscribed total RNA or without any cDNA or

RNA) were added to each experiment. The quantification was obtained using the relative standard curve method. The standard curve was created by amplification of 5 μl control total RNA extracted from the cells at different dilutions (1.0–0.025 ng/μl by twofold dilution). The relative amount of each unknown sample was calculated using the linear regression from the standard curve. The relative Gal-3 gene expression value was normalized to percentage of the value of the housekeeping gene, β-actin. The primers of Gal-3 using in this study were: Forward: ggccactgattgtgccttat; reverse: gaagcgtgggttaaagtgga (NCBI: NM_001177388.1).

Western Blotting

A piece of the intestinal mucosa was processed for protein extraction. Protein extracts were subjected to electrophoresis on a 10% SDS-polyacrylamide electrophoresis gel. The proteins were transferred onto nitrocellulose membrane, which was then blocked with 5% bovine serum albumin (BSA) in Tris-buffered saline containing 0.05% Tween 20 (TBST) for 1 h. The blot was then incubated with the primary antibody (1:500) overnight at 4°C in 5% BSA/TBST. The blot was washed with TBST and further incubated with the horseradish peroxidase-conjugated secondary antibody (1:1000) for 1 h at room temperature. Subsequently, the blot was washed 3 times with TBST for 1 h, and developed with SuperSignal chemiluminescence reagent, and exposed to X-ray film to visualize the proteins.

Culture of Eo Cell Lines

The Eo cell line, EoL-1 cells, generated from a patient with acute myeloid leukemia following hypereosinophilic syndrome, was purchased from the RIKEN Cell Bank (Tsukuba, Japan). EoL-1 cells were maintained in RPMI 1640 medium supplemented with 10% fetal calf serum and antibiotics at 37°C and 5% CO_2.

RNA Interference

The gene expression of TLR5 in DCs and CD98 in EoL cells was knocked down by the transduction with shRNA reagent kits for TLR5 and CD98 respectively. The experiments were performed following the manufacturer's instruction. The efficiency of gene knockdown was over 90% as assessed by Western blotting (data not shown).

Induction of Intestinal Eosinophilia

A parasitic infection model was adopted to induce eosinophilia in the intestine. The maintenance of the *T. muris* parasite and the methods using for infection and large intestinal worm burden assessment were performed as previously described [16]. BALB/c mice were infected by oral gavage with 120–150 infective eggs/mouse and sacrificed or used for further experiments 45 days later. The cecum was removed and opened to count the number of parasites. The results showed the parasites were found in the cecum of all infected mice (5–11 parasites were found in each cecum. The colon was excised and processed for paraffin sections and stained with the H&E method. The number of Eos was counted under a light microscope. The results showed that the number of Eos was 38.5±5.8/mm^2 in infected mice in contrast to 9.6±2.5/mm^2 in saline control mice ($p<0.01$).

Induction of Colitis in Mice with Eosinophilia

BALB/c mice with intestinal eosinophilia (the eosinophilic status in the intestine was verified by examining sample mice) were intrarectally introduced with 0.1 ml 50% ethanol containing FGN 50 μg/mouse (control mice were introduced with ethanol alone) under light general anesthesia, twice a week for 3 weeks. The body weight of each mouse was recorded before the treatment and before the sacrifice. The mice were sacrificed by cervical dislocation. A segment of the colon was excised and processed for paraffin embedding and H&E staining. A piece of the colon was used to extract protein to measure the levels of myeloperoxidase (MPO).

DC Depletion

A group of mice was depleted DCs by ip injection with dichloromethylenediphosphonic acid-loaded or PBS-loaded liposomes (Encapsula NanoSciences) or intravenously into mice (200–300 μl per mouse) as previously described [17]. As checked by immunohistochemistry, CD11c$^+$ DCs were not observed in the intestine of the mice (data not shown).

Depletion of CD98 and Gal-3 in Mice

BALB/c mice were ip injected with neutralizing anti-CD98 antibody (0.2 mg/mouse) or neutralizing anti-Gal-3 (0.2 mg/mouse) antibody daily for 5 consecutive days. As shown by the results of Western blotting, the expression of CD98 or Gal-3 was below the detectable levels in the intestine of the mice (data not shown).

Measurement of MPO Levels

A piece of the colon tissue was excised and homogenized in lysis buffer (200 mM NaCl, 5 mM EDTA, 10 mM Tris, 10% glycerin, 1 mM PMSF, 1 μg/mL leupeptin, and 28 μg/mL aprotinin (pH 7.4); 200 μL). Samples were centrifuged at 15000 ×g at 4°C for 15 minutes. The supernatants were collected; the MPO activity was assayed by mixing the supernatants with citric phosphate buffer (pH 5.0) containing 0.4 mg/ml O-phenylene diamine and 0.015% hydrogen peroxide. The optical density value of the samples were measured with a spectrophotometer at 450 nm.

Statistics

The values were expressed as the means with the SEM of at least three independent experiments. The data were analyzed using the two-tailed unpaired Student t test when the data were consisted of two groups or by ANOVA when three or more groups were compared. A value of $p<0.05$ was accepted as statistically significant.

Results

Frequency of CD98+ Eos was Increased in IBD Intestinal Mucosa

Previous studies suggested that the CD98 might play a role in the pathogenesis of IBD [9,10]. In the present study, we observed that the expression of CD98 was not only expressed on the epithelial cells, but also expressed on some cells in the lamina propria; most of the CD98$^+$ cells are polynuclear cells. The staining with eosin revealed that the cells were Eos. Immune staining revealed that more than 80% CD98$^+$ cells in the lamina propria were Eos (MBP$^+$); the frequency of CD98$^+$ Eos was not significantly different between UC and CD (Fig. 1). Eos were also detected in the non-IBD intestinal mucosa; but the frequency (11.6% ±2.2%;) of CD98$^+$ Eos was significantly lower in the non-IBD specimens than that in the IBD intestinal mucosa.

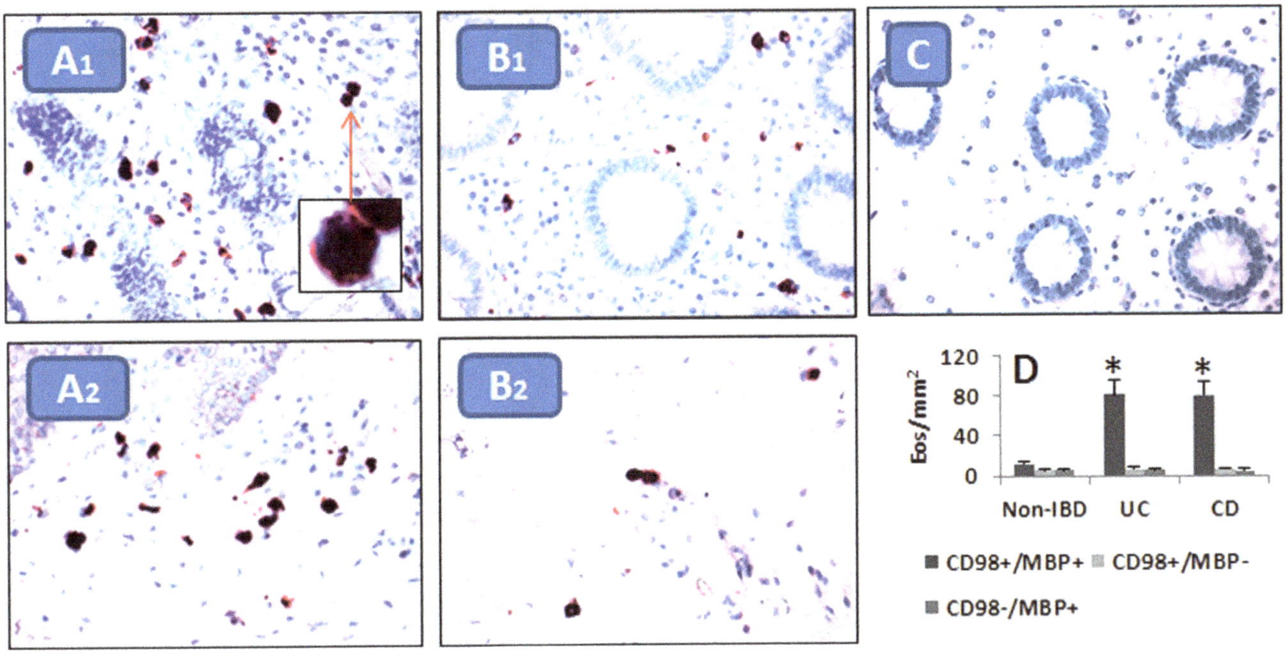

Figure 1. Intestinal Eos express CD98. Colon biopsies were obtained from 60 IBD patients (30 UC; 30 CD). The bioptic specimens were processed for cryosections and stained with antibodies of CD98 and MBP by a combination of peroxidase-nickel and alkaline phosphate methods. A-B, representative images show CD98$^+$ (in red) and MBP$^+$ (in black) Eos in the colon mucosa of IBD (A) and non-IBD (B; from 6 patients with colon polyps). Original magnification: ×400. Panel C is an isotype control. D, the bars indicate the frequency of CD98$^+$ or/and MBP$^+$ Eos (mean ± SEM). *, $p<0.01$, compared with non-IBD samples. The sections were contrast-stained with hematoxylin (no eosin staining). A1 and B1 were stained with anti-CD98 C-terminus antibody; A2 and B2 were stained with anti-N-terminus antibody.

Flagellin Induces Expression of Gal-3 in DCs

We next investigated the ligands of CD98. Gal-3 is the ligand of CD98 [12]. DCs express Gal-3 in response to appropriate stimulation [13]. DCs may be activated by the interaction of microbial products and Toll-like receptors (TLR). We then prepared DCs and exposed the DCs to microbial products, FGN, PolyI:C and LPS in the culture. The expression of Gal-3 in DCs was examined. The results showed that the exposure to FGN in the culture increased the expression of Gal-3 on DCs in a FGN dose-dependent manner while the exposures to LPS or PolyI:C did not. To confirm the results, we knocked down the TLR5 in DCs by the gene silence; the TLR5-deficient DCs were then exposed to FGN in the culture. As expected, the increase in the expression of Gal-3 was abolished (Fig. 2). The results indicate that exposure to FGN can upregulate the expression of Gal-3 on DCs.

DC-derived Gal-3 Activates CD98$^+$ Eos

As shown in Fig. 1, high frequency of CD98$^+$ Eos was observed in the IBD intestinal mucosa; Gal-3 is the ligand of CD98 [12], we inferred that the interaction of Gal-3 and CD98 might activate Eos. To test the hypothesis, we cultured DCs and an Eo cell line, the EoL-1 cells, in the presence of FGN for 24 h. Then, the levels of the Eo-derived chemical mediators in the culture supernatant were assessed by ELISA. The results showed that the exposure to FGN markedly increased the levels of the chemical mediators, including ECP, EPO, EDN and MBP, in the supernatant, that was abolished by knocking down the gene of CD98 in EoL-1 cells or in the absence of DCs. Cultured with the supernatant of FGN-treated DCs or addition of recombinant Gal-3 to the culture also increased the Eo-derived mediators in the culture supernatant (Fig. 3). The results indicate that the interaction of Gal-3 and CD98 can activate Eos to release proinflammatory mediators.

Serum Levels of FGN Ab in IBD Patients are Correlated with the Frequency of CD98$^+$ Eos

Prompted by the results of Fig. 2 and Fig. 3, we measured the serum levels of FGN antibody in 60 IBD patients and 30 healthy subjects. As shown by ELISA, the serum levels of FGN Ab were significantly higher in IBD patients than that in healthy controls (Fig. 4; $p<0.01$). Furthermore, a positive correlation was identified between the frequency of CD98$^+$ Eos in the intestinal biopsies and the serum levels of FGN Ab ($r=0.548$, $p<0.05$). In addition, FGN was detected in the colon biopsy specimens by Western blotting that was markedly higher in IBD samples than that in controls (10 patients with colon polyps).

Exposure to FGN Induces Colitis in Mice with Intestinal Eosinophilia

Finally we developed the eosinophilia in the mouse intestine by the parasitic infection. The mice were intrarectally introduced with FGN for 5 days. The histology of the colon showed that colitis was induced manifesting abundant inflammatory cell infiltration, tissue edema, intra-tissue bleeding and deformation of crypts (Fig. 5A). High frequency of Eos was also observed in the intestine (Fig. 5A). In addition, the body weight loss (Fig. 5B), high levels of MPO of the colon extracts (Fig. 5C) and bleeding stool were recorded. These pathological changes were abolished in mice pretreated with either anti-CD98 antibody, or anti-Gal-3 antibody, or depletion of DC (Fig. 5D). The serum levels of Eo-derived mediators were significantly higher only in mice with eosinophilia and exposure to FGN (Fig. 6).

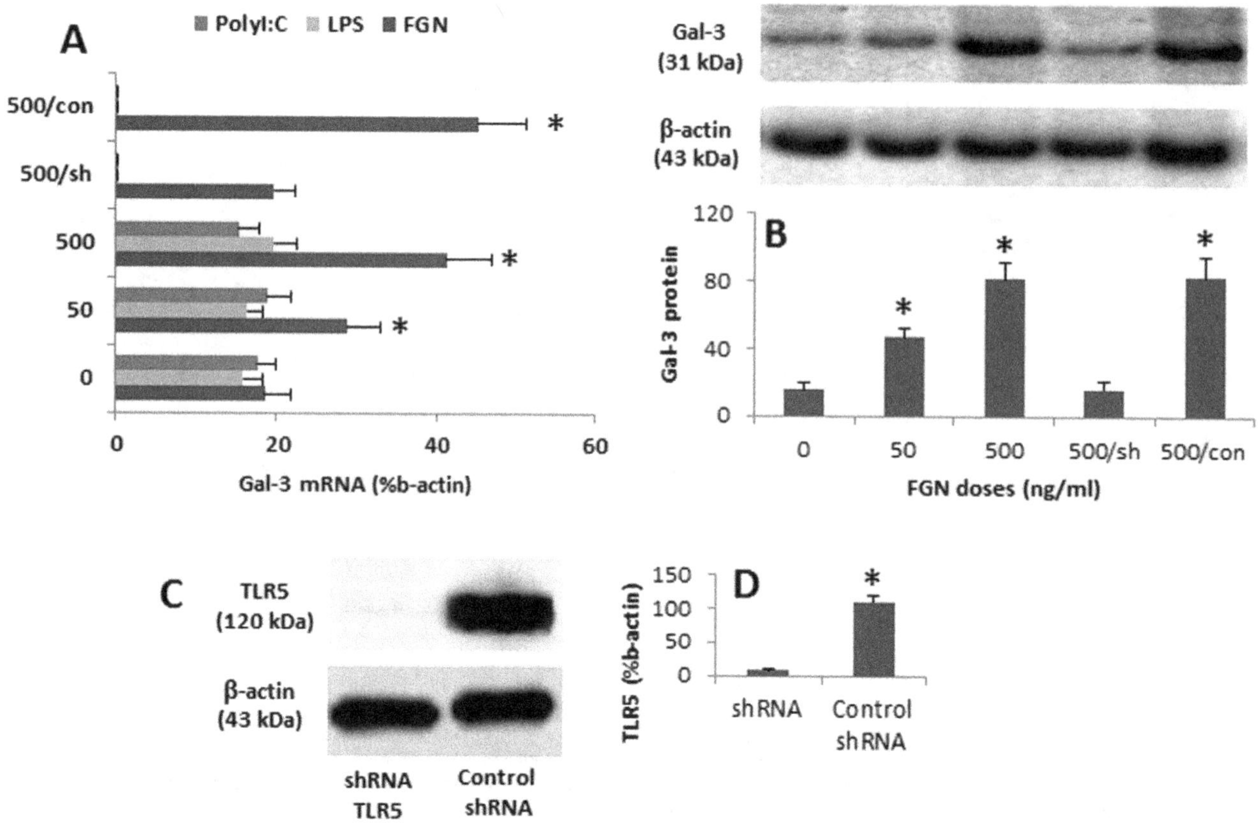

Figure 2. FGN induces the expression of gal-3 in DCs. DCs were generated from human PBMC and cultured in the presence of FGN, or LPS, or Polyl:C, at the indicated doses for 48 h. The expression of gal-3 in DCs was determined by qRT-PCR (A) and Western blotting (B). A, the bars indicate the mRNA levels of Gal-3 that were normalized to the percentage of β-actin. B, the immune blots shows the levels of Gal-3. The bars below the immune blots indicate the summarized integrated density of the immune blots. The data in bar graphs were expressed as mean ± SEM. *, $p<0.05$, compared with dose "0" group. sh: DCs were pre-treated with shRNA of TLR5 (for FGN group) for 48 h before using in the experiments. Con: DCs were pre-treated with control shRNA. C–D, the immune blots show the levels of TLR5 in DCs treated with shRNA of TLR5 or control shRNA (C); the bars indicate the summarized integrated density of the immune blots (D). The data represent 6 experiments.

Discussion

The present paper reports that the intestinal Eos express CD98, which is significantly higher in the intestinal mucosa of patients with IBD that non-IBD intestinal mucosa. The frequency of $CD98^+$ Eos is positively correlated with the serum level of FGN antibody in IBD patients. The data also indicate that FGN can induce DCs to release Gal-3; the latter ligates CD98 on Eos to induce Eos to release the chemical mediators, the latter contribute to the initiation of inflammation in the intestine. Thus, in addition to the well characterized IL-5 on activation of Eos [18], the present data provide a novel pathway to activate Eos in the intestine.

Eos are the residential cells in the intestine. The cells contribute to the innate immunity by inhibiting parasitic infection in the intestine [2]. Because of containing a number of chemical mediators, it is suggested that the activation of Eos is involved in the initiation of inflammation in the intestine. High levels of Eo-derived mediators can be detected in feces [19] or colon perfusion fluids [20] of patients with chronic colitis that are positively correlated with the infiltration of Eos in the colon. The present data are in line with these reports by showing a significant increase in the frequency of Eos in IBD intestinal biopsies.

A novel finding of the present study is that Eos express CD98. The data show that the $CD98^+$ Eos were detected in both IBD colon biopsies and non-IBD colon tissue; the frequency of $CD98^+$ Eos was significantly higher in the IBD specimens than that in the non-IBD samples. The underlying mechanism might be that there is a high level of IFN-γ in IBD intestinal tissue; IFN-γ can upregulate the expression of CD98 [9], which may induce Eos to express high levels of CD98. A recent report [10] indicates that the over-expressing CD98 results in inflammation in the intestine or promotes the carcinogenesis in the intestine. To date, previous reports only mentioned that intestinal epithelial cells express CD98. In line with the report [10], our results not only show that the expression of CD98 in the intestinal epithelial layer (data not shown), but also reveal a high frequency of $CD98^+$ Eos in the intestine of patients with IBD. The present data show that the activation of $CD98^+$ Eos can compromise the epithelial barrier function, which results in more macromolecular antigens to be absorbed into the deep tissue of the intestine. The data further demonstrate that the activation of CD98 causes Eos to release the chemical mediators; the mediators may attribute to the inflammation in IBD. The inference is supported by the subsequent data from the animal model study. The exposure to FGN induced severe colitis in mice with eosinophilia. Previous study also demonstrated that FGN was associated with intestinal inflammation [21]. Although several control groups, including those treated with anti-CD98, anti-Gal-3 and ethanol, also had intestinal eosinophilia, those mice did not have apparent signs of colitis.

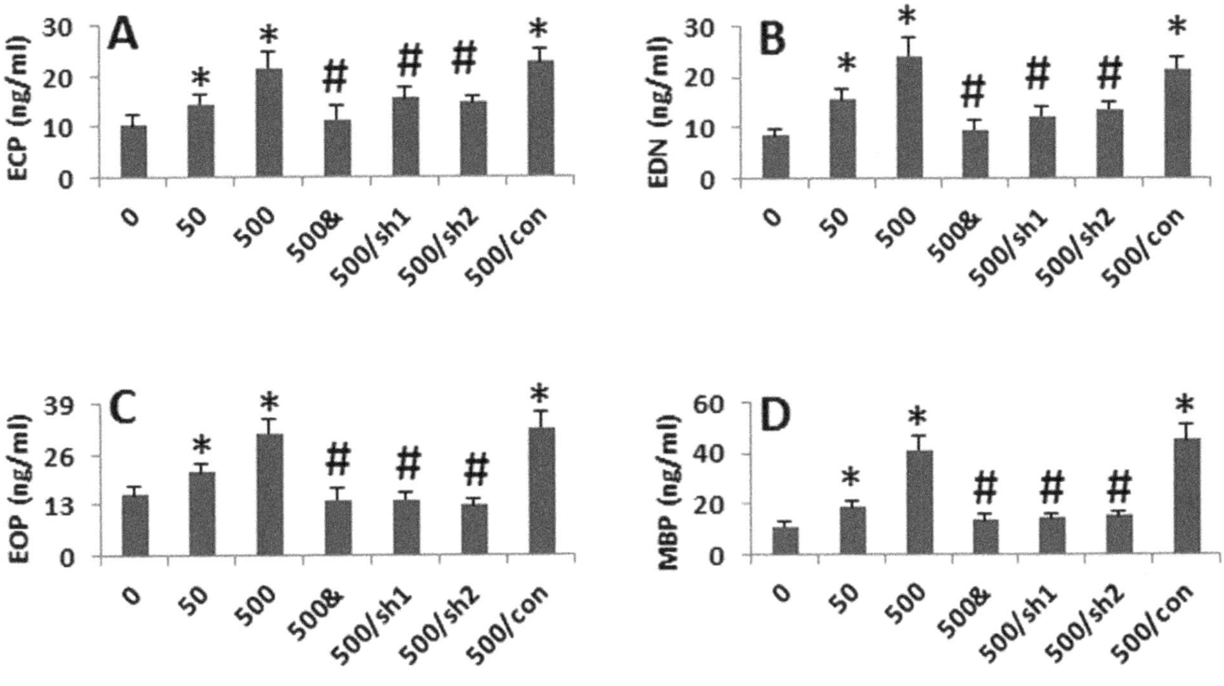

Figure 3. Levels of the Eo-derived chemical mediators in culture supernatant. DCs and EoL cells were cultured in the presence of FGN at graded doses for 24 h. The bars indicate the levels of the Eo-derived mediators that were determined by ELISA. The data were presented as mean ± SEM. *, p<0.05, compared with group "0". #, p<0.01, compared with group "500". &: No DCs were added to the culture. sh1: EoL cells were pretreated with the shRNA of CD98. sh2: DCs were treated with shRNA of Gal-3. Con: EoL cells were pretreated with the control shRNA. Super: EoL cells were exposed to the supernatants of DC treated with FGN (500 ng/ml; 12 h). rhGal3: EoL cells were stimulated with rhGal-3. The data represent 6 experiments.

The fact indicates that the increase in the Eo number alone is insufficient to cause inflammation in the intestine until the Eos are activated somehow. Indeed, the serum levels of Eo-derived chemical mediators, one of the signs of Eo activation, were markedly increased in mice with eosinophilia and exposure to FGN but not in those control mice.

Gal-3 is the ligand of CD98 [12]. The expression of Gal-3 in macrophages has been well-documented [13]. Following published procedures [13], we also generated Gal-3 expressing DCs. The generated DCs express TLR5; the fact indicates that these DCs can recognize the FGN's stimulation. Our further data proved the inference by showing that exposure to FGN, abundant Gal-3 were detected in the DCs as well as in the culture supernatants. Gal-3 is also an adhering molecule that facilitates the Eo rolling and plays a role in allergic inflammation, cancer, inflammation and fibrosis, heart disease, and stroke [22–24]. Our data also demonstrate that Gal-3 is involved in facilitating the development of inflammation by showing an indirect effect that the interaction of Gal-3/CD98

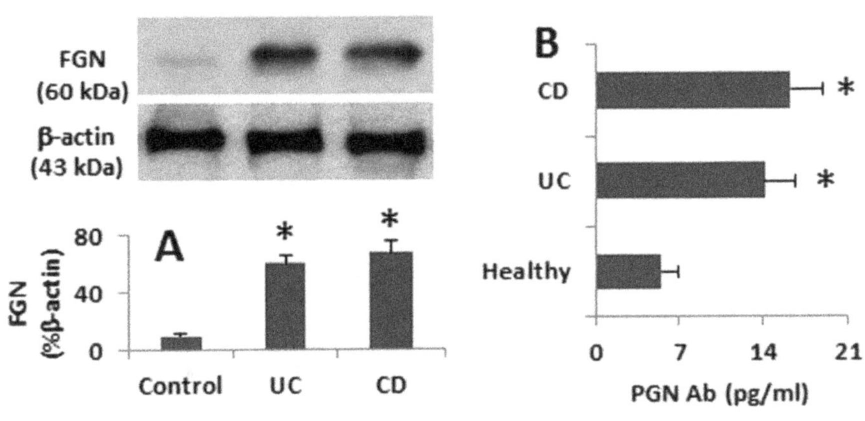

Figure 4. The levels of FGN antibody (Ab). A, one piece of the biopsies from each IBD patient was processed for Western blotting. The representative immune blots show FGN in the colon tissue. The bars show the summarized integrated density of the immune blots [mean ± SEM from 60 IBD specimens and 10 controls (the colon biopsies were obtained from patients with colon polyps)]. B, the sera were collected from 30 UC patients, 30 CD patients and 30 healthy subjects. The levels of FGN Ab were determined by ELISA. The bars indicate the levels of serum FGN Ab. The data were presented as mean ± SEM. *, p<0.01, compared with healthy controls.

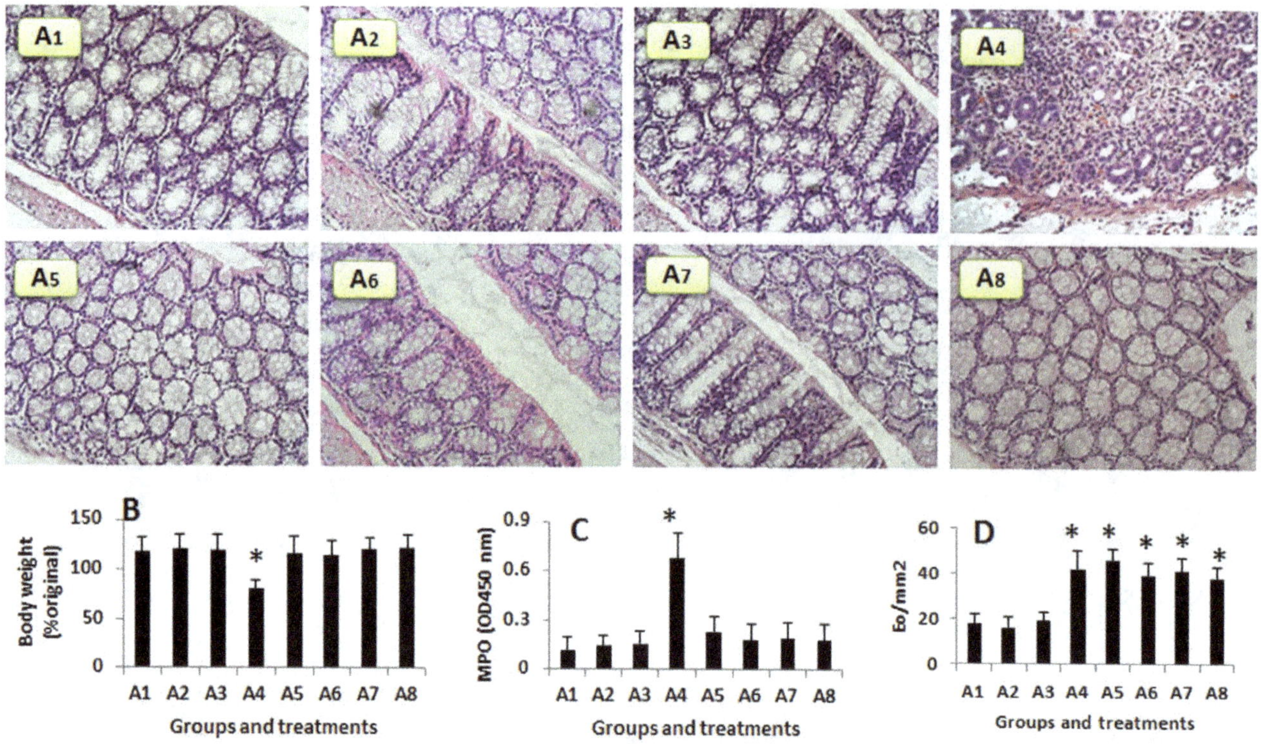

Figure 5. Exposure to FGN induces inflammation in the colon of mice with eosinophilia. Mice were induced the eosinophilia in the intestine by parasitic infections. Naïve mice (A1) did not have any specific treatment. A2–A3, naïve mice were treated with saline (A2) or FGN (A3) via the intrarectal route. A4–A7, mice with eosinophilia were exposed to FGN via intrarectal route and depletion of DCs (A5), or anti-CD98 antibody (A6), or anti-Gal-3 antibody (A7). A8, mice with intestinal eosinophilia were treated with 50% ethanol via the intrarectal route. Image magnification: ×200. B, the bars indicate the body weight records; the data were presented as a percentage of the original body weight. C, the bars indicate the MPO level in colon tissue extracts. D, the bars indicate the frequency of Eo in the colon mucosa (the counts were averaged from 20 fields per mouse). The data in B-D were expressed as mean ± SEM. *, $p<0.05$, compared with group A1. Each group had 6 mice.

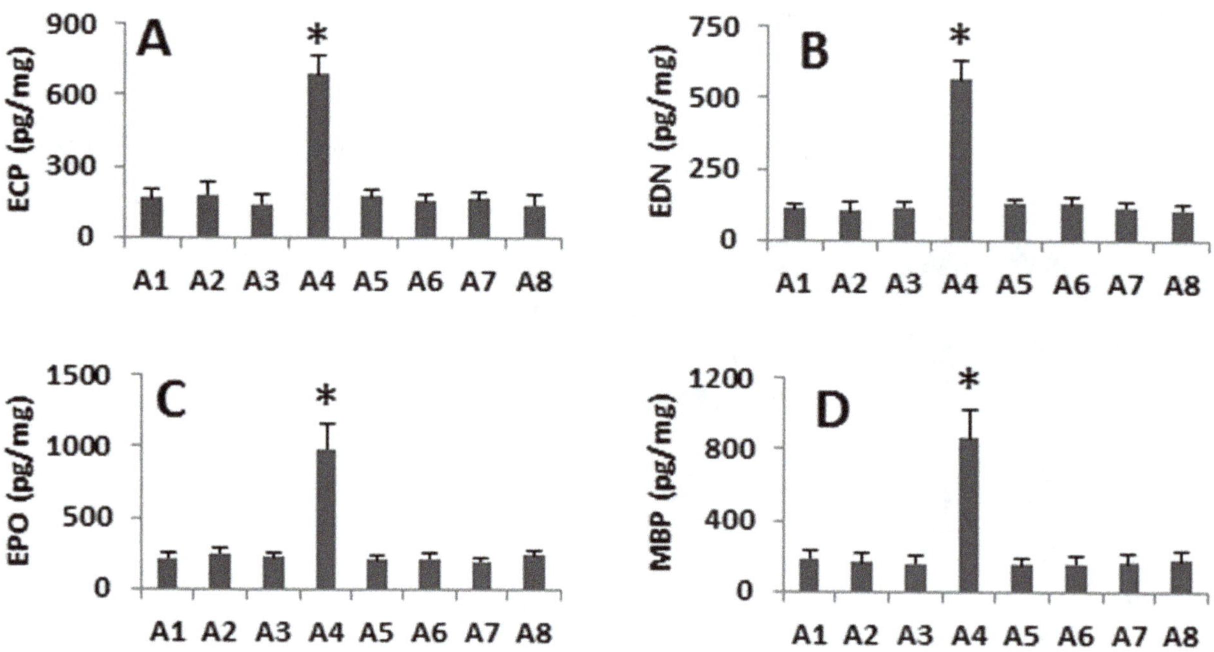

Figure 6. Levels of Eo-derived mediators in the intestine. The sera were collected from the mice in Fig. 5 and were analyzed for the levels of Eo-derived mediators by ELISA. The bars indicate the levels of ECP (A), END (B), EPO (C) and MBP (D). The data were presented as Eo mediators/mg serum protein (mean ± SEM from 6 mice per group). The X axes list the groups that are the same as those in Fig. 5. *, $p<0.01$, compared to the A1 group. Each group consisted of 6 mice.

induces Eos to release chemical mediators; the latter induces inflammation in the intestine.

In the present study, the eosinophilia and the presence of FGN are important factors in the induction of colitis. However, eosinophilia is common in the parasite infection; FGN is also a regular microbial product in the intestine, not all patients with parasite infections suffer from IBD. In the present study, that mice with eosinophilia were prone to colitis is based on a premise of breaking the epithelial barrier function after treating with ethanol. The fact emphasizes that the integrity of intestinal barrier function is important to maintain the homeostasis in the intestine. Our results are in line with a recent report that intestinal epithelial cells express CD98 is involved in the induction of colitis in mice [10]. A difference between our data and Nguyen's study [10] is that we observed that intestinal Eos expressed CD98 while they revealed that intestinal epithelial cells expressed CD98. The fact indicates that more than one cell types express CD98 in the intestine, which may be associated with the pathogenesis of intestinal inflammation.

To further confirm the role of CD98 in the induction of the intestinal inflammation in the present experimental system, we pretreated a group of mice with anti-CD98 antibody, which blocked the inflammation. However, as shown by histology, the number of Eos was not decreased in this group of mice. The fact indicates that administration with anti-CD98 did not cause the death of Eos in the intestine; only neutralized the CD98 on Eos. The underlying mechanism is to be further investigated. In fact, Eos are not the only cell type expressing CD98, many other cell types [25] also express CD98. Whether the anti-CD98 antibody interfered with other cells' function was not systematically observed, which needs to be further investigated.

In summary, our data indicate that Eos express CD98 in IBD intestinal tissue. Microbial product, FGN, can activate DCs to express Gal-3. The Gal-3 binds CD98 to activate Eos to release chemical mediators and induces inflammation in the intestine.

Author Contributions

Conceived and designed the experiments: BSF PCY. Performed the experiments: FMX HPZ HJH ZYS CZ. Analyzed the data: FMX HPZ HJH ZYS CZ. Contributed reagents/materials/analysis tools: FMX HPZ HJH ZYS CZ. Wrote the paper: PCY.

References

1. Podolsky DK (2003) The future of IBD treatment. J Gastroenterol 38 Suppl 15: 63–6.
2. Woodruff SA, Masterson JC, Fillon S, Robinson ZD, Furuta GT (2011) Role of eosinophils in inflammatory bowel and gastrointestinal diseases. J Pediatr Gastroenterol Nutr 52: 650–61.
3. Broide DH, Finkelman F, Bochner BS, Rothenberg ME (2011) Advances in mechanisms of asthma, allergy, and immunology in 2010. J Allergy Clin Immunol 127: 689–695. doi: 10.1016/j.jaci.2011.01.027.
4. Kargili A, Bavbek N, Kaya A, Koşar A, Karaaslan Y (2004) Eosinophilia in rheumatologic diseases: a prospective study of 1000 cases. Rheumatol Int 24: 321–324.
5. Qiu H, KuoLee R, Harris G, Zhou H, Miller H, et al (2011) Acinetobacter baumannii Infection Inhibits Airway Eosinophilia and Lung Pathology in a Mouse Model of Allergic Asthma. PLoS ONE 6: e22004.
6. von Wattenwyl F, Zimmermann A, Netzer P (2001) Synchronous first manifestation of an idiopathic eosinophilic gastroenteritis and bronchial asthma. Eur J Gastroenterol Hepatol 13: 721–5.
7. Lamousé-Smith ES, Furuta GT (2006) Eosinophils in the gastrointestinal tract. Current Gastroenterology Reports 8: 390–395.
8. Kucharzik T, Lugering A, Yan Y, Driss A, Charrier L, et al (2005) Activation of epithelial CD98 glycoprotein perpetuates colonic inflammation. Lab Invest 85: 932–941.
9. Yan Y, Vasudevan S, Nguyen HTT, Merlin D (2008) Intestinal epithelial CD98: An oligomeric and multifunctional protein. Biochim Biophys Acta 1780: 1087–1092. doi: 10.1016/j.bbagen.2008.06.007.
10. Nguyen HTT, Dalmasso G, Torkvist L, Halfvarson J, Yan Y, et al (2011) CD98 expression modulates intestinal homeostasis, inflammation, and colitis-associated cancer in mice. J Clin Invest 121: 1733–1747.
11. Dumic J, Dabelic S, Flögel M (2006) Galectin-3: An open-ended story. Biochim Biophys Acta 1760: 616–635. doi: 10.1016/j.bbagen.2005.12.020.
12. Dalton P, Christian HC, Redman CWG, Sargent IL, Boyd CAR (2007) Membrane trafficking of CD98 and its ligand galectin 3 in BeWo cells-implication for placental cell fusion. FEBS J 274: 2715–2727. 10.1111/j.1742-4658.2007.05806.x.
13. van Stijn CMW, van den Broek M, van de Weerd R, Visser M, Tasdelen I, et al (2009) Regulation of expression and secretion of galectin-3 in human monocyte-derived dendritic cells. Mol Immunol 46: 3292–3299. doi: 10.1016/j.molimm.2009.07.026.
14. Podolsky DK (1991) Inflammatory Bowel Disease. N Engl J Med 325: 928–937. doi: 10.1056/NEJM199109263251306.
15. Podolsky DK (1991) Inflammatory Bowel Disease. N Engl J Med 325: 1008–1016. doi: 10.1056/NEJM199110033251406.
16. Motomura Y, Khan WI, El-Sharkawy RT, Verma-Gandhu M, Grencis RK, et al (2010) Mechanisms underlying gut dysfunction in a murine model of chronic parasitic infection. Am J Physiol Gastrointest Liver Physiol 299: G1354–G1360.
17. Perruche S, Zhang P, Liu Y, Saas P, Bluestone JA, et al (2008) CD3-specific antibody-induced immune tolerance involves transforming growth factor-[beta] from phagocytes digesting apoptotic T cells. Nat Med 14: 528–535. 10.1038/nm1749.
18. Lodes MJ, Cong Y, Elson CO, Mohamath R, Landers CJ, et al (2004) Bacterial flagellin is a dominant antigen in Crohn disease. J Clin Invest 113: 1296–1306.
19. Kouro T, Takatsu K (2009) IL-5- and eosinophil-mediated inflammation: from discovery to therapy. Int Immunol 21: 1303–1309.
20. Peterson CG, Eklund E, Taha Y, Raab Y, Carlson M (2002) A new method for the quantification of neutrophil and eosinophil cationic proteins in feces: establishment of normal levels and clinical application in patients with inflammatory bowel disease. Am J Gastroenterol 97: 1755–1762.
21. Taha Y, Carlson M, Thorn M, Loof L, Raab Y (2001) Evidence of Local Eosinophil Activation and Altered Mucosal Permeability in Collagenous Colitis. Dig Dis Sci 46: 888–897.
22. Rao SP, Wang Z, Zuberi RI, Sikora L, Bahaie NS, et al (2007) Galectin-3 Functions as an Adhesion Molecule to Support Eosinophil Rolling and Adhesion under Conditions of Flow. J Immunol 179: 7800–7807.
23. Yanavitski M, Givertz M (2011) Novel Biomarkers in Acute Heart Failure. Curr Heart Fail Rep 8: 206–211.
24. Chiu CG, Strugnell SS, Griffith OL, Jones SJM, Gown AM, et al (2010) Diagnostic Utility of Galectin-3 in Thyroid Cancer. Am J Pathol 176: 2067–2081. doi: 10.2353/ajpath.2010.090353.
25. Yan Y, Vasudevan S, Nguyen HTT, Merlin D (2008) Intestinal epithelial CD98: An oligomeric and multifunctional protein. Biochim Biophys Acta 1780: 1087–1092. doi: 10.1016/j.bbagen.2008.06.007.

Enhanced Transferrin Receptor Expression by Proinflammatory Cytokines in Enterocytes as a Means for Local Delivery of Drugs to Inflamed Gut Mucosa

Efrat Harel[1], Abraham Rubinstein[1], Aviram Nissan[2], Elena Khazanov[1], Mirela Nadler Milbauer[1], Yechezkel Barenholz[3], Boaz Tirosh[1]*

1 Institute for Drug Research, The Hebrew University of Jerusalem, Jerusalem, Israel, **2** Department of Surgery, Hadassah Hebrew University Medical Center, Mount Scopus, Jerusalem, Israel, **3** The Laboratory of Membrane and Liposome Research, The Hebrew University of Jerusalem, Jerusalem, Israel

Abstract

Therapeutic intervention in inflammatory bowel diseases (IBDs) is often associated with adverse effects related to drug distribution into non-diseased tissues, a situation which attracts a rational design of a targeted treatment confined to the inflamed mucosa. Upon activation of immune cells, transferrin receptor (TfR) expression increases at their surface. Because TfR is expressed in all cell types we hypothesized that its cell surface levels are regulated also in enterocytes. We, therefore, compared TfR expression in healthy and inflamed human colonic mucosa, as well as healthy and inflamed colonic mucosa of the DNBS-induced rat model. TfR expression was elevated in the colonic mucosa of IBD patients in both the basolateral and apical membranes of the enterocytes. Increased TfR expression was also observed in colonocytes of the induced colitis rats. To explore the underlying mechanism CaCo-2 cells were treated with various proinflammatory cytokines, which increased both TfR expression and transferrin cellular uptake in a mechanism that did not involve hyper proliferation. These findings were then exploited for the design of targetable carrier towards inflamed regions of the colon. Anti-TfR antibodies were conjugated to nano-liposomes. As expected, iron-starved Caco-2 cells internalized anti-TfR immunoliposomes better than controls. *Ex vivo* binding studies to inflamed mucosa showed that the anti-TfR immunoliposomes accumulated significantly better in the mucosa of DNBS-induced rats than the accumulation of non-specific immunoliposomes. It is concluded that targeting mucosal inflammation can be accomplished by nano-liposomes decorated with anti-TfR due to inflammation-dependent, apical, elevated expression of the receptor.

Editor: Guillaume Dalmasso, Emory Unviersity, United States of America

Funding: The study was supported in part by research grant number 01797 from the Chief Scientist Office of the Israeli Ministry of Health (AR). The funders had no role in study design, data collection and analysis, decision to publish, or preparation of the manuscript. No additional external funding was received for this study. BT and AR are affiliated with the David R. Bloom Center of Pharmacy. BT is affiliated with the Dr. Adolf and Klara Brettler Centre for Research in Molecular Pharmacology and Therapeutics at the Hebrew University.

Competing Interests: The authors have declared that no competing interests exist.

* E-mail: boazt@ekmd.huji.ac.il

Introduction

Ulcerative colitis and Crohn's disease, collectively termed inflammatory bowel disease (IBD), are the two main chronic relapsing inflammatory diseases of the intestines. While the former is confined to the large bowel, the latter involves the entire gut. The clinical presentation is largely dependent on the disease location and may include diarrhea, abdominal pain, fever, bowel obstruction and bloody stool. Typical complications associated with CD include strictures, abscesses, or fistulas [1,2]. The etiologies of both ulcerative colitis and Crohn's disease remain unclear and are presumed to result from inherited and environmental factors involving the immune system. Whether the immune system is activated intrinsically (constitutive activation or failure of down-regulatory mechanisms), or by a continuous, mucosal driven stimulation is still unknown [3,4].

Despite significant progress in IBD therapy, in particular after the introduction of biological drugs such as infliximab [5,6], patients often suffer disease relapse associated with impairments in their quality of life. This often necessitates a therapy with high doses of anti-inflammatory drugs (steroids or nonsteroidal anti-inflammatory drugs) [7,8], a regimen commonly accompanied by severe adverse effects. It was postulated by us and others that delivery of potent anti-inflammatory drugs in the closest proximity possible to the inflamed mucosal tissues would improve drug efficacy and reduce toxicity [9,10,11]. Still, a major drawback of such colonic delivery systems was their lack of specificity to the inflamed regions within the organ.

It has recently shown that drug enrichment in inflamed mucosa can be accomplished with negatively charged liposomes. Low and high molecular weight antioxidants that were delivered via anionic liposomes to the inflamed mucosa of experimental colitis-induced rats were more effective in attenuating the induced inflammation compared with aqueous solutions of the enzymes [12]. This was probably due to specific attachment of the negatively charged liposomes to the inflamed regions, which led to a prolonged residence time and a better uptake of the antioxidants into the inflamed epithelium. It was also observed that while positively charged liposomes exhibited enhanced adherence to both healthy and normal intestinal mucosa, negatively charged liposomes adhered preferentially to the inflamed (experimental colitis) epithelium of the rat colon [13]. A recent study, conducted in our laboratory, provided evidence that transferrin (Tf) at the luminal region of the inflamed colon, coupled with a typical low luminal pH may be related to the mechanism underlying this preferential adhesion [14]. This observation may also suggest a role for mucosal transferrin receptor (TfR) in IBD. It has already been reported that TfR levels are elevated in activated immune cells, lymphocytes and macrophages [15,16]. In this study we addressed the question whether TfR levels are subjected to similar regulation in epithelial cells of the colon.

TfR internalizes the serum glycoprotein Tf (80 kDa) by endocytosis [17]. Commonly, TfR is ubiquitously expressed at low levels [18]. Its expression is elevated, however, in rapidly dividing cells, including a variety of human cancers [19,20]. In addition to its role in iron metabolism it was suggested that TfR may play a role in cellular signaling and proliferation stimuli [21,22,23]. We have already shown that the luminal aspect of the inflamed colon epithelium of the rat was enriched with Tf [14], suggesting that the increase in both mucosal Tf levels and TfR expression is associated with the pathophysiology of IBD.

The objectives of the study were to: (***a***) measure the expression levels of TfR in normal mucosa and in IBD; (***b***) elucidate the relationship between typical IBD cytokines and mucosal TfR expression and function in IBD and (***c***) examine the possibility to preferentially target IBD mucosa with immuno-liposomes conjugated with anti-TfR.

Materials and Methods

Unless stated otherwise, all materials were purchased from Sigma (St. Louis, MO, USA). Solvents were of analytical grade or higher. Water was deionized and ultrafiltered by reverse osmosis (Barnstead Nanopure, Waltham, MA). For detection of human and rat TfR we used the monoclonal anti-TfR (H68.4, Abcam, Cambridge, MA). Goat anti-mouse IgG Alexa Fluor® 647 was purchased from Invitrogen (Carlsbad, CA, USA). For detection of human E-cadherin we used Mouse anti human E-cadherin BD Transduction Laboratories (NJ USA). Rabbit anti-GRP78 (BiP) antibody was obtained from Abcam (Cambridge, MA, USA). Horseradish peroxidase (HRP) - conjugated secondary antibodies were purchased from Jackson ImmunoResearch Laboratories (Suffolk, UK) and Santa Cruz Biotechnology (Santa Cruz, CA, USA). Hydrogenated soybean phosphatidylcholine (HSPC), phosphatidylglycerol (HSPG) and 1, 2-Dioleyl-sn-glycerol-3-phosphoethanolamine- N-carboxyfluorescein (PE-CF) were purchased from Avanti Polar Lipids (Alabaster, AL, USA). NHS-PEG-DSPE [3-(N-succinimidyloxyglutaryl) aminopropyl, polyethyleneglycol-carbamyl distearoylphosphatidyl-ethanolamine] was obtained from NOF Corporation (Tokyo, Japan). Elisa kit for rat TNFα was obtained from R&D Systems, Inc. (MN, USA) and the mouse Cytokine Screen ELISA from Quansys Biosciences (UT, USA).

Ethics statement

Inflamed and non-inflamed human colons were obtained as slides of paraffin embedded from the Department of Surgery, Hadassah - Hebrew University Medical Center, Mount Scopus. This part of the study was approved by the Independent Ethical Committee (IEC, Helsinki Committee)-Protocol # HMO-0512-08. Adult patients operated on for inflammatory bowel disease were offered participation in the trial. Eligible patients signed an IEC-approved consent form.

All animal studies were conducted in accord with the Principles of Laboratory Animal Care (NIH publication #85-23, revised1985) under protocol no. MD-10603-4. The joint ethics committee (IACUC) of the Hebrew University and Hadassah Medical Center approved the study protocol for animal welfare. The Hebrew University Animal Facility is an AAALAC international accredited institute (#1285).

Rats, maintenance and euthanasia

Male Sabra rats (200–225 g), obtained from Harlan Laboratories, Ein Kerem (Jerusalem, Israel) breeding farm, were kept under constant environmental conditions (22°C, 12 h light/dark cycles) and fed with standard laboratory chow and tap water. Anesthesia was performed by an intraperitoneal injection of a mixture of 100 mg/kg body weight of ketamine (Ketaset, 0.1 g/mL, Fort Dodge, IA, USA) and xylazine HCl (20 mg/mL). Euthanasia of anesthetized rats was carried out by chest wall puncturing.

Induction of experimental colitis in the rat and inflammation severity assessment

Twenty-four hours prior to colitis induction, the rats were deprived of food, but allowed free access to water. Experimental colitis was induced, under light anesthesia (isoflurane inhalation), by a rectal slow (20 seconds) instillation of 30 mg of dinitrobenzensulfonic acid (DNBS) dissolved in 1 mL of 50% v/v ethanol through a flexible, perforated foley catheter (0.3 mm outer diameter). Immediately after the hapten administration the catheter was removed and the rats were left in an inverted position for additional 40 seconds. Four days after colitis induction (maximal onset of inflammation as identified in preliminary studies) the rats were anesthetized as above, their abdomen was cut open and a 0.5 ml blood was withdrawn from the portal vein for hematological analysis (RBC, hematocrit and hemoglobin analyses). The colons were removed and rinsed with normal saline. Inflammation severity was scored (wet weight, dimensions, edema, hyperemia ulceration area and stool viscosity prior to the saline rinse) [12,24]. The control (healthy) group was treated similarly with a normal saline solution replacing the DNBS ethanolic solution. Homogenates of colon tissues obtained from of inflamed or non-inflamed regions one or four days after colitis induction were analyzed for TNFα by commercial ELISA kit (Eli-pair, Diaclone, France).

TfR immunofluorescence analysis in rat colon mucosal specimens and in human biopsies

Mucosal specimens from isolated rat colons (healthy or inflamed regions) were rinsed with a 4% w/v aqueous sucrose solution and fixated with 12% v/v formaldehyde in PBS. After a PBS rinse the fixated tissues were preserved in a 20% w/v sucrose solution until sectioning. Prior to sectioning the specimens were dehydrated (ethanol and PBS). Sectioning (10–12 μm) was performed by embedding in paraffin blocks and press-heating in 40 nM Tris/ 1 Mm EDTA buffer pH 9, at 125°C for 2.45 minutes, followed by 27 min at 90°C. Nonspecific staining was blocked by 2% BSA in PBS. Immunostaining of the fixed colonic specimens from the rat or human biopsies was performed by their incubation (overnight, 4°C) with diluted (1:500) mouse anti-human TfR followed by incubation (1 h, room temperature) with diluted (1:800) goat anti-mouse IgG- Alexa 647. Nuclei were stained with 0.1 mg/ml of Hoechst dye. Fluorescence was monitored by confocal microscopy (Carl Zeiss, Germany).

Western analysis of TfR expression in the colonic mucosa of the rat

Mucosal specimens from isolated rat colons from either DNBS-induced or saline-treated rats were scraped with glass slides, collected in a microcentrifuge test-tube containing a lysis buffer (RIPA), shaken vigorously (15 min, 4°C) and centrifuged (10 min, 14,000 rpm, 4°C). The clear supernatant was collected and its protein content was determination (Bradford). A volume equivalent to 15 µg of protein was boiled in reduced Laemmli sample buffer, analyzed by 12% SDS-PAGE and electrotransferred to a nitrocellulose membrane. Membranes were blocked with 5% non-fat milk in PBS containing 0.05% Tween 20 (PBST) for 1 hour at room temperature and stained with mouse anti human TfR. HRP-conjugated goat anti mouse was used as a secondary antibody. Rabbit anti BiP was used as loading control, followed by HRP-conjugated goat anti rabbit. Proteins were visualized by chemical luminescence (EZ-ECL, Biological Industries, Israel).

Preparation of cytokine rich medium (CRM)

Male C57BL/6 mice (20 g) or male Sabra rats (250 g) were sacrificed, their spleen was removed immediately into 10 ml of PBS (RT) pounded and sieved through a cell strainer. The sieved homogenate was centrifuged (5 min, 1,250 rpm) and red blood cells were removed by incubation in lysis buffer (20 ml, 5 min, RT). After centrifugation the supernatant was discarded and the cells-containing pellet was resuspended immediately in 10 ml of warm DMEM (no serum). 10×10^6 cells/ml were plated in the presence of 100 µg/µl of lipopolysaccharide (LPS) in a 96 wells plate. After incubation (24 h, 37°C, 5% CO_2) the content of each well was aspirated, centrifuged (4,000 rpm, 20 min, 4°C), the supernatants collected, and stored at −80°C until use for inflammation induction. The cytokine content of the CRM was characterized by multi cytokines elisa (QUANSYS) according to the manufacturer's protocol. CRM was positive for IL-1α, IL-1β, IL-3, IL-6, IL-10, Interferonγ, TNFα, MIP-1 α, RANTES and negative for IL-2, IL-4, IL-5, IL-12p70, IL-17, MCP-1, GM-CSF.

Preparation and characterization of negatively charged fluorescently-tagged PEGylated immunoliposomes

Seven different liposomal formulations were prepared by the ethanol injection method [14]. Lipid composition is specified in **Table 1**. The formulations differed from each other by the amount of antibodies (Ab) on their surface. All liposomes were tagged fluorescently with 0.5 mole% of 18:1, 1,2-dioleoyl-sn-glycero-3-phosphoethanolamine-*N*-(carboxyfluorescein). After dialysis against PBS, the liposomes were extruded stepwise with a final extrusion through 100 nm pore polycarbonate filter and kept in PBS at 4°C until use. The Ab was either mouse anti human TfR (anti-TfR) or goat anti-mouse IgG (Anti IgG, served as non-specific controls). The Ab was conjugated to the liposomes, immediately after their preparation, with the aid of 3-(N-succinimidyloxyglutaryl) aminopropyl, polyethyleneglycol-carbamyl distearoylphosphatidyl-ethanolamine (NHS-PEG-DSPE) spacers, which was added to the lipids before hydration preincorporated into the liposomal formulation, at a ratio of 5 Mol% (**Scheme S1**). The coupling reaction was terminated with 100 mM of TRIS buffer.

Since the functional group for attaching the antibody (NHS coupled to PEG-DSPE) is prone to hydrolysis prior to antibody conjugation, we evaluated two pH conditions acidic (pH = 5) and neutral (pH = 7.4) for liposome preparation. After liposome extrusion, the antibody was coupled at pH value same as for liposome fabrication (overnight, room temperature). Following quenching of non reacting NHS groups with TRIS, non-bound Ab was removed by ultracentrifugation (55,000 RPM, 2 h). Ultracentrifugation did not affect liposome size (data not shown). The pellet containing the immunoliposomes was resuspended in PBS and kept at 4°C until use. After resuspension of the liposomal pellet, an aliquot was removed and immediately boiled in reduced Laemmli sample buffer. An equivalent portion of the supernatant, which contains unconjugated Ab as well as non-precipitated immunoliposomes, was also boiled in reduced Laemmli sample buffer. Western blotting analysis for the presence of antibody heavy and light chains indicated similar efficiency of antibody coupling at either pH = 7.4 or pH = 5.0. We estimate the recovery of the immunoliposomes by precipitation at approximately 50%, as the antibody amount in the pellet (labeled as Pellet) or the supernatant (labeled as Sup) was similar (**figure 1A**).

To further evaluate the effect of pH on the conjugation reaction, we incorporated into the liposomes a carboxyfluorescein-tagged lipid and used Alexa 647-tagged Ab. This double staining with orthogonal fluorophores allowed a single step quantitation of the conjugated Ab and the liposomes. Increasing amounts (1, 10 or 100 µg) of Alexa 647-labeled antibodies were incubated with the carboxyfluorescein-tagged liposomes at pH = 7.4 or pH = 8.5. Unbound Ab was removed by ultracentrifugation and the fluorescence of either of the two fluorophores was determined in the pellet and the supernatant. The Alexa 647 concentration-dependent increase in the pellet's fluorescence at λ = 647 nm, at two pH values is shown in **Figure 1B**, indication on an Ab increase in the pellet. Again, we observed a yield of ~50% regardless the antibody

Table 1. Materials used for the various liposomal formulations.

Liposomal Formulation Name →	No Ab		Anti TfR 50		Anti TfR 5		Anti TfR 1		Anti IgG 100		Anti IgG 10		Anti IgG 1	
Composition	**Mol%**	**mM**	**Mol%**	**mM**	**Mol%**	**mM**	**Mol%**	**mM**	**Mol%**	**mM**	**Mol%**	**mM**	**Mol%**	**mM**
HSPC	64.5	12.9	64.5	12.9	64.5	12.9	64.5	12.9	64.5	12.9	64.5	12.9	64.5	12.9
HSPG	30	6	30	6	30	6	30	6	30	6	30	6	30	6
NHS- PEG-DSPE	5	1	5	1	5	1	5	1	5	1	5	1	5	1
FC-PE	0.5	0.1	0.5	0.1	0.5	0.1	0.5	0.1	0.5	0.1	0.5	0.1	0.5	0.1
Ab amount (µg) -theoretical	-		50 µg		5 µg		1 µg		100 µg		10 µg		1 µg	

Abbreviations:
CRM: cytokine rich medium.
HSPC: Hydrogenated soy phosphatidylcholine.
HSPG: Hydrogenated soy phosphoglycerol (HSPG).
NHS-PEG-DSPE: 3-(N-succinimidyloxyglutaryl) aminopropyl, polyethyleneglycol-carbamyl distearoylphosphatidyl-ethanolamine.
FC-PE: 18:1, 1,2-dioleoyl-sn-glycero-3-phosphoethanolamine-N-(carboxyfluorescein).

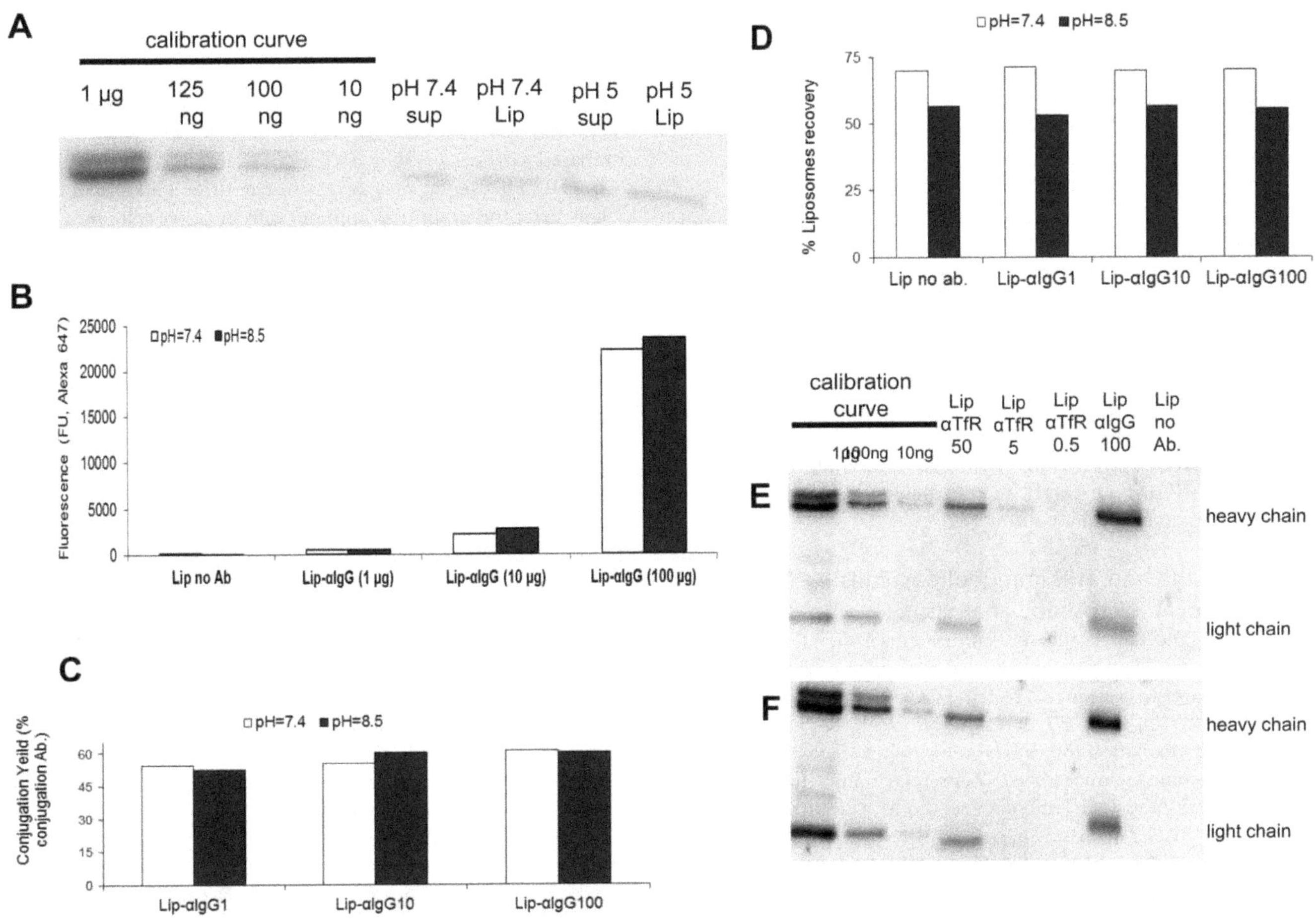

Figure 1. Optimization of anti-TfR conjugation to the liposomes. (A) Identifying the optimal pH (5 or 7.4) for the imunoliposomal preparation by Western blot analysis; (B) Fluorescence measurements of Alexa 647 (anti IgG) at different concentrations (1, 10,100 µg) conjugated to liposomes in pH = 7.4 or pH = 8.5; (C) Fluorescence assessments of the conjugation yield of the anti IgG antibodies to the liposomes at pH = 7.4 or pH = 8.5; (D) Recovery of liposomes after ultracentrifugation following antibody conjugation reaction at pH = 7.4 or pH = 8.5; (E, F) Western blot analysis for anti-TfR or anti-IgG conjugated antibodies (E, upper blot) and antibody content in the supernatant (F, lower blot) after ultracentrifugation (pH = 7.4).

amount or the pH conditions (**Figure 1C**). However, the efficiency of ultracentrifugation was better at pH 7.4 than 8.5 (70% and 55%, respectively) (**Figure 1D**). Therefore all liposomal preparations were conducted at pH = 7.4. Similar results were obtained for the mouse anti human TfR (**Figures 1E and 1F**). Based on the ultracentrifugation recovery values, the conjugation efficacy was estimated to be approximately 100%, as the amounts of Ab in both liposomal pellet and supernatant were similar to the amounts of the liposomes themselves in the corresponding fractions. This indicated that the vast majority of Ab molecules in the supernatants were conjugated to liposomes that failed to precipitate. Thus, the ultracentrifugation step was the main limitation in the preparation of the immunoliposomes.

Physical characterization of the immunoliposomes

Size distribution and zeta potential were analyzed after dilution (1:100) with sodium nitrite 0.15 M by Zetasizer (3000 HS, Nano-ZS, Malvern, UK). The size and zeta potential of the seven formulations (**Table 1**) were similar, with an average size of 105.6±7 nm and a zeta potential of −14.1±3.3 mV. Fluorescence level of the liposome was measured (Synergy HT, BioTek, VI, USA) at $\lambda ex = 485$ nm and $\lambda em = 528$ nm. Liposomes phospholipids content was measured by determining their phospholipid phosphorus concentration as described elsewhere [25].

Liposomal antibody load quantification by Western blot

Twenty µl of the immunoliposomes were boiled in a reduced Laemmli sample buffer and loaded onto 12% SDS-PAGE resolution gel. Following electrotransfer to a nitrocellulose membrane, Ab heavy and light chains were detected by HRP-conjugated antibodies. Their amounts were assessed with the aid of a 4-points calibration curve, prepared in a similar manner, using known amounts of purified Ab.

Cell proliferation and TfR levels analysis by flow cytometry

Low passage Caco-2 cells were purchased from the ATCC (Manassas, VA). Cell proliferation was measured by carboxyfluorescein diacetate succinilimide ester (CFSE, Invitrogen, Merelbeke, Belgium) dilution assay. In this assay, as the cell proliferates the entrapped CFSE is diluted. Hence, proliferation is indicated by low CFSE levels. Caco-2 cells, harvested by 2 mM of EDTA in PBS, were resuspended in PBS containing 1% BSA and incubated (7 min, 37°C) with 10 µm of CFSE, after which the cells were washed and resuspended in a culture medium. The cells were cultured for 24 h and the medium was replaced by a fresh one containing the following recombinant human cytokines TNFα, IL1β and IL-6 (Peprotech, Israel), separately, mixed together or CRM and incubated for additional 24 h. Because CRM contained

LPS, LPS was added to the incubation medium of the control studies involving Caco-2. TfR was stained with mouse anti-human TfR following by Alexa 647 labeled goat anti-mouse IgG. TfR expression and proliferation analysis was performed by flow cytometry (LSR II, Becton, Dickinson Biosciences, ON, Canada).

Tf uptake by iron-starved Caco-2 cells

Low passage Caco-2 cells were cultured in DMEM containing 10% fetal bovine serum (FBS), 100 IU/ml of penicillin, 1% L-glutamine, 1 mM sodium pyruvate and 1% non essential amino acids. Cells were plated on μ- slide 8 wells (Ibdi, Germany) at a concentration of 3×10^4 cells/well. After the addition of CRM the plates were incubated for 24 h at 37°C. Fifty μg of Alexa 594-labeled Tf (Tf-594, Invitrogen, CA, USA) was added and plates incubated for additional 24 h. The cells were then rinsed twice with PBS and Tf uptake was visualized by confocal microscopy (Zeiss, Germany). Iron starvation was accomplished by the addition of 10 μM Desferal® to the incubation medium. Non-starved cells served in the control studies.

Uptake of the anti TfR- immunoliposomes by Caco-2 cells- confocal microscopy analysis

Iron-starved Caco-2 cells were cultured on μ-slide 8 wells plates (Ibdi, Germany) and incubated in the presence or absence of proinflammatory cytokines (24 h, 37°C), followed by a 4 h incubation (37°C) with 20 or100 μl of anti-TfR- immunoliposomes. After incubation the cells were washed twice with PBS and imaged by confocal microscopy (Zeiss, Germany). Immunoliposomes carrying anti IgG antibodies served as a negative control.

Flow cytometry analyses for the uptake of Anti-TfR liposomes by Caco-2 cells

CaCo-2 cells, pretreated with CRM and desferal for 24 hours were incubation for 6 h with naked (no Ab.) liposomes, Lip-αIgG100, lip-αTfR50, all fluorescently labeled formulations were of equivalent florescence level. Flow cytometry analysis was performed on LSR II instrument (Becton-Dickinson).

Uptake of the anti TfR- immunoliposomes by colon mucosa

The colons specimens of either anesthetized DNBS-induced or healthy rats were removed and rinsed with normal saline and incubate (30 min, 37°C) with 2 mM of dithiothreitol to remove the mucous lining which covers the epithelium. Everted sacs (1 cm) were prepared and incubated (3 h, 37°C, while shaking) in 100 μl of the immunoliposomes, or liposomes without Ab (**Table 1**), suspended in 1 ml of PBS. The sacs were then washed twice with PBS and homogenized, on ice in 1 mL of acidic isopropanol. The homogenates were centrifuged (25,000 g, 30 min, 4°C), and the clear supernatant was collected. After the addition of a borate buffer (pH = 9), fluorescence was measured (excitation: 485 nm, emission:521 nm) and liposomes concentrations were calculated with the aid of a 5 points calibration curve which was made of increasing amounts of the liposomes in acidic isopropanol.

Results

TfR expression was elevated in human specimens from IBD patients and in the colonic epithelium of rats induced with experimental colitis

To examine the relationship between epithelial inflammation in the colon and TfR expression, we analyzed human colon biopsies from Crohn's disease patients. Specimens were taken from active inflamed areas and compared to histological normal colonic mucosa form patients with diseases other than IBD. Inflammation was verified histologically by standard H&E staining (**Figure 2A**). In 7 of 9 IBD patients elevated signal for TfR was obtained compared to normal tissues (a total of 12 samples) (**Figure 2B, 2C and 2D**). This signal may originate from the epithelial lining as well as from the infiltrated immune cells or other cell types in the specimen. Costaining with the specific epithelial marker E-cadherin demonstrated that the vast majority of the TfR signal emanates from the epithelial lining (**Figure 2E**), suggesting an increased expression of TfR in the epithelial cells under conditions of inflammation. Interestingly, while in the normal colonic mucosa TfR expression was observed at the basolateral surface, in the biopsies taken from active IBD patients TfR was clearly confined also to the apical aspect of the mucosa (**Figure 3**).

To further examine whether TfR expression is affected by inflammation conditions we established a DNBS-induced colitis in rats. TfR expression was also measured in the colonic epithelium of rats 4 days after experimental colitis induction (a period of time which was required for the mucosa to recover from the local damage caused by the ethanolic vehicle of the control group). Inflammation was verified by H&E staining (**Figure 4A**) and further characterized directly by measuring colon mucosa edema ulceration and change in colon weight and length, and indirectly by monitoring diarrhea, rat weight and hyperemia (Figure S1, A). An elevation in mucosal TfR expression accompanied the DNBS induced inflammation, compared with the sham treatment with highest levels in the ulcerated regions of the mucosa (**Figure 4B, 3C and 3D**). This observation was verified by a Western blot of total protein extraction from the inflamed and vehicle-treated rat mucosa. As seen in **Figure 4 (panels E and F)**, higher TfR levels were observed in the former.

The elevated mucosal TfR level in the inflamed colons was expected due to the inflammation-driven bleeding. This theoretically should lead to the dwindling of iron depots, which signal via RNA-binding iron regulatory proteins (IRP) signaling to increase TfR translation [26,27]. To account for this possibility blood samples of 3 vehicle-treated and 4 colitis-induced rats were collected, sera was separated and tested, hematologically, for anemia. Surprisingly, no difference between the two groups could be observed for both red blood cells count and hemoglobin and hematocrit levels (see **Figures S1 and S2**), suggesting a direct impairment involved in the mucosal TfR elevated expression.

Proinflammatory cytokines promotes TfR expression in Caco-2 cells

To better understand the involvement of induced inflammation on TfR expression, we decided to explore, at the cellular level, the role of proinflammatory mediators in TfR expression. The human colon carcinoma Caco-2 cell line is a widely used model for colon epithelium. Flow cytometry analysis of the Caco-2 cells incubated with CRM revealed elevated cell surface TfR levels (**Figure 5A, 5B**). It has been shown that the exposure of Caco-2 cells to TNFα (a proinflammatory cytokine, playing a major role in the pathogenesis of IBD) increased iron ions uptake from the incubation medium [28]. We therefore speculated that TNFα was responsible, at least in part, for the CRM-induced increase in TfR expression. Indeed incubation of the Caco-2 cells with recombinant TNFα resulted in a similar increase in TfR expression (**Figure 5C**). We conclude that proinflammatory cytokines promote the cell surface expression of TfR in colon epithelium.

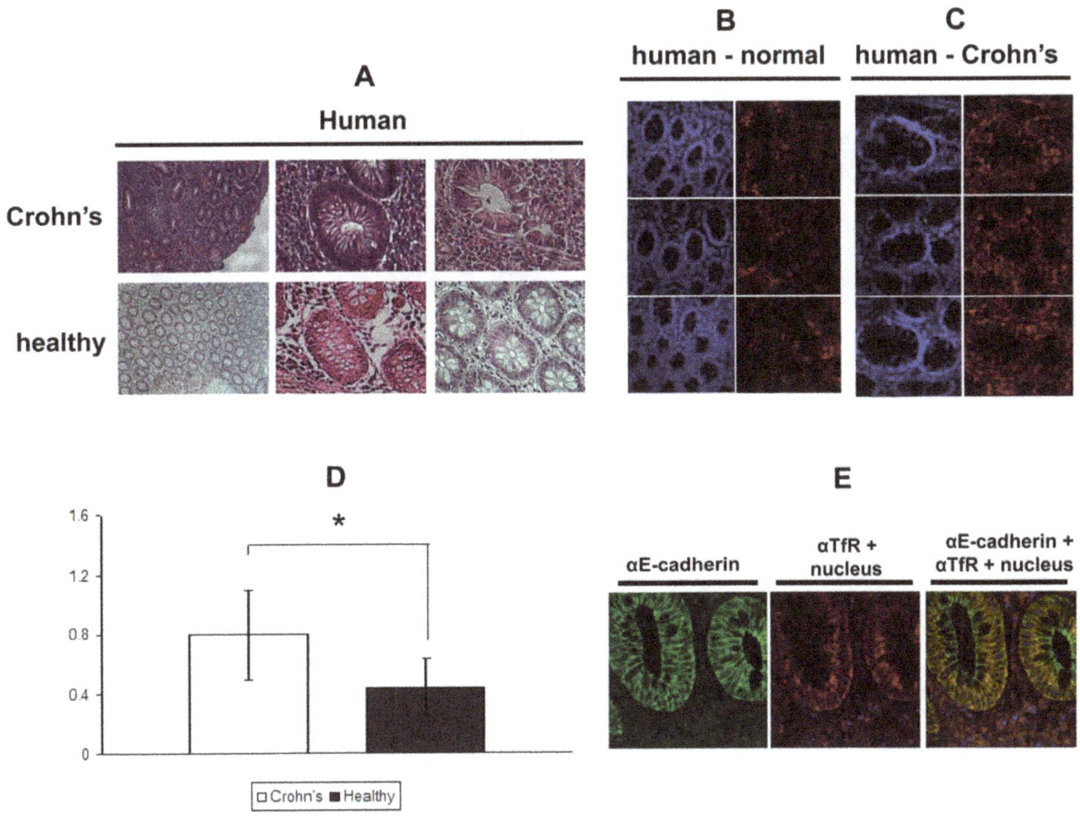

Figure 2. Enhanced expression of TfR in inflamed colonic epithelium in humans. (A) Typical hematoxylin and eosin staining of human biopsies taken from Crohn's disease patients and patients with non-inflamed colonic mucosa.TfR immunostaining of transverse sections from human biopsies taken from non-inflamed colonic mucosa (B) and from lesions of Crohn's disease patients (C). Left panels (of B and C): nucleus staining (blue). Right panels (of B and C): TfR staining (red). Magnification: ×25; (D) Quantification of the fluorescence intensity (Image Pro Plus) in the specimens taken from the Crohn's patients (N = 9) and non-inflamed ("normal") patients (N = 12) is shown on the left; (E) Anti-E-cadherin (left panel, green) staining of inflamed tissue, staining of TfR (red) and nuclei (blue) (middle panel), merge (right panel).

Higher levels of TfR are not necessary associated with Tf uptake enhancement. For that purpose we imaged by confocal microscopy the uptake of fluorescent Tf by Caco-2 cells. **Figure 6** shows an enhanced Tf uptake caused by the presence of the CRM cocktail, an effect which was even augmented when the cells were deprived of iron by the addition of 100 μM of Desferal to the incubation medium. Similar observation was obtained when the study was repeated with IEC-6 cells (resemble normal, intestinal

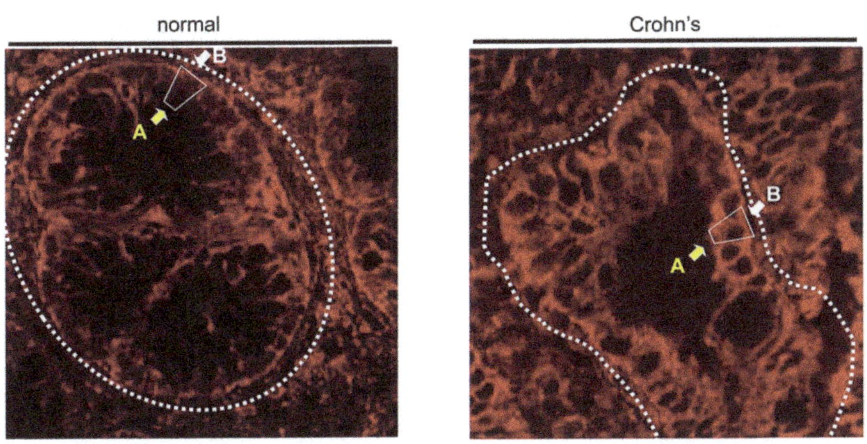

Figure 3. TfR is expressed at the apical aspect of the inflamed colonic epithelium in humans. Larger magnification (×63) of (Figure 2B) immunostained for TfR. Left: a transverse section from non-inflamed colonic mucosa. Right: a transverse section from a Crohn's disease patients, the basolateral membrane of the colon crypts is marked with white arrows, while the apical membrane is marked with yellow arrows.

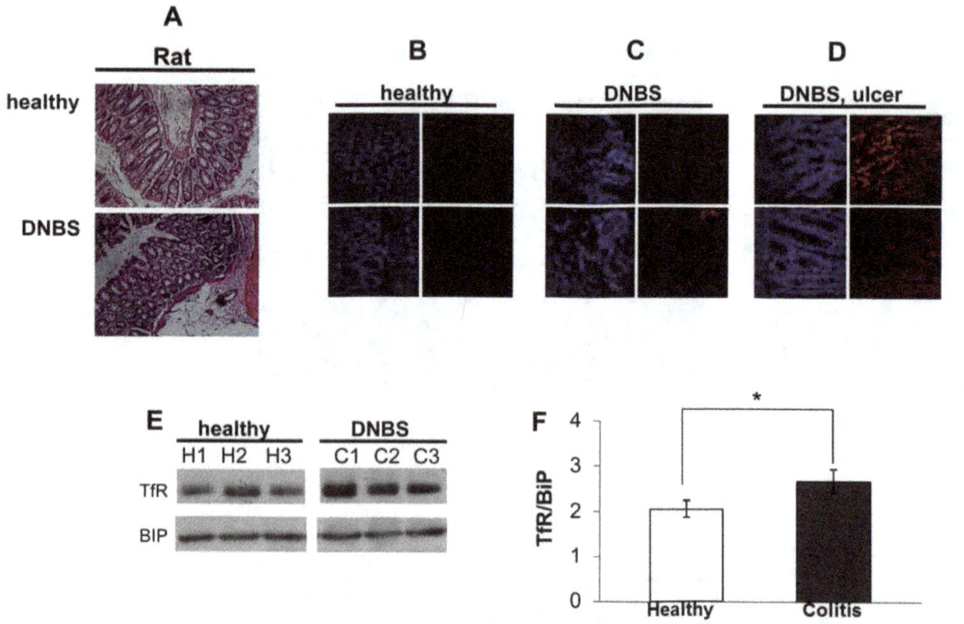

Figure 4. TfR expression is elevated in the mucosa of DNBS induced rats. (A) Hematoxylin and eosin staining of rat colon specimens taken from DNBS-induced rats 4 days after colitis induction and from healthy rat colonic mucosa.TfR immunostaining of transverse sections taken from the mucosa of vehicle treated (B), DNBS-induced (C) and ulcerated region in the DNBS-induced (D) rats. Left panels: nucleus staining (blue). Right panels: TfR staining (red). Magnification: ×25; (E) immunoblot analysis of protein extracts (40 μg per lane) taken from the colon mucosa of sham treated ("healthy") or inflamed mucosa from DNBS-induced rats. Anti-TfR (95 kDa) was used for staining. (F) Blots quantification was performed by densitometry and normalized to BiP (78 kDa). *P-value* <0.05 was obtained by Mann-Whitney test.

epithelium, data not shown). These observations support the assumption that iron uptake in the colon epithelium is affected by local inflammation due to the increase in cell surface TfR.

Hyper proliferation was not involved in the cell-surface TfR expression

In immune cells activation often triggers proliferation, which necessitates higher uptake of iron. Therefore, we tested whether cytokine-driven enhanced TfR expression was a consequence of hyper proliferation, rather than a direct effect on TfR synthesis. To address this, we monitored Caco-2 cell proliferation by the carboxyfluorescein succinimidyl ester (CFSE) dilution assay. A double staining of the cells in the presence or absence of human TNFα, IL1β, IL-6, mix thereof or CRM, revealed a reduction in the fraction of proliferating cells (**Figure 7**). Interestingly, TfR levels were higher in the non-proliferating cells (CFSE high), compared with the CFSE low population, indicating that the proinflammatory cytokines had a net effect on the elevation in cellular TfR expression, which was not related to their proliferation.

Cellular uptake of immunoliposomes is increased compared with naked liposomes with and without cytokine

Flow cytometry was also used for comparing the ability of the immunoliposomes to direct themselves to CaCo-2 and IEC-6 cells compared to the uptake of immunoliposomes bearing a nonspecific Ab and with that of naked (no Ab) negatively charged liposomes. Caco-2 cells were incubated with the various preparations at equivalent fluorescence level. **Figure 8** shows that anti-TfR immunoliposomes accumulated to a higher level in Caco-2 cells. Since the interaction between membrane TfR and anti-TfR (either free or conjugated to the liposomal vehicle) should induce endocytosis, it was expected that targeting the cellular TfR would facilitate not only liposomal adherence, but also provoke their

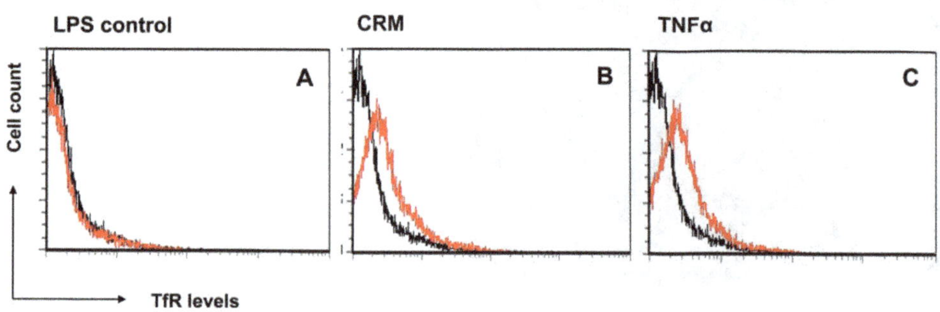

Figure 5. Proinflammatory cytokines increase TfR levels in Caco-2 cells. Flow cytometry analysis of Caco-2 cells following 48 h incubation with LPS (negative control, A), CRM (B), or TNFα (C).

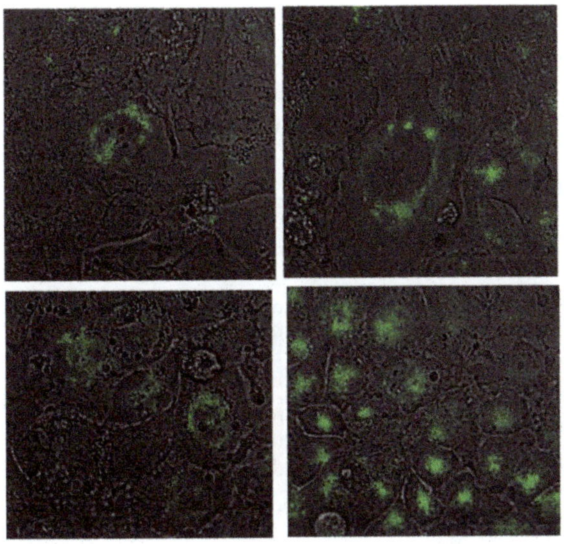

Figure 6. Proinflammatory cytokines promote Tf uptake by CaCo-2 cells. The effect of CRM (lower panel) and iron starvation (100 μM Desferal, right panel) on tagged (Alexa 594) Tf uptake by Caco-2 cells as imaged by confocal microscopy (×25).

intracellular uptake. To demonstrate this directly we incubated either fluorescently-labeled immunoliposomes or naked liposomes with Caco-2 or IEC-6 cells at equivalent fluorescence level. The incubation was conducted in the presence or absence of CRM. Liposome uptake was assessed by confocal microscopy. When uptake was compared, the anti-TfR liposomes entered the endocytic pathway to higher efficiency than of the naked liposomes (**Figure 9A and B, left and middle panels**). Increase of the amount of liposomes was resulted in increased uptake, indicating that the experiment was not performed under saturation conditions (**Figure 9A and B, right panel**). Anti-TfR liposomes were also found to be superior in their intracellular uptake when compared to liposomes equipped with non-specific antibody (**Figure 9C**).

Lastly, the targeting capability of the novel immunoliposomes was tested in everted gut-sac preparations, taken from inflamed colon of the DNBS induced rat and from vehicle treated control rats. For that purpose 5 formulations were prepared: two formulation of immunoliposomes bearing 5 or 50 μg anti-TfR antibody, two negative control formulations, bearing 10 or 100 μg non-specific antibody and naked liposomes (no antibody). We observed that the anti-TfR immunoliposomes formulation adhered significantly better (up to 4.5-fold) to the inflamed colon epithelium compared with the three non specific formulations (**Figure 10A**). This was in good agreement with the local TNFα concentration in the mucosa (**Figure 10B**).We conclude that immunoliposomes directed to the TfR may provide a means for apical targeting to inflamed colon mucosa.

Discussion

In recent years, major improvements were achieved in the management of IBD. The incorporation of immunosuppressive agents as well as anti-TNFα antibodies improved IBD outcomes and quality of life. However, toxicity and treatment failure resulting in surgery are still major issues in the management of IBD. Ferrying drugs directly to the colon ("colonic delivery systems") lacks the ability to target the inflamed mucosa and new approaches that will allow mucosal accumulation of antiinflammatory drugs after oral or rectal administration are sought after [9,29]. Employing a proteomic approach, in the search for suitable mucosal targets, we identified recently that Tf accumulates at the apical side of the inflamed gut mucosa [14]. This observation impelled us to investigate whether Tf plays a physiological or pathological role in regulating iron metabolism during colonic inflammation. An obvious notion was to explore a possible linkage between inflammation and local TfR expression. Moreover, because TfR levels are elevated along with the local accumulation of immune cells [16], we addressed the question whether similar TfR increase, with potential medical merit, is observed in epithelial cells, in addition to its systemic elevation.

TfR is encoded by two genes producing two types of the receptor - TfR1 and TfR2. The affinity of the former to Tf is 25-fold higher that the affinity of the latter. At the transcriptional level TfR1 expression is controlled by the intracellular level of iron. When the levels of iron drop, RNA- binding iron regulatory proteins (IRPs) become active and bind to an IRE element in the mRNA of TfR1. This IRP/IRE interaction stabilizes TfR1 mRNA and increases TfR1 production. Unlike TfR1, the expression of TfR2 is not expressed ubiquitously and is not influenced by intracellular iron levels [19,26,30]. The monoclonal antibodies used in the course of this study were those against TfR1.

In the present study, quantitative analysis of IF images of human specimens from the colon epithelium of Crohn's patients and normal specimens showed that TfR expression was higher at the membrane of colonocytes in IBD patients (**Figures 2 and 3**) and in colitis-induced rats (**Figure 4**). Extracting the mucosal proteins from the rat colons, followed by immunoblotting showed a lesser difference in TfR levels (1.4-fold, **Figure 5**). The observation that the relative expression of TfR in the mucosa of the inflamed colon of the rat was lower than that of human specimens compared with normal mucosa, suggests that the manner by which inflammation is induced involves membrane trafficking of TfR1, while the total intracellular pool of the receptor is less affected. Interestingly, a 4-fold enrichment of cell surface TfR levels was reported in malignant breast cells when compared to non-neoplastic breast cells [19]. Thus, under harsh inflammatory conditions TfR may serve as a therapeutic target similar to its use in cancer. Because TfR is upregulated in proliferating cells it is not surprising that both T and B lymphocytes express high levels of TfR in DSS-induced mice [31]. Nonetheless, the regulation of TfR1 expression in macrophages is more complicated. While exposure of macrophages to LPS and IFNγ causes down regulation of surface TfR1 [32], downstream signals, independent of IRP, enhance TfR transcription and promotes its expression [16,33]. Only a small number of studies addressed TfR expression in gut mucosal cells in IBD. In a series of studies, Pallone et al showed that HLA-DR, 4F2 antigen and TfR are upregulated in IBD. Sixteen of 24 mucosal specimens from colitis patients (compared with none of 7 normal biopsies) were stained positively to TfR [15,34,35,36,37]. However, because of technical limitations related to the year in which these studies were conducted, the quality of the images and lack of quantification precluded a clear conclusion to whether TfR expression is elevated on colonocytes themselves in colitis. Here, two decades later, with improved imaging technology, we clearly show that TfR is expressed on both the apical and the basolateral membranes of the colonocytes in a manner directly correlated with the severity of the disease (**Figure 2**). While in the non-inflamed controls TfR was confined to the basolateral membrane, in the biopsies taken from the colonic mucosa of Crohn's patients TfR was

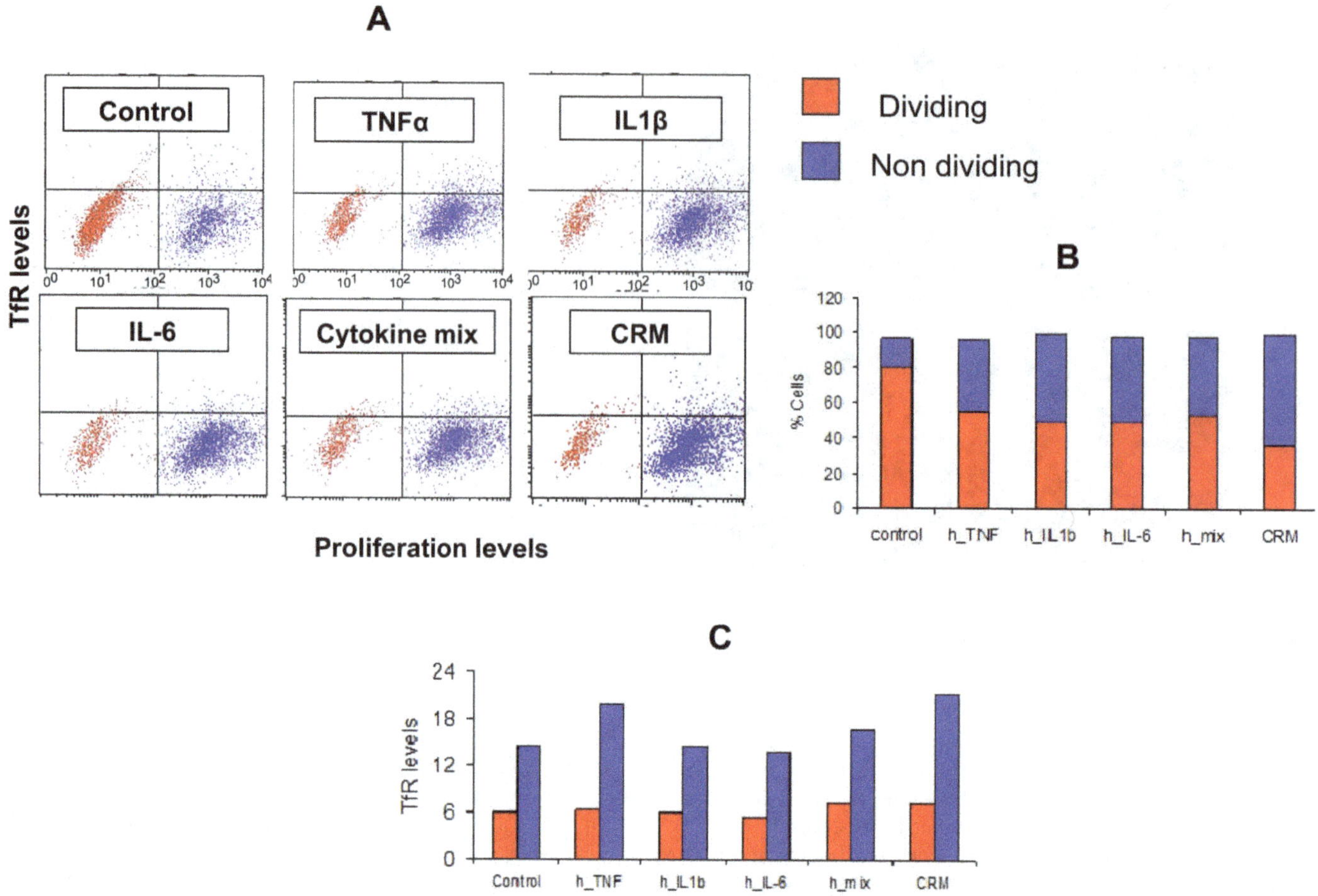

Figure 7. Increased TfR expression in CaCo-2 cells is not due to enhanced proliferation. Flow cytometry analysis of CaCo-2 cells double stained for CFSE dilution assay and TfR (mouse anti-human TfR stain), after incubation with the following inflammation mediators: TNFα, IL1β, IL-6, a mixture of the three, or CRM from mouse source. (A) Dot plot of stained TfR levels and the proliferation marker, CFSE. Dividing cells are marked in red, non-dividing cells are marked in blue; (B) Quantification of the dot plot shown in A; (C) TfR quantification in the dividing (red) and non-dividing (blue) cell populations.

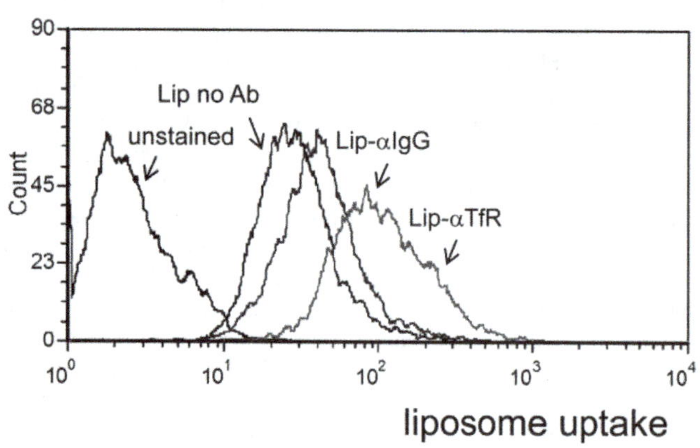

Figure 8. Anti-TfR antibodies maintain functionality when conjugated to the liposomes. Flow cytometry analysis of CaCo-2 cells pretreated with CRM and desferal for 24 hours following 6 h incubation with fluorescently-labeled negative liposomes.

enriched also at the apical surface (**Figure 3**). This is in contradiction to previous reports dealing with Madin-Darby canine kidney (MDCK) cells and Caco-2 cells, in which TfR expression was 40-fold higher in the basolateral than in the apical membranes. The sorting signal of TfR to the basolateral surface was ascribed to tyrosine motifs in its cytoplasmic tail [38,39,40]. A possible explanation to the findings in our models is the injury caused by the inflammation which may perturb the integrity of the tight junctions separating the basolateral from the apical membranes, allowing basolateral TfR to diffuse apically across the tight junctions. Indeed, proinflammatory mediators, such as IL-13, IFNγ and TNFα have been shown to disrupt and dysfunction tight junctions [41]. It remains to determine whether, in IBD, other typical basolateral proteins relocalize towards the apical side of the cells, indicating a general fault in cell polarity.

Another concern we had was that the increased level of TfR was perhaps secondary to the development of anemia and not due to direct effect on TfR regulation. Of the 9 specimens from Crohn's patients, at least four had overt clinical signs of anemia. Nevertheless, no signs of anemia were observed in colonic mucosa specimens from the colitis-induced rats, as indicated by various hematological parameters, despite clear elevation in TfR expression (**Figure S1 and S2**). To further explore the inflammation-mediated TfR regulation, we tested whether proinflammatory

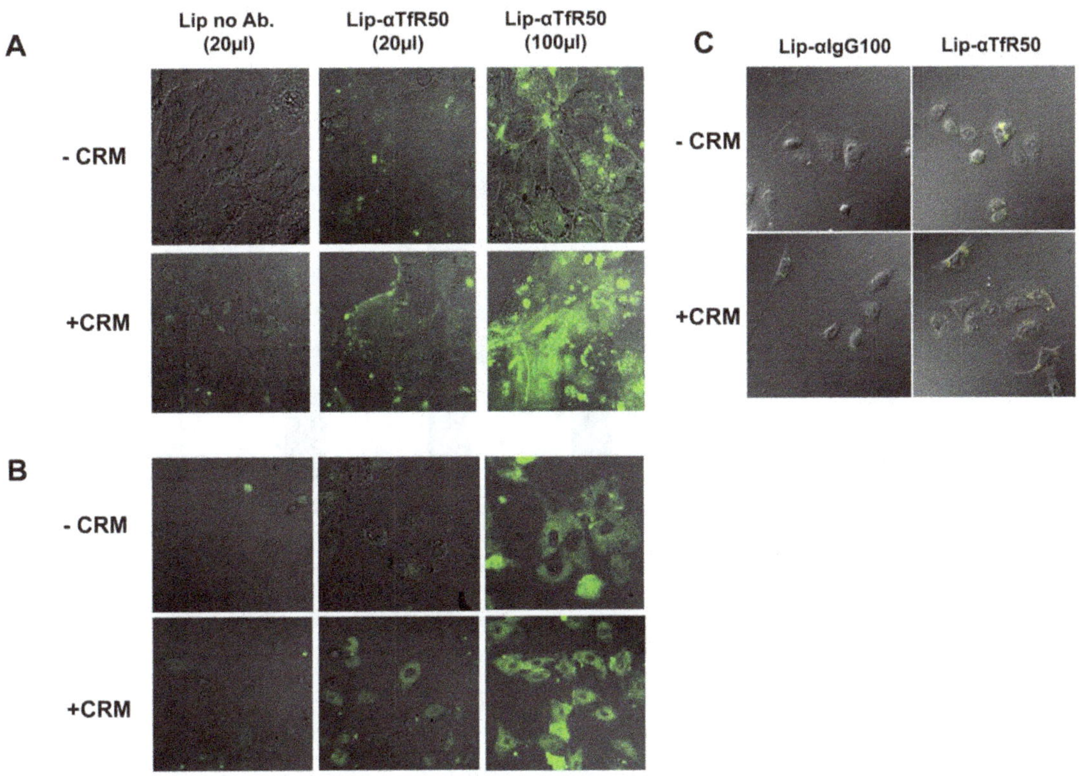

Figure 9. Cytokine treated CaCo-2 cells uptake better the immunoliposomes than naked liposomes. Representative images of confocal scan microscopy of fluorescently-tagged immunoliposomes conjugated to anti-TfR Ab (center and right panels) or naked (no Ab) negative liposomes (left panel) after 24 h of incubation with non stimulated (upper panels) or pre-incubated (lower panels) with CRM. Caco-2 cells are in panel A; IEC-6 cell are in panel B. Epifluorescence images following 10 h incubation of Lip-αIgG or Lip-αTfR in the presence or absence of CRM (C).

cytokines affect TfR levels *in vitro*. TNFα is most likely the most important proinflammatory cytokine in the pathogenesis of Crohn's disease as evident by the efficacy of anti-TNFα therapy in the clinics [1,10,42]. Furthermore, it has been reported that the exposure of Caco-2 cells to a mixture of TNFα, IL1β and IL-6 increased transferrin-iron uptake by 70%, inferring that proinflammatory cytokines are capable of modulating iron homeostasis in intestinal epithelial cells [28]. For this reason we analyzed TfR levels in Caco-2 cells subjected to cytokines treatment. We found that TNFα was capable of increasing TfR levels *in vitro* in a mechanism which does not involve hyper proliferation. In our hands IL-6 and IL-1β did not affect TfR (**Figures 5 and 7**). It would be interesting to test whether this effect of TNFα can be subverted by anti-inflammatory cytokines. Regardless, our data demonstrate a direct role of inflammation in the regulation of TfR expression level.

Does apical TfR play a functional role in retrieving iron? One third of IBD patients suffer from recurrent anemia due to iron deficiency [30,43]. Physiologically, TfR is not involved in iron absorption from the gut. However, because transferrin is accumulated at the apical side of colonocytes in IBD, the simultaneous enhancement in apical TfR levels could lead to reabsorbtion of the leaked transferrin. If true, apical TfR could serve as a targeting molecule in the design of specific drug delivery vehicles for the treatment of IBD, owing to its location at the inflamed sites and the possibility that it may trigger endocytosis upon ligation. TfR targeting has been extensively studied in the context of cancer therapy [26,27]. To this end TfR was targeted by virtue of its ligand Tf, as well as by specific monoclonal antibodies or single chain antibody fragments directed to its extracellular domain [27,44,45].

To explore the potential of TfR as a means to direct drug vehicles to the inflamed mucosa we prepared negatively charged liposomes and conjugated them with anti-TfR antibodies. Anti-TfR was favored over Tf due to three reasons: first, endogenous Tf which accumulate in the inflamed mucosa [14] may compete with Tf-bound liposomes for TfR binding. In contrast, anti- TfR does not bind to the Tf binding site and therefore less susceptible to direct competition. Secondly, the pH of inflamed tissue becomes acidic. At pH lower than 5, Tf acquires a positive charge which may form electrostatic interactions with the negatively charged liposomes. The antibody is most likely more resilient to changes in pH values. Lastly, at acidic pH, typical to the colon lumen in IBD, Tf forms a stable complex with TfR, which enable the release of iron and recycling Tf back to the cell surface [26]. The acidic ambience in the inflamed colon could potentially cause Tf to release the ferric ions and lose affinity to the receptor.

Although not directly addressed in this study, we decided to generate immunoliposomes as our model for drug delivery vehicle owing to their capability to entrap a variety of drugs for the topical treatment of IBD. In addition, if made at the right size, they could adhere to the cellular membranes and deliver the drug payload by endocytosis [46]. Since the immunoliposomes are aimed at targeting mucosal tissues, the mucus barrier should not be underestimated. To overcome this, PEG was used as a spacer for the conjugation of the anti-TfR [47]. It has been reported that PEG effectively minimizes adhesive interactions between mucin mesh fibers and particles' surface [48,49,50]. Preparation of the liposomes at acidic conditions, which should theoretically increase their stability, did not improve the conjugation yield (**Figure** 1).

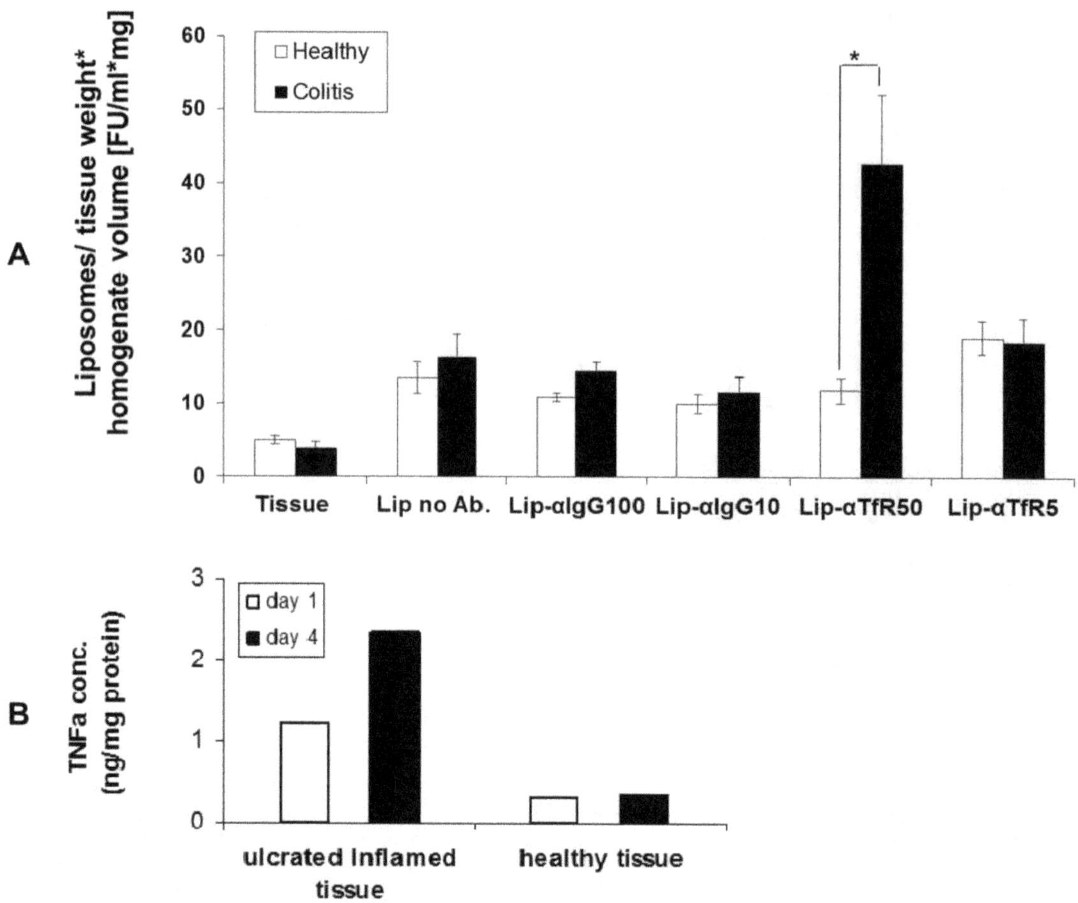

Figure 10. Anti-TfR immunoliposomes adhere preferentially to inflamed mucosa. (A) Ex vivo adherence of two formulation bearing anti-TfR antibody ("Lip-αTfR5 " and "lip-αTfR50" respectively), two negative control formulations, bearing non-specific antibody ("Lip-αIgG10" and "Lip-αIgG100" respectively) and naked liposomes (no antibody, "lip no Ab") to everted gut-sacs taken from DNBS-treated or vehicle treated rats. Shown are the averages of 3 independent experiments ± S.E.M. * *P-value*<0.05 was obtained by t- test. (B) TNFα levels analyzed by ELISA of inflamed and non-inflamed homogenate tissue obtained from experimental induced colitis one or four days after colitis induction.

Upon incubation with Caco-2 and IEC-6 cells, the immunoliposomes were internalized (**Figures 8 and 9**), indicating that the liposomes were recognized by membrane TfR. Moreover, anti-TfR facilitated the apical uptake to the rat inflamed mucosa by more than 4-fold compared to their uptake by healthy mucosa (**Figures 10**). TfR expression may rise globally due to development of anemia or locally in healthy mucosal areas adjacent to the inflamed regions, owing to leakage of proinflammatory cytokines from the site of active inflammation to neighboring cells. If occurs, it may allow preferential delivery of drugs to areas prone to exert inflammation as the disease progresses. Obviously, because of these reasons and because basal levels of TfR are expressed in the healthy duodenum and proximal small intestine [27], liposomes equipped with anti-TfR antibody are not suitable for drug delivery via the oral route as is. However, once delivered to the distal organs of the alimentary canal by either colonic delivery systems or by enema, their homing to the sites of injury will be facilitated. This assumption requires further verification. Inasmuch, we do not know at this point whether at an in vivo setting anti-TfR immunoliposomes will penetrate the enterocytes by transcytosis, as suggested by Widera et al [26], or remain confined to the apical site.

Overall, our findings delineate, for the first time that mucosal TfR is directly regulated by proinflammatory cytokines and that this regulation could be exploited for colon-specific delivery of drugs, for the local treatment of IBD.

Supporting Information

Scheme S1 Preparation of the αTfR immunoliposomes. The antibody solution was added to an aqueous dispersion of negatively charged liposomes, bearing NHS-PEG-DSPE handle and tagged with carboxyfluorescein (CF), right after their preparation. Conjugation was accomplished by an overnight agitation at room temperature, after which the reaction was stopped by the addition of a TRIS buffer.

Figure S1 Characterization of DNBS induced colitis. Scoring of the colon of saline treated or DNBS induced colitis. The induced rats showed high score (total score of 4) as measured by weight lost, diarrhea, colon weight, hyperemia, edema, ulcerated areas and shorten of the colon length.

Figure S2 DNBS induced colitis do not develop anemia. Blood count: blood count for healthy and inflamed rats: (a) white blood cells count. (b) Red blood cells count. (c) Hemoglobin (d) Hematocrit. (e) Mean corpuscular volume. (f) Mean Cell Hemoglobin.

(g) Platelets. The tests were performed in veterinary division of American medical Laboratories, AML, ISREAL, LTD. Healthy (N = 3), Inflammation (N = 4).

Acknowledgments

The skilful assistance of Ms. Irena Djavsarov is greatly acknowledged.

Author Contributions

Conceived and designed the experiments: BT AR. Performed the experiments: EH MNM BT. Analyzed the data: EH BT AN. Contributed reagents/materials/analysis tools: EH AR AN EK YB. Wrote the paper: BT EH AR. Performed the experiments: EH BT. Contributed reagents/materials/analysis tools: EH AR AN YB.

References

1. Baumgart DC, Sandborn WJ (2007) Inflammatory bowel disease: clinical aspects and established and evolving therapies. Lancet 369: 1641–1657.
2. Targan SR, Shanahan F, Karp LC (2005) Inflammatory Bowel Disease: From Bench to Bedside. New York: Springer. 903 p.
3. Carter MJ, Lobo AJ, Travis SPL (2004) Guidelines for the management of inflammatory bowel disease in adults. Gut 53: v1–v16.
4. Fiocchi C (1998) Inflammatory bowel disease: etiology and pathogenesis. Gastroenterology 115: 182–205.
5. Kurtovic J, Segal I (2004) Recent advances in biological therapy for inflammatory bowel disease. Trop Gastroenterol 25: 9–14.
6. Scholmerich J, Huber G (2003) Biological therapy in IBD. Anti-tumor necrosis factor-alpha and others. Dig Dis 21: 180–191.
7. Campieri M (2002) New steroids and new salicylates in inflammatory bowel disease: a critical appraisal. Gut 50 Suppl 3: III43–III46.
8. Hanauer SB (2008) Review article: evolving concepts in treatment and disease modification in ulcerative colitis. Aliment Pharmacol Ther 27 Suppl 1: 15–21.
9. Jubeh TT, Antler S, Haupt S, Barenholz Y, Rubinstein A (2005) Local prevention of oxidative stress in the intestinal epithelium of the rat by adhesive liposomes of superoxide dismutase and tempamine. Mol Pharm 2: 2–11.
10. Kesisoglou F, Zimmermann EM (2005) Novel drug delivery strategies for the treatment of inflammatory bowel disease. Expert Opin Drug Deliv 2: 451–463.
11. Steidler L, Hans W, Schotte L, Neirynck S, Obermeier F, et al. (2000) Treatment of murine colitis by Lactococcus lactis secreting interleukin-10. Science 289: 1352–1355.
12. Jubeh TT, Nadler-Milbauer M, Barenholz Y, Rubinstein A (2006) Local treatment of experimental colitis in the rat by negatively charged liposomes of catalase, TMN and SOD. J Drug Target 14: 155–163.
13. Jubeh TT, Barenholz Y, Rubinstein A (2004) Differential adhesion of normal and inflamed rat colonic mucosa by charged liposomes. Pharm Res 21: 447–453.
14. Tirosh B, Khatib N, Barenholz Y, Nissan A, Rubinstein A (2009) Transferrin as a luminal target for negatively charged liposomes in the inflamed colonic mucosa. Mol Pharm 6: 1083–1091.
15. Pallone F, Fais S, Squarcia O, Biancone L, Pozzilli P, et al. (1987) Activation of peripheral blood and intestinal lamina propria lymphocytes in Crohn's disease. In vivo state of activation and in vitro response to stimulation as defined by the expression of early activation antigens. Gut 28: 745–753.
16. Tacchini L, Gammella E, De Ponti C, Recalcati S, Cairo G (2008) Role of HIF-1 and NF-kappaB transcription factors in the modulation of transferrin receptor by inflammatory and anti-inflammatory signals. J Biol Chem 283: 20674–20686.
17. Huebers HA, Finch CA (1987) The physiology of transferrin and transferrin receptors. Physiol Rev 67: 520–582.
18. Kawabata H, Yang R, Hirama T, Vuong PT, Kawano S, et al. (1999) Molecular cloning of transferrin receptor 2. A new member of the transferrin receptor-like family. J Biol Chem 274: 20826–20832.
19. Daniels TR, Delgado T, Rodriguez JA, Helguera G, Penichet ML (2006) The transferrin receptor part I: Biology and targeting with cytotoxic antibodies for the treatment of cancer. Clin Immunol 121: 144–158.
20. Rodriguez JA, Helguera G, Daniels TR, Neacato II, Lopez-Valdes HE, et al. (2007) Binding specificity and internalization properties of an antibody-avidin fusion protein targeting the human transferrin receptor. J Contr Rel 124: 35–42.
21. Cano E, Pizarro A, Redondo JM, Sanchez-Madrid F, Bernabeu C, et al. (1990) Induction of T cell activation by monoclonal antibodies specific for the transferrin receptor. Eur J Immunol 20: 765–770.
22. Levy JE, Jin O, Fujiwara Y, Kuo F, Andrews NC (1999) Transferrin receptor is necessary for development of erythrocytes and the nervous system. Nat Genet 21: 396–399.
23. Manger B, Weiss A, Hardy KJ, Stobo JD (1986) A transferrin receptor antibody represents one signal for the induction of IL 2 production by a human T cell line. J Immunol 136: 532–538.
24. Wallace JL, Le T, Carter L, Appleyard CB, Beck PL (1995) Heptan-induced chronic colitis in the rat: alternatives to trinitrobenzene sulfonic acid. J Pharmacol Tox Meth 33: 237–239.
25. Barenholz Y, Amselem S (1993) Quality control assays in the development and clinical use of liposome-based formulations. In: Gregoriadis G, ed. Liposome Technology 2ed. Boca Raton: CRC. pp 527–616.
26. Widera A, Norouziyan F, Shen WC (2003) Mechanisms of TfR-mediated transcytosis and sorting in epithelial cells and applications toward drug delivery. Adv Drug Deliv Rev 55: 1439–1466.
27. Daniels TR, Delgado T, Helguera G, Penichet ML (2006) The transferrin receptor part II: targeted delivery of therapeutic agents into cancer cells. Clin Immunol 121: 159–176.
28. Han O, Failla ML, Smith JC (1997) Transferrin-iron and proinflammatory cytokines influence iron status and apical iron transport efficiency of Caco-2 intestinal cell line. J Nutr Biochem 8: 585–591.
29. Kohen R, Kakunda A, Rubinstein A (1992) The role of cationized catalase and cationized glucose oxidase in mucosal oxidative damage induced in the rat jejunum. J Biol Chem 267: 21349–21354.
30. Hentze MW, Muckenthaler MU, Galy B, Camaschella C (2010) Two to tango: regulation of mammalian iron metabolism. Cell 142: 24–38.
31. Kucharzik T, Lugering A, Yan Y, Driss A, Charrier L, et al. (2005) Activation of epithelial CD98 glycoprotein perpetuates colonic inflammation. Lab Invest 85: 932–941.
32. Kim S, Ponka P (2000) Effects of interferon-gamma and lipopolysaccharide on macrophage iron metabolism are mediated by nitric oxide-induced degradation of iron regulatory protein 2. J Biol Chem 275: 6220–6226.
33. Taetle R, Honeysett JM (1988) Gamma-interferon modulates human monocyte/macrophage transferrin receptor expression. Blood 71: 1590–1595.
34. Fais S, Delle Fratte F, Mancini F, Cioni V, Guadagno M, et al. (1991) Human cervical epithelial cells that express HLA-DR associated with viral infection and activated mononuclear cell infiltrate. J Clin Pathol 44: 290–292.
35. Fais S, Pallone F (1989) Ability of human colonic epithelium to express the 4F2 antigen, the common acute lymphoblastic leukemia antigen, and the transferrin receptor. Studies in inflammatory bowel disease and after in vitro exposure to different stimuli. Gastroenterology 97: 1435–1441.
36. Pallone F, Fais S, Capobianchi MR (1988) HLA-D region antigens on isolated human colonic epithelial cells: enhanced expression in inflammatory bowel disease and in vitro induction by different stimuli. Clin Exp Immunol 74: 75–79.
37. Fais S, Pallone F, Squarcia O, Biancone L, Ricci F, et al. (1987) HLA-DR antigens on colonic epithelial cells in inflammatory bowel disease: I. Relation to the state of activation of lamina propria lymphocytes and to the epithelial expression of other surface markers. Clin Exp Immunol 68: 605–612.
38. Shah D, Shen WC (1994) The establishment of polarity and enhanced transcytosis of transferrin receptors in enterocyte-like Caco-2 cells. J Drug Target 2: 93–99.
39. Gravotta D, Deora A, Perret E, Oyanadel C, Soza A, et al. (2007) AP1B sorts basolateral proteins in recycling and biosynthetic routes of MDCK cells. Proc Natl Acad Sci U S A 104: 1564–1569.
40. Odorizzi G, Trowbridge IS (1997) Structural requirements for basolateral sorting of the human transferrin receptor in the biosynthetic and endocytic pathways of Madin-Darby canine kidney cells. J Cell Biol 137: 1255–1264.
41. Forster C (2008) Tight junctions and the modulation of barrier function in disease. Histochem Cell Biol 130: 55–70.
42. Korzenik JR, Podolsky DK (2006) Evolving knowledge and therapy of inflammatory bowel disease. Nat Rev Drug Discov 5: 197–209.
43. Erichsen K, Ulvik RJ, Nysaeter G, Johansen J, Ostborg J, et al. (2005) Oral ferrous fumarate or intravenous iron sucrose for patients with inflammatory bowel disease. Scand J Gastroenterol 40: 1058–1065.
44. Krishna AD, Mandraju RK, Kishore G, Kondapi AK (2009) An efficient targeted drug delivery through apotransferrin loaded nanoparticles. PLoS One 4: e7240.
45. Barth BM, Sharma R, Altinoglu EI, Morgan TT, Shanmugavelandy SS, et al. (2010) Bioconjugation of calcium phosphosilicate composite nanoparticles for selective targeting of human breast and pancreatic cancers in vivo. ACS Nano 4: 1279–1287.
46. Faraji AH, Wipf P (2009) Nanoparticles in cellular drug delivery. Bioorg Med Chem 17: 2950–2962.
47. Ravi Shankaran R, Miura N (2007) Trends in interfacial design for surface plasmon resonance based immunoassays. J Phys D: Appl Phys 40: 7187–7200.
48. Lai SK, Wang YY, Hanes J (2009) Mucus-penetrating nanoparticles for drug and gene delivery to mucosal tissues. Adv Drug Deliv Rev 61: 158–171.
49. Cu Y, Saltzman WM (2009) Drug delivery: Stealth particles give mucus the slip. Nat Mater 8: 11–13.
50. Tang BC, Dawson M, Lai SK, Wang YY, Suk JS, et al. (2009) Biodegradable polymer nanoparticles that rapidly penetrate the human mucus barrier. Proc Natl Acad Sci U S A 106: 19268–19273.

15

The Complement Anaphylatoxin C3a Receptor (C3aR) Contributes to the Inflammatory Response in Dextran Sulfate Sodium (DSS)-Induced Colitis in Mice

Elisabeth Wende[1], Robert Laudeley[1], André Bleich[2], Eva Bleich[2], Rick A. Wetsel[3], Silke Glage[2], Andreas Klos[1]*

1 Institute for Medical Microbiology and Hospital Epidemiology, Hannover Medical School, Hannover, Germany, **2** Institute for Laboratory Animal Science, Hannover Medical School, Hannover, Germany, **3** Brown Foundation Institute of Molecular Medicine, University of Texas, Health Science Center, Houston, Texas, United States of America

Abstract

Inflammatory bowel diseases are a critical public health issue, and as treatment options remain limited, there is a need to unravel the underlying pathomechanisms in order to identify new therapeutic targets. Complement activation was found in patients suffering from inflammatory bowel disease, and the complement anaphylatoxin C5a and its receptor C5aR have been implicated in disease pathogenesis in animal models of bowel inflammation. To further characterize complement-related pathomechanisms in inflammatory bowel disease, we have investigated the role of the anaphylatoxin C3a receptor in acute dextran sulfate sodium-induced colitis in mice. For this, colitis was induced in C3a receptor-deficient BALB/c and C57BL/6 mice, and disease severity was evaluated by clinical and histological examination, and by measuring the mRNA expression or protein levels of inflammatory mediators in the tissue. C3a receptor deficiency was partially protective in BALB/c mice, which had significantly reduced weight loss, clinical and histological scores, colon shortening, and CXCL-1/KC mRNA, myeloperoxidase and interleukin-6 tissue levels compared to the corresponding wild type mice. In C57BL/6 mice the differences between wild type and C3a receptor-deficient animals were much smaller and reached no significance. Our data demonstrate that the contribution of C3a receptor to disease pathogenesis and severity of dextran sulfate sodium-induced colitis in mice depends on the genetic background. Further studies will be required to clarify whether targeting of C3a receptor, possibly in combination with C5a receptor, might be considered as a therapeutic strategy for inflammatory bowel disease.

Editor: Stefan Bereswill, Charité-University Medicine Berlin, Germany

Funding: This work was supported by the Deutsche Forschungsgemeinschaft through a Collaborative Research Centre Grant (SFB566/A04 "Cytokine Receptors and Cytokine-Dependent Signalling"), and by a scholarship of the Hannover Biomedical Research School and the Helmholtz International Research School for Infection Biology. The funders had no role in study design, data collection and analysis, decision to publish, or preparation of the manuscript.

* E-mail: klos.andreas@mh-hannover.de

Introduction

Inflammatory bowel diseases (IBD), which in humans comprise Crohn's disease and ulcerative colitis, are chronic recurring inflammatory disorders of the gastrointestinal tract. As they impose a serious burden of suffering on affected individuals and frequently lead to inability to work, IBD are a critical public health issue. The incidence of IBD is increasing, but treatment options remain limited. Much effort has been made to identify the pathomechanisms underlying IBD, and it is believed that inflammation is caused by dysregulated mucosal immune responses to luminal antigens, triggered in susceptible individuals by as yet unidentified environmental factors. Histopathologically, IBD is characterized by mucosal inflammation with crypt distortion and abscesses, ulceration, edema, and recruitment of neutrophils and lymphocytes. The infiltrating immune cells release chemokines and cytokines, which amplify the inflammatory reaction and play a key role in IBD pathogenesis. This issue has been addressed by the development of tumor necrosis factor (TNF)-α-blocking antibodies, which are used in IBD that does not respond to conventional treatment. However, anti-TNF-α therapy is not beneficial for all patients, and may cause immunological side effects [1]. Efforts to block other cytokines have yielded some promising results but their efficacy remains to be validated (reviewed in [2]). To improve the overall treatment options for IBD, the identification of novel therapeutic targets is needed, and in this context, pro-inflammatory components of the complement system might be considered.

Complement is an integral part of the immune system and is activated by contact with foreign surface structures like lipopolysaccharide, mannose, necrotic cells, or by immune complexes. Upon complement activation, a proteolytic cascade is initiated and results in the release of components that contribute to host defense and inflammation. These include the anaphylatoxic peptides C3a and C5a, which mediate pro-inflammatory and immunemodulatory signals via their corresponding seven-transmembrane domain receptors, C3a receptor (C3aR) and C5a receptor (C5aR). The anaphylatoxin receptors are found on myeloid cells like granulo-

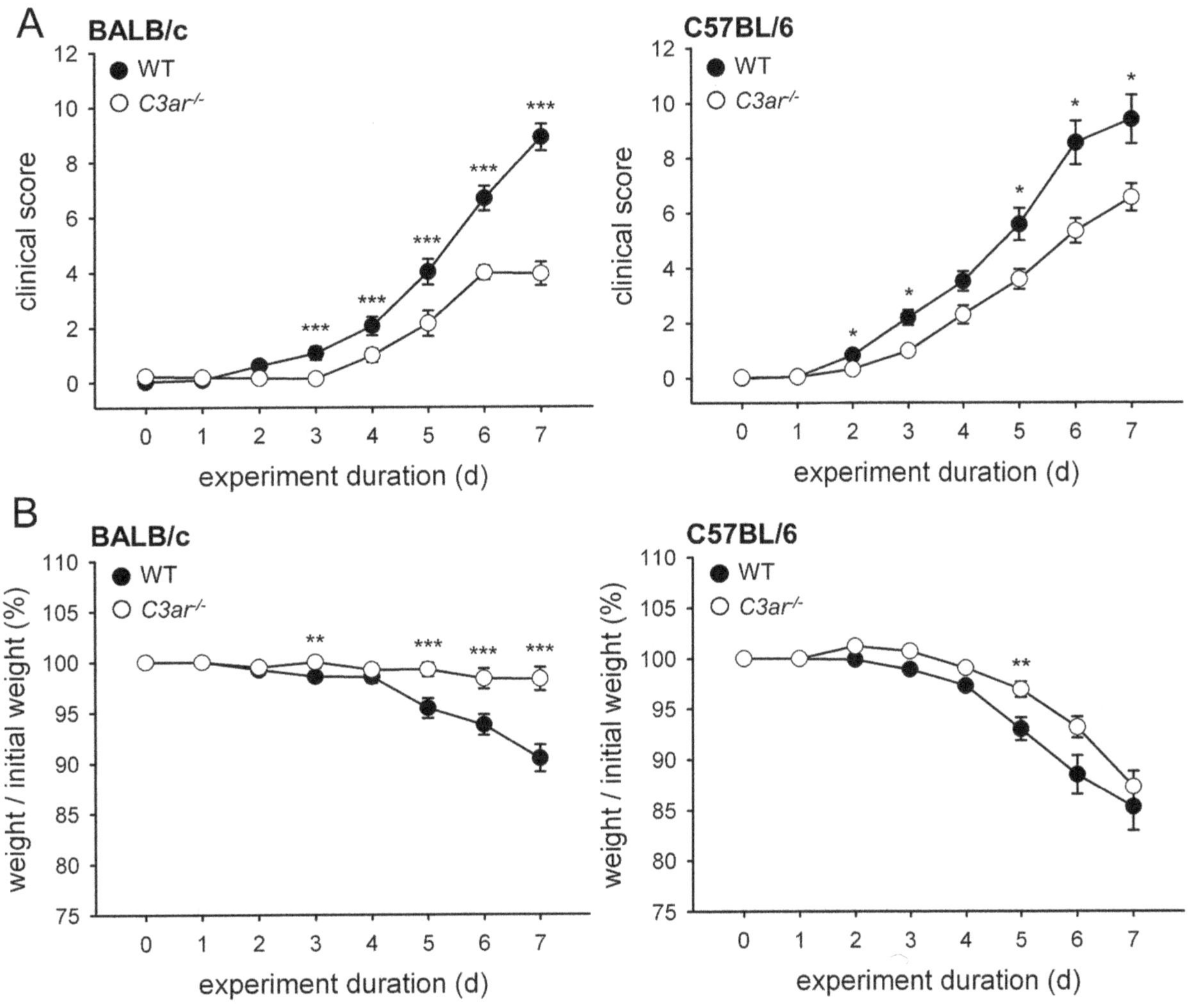

Figure 1. Clinical course of DSS-induced colitis in *$C3ar^{-/-}$* *vs.* WT BALB/c and B6 mice. Mice were given 3% DSS with the drinking water from day 0–7. Clinical score and weight were determined daily, starting on day −1. Control animals fed with water did not have any clinical signs or weight loss (data not shown). **A**, Time course of clinical score and **B**, Time course of body weight. To minimize suffering, three out of 25 B6 WT animals had to be sacrificed on day 6, leading to a seemingly smaller increase of the clinical score, and to a seemingly smaller weight loss, from day 6 to day 7, as compared to the preceding days. The data shown are means ± SEM of two independent trials with a total of n = 33 WT mice and n = 32 *$C3ar^{-/-}$* mice for BALB/c, and of four independent trials with a total of n = 25 (day 0–6) or n = 22 (day 7) WT mice and n = 21 *$C3ar^{-/-}$* mice for C57BL/6. *, $p<0.05$; **, $p<0.01$; ***, $p<0.001$.

cytes, mast cells, dendritic cells, monocytes and macrophages, and on non-myeloid cells such as neurons. In inflammation, they induce cytokine production, degranulation and chemotaxis of leukocytes, and vascular permeability (reviewed in [3;4]).

Although the primary functions of the anaphylatoxins are in host defense, their excessive or sustained generation causes tissue damage and adversely affects the course of inflammatory conditions. C3aR is a well-established player in airway hyperresponsiveness, where it aggravates inflammation by promoting a T helper cell (Th)2-polarized response [5;6]. Moreover, C3aR has been found harmful in *P. aeruginosa* pneumonia, whereas its functions in sepsis may vary depending on the tissue. C5aR has been shown to play deleterious roles in sepsis, airway hyperresponsiveness, rheumatoid arthritis, neurodegenerative diseases, and ischemia-reperfusion injury (reviewed in [3]). Animal experiments and observations in patients provide evidence for complement activation in IBD, and for its participation in pathogenesis with mainly adverse effects [7–10]. Mice deficient in the complement regulatory protein decay-accelerating factor, which protects host cells against assembly of C3 convertases early in the complement cascade, exhibit aggravated dextran sulfate sodium (DSS)-induced colitis [11]. This indicates that downstream complement effectors are involved in bowel inflammation. To this effect, our group has previously investigated the role of C5a/C5aR in a mouse model of IBD, dextran sulfate sodium (DSS)-induced colitis, and found that targeted deletion of C5aR is protective in acute but disadvantageous in chronic colitis [12]. Others have found C5aR antagonists or C5a antibodies to ameliorate trinitrobenzenesulfonic acid (TNBS)-induced colitis in rats or mice [13–15].

Here, we focused on the role of C3aR in IBD, and gave special attention to the influence of the genetic background, by examining C3aR-deficient BALB/c as well as C57BL/6 mice in DSS-induced colitis. We found that C3aR deficiency was partially protective in BALB/c mice but not significantly protective in C57BL/6 mice, showing that the effect of C3aR on bowel inflammation depends on the genetic background.

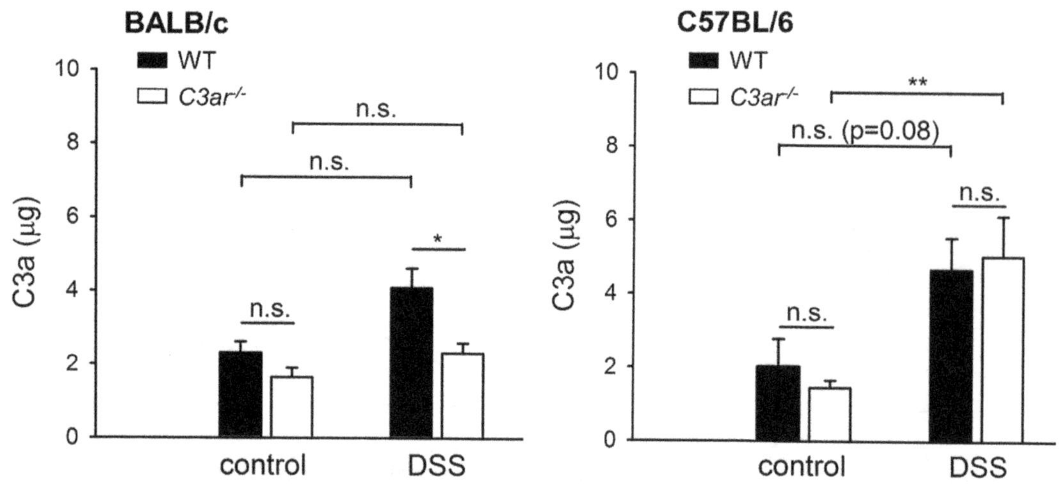

Figure 2. Plasma C3a/C3a-desArg levels in *C3ar$^{-/-}$* vs. WT BALB/c and B6 mice in DSS colitis. C3a/C3a-desArg was measured by enzyme-linked immunosorbent assay (ELISA) in EDTA plasma samples withdrawn by cardiac puncture. Of note, the calculated and depicted values are most likely too high because purified murine C3a had to be used as standard (see Materials and Methods). The data shown are means ± SEM from n = 4 (WT, H_2O), n = 21 (WT, DSS), n = 4 (*C3ar$^{-/-}$*, H_2O), and n = 21 (*C3ar$^{-/-}$*, DSS) mice for BALB/c, and n = 4 (WT, H_2O), n = 11 (WT, DSS), n = 4 (*C3ar$^{-/-}$*, H_2O) and n = 12 (*C3ar$^{-/-}$*, DSS) mice for C57BL/6. n.s., not significant; *, $p<0.05$.

Materials and Methods

Animals and Housing

Wild type BALB/c (BALB/c WT) and C57BL/6 (B6 WT) mice were obtained from Janvier SAS (Le Genest-Saint-Isle, France) and Charles River Laboratories (Wilmington, MA, USA), respectively. Breeding pairs of C3aR-deficient mice (C.129S4-C3ar1^{tm1}Cge/J; BALB/c *C3ar$^{-/-}$*) were purchased from The Jackson Laboratory (Bar Harbor, ME, USA). Breeding pairs of C3aR-deficient C57BL/6 mice (B6.129X1-C3ar1^{tm1}Raw, B6 *C3ar$^{-/-}$*) were provided by Prof. Dr. R. A. Wetsel (Institute of Molecular Medicine, The University of Texas, Houston, TX, USA). Mice were housed and bred under specific pathogen-free conditions. Routine microbiological monitoring was carried out according to FELASA recommendations [16]. This study was conducted in accordance with the German Animal Protection Law and with the European Communities Council Directive 86/609/EEC for the protection of animals used for experimental purposes. All experiments were approved by the Local Institutional Animal Care and Research Advisory Committee and permitted by the local authority (Lower Saxony State Office for Consumer Protection, Food Safety, and Animal Welfare Service, AZ/permit number: 33.9-42502-04-09/1705).

DSS-induced Colitis

Male mice aged 8–10 weeks were used. Starting four weeks before colitis induction, litter was exchanged weekly between all involved cages to distribute the specific pathogens present in the facility to all mouse strains and to avoid acute infections as confounding variables during the experiment. Group sizes for each independent experiment were between 4–10 per mouse line, limited by the number of offspring available at any one time. In parallel to B6 *C3ar$^{-/-}$* other C57BL/6 lines without relevance to this manuscript were tested, and B6 WT mice were always included as controls. For this reason, the overall number of mice tested was larger for B6 WT than for the other mouse lines. To induce intestinal inflammation, mice were fed 3% DSS, M_W 36–50 kDa (MP Biomedicals, Illkirch, France) *ad libitum* with the drinking water from day 0 through day 7. Body weight and clinical signs of disease were recorded beginning on day -1. To account for inaccuracies in weight determination, a mean initial weight was calculated from the first three measurements on days -1, 0, and 1, during which the values were stable, and the body weight for days 2–7 was determined relative to the mean initial weight (in %) for each individual. The following criteria contributed to the clinical score (score points in brackets): coat (0–3); posture (0–3), spontaneous behavior (0–3), induced behavior (0–3), feces (0–2), hygiene of the perianal region (0–2), overall health appearance (0–3). According to the research permit, a DSS concentration was chosen that should not lead to clinical scores ≥15. If on rare occasions individual mice scored ≥15, they were euthanized before the end of the experiment to minimize suffering. On day 7, mice were sacrificed, blood was withdrawn by cardiac puncture, colon length was determined, and mesenteric lymph nodes (mLN), cecum, and colon tissue samples were collected for further analysis.

Determination of Colon Length

Mean colon length differed between C57BL/6 and BALB/c ($p<0.001$ for all groups with t-test): 10.6 cm or 0.46 cm/kg body weight for BALB/c WT, 8.0 cm or 0.34 cm/kg body weight for B6 WT mice. To make the degree of DSS-induced colon shortening directly comparable between the two strains, colon length was expressed as a percentage. For this, colon length, measured from the distal end of the caecum to the anus, was put in relation to the initial weight for each mouse, to account for length variations that might be due to individual body size. To compare DSS-treated WT and *C3ar$^{-/-}$* groups, the mean colon length from the respective H2O-treated control groups was set to 100%. For each of the DSS-treated mice, the colon length was then calculated as percentage of the control group mean, and the means and SD were determined of those percentage values.

Histology

The cecum and colon were fixed in 4% formaldehyde, embedded in paraffin, cut into 4–6 µm sections, and stained with hematoxylin and eosin. Histological scoring was done in a blinded fashion and followed a scheme adapted from Cooper *et al.* [17]

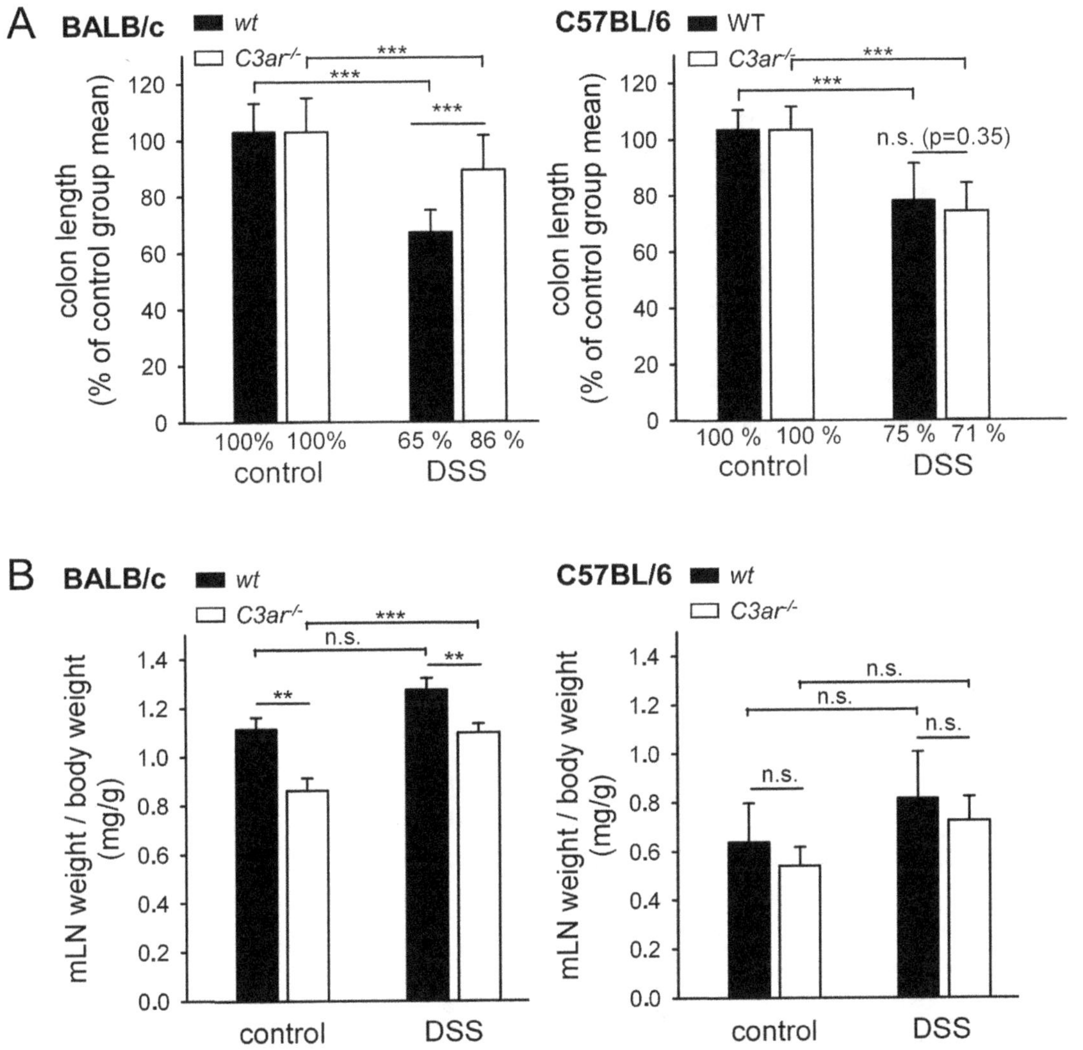

Figure 3. Macroscopic findings in *C3ar$^{-/-}$ vs.* WT BALB/c and B6 mice in DSS colitis. To account for individual variations in body size, colon length and mLN weight were calculated relative to the body weight for each mouse. **A**, Colon shortening. To compare DSS-treated WT and *C3ar$^{-/-}$* mice, the mean colon length from the H_2O-treated control groups was set to 100%, and used as a relative measure. **B**, Mesenteric lymph node (mLN) weight. The data shown are means ± SD (colon shortening) or ± SEM (mLN weight) of two independent trials with a total of n = 16 (WT, H_2O), n = 33 (WT, DSS), n = 16 (*C3ar$^{-/-}$*, H_2O), and n = 32 (*C3ar$^{-/-}$*, DSS) mice for BALB/c, and of four independent trials with a total of n = 15 (WT, H_2O), n = 25 (WT, DSS, day 0–6) or n = 22 (WT, DSS, day 7), n = 12 (*C3ar$^{-/-}$*, H_2O), and n = 21 (*C3ar$^{-/-}$*, DSS) mice for C57BL/6. n.s., not significant; ***, $p<0.001$.

and Bleich *et al.* [18], including the following criteria: epithelial changes (crypts unchanged: 0, loss of basal ⅓: 1, basal ⅔: 2, complete: 3, loss of crypts plus ulceration: 4), cellular infiltration (none: 0, infiltrates in lamina propria: 1, in lamina propria plus edema formation: 2, in lamina propria and submucosa: 3), area involved (none: 0, 10–30%: 1, 40–60%: 2, >60%: 3; applied to each of the parameters). This scheme yielded scores from 0–13 for each segment (cecum; proximal, medial, and distal colon), i.e. 0–39 for total colon and 0–52 for colon plus cecum. Images of histological sections were taken on an Axioskop 40 microscope (Carl Zeiss AG, Oberkochen, Germany).

Quantitative Real Time PCR

For RNA extraction, the RNAII kit (Macherey Nagel, Duren, Germany) was used. Colon tissue samples were preserved in RNAlater™ (Qiagen, Hilden, Germany) and homogenized with ¼" ceramic spheres in Fastprep® tubes (MP Biomedicals, Illkirch, France) in the supplied buffer on a Ribolyzer instrument (Hybaid, Middlesex, UK). For reverse transcription with Superscript™ II (Invitrogen, Darmstadt, Germany), 5 µg of total RNA and 250 ng random hexamer oligonucleotides (Roche, Mannheim, Germany) were used. Gene expression was analysed with the qPCR Core kit for SYBR®-Green (Eurogentec, Köln, Germany) using the following primers: forward 5′-CTGGTGAAAAG-GACCTCTCG-3′, reverse 5′-GTCAAGGGCATATCCAA-CAAC-3′ for Hprt-1 (*Hprt1*, NM013556.1); forward 5′-GCACC-CAAACCGAAGTCATA-3′, reverse 5′-TGGGGACACCTTT-TAGCATC-3′ for CXCL-1/KC (*Cxcl1*, NM008176); forward 5′-GGGTATGTCTCTCTGTGTAG-3′, reverse 5′-GGAGAA-GATTAGGGGAGAAC-3′ for CCL-8 (*Ccl8*, NM021443.1); forward 5′-CAAATCCCTCAAAGACCTCAA-3′, reverse 5′-CTTTTGCTTTTTCTTTTGGCTG-3′ for CXCL-9 (*Cxcl9*, NM008599.2); and forward 5′-GAGATGCTCACTTTGAC-GATG-30, reverse 5′-CCTTGGCTGAGTGGTAGAG-3′ for matrix metalloproteinase 3 (*Mmp3*, NM010809.1). A serial dilution of pooled cDNA was used as a standard, and expression of all

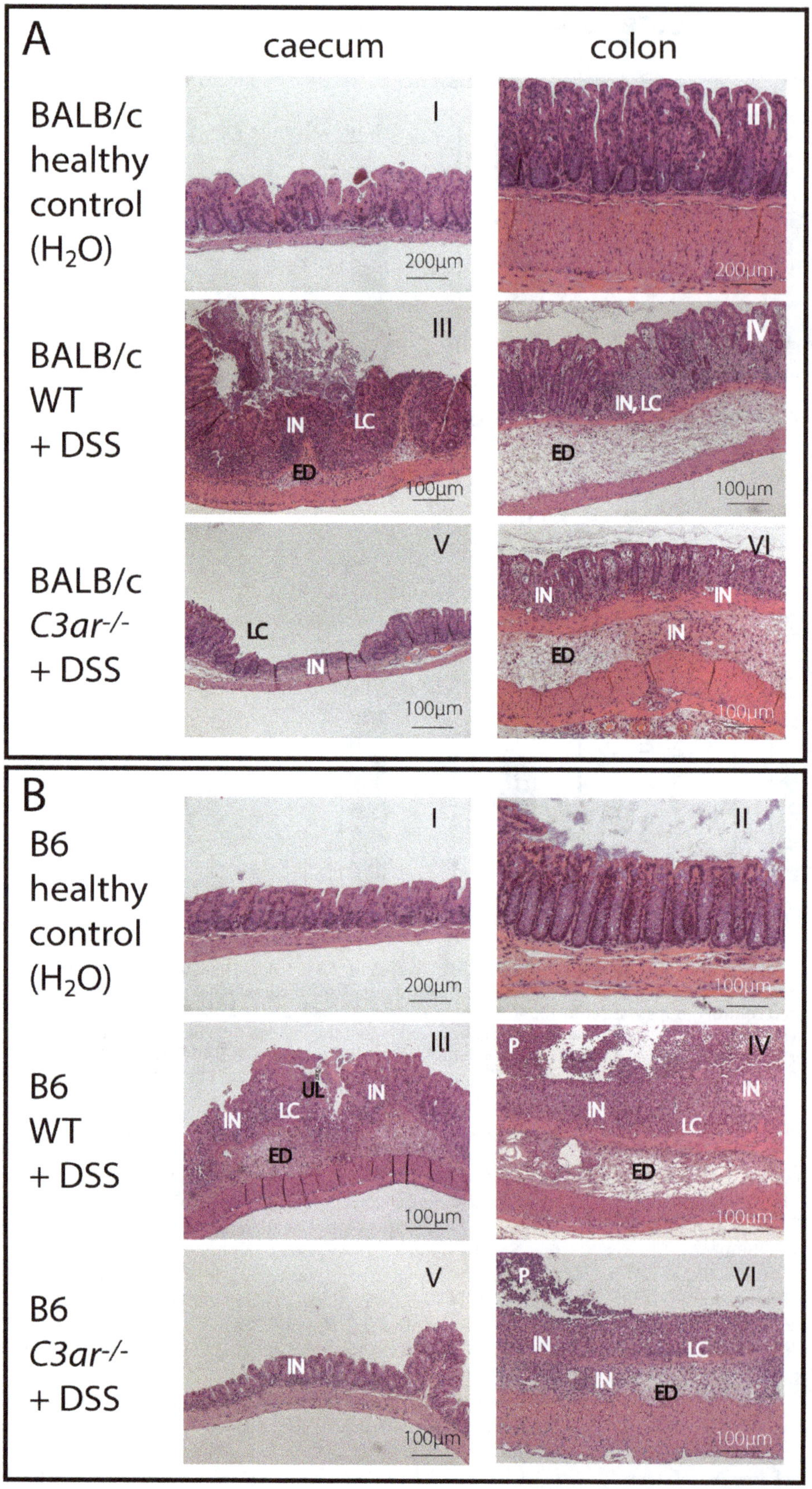

Figure 4. Histological evaluation of *C3ar$^{-/-}$ vs.* WT BALB/c and B6 mice in DSS colitis (first part). A (BALB/c) and **B** (C57BL/6), Representative sections of the cecum and colon stained with hematoxylin and eosin. Enlargement of the keratinized epithelium was found exclusively and epithelial hyperplasia was more frequent in BALB/c WT mice. ED = edema, HY = epithelial hyperplasia, IN = inflammatory cell infiltrate,

KE = enlargement of keratinized epithelium, LC = loss of crypts, P = pus, UL = ulceration. See also Fig. **5 C** for histological score based on the severity and extent of inflammatory changes in the cecum and colon. No histological abnormalities were found in control animals fed with water (data not shown).

genes was normalized to expression of the housekeeping gene *Hprt1*. Gene induction in DSS-treated mice was calculated as -fold change in expression compared to the control group.

Quantification of Inflammatory Mediators

Colon tissue samples were snap-frozen in liquid nitrogen and homogenized as described above, in 10 µL/mg tissue of sample buffer (200 mM NaCl, 4 mM EDTA, 10 mM Tris, 10% [w/v] glycine, cOmplete Protease Inhibitor Cocktail (Roche), pH 7.4). To determine myeloperoxidase (MPO), an enzyme-linked immunosorbent assay (ELISA) kit for mouse myeloperoxidase (HyCult Biotechnology, Uden, Netherlands) was used. Cytokine levels were measured with a Mouse Th1/Th2/Th17 Cytokine Cytometric Bead Array™ (CBA) Kit (BD, Heidelberg, Germany) on a FACSCalibur™ flow cytometer (BD), and data was analysed using FCAP Array software (BD).

C3a ELISA

For the detection of C3a/C3a-desArg by ELISA, purified rat anti-mouse C3a antibody (clone I87–1162, BD), and biotinylated rat anti-mouse C3a (clone I87–419, BD) antibody were employed as described elsewhere [12]. As a standard sample, zymosan-activated EGTA plasma was included in each run. Additionally, purified murine C3a (BD Pharmingen, Heidelberg, Germany) was used as a standard to calculate actual peptide concentrations. Of note, neoepitope-specific antibodies directed against C3 cleavage products (here: ELISA capture antibody) are usually much less sensitive for C3a than for C3a-desArg (as discussed in [3]). In contrast to the standard of C3a, the zymosan-activated standard plasma as well as the plasma samples mainly contain C3a-desArg. Thus, the calculated and depicted concentrations for C3a are most likely (10–100 fold?) false high. Specificity of the C3a/C3a-desArg ELISA was confirmed using zymosan-activated EGTA plasma from C3-deficient mice as a negative control.

Statistical Analysis

For statistical analyses, SigmaStat 3.5 (Systat Software, Chicago, IL, USA) was used. Clinical and histological scores were evaluated by Mann-Whitney *U*-test. Differences in parametric data were analysed by Student's *t*-test where applicable, otherwise by Mann-Whitney *U*-test. Differences of $P<0.05$ were considered significant.

Results

Partially Protective Effect of C3aR Deficiency in BALB/c Mice in Acute DSS-induced Colitis

To gain insight into the role of C3aR in bowel inflammation on different genetic backgrounds, BALB/c and B6 mice deficient in C3aR were subjected to DSS-induced colitis. Clinical signs of illness appeared from day 2 on (Fig. 1A), starting with traces of blood in the feces, next followed by diarrhoea, coat aberrances, bent posture, and later also by reduced spontaneous agility, and weak resistance to provocation. In BALB/c *C3ar*$^{-/-}$ mice, the appearance of first disease signs was delayed until day 4, and in both B6 *C3ar*$^{-/-}$ and BALB/c *C3ar*$^{-/-}$ mice, clinical scores from day 2 to day 7 were lower than in the corresponding WT animals. From day 3–4 on, clinical signs were accompanied by weight loss, reaching ~15% in B6 WT, and ~10% in BALB/c WT on day 7 (Fig. 1B). In contrast, the body weight of BALB/c *C3ar*$^{-/-}$ mice remained nearly stable, and was significantly higher than in BALB/c WT mice on days 5–7. Between B6 *C3ar*$^{-/-}$ and B6 WT animals, no significant differences in body weight were found. Due to a clinical score >15 and/or weight loss >30%, three out of 25 B6 WT animals had to be sacrificed on day 6, so they were not available for scoring and weighing on day 7, and their tissues were excluded from analysis. In the graphical representation, this appears as a seemingly smaller increase of the clinical score from day 6 to day 7, as compared to the preceding days (Fig. 1A), and a seemingly smaller weight loss, respectively (Fig. 1B). Consequently, the determinable differences between B6 WT and the less affected B6 *C3ar*$^{-/-}$ mice were smaller in these and probably also in other parameters. Taken together, these data indicated that in DSS-induced colitis, C3aR deficiency is moderately protective, which was more apparent in BALB/c than in B6 mice.

Reduced Complement Activation in BALB/c C3ar$^{-/-}$ Mice in DSS-induced Colitis

To assess complement activation, C3a and its degradation product C3a-desArg were measured in plasma samples taken on day 7. After DSS-induced colitis, C3a plasma levels were moderately elevated in B6 *C3ar*$^{-/-}$ mice only (Fig. 2). This excludes high systemic activation and suggests that complement activation was mainly restricted to the inflamed bowel. Measurement of C3a/C3a-desArg in colon tissue homogenate returned equally elevated high levels for all groups including H_2O controls and thus did not provide additional information, probably attributable to complement activation during the preparation of this tissue.

C3aR Deficiency Slightly Reduces Macroscopic Pathology, Histological Alterations, and Tissue Myeloperoxidase Content in BALB/c Mice

In DSS-induced colitis, colon shortening is regarded as a macroscopic measure of disease pathology and tissue remodelling in inflammation [19;20]. As shown in Fig. 3A, DSS treatment led to shortening of the colon in all four mouse lines. In BALB/c WT mice, this was significantly more pronounced than in BALB/c *C3ar*$^{-/-}$ mice, whereas no difference was seen between B6 WT and B6 *C3ar*$^{-/-}$. Along with the colon, the mesenteric lymph nodes (mLN) were removed, and their weight was determined. BALB/c *C3ar*$^{-/-}$ mice had smaller mLN than their WT counterparts, both without and with DSS treatment. In B6 mice there were only non-significant differences in mLN size between WT and *C3ar*$^{-/-}$. After DSS colitis mLN size was significantly increased in BALB/c *C3ar*$^{-/-}$ mice and non-significantly increased in the other three lines (Fig. 3B).

Histological examination of the cecum and colon revealed inflammatory tissue damage in all DSS-treated animals (Fig. 4 and 5). The epithelium was affected by loss of crypt architecture, crypt abscesses, and ulcerations (Fig. 4A and 4B, panels III-VI, and Fig. 5A). In the lamina propria and in the submucosal tissue, edema formation and infiltrates of mononuclear (*i.e.* lymphocytes and macrophages) and polymorphonuclear cells (*i.e.* granulocytes) were frequent (Fig. 5A). In all mouse lines, epithelial alterations, cellular infiltrates and ulcerations were most pronounced in the medial colon, followed by the distal colon and cecum, and finally by fewer and less extensive lesions in the proximal colon.

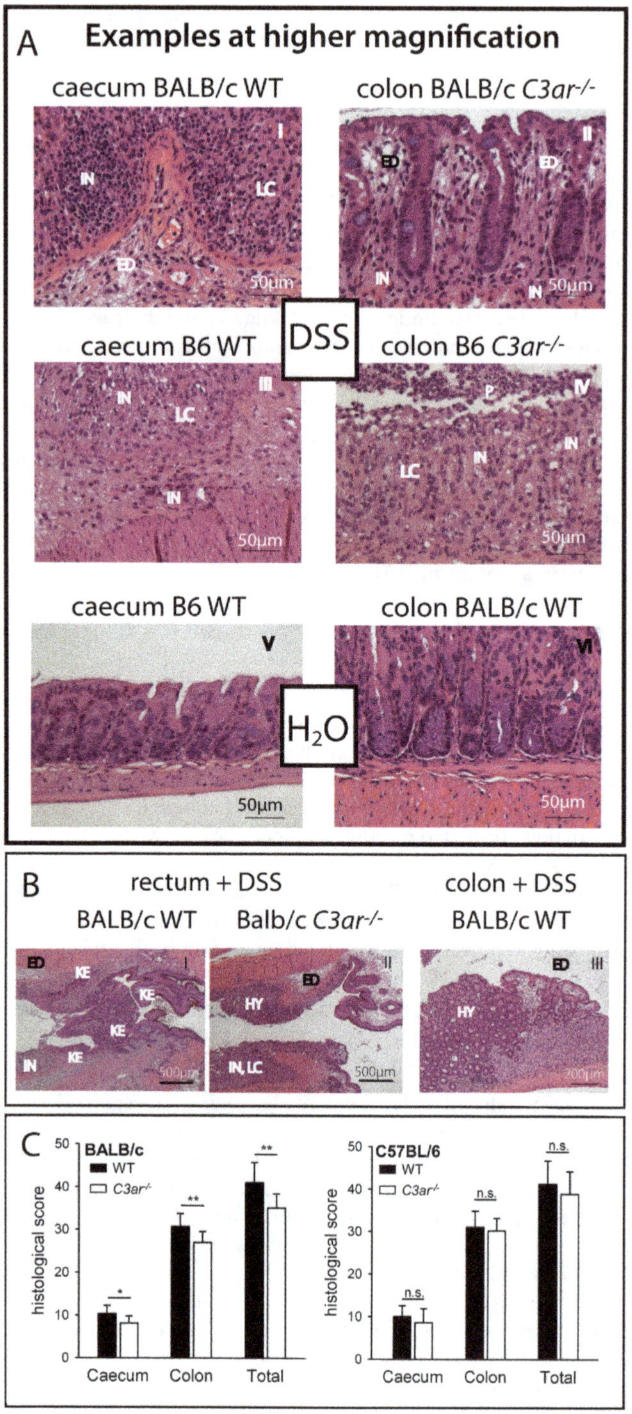

Figure 5. Histological evaluation of *C3ar$^{-/-}$* vs. WT BALB/c and B6 mice in DSS colitis (second part). Sections of the cecum, colon and rectum stained with hematoxylin and eosin, and histological score, as indicated. **A**, Exemplary lesions (edema, cellular infiltrates, loss of crypts) found in DSS-treated animals. Note that the details are not representative of the overall severity or the frequency of the lesions in the respective treatment group. **B**, Exemplary sections of the rectum of DSS-treated BALB/c WT and *C3ar$^{-/-}$* mice. Enlargement of the keratinized epithelium was found exclusively and epithelial hyperplasia was more frequent in BALB/c WT mice. ED = edema, HY = epithelial hyperplasia, IN = inflammatory cell infiltrate, KE = enlargement of keratinized epithelium, LC = loss of crypts, P = pus, UL = ulceration. **C**, Histological score (as depicted in Fig. 4 and 5A and 5B) based on the severity and extent of inflammatory changes in the cecum and colon. For each specimen, the colon score is the sum of the scores for the proximal, medial and distal parts, and the total score is the combined score of the cecum and colon. The data shown are means ± SD of specimens from n = 11 (WT, DSS) and n = 10 (*C3ar$^{-/-}$*, DSS) mice for BALB/c, and n = 24 (WT, DSS) and n = 10 (*C3ar$^{-/-}$*, DSS) mice for C57BL/6. No histological abnormalities were found in control animals fed with water (data not shown). n.s., not significant; *, $p<0.05$; **, $p<0.01$.

Especially in BALB/c WT mice, areas of mucosal hyperplasia and intramucosal edema in the colon were observed (Fig. 5B, panel III), together with a dense infiltrate of inflammatory cells even into the submucosal muscular layer (not shown). Notably, the rectum sections of six out of the 11 examined BALB/c WT animals displayed enlargement of the keratinized epithelium, which was neither found in BALB/c *C3ar$^{-/-}$* mice (Fig. 5B, panels I and II), nor in C57BL/6 mice (not shown). Overall, BALB/c *C3ar$^{-/-}$* mice were slightly but significantly less affected than BALB/c WT mice (Fig. 5C), whereas between B6 WT and *C3ar$^{-/-}$* mice, no differences were found.

To quantify the degree of inflammatory cell infiltration, the levels of myeloperoxidase, an enzyme produced mainly by neutrophil granulocytes, were measured in the colon tissue. After DSS treatment, BALB/c *C3ar$^{-/-}$* mice had significantly lower tissue MPO concentrations than BALB/c WT mice (Fig. 6), and B6 *C3ar$^{-/-}$* had slightly lower MPO levels than B6 WT mice, but without significance. Remarkably, DSS-treated B6 WT and *C3ar$^{-/-}$* mice had about 2.5– and 4.5–fold higher colon tissue MPO levels than the respective BALB/c groups. Flow cytometric analysis of whole blood samples from healthy WT mice showed that this was not due to strain differences in circulating granulocyte levels: BALB/c WT even had slightly higher numbers of circulating granulocytes than B6 WT mice (data not shown).

Overall, C3aR deficiency significantly reduced disease pathology in BALB/c mice, while in B6 mice, no significant effects of C3aR were observed.

Differential Cytokine Profile in the Colon Tissue of BALB/c and B6 Mice, and Differential Effects of C3aR Deficiency

To further characterize the inflammatory response, colon tissue homogenates were analysed for protein and transcript levels of inflammatory mediators that may be regulated during DSS-induced colitis [12].

On the protein level, the pro-inflammatory cytokines TNF-α and interleukin (IL)-6 were elevated in DSS-treated BALB/c WT, B6 WT, and B6 *C3ar$^{-/-}$* mice (Fig. 7). In BALB/c *C3ar$^{-/-}$* mice, TNF-α levels but not IL-6 levels were elevated, leading to significantly lower levels of IL-6 in DSS-treated BALB/c *C3ar$^{-/-}$* *vs.* WT mice. In B6 *C3ar$^{-/-}$*, IL-6 levels were non-significantly lower than in B6 WT, and in both BALB/c *C3ar$^{-/-}$* and B6 *C3ar$^{-/-}$*, TNF-α levels were slightly yet non-significantly lower than in the respective WT mice. The cytokine IL-2, which induces T cell proliferation, was slightly increased in all DSS-treated groups except B6 WT, but there were no differences between WT and *C3ar$^{-/-}$* animals. To assess the induction of Th1, Th2, and Th17 cells during colitis, the levels of the corresponding cytokines interferon (IFN)-γ, IL-4, and IL-17A were determined. After DSS treatment, IFN-γ was comparably increased in BALB/c WT and *C3ar$^{-/-}$* mice, but not significantly increased in B6 mice (Fig. 7). DSS-treated B6 *C3ar$^{-/-}$* had slightly lower IFN-γ levels than B6 WT mice. IL-4 levels were not elevated in any of the DSS-treated groups. IL-17A was not elevated in BALB/c mice, but in B6 mice, and B6 *C3ar$^{-/-}$* had lower IL-17A levels than B6 WT mice after DSS-induced colitis. The levels of the immunomodulatory

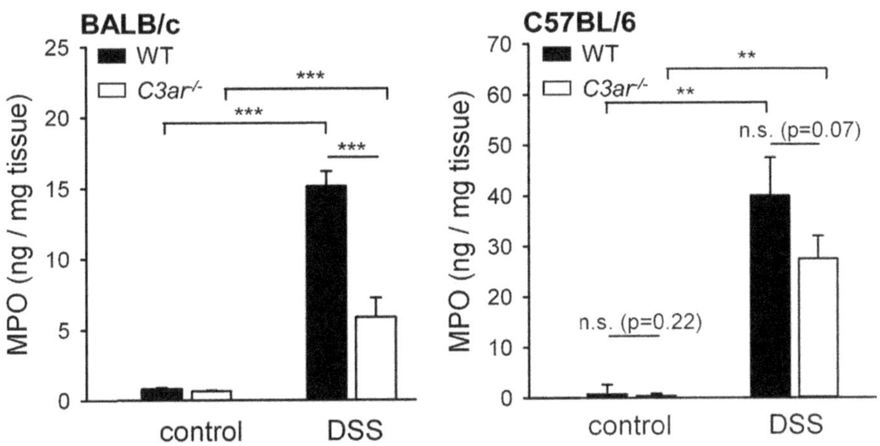

Figure 6. Myeloperoxidase (MPO) levels in the colonic tissue of *C3ar*$^{-/-}$ *vs.* WT BALB/c and B6 mice in DSS colitis. Levels of the granulocyte marker enzyme MPO were measured by enzyme-linked immunosorbent assay (ELISA) in tissue homogenates. The data shown are means ± SEM from n = 7 (WT, H_2O), n = 21 (WT, DSS), n = 5 (*C3ar*$^{-/-}$, H_2O), and n = 21 (*C3ar*$^{-/-}$, DSS) mice for BALB/c, and n = 5 (WT, H_2O), n = 11 (WT, DSS), n = 5 (*C3ar*$^{-/-}$, H_2O) and n = 12 (*C3ar*$^{-/-}$, DSS) mice for C57BL/6. n.s., not significant; ***, p<0.001.

cytokine IL-10 were below the detection limit in all groups (data not shown).

TNF-α and IFN-γ are known to induce the expression of other pro-inflammatory mediators, including CXCL-1/KC, CCL-8, CXCL-9 and MMP-3, through transcriptional regulation. In DSS-treated BALB/c WT and *C3ar*$^{-/-}$ mice, quantitative real time PCR analysis revealed slight upregulation of mRNA for CCL-8, a chemoattractant for various types of immune cells that is implicated in IBD [21], and unchanged levels of mRNA for MMP-3, a protease in tissue remodelling, including during bowel inflammation [22;23] (Fig. 8). There were significant differences in the regulation of mRNA for the neutrophil chemotaxin CXCL-1/KC, which was substantially elevated in BALB/c WT but not in BALB/c *C3ar*$^{-/-}$ mice after DSS administration. Minor upregulation of T cell chemoattractant CXCL-9 mRNA [24] was found in DSS-treated BALB/c *C3ar*$^{-/-}$ but not in WT mice. In both DSS-treated B6 WT and *C3ar*$^{-/-}$ mice, there were moderate increases in CCL-8 mRNA, and in CXCL-1/KC mRNA (Fig. 8). Unlike BALB/c mice, both B6 wt and *C3ar*$^{-/-}$ mice showed substantial upregulation of MMP-3 mRNA after DSS-induced colitis. CXCL-9 mRNA was upregulated in colitis in B6 mice, but the effect of C3aR on the expression of this cytokine was difficult to interpret, as B6 WT and *C3ar*$^{-/-}$ mice had different basal levels of CXCL-9 mRNA.

Thus, BALB/c and B6 mice develop partially different cytokine profiles during DSS-induced colitis, and C3aR appears to differentially contribute to their regulation.

Discussion

Crohn's disease and ulcerative colitis, the two major forms of IBD in humans, have a severe impact on health and quality of life of the affected individuals. In many cases, the currently available treatments cannot ameliorate the disease for lasting periods of time, or cause serious side effects. To establish novel therapeutic strategies in the long run, a broader knowledge of the pathomechanisms underlying intestinal inflammation is needed. These are now widely accepted to include a barrier dysfunction of the intestinal epithelium, and an overdriven immune response to luminal antigens.

Among the diverse rodent models of bowel inflammation, none may reflect all aspects of human IBD pathogenesis, but still many of them have proven useful to elucidate involved pathways and have contributed to the development of novel therapeutics. In several murine models of colitis, T cells were identified as the driving force of inflammation, and those models are highly suitable to investigate therapeutics that target T cell function [25].

In contrast, DSS-induced colitis is initiated by epithelial damage and independently of T or B cells [26]. However, innate immune mechanisms and cells that contribute to human IBD are activated early in DSS-induced colitis, and T cells are involved later in the inflammation process [12;27–29]. The DSS-induced colitis model has contributed to identify candidate drugs and drug targets, including TNF-α, which is now an established therapeutic target in human IBD [30;31]. In our group, the DSS-induced colitis model was previously employed to demonstrate an adverse role for C5aR, and the resulting data were in good accordance with those that other investigators obtained from TNBS-induced colitis, and from tissue samples of IBD patients [12;15]. In acute DSS-induced colitis in mice, the complement anaphylatoxin receptor C5aR has detrimental functions, and C3aR, C5aR, and the alternative receptor for C5a, C5L2, are upregulated in the colon tissue [12].

Here, we investigated the role of C3aR in experimental IBD, and the influence of the genetic background, by comparing BALB/c and B6 WT and *C3ar*$^{-/-}$ mice in acute DSS-induced colitis. We found that the complement system was activated in both mouse strains during DSS-induced colitis. After DSS treatment, BALB/c *C3ar*$^{-/-}$ had significantly lower plasma C3a levels than BALB/c WT mice. This may be attributable to an attenuation of a positive feedback loop of local inflammation and tissue damage, partially driven by the anaphylatoxins and their receptors, on complement activation. On the C57BL/6 background, where markers of inflammation were less influenced by the gene knockout, plasma C3a levels did not differ between DSS-treated WT and *C3ar*$^{-/-}$ mice.

Clinical and histological scores were similar in B6 WT and BALB/c WT mice, while complement activation and tissue levels of the pro-inflammatory cytokines TNF-α and IL-6 were slightly higher in B6 WT than in BALB/c WT mice. In the colonic tissue of DSS-treated BALB/c WT mice, we found an increase in IFN-γ, and in B6 WT there was non-significant upregulation of IFN-γ as well as significant upregulation of IL-17A. This is in accordance with other studies that have reported a Th1-polarized immune

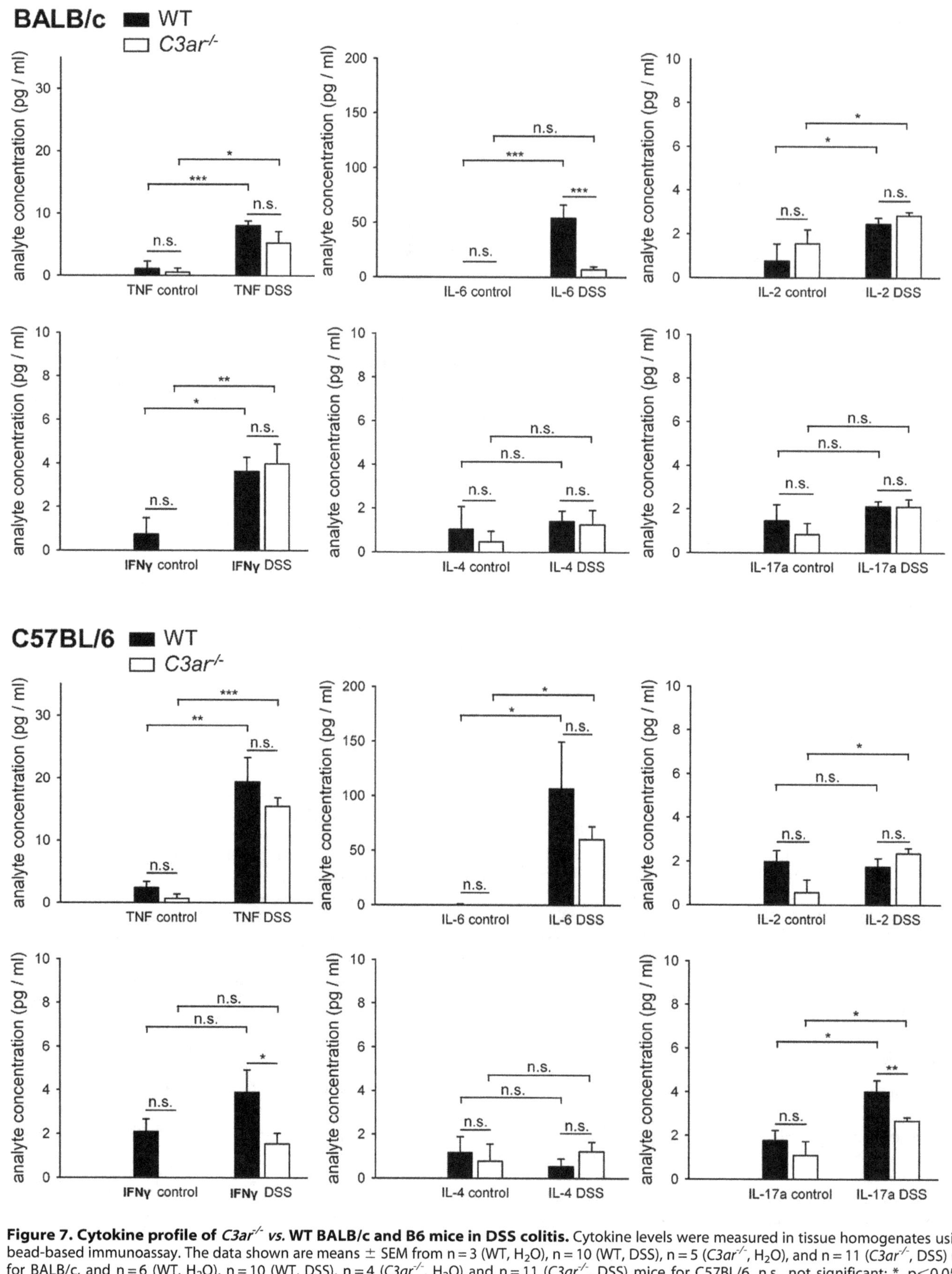

Figure 7. Cytokine profile of *C3ar*$^{-/-}$ *vs.* WT BALB/c and B6 mice in DSS colitis. Cytokine levels were measured in tissue homogenates using a bead-based immunoassay. The data shown are means ± SEM from n = 3 (WT, H_2O), n = 10 (WT, DSS), n = 5 (*C3ar*$^{-/-}$, H_2O), and n = 11 (*C3ar*$^{-/-}$, DSS) mice for BALB/c, and n = 6 (WT, H_2O), n = 10 (WT, DSS), n = 4 (*C3ar*$^{-/-}$, H_2O) and n = 11 (*C3ar*$^{-/-}$, DSS) mice for C57BL/6. n.s., not significant; *, $p<0.05$; **, $p<0.01$; ***, $p<0.001$.

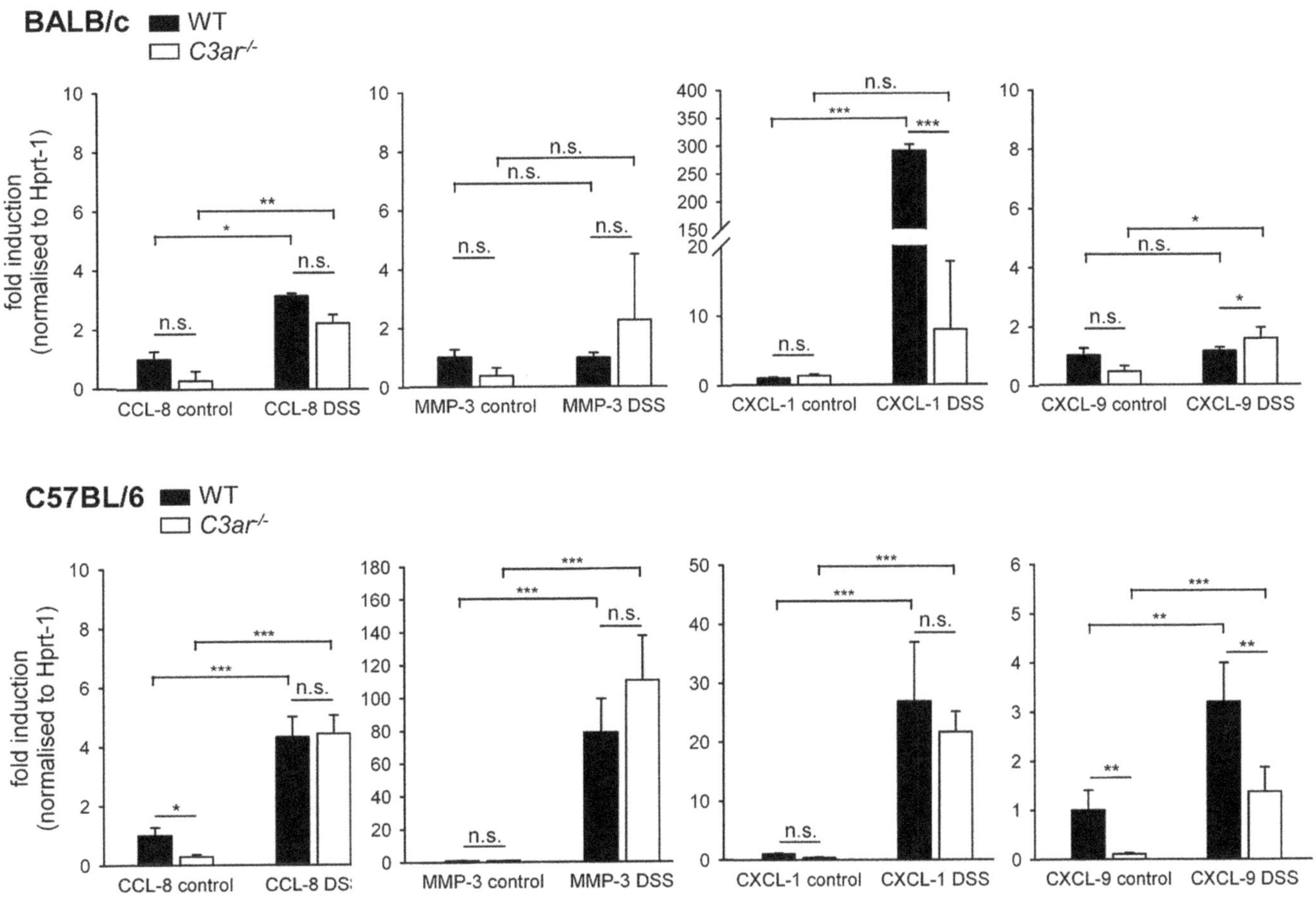

Figure 8. Regulation of mRNA expression in *C3ar^-/-^* *vs.* WT BALB/c and B6 mice in DSS colitis. RNA was isolated from colon tissue homogenates, and mRNA levels were measured by quantitative real time PCR and normalized to the expression of the housekeeping gene *Hprt-1*. For each gene, mRNA expression is shown relative to its expression in the WT control group. The data shown are means ± SEM from n = 12 (WT, H_2O), n = 22 (WT, DSS), n = 12 (*C3ar*$^{-/-}$, H_2O), and n = 21 (*C3ar*$^{-/-}$, DSS) mice for BALB/c, and n = 10 (WT, DSS), n = 12 (WT, H_2O), n = 12 (*C3ar*$^{-/-}$, H_2O), and n = 14 (*C3ar*$^{-/-}$, DSS) mice for C57BL/6. *, $p<0.05$; **, $p<0.01$; ***, $p<0.001$.

response in BALB/c mice [26;32], and a mixed Th1/Th17 profile for C57BL/6 mice [29] in acute DSS-induced colitis.

In BALB/c mice, the absence of C3aR was protective, as evidenced by a delayed onset of clinical signs, less weight loss, and reduced histological damage in BALB/c *C3ar*$^{-/-}$ mice after colitis. In BALB/c *C3ar*$^{-/-}$, the tissue levels of the granulocyte marker enzyme MPO, and of the inflammatory cytokine IL-6, were lower than those in BALB/c WT animals. However, in B6 mice treated with DSS, there were no obvious differences between *wt* and *C3ar*$^{-/-}$ animals. B6 *C3ar*$^{-/-}$ had improved clinical scores over B6 WT mice, but regarding weight loss, histology, and MPO and IL-6 levels, there was no amelioration.

Notably, neutrophil influx in terms of MPO levels in the colonic tissue was higher in B6 WT than in BALB/c WT mice, despite BALB/c WT having slightly higher levels of circulating granulocytes. However, mRNA levels of the neutrophil chemoattractant CXCL-1/KC were much more abundant in BALB/c WT mice. This might indicate that in BALB/c mice, CXCL-1/KC is less efficient in neutrophil recruitment, or that in C57BL/6 mice, other compensating chemoattractants make greater contributions. Neutrophils are critically involved in tissue damage in DSS-induced colitis, as shown by a study in which the exacerbated phenotype of macrophage- and/or dendritic cell-depleted mice in DSS-induced colitis was rescued by antibody-mediated neutrophil removal [28]. However, in CXCL-1/KC-deficient mice, where tissue infiltration is dominated by mononuclear cells, the inflammatory response in DSS-induced colitis is increased [33], suggesting that a certain amount of neutrophil recruitment is required for adequate inflammatory and regenerative responses in this disease model. We found significantly reduced levels of CXCL-1/KC mRNA and of MPO in BALB/c *C3ar*$^{-/-}$ *vs.* WT mice after DSS administration, and a non-significant reduction of MPO in B6 *C3ar*$^{-/-}$ *vs.* WT mice. C3a/C3aR thus appears to contribute to CXCL-1/KC mRNA production in acute DSS-induced colitis, and to augment neutrophil infiltration. Neutrophil recruitment might be more dependent on CXCL-1/KC in BALB/c mice than in B6 mice, which could explain why the impact of C3aR deficiency becomes apparent on the BALB/c background only.

Levels of CCL-8 mRNA were upregulated in all DSS-treated groups, suggesting that this chemotaxin for various immune cells contributes to DSS-induced bowel inflammation but is not influenced by C3a/C3aR. MMP-3 mRNA levels were not affected by DSS in BALB/c mice, whereas in DSS-treated C57BL/6 mice they were substantially elevated without significant difference of WT *vs.* *C3ar*$^{-/-}$. This may correlate with the higher levels of neutrophils and inflammatory cytokines in C57BL/6, reflecting a strain-specific inflammatory reaction. In BALB/c, other metalloproteases that were not examined here may participate in tissue remodelling.

Apart from direct inflammatory effector cells such as granulocytes and phagocytes, Th cell subsets play an important role in orchestrating the immune response in IBD models (reviewed in [25;34]). We observed that BALB/c *C3ar*$^{-/-}$ mice had smaller mLN than BALB/c WT independent of DSS treatment, which might be due to lower numbers of lymphocytes residing in the mLN. Others reported that B6 *C3ar*$^{-/-}$ mice had fewer and less viable T cells in their spleens than B6 WT mice, and attributed this to the lack of co-stimulatory C3a/C3aR signals for naïve T cells [35]. However, we did not find any significant differences in mLN size between B6 *C3ar*$^{-/-}$ and WT mice. After DSS treatment, mLN were significantly enlarged in BALB/c *C3ar*$^{-/-}$, and non-significantly enlarged in B6 *C3ar*$^{-/-}$, suggesting that substantial expansion of lymphocytes does occur in C3aR-deficient mice. Accordingly, the levels of the T cell cytokine IL-2 were elevated in both BALB/c *C3ar*$^{-/-}$ and B6 *C3ar*$^{-/-}$ mice after colitis induction. Another study by Strainic *et al.* reports that C3aR and C5aR signalling is involved in the differentiation of Th17 *vs.* regulatory T cells, and that the functions of the two receptors are overlapping but not redundant [36]. As C5aR plays a prominent role in DSS colitis, it is conceivable that generation of C5a during bowel inflammation is able to partly compensate for the lack of C3a/C3aR signalling, leading to T cell recruitment and activation. Still, signalling by C3a/C3aR might influence the relative abundance of T cell subsets, thus leading to different outcomes in WT *vs.* *C3ar*$^{-/-}$ in DSS colitis. An effect of C3aR on the steady state abundance or distribution of immune cells might also underlie the reduced background of some cytokines (mRNA or protein) in *C3ar*$^{-/-}$ *vs.* WT mice in the absence of disease.

A study that monitored BALB/c and C57BL/6 mice for 4 weeks after 5 days of DSS administration found that BALB/c mice quickly recovered, whereas C57BL/6 mice developed chronic inflammation [37], and in another study, chronification of DSS-induced colitis in C57BL/6 mice was associated with a switch from a Th1/Th17 phenotype to a predominantly Th2-mediated immune response [29]. In our study, DSS-treated B6 *C3ar*$^{-/-}$ mice had lower IL-17A and IFN-γ levels than B6 WT, indicating that C3aR participates in the regulation of T cell-mediated responses in DSS-induced colitis. In accordance with their lower IFN-γ levels, B6 *C3ar*$^{-/-}$ also had lower mRNA levels than B6 WT mice of the macrophage-derived IFN-γ-inducible T cell chemoattractant CXCL-9. Whether the absence of C3aR might facilitate the Th phenotype switch that initiates the chronic phase of disease in C57BL/6 mice can only be speculated about, as there was no concomitant increase in the Th2 cytokine IL-4, and the lower IL-17A and IFN-γ cytokine levels may simply reflect an overall lower degree of inflammation. However, in BALB/c *C3ar*$^{-/-}$ mice, we saw no influence on IL-17A and IFN-γ levels of C3aR, despite its overall more distinctive effect.

In analogy to C5aR, which was shown to modify Th cell polarization in chronic DSS-induced colitis [12], effects of C3aR on cytokine expression may also play a role in chronic disease. For the present study, we initially intended to apply the chronic disease model, but the effects of C3aR found in the acute model are rather small. At present, we therefore consider the chronic model not justifiable in terms of animal welfare.

In conclusion, C3aR contributes to disease pathogenesis in acute DSS-induced colitis in BALB/c mice, although the effect of C5aR may be more prominent [12]. Moreover, the C3aR-induced effects depend on the genetic background, as they are not obvious in C57BL/6 mice. This may be attributable to the different inflammatory profiles that have been reported for the two mouse strains [26;29;32], and that were also observed by us. Variations in DSS susceptibility between different inbred strains of mice [37;38] might also modulate the impact of C3aR on the disease. Given the well-established disadvantageous role for C5aR, and the efficacy of C5aR antagonists and anti-C5a antibodies in acute DSS- and TNBS-induced colitis in rodents [12–15], it may be of interest to assess if C3aR and C5aR co-operate in IBD pathogenesis.

Although it is difficult to predict the relevance and therapeutic value of C3aR in human IBD patients with a highly heterogeneous genetic background, it might be worthwhile to assess in the animal model if blockade of C3aR along with C5aR in intestinal inflammation could improve the effect of targeting C5aR alone.

Acknowledgments

We would like to thank the head of the Institute for Medical Microbiology and Hospital Epidemiology at Hannover Medical School, Prof. S. Suerbaum, for his support, and C. Rheinheimer for excellent technical assistance.

Author Contributions

Conceived and designed the experiments: EW AK. Performed the experiments: EW RL AB EB SG. Analyzed the data: EW AB AK. Contributed reagents/materials/analysis tools: RAW. Wrote the paper: EW AK.

References

1. Sandborn WJ, Faubion WA (2004) Biologics in inflammatory bowel disease: how much progress have we made? Gut 53: 1366–73.
2. Perrier C, Rutgeerts P (2011) Cytokine blockade in inflammatory bowel diseases. Immunotherapy. 3: 1341–52.
3. Klos A, Wende E, Wareham KJ, Monk PN (2013) International Union of Pharmacology. LXXXVII. Complement Peptide C5a, C4a, and C3a Receptors. Pharmacol Rev 65: 500–43.
4. Heeger PS, Kemper C (2012) Novel roles of complement in T effector cell regulation. Immunobiology 217: 216–24.
5. Drouin SM, Corry DB, Hollman TJ, Kildsgaard J, Wetsel RA (2002) Absence of the complement anaphylatoxin C3a receptor suppresses Th2 effector functions in a murine model of pulmonary allergy. J Immunol 169: 5926–33.
6. Lajoie S, Lewkowich IP, Suzuki Y, Clark JR, Sproles AA, et al. (2010) Complement-mediated regulation of the IL-17A axis is a central genetic determinant of the severity of experimental allergic asthma. Nat Immunol 11: 928–35.
7. Halstensen TS, Mollnes TE, Garred P, Fausa O, Brandtzaeg P (1992) Surface epithelium related activation of complement differs in Crohn's disease and ulcerative colitis. Gut 33: 902–8.
8. Ueki T, Mizuno M, Uesu T, Kiso T, Nasu J, et al. (1996) Distribution of activated complement, C3b, and its degraded fragments, iC3b/C3dg, in the colonic mucosa of ulcerative colitis (UC). Clin Exp Immunol 104: 286–92.
9. Scheinin T, Bohling T, Halme L, Kontiainen S, Bjorge L, et al. (1999) Decreased expression of protectin (CD59) in gut epithelium in ulcerative colitis and Crohn's disease. Hum Pathol 30: 1427–30.
10. Deguchi Y, Andoh A, Inatomi O, Araki Y, Hata K, et al. (2005) Development of dextran sulfate sodium-induced colitis is aggravated in mice genetically deficient for complement C5. Int J Mol Med 16: 605–8.
11. Lin F, Spencer D, Hatala DA, Levine AD, Medof ME (2004) Decay-accelerating factor deficiency increases susceptibility to dextran sulfate sodium-induced colitis: role for complement in inflammatory bowel disease. J Immunol 172: 3836–41.
12. Johswich K, Martin M, Bleich A, Kracht M, Dittrich-Breiholz O, et al. (2009) Role of the C5a receptor (C5aR) in acute and chronic dextran sulfate-induced models of inflammatory bowel disease. Inflamm Bowel Dis 15: 1812–23.
13. Woodruff TM, Arumugam TV, Shiels IA, Reid RC, Fairlie DP, et al. (2003) A potent human C5a receptor antagonist protects against disease pathology in a rat model of inflammatory bowel disease. J Immunol 171: 5514–20.
14. Woodruff TM, Pollitt S, Proctor LM, Stocks SZ, Manthey HD, et al. (2005) Increased potency of a novel complement factor 5a receptor antagonist in a rat model of inflammatory bowel disease. J Pharmacol Exp Ther 314: 811–7.
15. Chen G, Yang Y, Gao X, Dou Y, Wang H, et al. (2010) Blockade of complement activation product C5a activity using specific antibody attenuates

intestinal damage in trinitrobenzene sulfonic acid induced model of colitis. Lab Invest 91(3): 472–83.
16. Nicklas W, Deeny A, Diercks P, Gobbi A, Illgen-Wilcke B, et al. (2010) FELASA guidelines for the accreditation of health monitoring programs and testing laboratories involved in health monitoring. Lab Anim (NY) 39: 43–8.
17. Cooper HS, Murthy SN, Shah RS, Sedergran DJ (1993) Clinicopathologic study of dextran sulfate sodium experimental murine colitis. Lab Invest 69: 238–49.
18. Bleich A, Mahler M, Most C, Leiter EH, Liebler-Tenorio E, et al. (2004) Refined histopathologic scoring system improves power to detect colitis QTL in mice. Mamm Genome 15: 865–71.
19. Siegmund B, Fantuzzi G, Rieder F, Gamboni-Robertson F, Lehr HA, et al. (2001) Neutralization of interleukin-18 reduces severity in murine colitis and intestinal IFN-gamma and TNF-alpha production. Am J Physiol Regul Integr Comp Physiol 281: R1264–R1273.
20. Mennigen R, Nolte K, Rijcken E, Utech M, Loeffler B, et al. (2009) Probiotic mixture VSL#3 protects the epithelial barrier by maintaining tight junction protein expression and preventing apoptosis in a murine model of colitis. Am J Physiol Gastrointest Liver Physiol 296: G1140–G1149.
21. Banks C, Bateman A, Payne R, Johnson P, Sheron N (2003) Mucosal chemokine expression is unselectively increased in both ulcerative colitis and Crohn's disease. J Pathol 199: 28–35.
22. von Lampe B, Barthel B, Coupland SE, Riecken EO, Rosewicz S (2000) Differential expression of matrix metalloproteinases and their tissue inhibitors in colon mucosa of patients with inflammatory bowel disease. Gut 47: 63–73.
23. Kobayashi K, Arimura Y, Goto A, Okahara S, Endo T, et al. (2006) Therapeutic implications of the specific inhibition of causative matrix metalloproteinases in experimental colitis induced by dextran sulphate sodium. J Pathol 209: 376–83.
24. Park MK, Amichay D, Love P, Wick E, Liao F, et al. (2002) The CXC chemokine murine monokine induced by IFN-gamma (CXC chemokine ligand 9) is made by APCs, targets lymphocytes including activated B cells, and supports antibody responses to a bacterial pathogen in vivo. J Immunol 169: 1433–43.
25. Bouma G, Strober W (2003) The immunological and genetic basis of inflammatory bowel disease. Nat Rev Immunol 3: 521–33.
26. Dieleman LA, Ridwan BU, Tennyson GS, Beagley KW, Bucy RP, et al. (1994) Dextran sulfate sodium-induced colitis occurs in severe combined immunodeficient mice. Gastroenterology 107: 1643–52.
27. Dieleman LA, Palmen MJ, Akol H, Bloemena E, Pena AS, et al. (1998) Chronic experimental colitis induced by dextran sulphate sodium (DSS) is characterized by Th1 and Th2 cytokines. Clin Exp Immunol 114: 385–91.
28. Qualls JE, Kaplan AM, Van Rooijen N, Cohen DA (2006) Suppression of experimental colitis by intestinal mononuclear phagocytes. J Leukoc Biol 80: 802–15.
29. Alex P, Zachos NC, Nguyen T, Gonzales L, Chen TE, et al. (2009) Distinct cytokine patterns identified from multiplex profiles of murine DSS and TNBS-induced colitis. Inflamm Bowel Dis 15: 341–52.
30. Myers KJ, Murthy S, Flanigan A, Witchell DR, Butler M, et al. (2003) Antisense oligonucleotide blockade of tumor necrosis factor-alpha in two murine models of colitis. J Pharmacol Exp Ther 304: 411–24.
31. Naito Y, Takagi T, Handa O, Ishikawa T, Nakagawa S, et al. (2003) Enhanced intestinal inflammation induced by dextran sulfate sodium in tumor necrosis factor-alpha deficient mice. J Gastroenterol Hepatol 18: 560–9.
32. Egger B, Bajaj-Elliott M, MacDonald TT, Inglin R, Eysselein VE, et al. (2000) Characterisation of acute murine dextran sodium sulphate colitis: cytokine profile and dose dependency. Digestion 62: 240–8.
33. Shea-Donohue T, Thomas K, Cody MJ, Aiping Z, Detolla LJ, et al. (2008) Mice deficient in the CXCR2 ligand, CXCL1 (KC/GRO-alpha), exhibit increased susceptibility to dextran sodium sulfate (DSS)-induced colitis. Innate Immun 14: 117–24.
34. Zenewicz LA, Antov A, Flavell RA (2009) CD4 T-cell differentiation and inflammatory bowel disease. Trends Mol Med 15: 199–207.
35. Strainic MG, Liu J, Huang D, An F, Lalli PN, et al. (2008) Locally produced complement fragments C5a and C3a provide both costimulatory and survival signals to naive CD4+ T cells. Immunity 28: 425–35.
36. Strainic MG, Shevach EM, An F, Lin F, Medof ME (2012) Absence of signaling into CD4(+) cells via C3aR and C5aR enables autoinductive TGF-beta1 signaling and induction of Foxp3(+) regulatory T cells. Nat Immunol 14: 162–71.
37. Melgar S, Karlsson A, Michaelsson E (2005) Acute colitis induced by dextran sulfate sodium progresses to chronicity in C57BL/6 but not in BALB/c mice: correlation between symptoms and inflammation. Am J Physiol Gastrointest Liver Physiol 288: G1328–G1338.
38. Mahler M, Bristol IJ, Leiter EH, Workman AE, Birkenmeier EH, et al. (1998) Differential susceptibility of inbred mouse strains to dextran sulfate sodium-induced colitis. Am J Physiol 274: G544–G551.

16

Downregulation of the NHE3-Binding PDZ-Adaptor Protein PDZK1 Expression during Cytokine-Induced Inflammation in Interleukin-10–Deficient Mice

Henrike Lenzen[1]*, Maria Lünnemann[1], Andre Bleich[2], Michael P Manns[1], Ursula Seidler[1], Anne Jörns[3,4]

1 Department of Gastroenterology, Hepatology and Endocrinology, Hannover Medical School, Hannover, Germany, **2** Institute of Laboratory Animal Science, Hannover Medical School, Hannover, Germany, **3** Institute of Clinical Biochemistry, Hannover Medical School, Hannover, Germany, **4** Center of Anatomy, Hannover Medical School, Hannover, Germany

Abstract

Background: Impaired salt and water absorption is an important feature in the pathogenesis of diarrhea in inflammatory bowel disease (IBD). We analyzed the expression of proinflammatory cytokines in the infiltrating immune cells and the function and expression of the Na^+/H^+ exchanger isoform 3 (NHE3) and its regulatory PDZ-adaptor proteins NHERF1, NHERF2, and PDZK1 in the colon of interleukin-10–deficient (IL-$10^{-/-}$) mice.

Methodology/Principal Findings: Gene and protein expression were analyzed by real-time reverse transcription polymerase chain reaction (*q*RT-PCR), *in situ* RT-PCR, and immunohistochemistry. NHE3 activity was measured fluorometrically in apical enterocytes within isolated colonic crypts. Mice developed chronic colitis characterized by a typical immune cell infiltration composed of T-lymphocytes and macrophages, with high levels of gene and protein expression of the proinflammatory cytokines interleukin-1β and tumor necrosis factor-α. In parallel, inducible nitric oxide synthase expression was increased while procaspase 3 expression was unaffected. Interferon-γ expression remained low. Although acid-activated NHE3 activity was significantly decreased, the inflammatory process did not affect its gene and protein expression or its abundance and localization in the apical membrane. However, expression of the PDZ-adaptor proteins NHERF2 and PDZK1 was downregulated. NHERF1 expression was unchanged. In a comparative analysis we observed the PDZK1 downregulation also in the DSS (dextran sulphate sodium) model of colitis.

Conclusions/Significance: The impairment of the absorptive function of the inflamed colon in the IL-$10^{-/-}$mouse, in spite of unaltered NHE3 expression and localization, is accompanied by the downregulation of the NHE3-regulatory PDZ adaptors NHERF2 and PDZK1. We propose that the downregulation of PDZ-adaptor proteins may be an important factor leading to NHE3 dysfunction and diarrhea in the course of the cytokine-mediated inflammatory process in these animal models of IBD.

Editor: Yoshiro Ishimaru, University of Tokyo, Japan

Funding: This work was supported by grants Se460/9-5, S460/9-6 and SFB621-C9 from the Deutsche Forschungsgemeinschaft (to US). Publication charges for this article were supported by the Deutsche Forschungsgemeinschaft in the framework of the program "Open Access Publishing". The funders had no role in study design, data collection and analysis, decision to publish, or preparation of the manuscript.

Competing Interests: The authors have declared that no competing interests exist.

* E-mail: Lenzen.Henrike@mh-hannover.de

Introduction

Inflammatory bowel disease (IBD) is a cytokine-mediated chronic inflammatory disease [1] with diarrhea attributable to intestinal inflammation-mediated dysregulation in salt and water transport as well as leaky tight junctions. [2]. However, the pathogenesis of inflammatory diarrhea is only partially understood, and the proinflammatory cytokines and their role in inflammation-associated diarrhea are not known in detail. Different proinflammatory cytokines, in particular tumor necrosis factor (TNF)-α, interferon (IFN)-γ, and interleukin (IL)-1β, have been implicated as key mediators of inflammatory diarrhea in IBD [3,4]. However, results have been inconsistent. A crucial contribution to the inflammatory disease process has been documented in particular for the proinflammatory cytokine TNF-α [5–7]. This is supported in particular by the observation of a significant improvement of IBD through anti–TNF-α antibody treatment in many patients [8,9].

The action of a defined set of ion transport proteins dominates transmucosal ion and fluid movement [2], and the inhibition of electroneutral NaCl absorption plays a key role in the pathogenesis of inflammatory diarrhea [10]. In the intestinal tract, the Na^+/H^+ exchanger isoform 3 (NHE3) is the most important transport protein for Na^+ and water absorption [11]. NHE3 is expressed in the whole intestine [12], and it exists in dynamic multiple large multiprotein complexes [13]. The regulation of NHE3 involves direct linkage to PDZ-domain–containing proteins, including NHERF1, NHERF2, and PDZK1 (NHERF3) members of the NHERF family [14–16]. These PDZ-domain–containing proteins are involved in a wide range of biological functions, including multiprotein complex formation, interaction with other transporters, and signal transduction [13].

The IL-10$^{-/-}$ mouse model, which under conventional housing conditions spontaneously develops a generalized enterocolitis similar to human IBD [17], is an interesting animal model to characterize the relationships between cytokine-mediated immune responses and dysfunction of the intestinal mucosa. Using the IL-10$^{-/-}$ mouse model and for comparison also the DSS (dextran sulphate sodium) model, we analyzed the expression of different proinflammatory cytokines as well as of the Na^+ absorptive ion transporter NHE3 and the regulatory PDZ-adaptor proteins NHERF1, NHERF2, and PDZK1. When we found a strong alteration in the mRNA and protein expression of the PDZ-adaptor protein PDZK1, but not of NHE3, we wondered whether the normal NHE3 expression is accompanied by normal NHE3 function in this mouse model of IBD.

Results

Histopathological Alterations in the Inflamed Colonic Mucosa of IL-10$^{-/-}$ Mice

H&E staining of the inflamed colon of IL-10$^{-/-}$ mice showed clear signs of inflammation, characterized by an increase in mononuclear cells, infiltrating all layers of the mucosa with the highest accumulation in the submucosal layer. The mucosal layer in the inflamed colon analyzed in this chronic stage was intact but hyperplastic. In the colon of WT mice, mononuclear cells were only occasionally observed, mostly in the mucosal layer. The appearance of H&E sections of the colon from IL-10$^{-/-}$ mice kept under SPF conditions did not differ from those of the WT controls (H&E sections not shown). A histopathological scoring yielded for colon from control WT and IL-10$^{-/-}$ SPF mice scores of 0 and 0.3±0.3, respectively, while the score was 3.1±0.1 in the colon of IL-10$^{-/-}$ mice under conventional housing conditions (n = 4 mice in each group).

Pattern of Proinflammatory Cytokines and iNOS Gene Expression in IL-10$^{-/-}$ Mice

To further assess the chronic inflammatory state in the colon of IL-10$^{-/-}$ mice, we measured mRNA expression profiles by *q*RT-PCR of different proinflammatory cytokines and cell death markers. IL-1β and TNF-α were more than 10 times and 5 times, respectively, increased in the inflamed colonic mucosa of IL-10$^{-/-}$ mice as compared to the non-inflamed colonic mucosa of WT mice (Table 1). In contrast, IFN-γ gene expression was very low in the colonic mucosa of WT controls and was not significantly increased in the inflamed colonic mucosa of IL-10$^{-/-}$ mice (Table 1). The iNOS gene expression was significantly induced in the inflamed colonic mucosa of IL-10$^{-/-}$ mice (Table 1). Procaspase 3 gene expression was not increased in the cells in the colonic mucosa. In the colon of IL-10$^{-/-}$ SPF mice IL-1ß and TNF-α gene expression were not increased in comparison to WT mice. Also, IFN-γ gene expression was very low in the colonic mucosa of IL-10$^{-/-}$ SPF mice like in WT mice. iNOS and procaspase 3 gene expression were also not affected in the IL-10$^{-/-}$ SPF mice (Table S1).

In situ RT-PCR Measurements of Proinflammatory Cytokine and iNOS Gene Expression

To specify the cell types that produced the proinflammatory cytokines and induced iNOS, we performed *in situ* RT-PCR experiments. We identified a very high gene expression for the proinflammatory cytokines IL-1ß (Figure 1A) and TNF-α (Figure 1B) in the infiltrating immune cells in the mucosal (Figure 1) and submucosal (not shown) layers of the inflamed colonic mucosa of IL-10$^{-/-}$ mice. No mRNA expression was observed in any other cell type of the colon, in particular not in enterocytes, goblet cells, muscle, or connective tissue. Only single immune cells with cytokine positivity were observed occasionally in the different layers of the colon from WT mice (Figure 1A and 1B). Faint mRNA expression of IFN-γ was detected only in a very few immune cells in the inflamed mucosa of IL-10$^{-/-}$ mice and in the mucosa of WT mice (Figure 1C). The mRNA transcripts of the IL-1β–inducible enzyme iNOS, as measured by *in situ* RT-PCR, were found at very high expression levels only in infiltrating immune cells in the mucosal (Figure 1D) and submucosal (not shown) layers in the inflamed colon of IL-10$^{-/-}$ mice. Interestingly, the iNOS-expressing immune cells were located close to the epithelial layer. Only faint mRNA expression for iNOS was observed occasionally in the immune cells of the colon under control conditions (Figure 1D). Faint procaspase 3 gene expression was observed occasionally in enterocytes as well as in infiltrating immune cells in healthy WT mice without any indication of an increase in these cell types in IL-10$^{-/-}$ samples (Figure 1E).

Table 1. Gene expression profile of the proinflammatory cytokines IL-1β, TNF-α, IFN-γ and iNOS and the cell death marker procaspase 3 in the colonic mucosa of WT and IL-10$^{-/-}$ mice.

Gene	WT control	IL-10$^{-/-}$	Fold change against WT control
IL-1β	3.4±1.0	34.6±5.1*	10.2
TNF-α	1.3±0.3	7.9±2.1*	6.1
IFN-γ	0.007±0.0	0.008±0.01	1.2
iNOS	4.7±3.3	71.9±22.8*	15.3
Procaspase 3	36.9±12.6	24.9±12.4	0.7

Results are expressed as the mean normalized expression and fold change of IL-10$^{-/-}$ mice against WT controls. mRNA was quantified in relation to β-actin. Data are mean values ± SEM (from 5–6 experiments in each group).
*$p<0.05$ versus control.

Protein Expression of Proinflammatory Cytokines by Double Immunofluorescence

To characterize the immune cell subtypes that express the cytokines also at the protein level, we used double immunofluorescence staining. The colonic mucosa of IL-10$^{-/-}$ mice showed signs of inflammation with strong accumulation of IL-1β–positive (Figure 2A and 2B) and TNF-α–positive (Figure 2C and 2D) CD3 T-lymphocytes and macrophages in the mucosal and submucosal layers, whereas CD3 T-lymphocyte infiltration was more pronounced than the macrophage infiltration in comparison to healthy WT mice (Figure 2A and C versus Figure 2B and D). No protein expression was observed in enterocytes or goblet cells or in muscle and connective tissue (Figure 2). Single immune cells with cytokine positivity were observed occasionally in the different layers of the colon from WT controls.

Gene Expression of NHE3 and PDZ-adaptor Proteins

Since the mice developed a pasty stool which is a sign of murine diarrheal disease, we measured the expression of NHE3, the dominant salt-absorptive transporter in the proximal part of the colon in IL-10$^{-/-}$ mice. NHE3 gene expression by *q*RT-PCR was not affected by the inflammatory process in the colonic mucosa of IL-10$^{-/-}$ mice (Figure 3C). Because of the reduced NHE3 activity

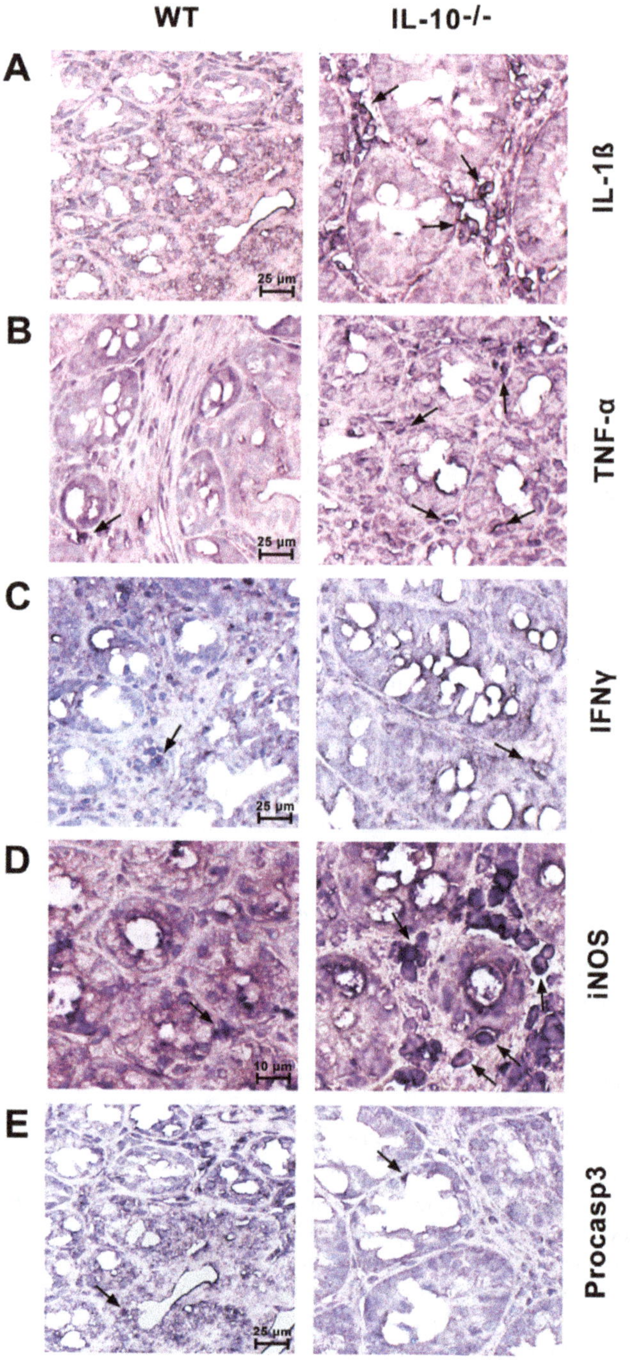

Figure 1. Gene expression by *in situ* RT-PCR of proinflammatory cytokines, iNOS, and procaspase 3 in the colonic mucosa. (A) and (B) High expression levels of IL-1β and TNF-α in infiltrating immune cells of IL-$10^{-/-}$ mice. (C) IFN-γ exhibited scant expression in only single immune cells of IL-$10^{-/-}$ mice and healthy WT mice. (D) High expression of iNOS in the immune cells surrounding the epithelial cells and in single immune cells in the connective tissue of the mucosa compared to WT mice. (E) Comparable procaspase 3 expression in WT and IL-$10^{-/-}$ mice. Arrows show representative mononuclear cells. Representative images of three independent experiments.

despite normal gene expression, we further studied expression levels of the PDZ-adaptor proteins of the NHERF family, which play an important role for acid-activated NHE3 activity in the murine colon [18,19]. We found that the gene expression of the two PDZ-adaptor proteins NHERF2 and PDZK1 was significantly reduced in the inflamed colonic mucosa of IL-$10^{-/-}$ mice (Figure 3C) while, on the other hand, the inflammation did not affect NHERF1 expression. In the colon of IL-$10^{-/-}$ SPF mice gene expression of NHE3 and the PDZ-adaptor proteins of the NHERF family did not differ from WT mice (Table S1).

Unaltered NHE3 and Downregulation of NHERF2 and PDZK1 Gene Expression

In situ RT-PCR was performed to further assess mRNA expression levels of NHE3 and the PDZ-adaptor proteins NHERF1, NHERF2, and PDZK1 in the epithelial cells of the colonic mucosa. Gene expression of NHE3 (Figure 4A) was localized only in the cytoplasm of enterocytes of the epithelial layer and showed no differences in expression between enterocytes of IL-$10^{-/-}$ and WT mice. The gene expression of NHERF2 (Figure 4B) and PDZK1 (Figure 4C) was reduced in enterocytes of IL-$10^{-/-}$ mice in comparison to WT controls. NHERF1 gene expression did not differ in enterocytes of the epithelial layer in IL-$10^{-/-}$ and WT mice (data not shown). No mRNA expression for NHE3, NHERF1, NHERF2, or PDZK1 was observed in any cell type other than enterocytes in the colon.

Protein Expression by Double Immunofluorescence of NHE3, NHERF2 and PDZK1

To further investigate the functional NHE3 transport defect, we also studied the protein expression of NHE3 and the PDZ-adaptor proteins NHERF2 and PDZK1 by double immunofluorescence. NHE3 protein expression in the colonic mucosa of IL-$10^{-/-}$ and WT mice was restricted to the apical membrane of the enterocytes without differences in localization and staining intensity (Figure 5A in green and Figure 5B in red). NHE3 immunostaining was not detected in other intestinal cell types in the epithelial layer of the mucosa. NHERF2 protein expression (Figure 5A in red) in the form of dotted areas, located in close vicinity to the NHE3 staining in the apical region of the enterocytes, was strongly reduced in the inflamed colon. PDZK1 staining in the enterocytes showed a more diffuse distribution in the cytoplasm, but the protein expression was also strongly reduced in the inflamed colon compared to the control samples (Figure 5B in green).

Densitometric Quantification of NHE3, NHERF2, and PDZK1 Protein Expression

Changes in NHE3, NHERF2, and PDZK1 protein expression in the enterocytes of IL-$10^{-/-}$ and WT mice were quantified by a computer-assisted densitometric method using microscopic fluorescence illumination (Figure 5C). NHE3 expression did not differ in IL-$10^{-/-}$ mice compared to WT mice. NHERF2 expression was significantly reduced by 62% in the inflamed colon. PDZK1 expression in the enterocytes of the inflamed colon was also significantly reduced by 81% compared to the control samples.

Fluorometric Measurements of NHE3 Transport Activity in Colonic Enterocytes

NHE3 mRNA and protein expression was not altered in the inflamed colon of IL-$10^{-/-}$ mice and the brush border membrane localization was unaltered. The mRNA and protein expression of two of the NHE3 regulatory PDZ proteins of the NHERF family (PDZK1 and NHERF2) were downregulated in the inflamed colonic epithelium. Since PDZK1 reduction but not NHERF2 reduction has been shown to reduce acid-activated NHE3 activity,

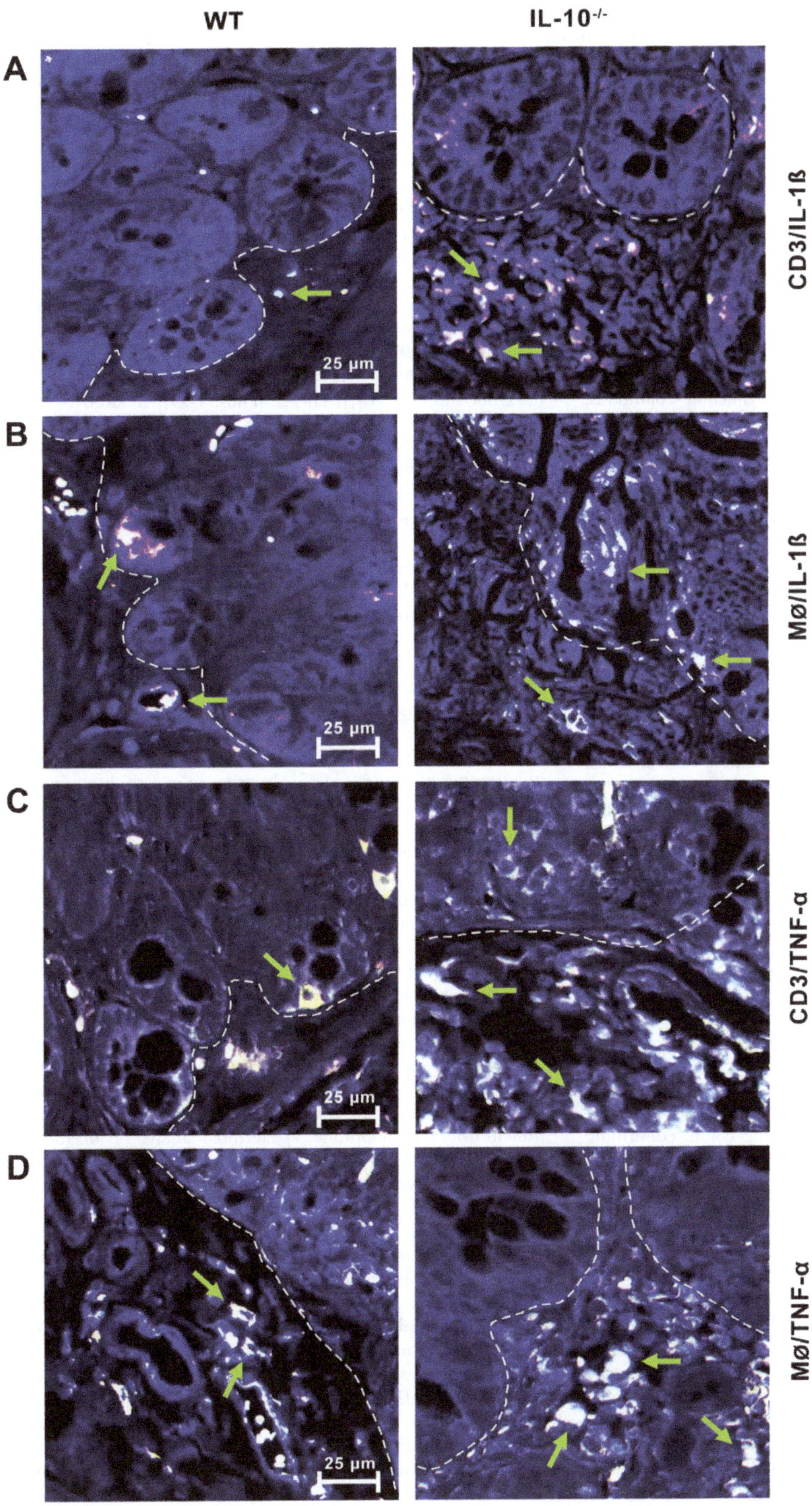
WT
IL-10-/-
A
B
C
D
CD3/IL-1ß
Mø/IL-1ß
CD3/TNF-α
Mø/TNF-α
25 µm

Figure 2. Double immunofluorescence staining of the proinflammatory cytokines IL-1β and TNF-α in infiltrating CD3 T-lymphocytes and macrophages. IL-10$^{-/-}$ mice showed signs of inflammation with strong accumulation of CD3 T-lymphocytes and macrophages (Mø) in the mucosal and submucosal layer in the colon with high expression of the proinflammatory cytokines IL-1β and TNF-α. Only single-cytokine–positive CD3 T-lymphocytes and macrophages were observed in the layers of the colon from WT mice. The dashed line separates the epithelial layer from the connective tissue of the submucosal layer. Double immunofluorescence staining presents as mostly white in the overlay (instead of yellow) as an amalgamation of green and red due to the background staining with DAPI (blue). Representative cells are marked with arrows. Shown are representative images of three independent experiments.

we analyzed NHE3 transport function in IL-10$^{-/-}$ and WT colonic enterocytes. To assess the NHE3 transport activity, we measured acid-activated, Hoe642-insensitive, Na^+-dependent proton flux in isolated colonic enterocytes (Figure 3A). The experimentally created transmembrane H^+ and Na^+ gradient was used as the driving force in this fluorometric measurement. In the presence of Hoe642, NHE1 and NHE2 were inhibited so that NHE3 almost completely mediated the acid-activated sodium-dependent proton flux. Under these experimental conditions, NHE3 activity was significantly reduced in the apical region of isolated colonic enterocytes from IL-10$^{-/-}$ mice as compared to WT mice (Figure 3B).

Comparison of the IL-10$^{-/-}$ Mouse Model with the DSS Mouse, Another Model of IBD

To confirm the results in another mouse model of chronic colonic inflammation, we performed a comparison with the chronic DSS mouse model of IBD. In the colon of DSS treated mice H&E staining showed clear signs of inflammation characterized by an increase in mononuclear cells, infiltrating the mucosal and submucosal layer and some single cells migrating into the muscularis layer (H&E sections not shown). The mucosal layer in the inflamed colon analyzed in this chronic stage was intact but mildly hyperplastic. In the colon of non-treated control mice, mononuclear cells were only occasionally observed, mostly in the mucosal layer. A semiquantitative analysis yielded for the colon from control and DSS treated mice histopathological scores of 0 and 2.7±0.3, respectively (n = 3 mice in each group). Changes of mRNA expression profiles by *q*RT-PCR were comparable (Table S2). The expression of IL-1β and TNF-α as well as of iNOS, but not of IFN-γ and procaspase 3, were significantly increased. Gene expression of PDZK1 was also significantly decreased while that of NHE3 as well as of NHERF1 and NHERF2 were not changed (Table S2).

Discussion

IBD in the IL-10$^{-/-}$ mouse model was characterized by an immune cell infiltration comprising T-lymphocytes and macrophages in the mucosa and submucosa of the colon, confirming earlier observations [20,21]. We show here that these immune cells were activated and produced proinflammatory cytokines, a combination of high levels of IL-1β and TNF-α, as documented at both the gene and protein expression levels by *q*RT-PCR, *in situ* RT-PCR, and immunohistochemistry. These parallel analyses of the gene and protein expression of proinflammatory cytokines allowed reliable identification of the immune cell activation status [22–24]. The results show that in contrast to the infiltrating immune cells, epithelial cells did not express the proinflammatory cytokines IL-1β and TNF-α, neither at the gene nor protein level. IFN-γ gene expression, originating from single activated infiltrating immune cells, was not increased in this chronic inflammatory state, confirming reports in other autoimmune diseases [22,25]. IL-1β typically induces iNOS expression in activated infiltrating immune cells [26], as documented through expression of this inducible nitric oxide (NO) generating enzyme in the present study. In addition, very high expression levels of the proinflammatory cytokine TNF-α were detected at both the gene and protein expression levels in the immune cells. The additional presence of TNF-α potentiates the toxicity of IL-1β by fostering superoxide radical formation [27]. Treatment with anti–TNF-α antibody ameliorates mucosal inflammation and diarrhea in the IL-10$^{-/-}$ mouse model [28], as well as in humans [8,9], indicating that this proinflammatory cytokine is critical for the disease process; however, TNF-α antibody therapy does not suppress IL-1β effects. Thus, IL-1β–induced NO production alone, without concomitant superoxide radical formation resulting from TNF-α activity, is apparently not sufficient to cause intestinal dysfunction.

Many studies in humans and mice have shown that intestinal inflammation causes a functional disturbance of electroneutral sodium absorption [10]. NHE3 is the most important sodium absorptive transporter and responsible for the majority of electroneutral salt absorption in the intestine [11], and is the only functionally recognized sodium absorptive transporter in the proximal-mid colon, the area most affected by IL-10$^{-/-}$ colitis [17]. Data on NHE3 expression in chronic intestinal inflammation are inconsistent, with both up- and downregulation as well as unchanged expression having been reported [29–33]. In addition, salt absorption in the intestinal mucosa may be disturbed because of a backflux of Na^+ through leaky tight junctions, as demonstrated in a number of studies [34,35]. In order to selectively study NHE activity in colonocytes, we therefore isolated colonic crypts and assessed fluorometrically acid-activated Na^+/H^+ exchange activity in the surface colonocytes in the mouths of the cryptal opening, which is >85% due to NHE3, as demonstrated before [18]. The present study shows that NHE3 transport activity in this mouse model of chronic intestinal inflammation was dysfunctional, as evidenced by reduced acid-activated NHE3 transport activity. This dysfunction was observed in spite of constitutive NHE3 gene expression as documented by *q*RT-PCR and for the first time by *in situ* RT-PCR, allowing a cell type specific identification of gene expression changes. Protein expression of NHE3 in the plasma membrane of the epithelial cells, as measured by immunofluorescence combined with quantitative densitometric analysis, was also not significantly affected without evidence for internalization of the protein from the membrane. Western blot analyses confirmed this observation (data not shown). This observation is in accordance with recent functional analyses in human colon biopsies of ulcerative colitis, which also revealed NHE3 dysfunction despite unchanged NHE3 expression [33].

So far, little is known about NHE3 transport regulation in the chronically inflamed intestine. PDZ-adaptors are scaffolding proteins, playing a central role in targeting, membrane retention, and signal complex formation of membrane proteins, including NHE3 [14]. Transgenic animal studies have shown that not only NHE3 deficiency [36] but also PDZ-adaptor protein deficiency as observed in NHERF1- [19,37], NHERF2- [38], and PDZK1- [18,39] knockout mice, can cause intestinal NHE3 dysfunction. To further investigate the NHE3 transport dysfunction in this animal model of chronic IBD, we therefore measured the expression of PDZ-adaptor proteins of the NHERF family. Indeed, we found that in IL-10$^{-/-}$ mice, NHERF2 and PDZK1 expression at both

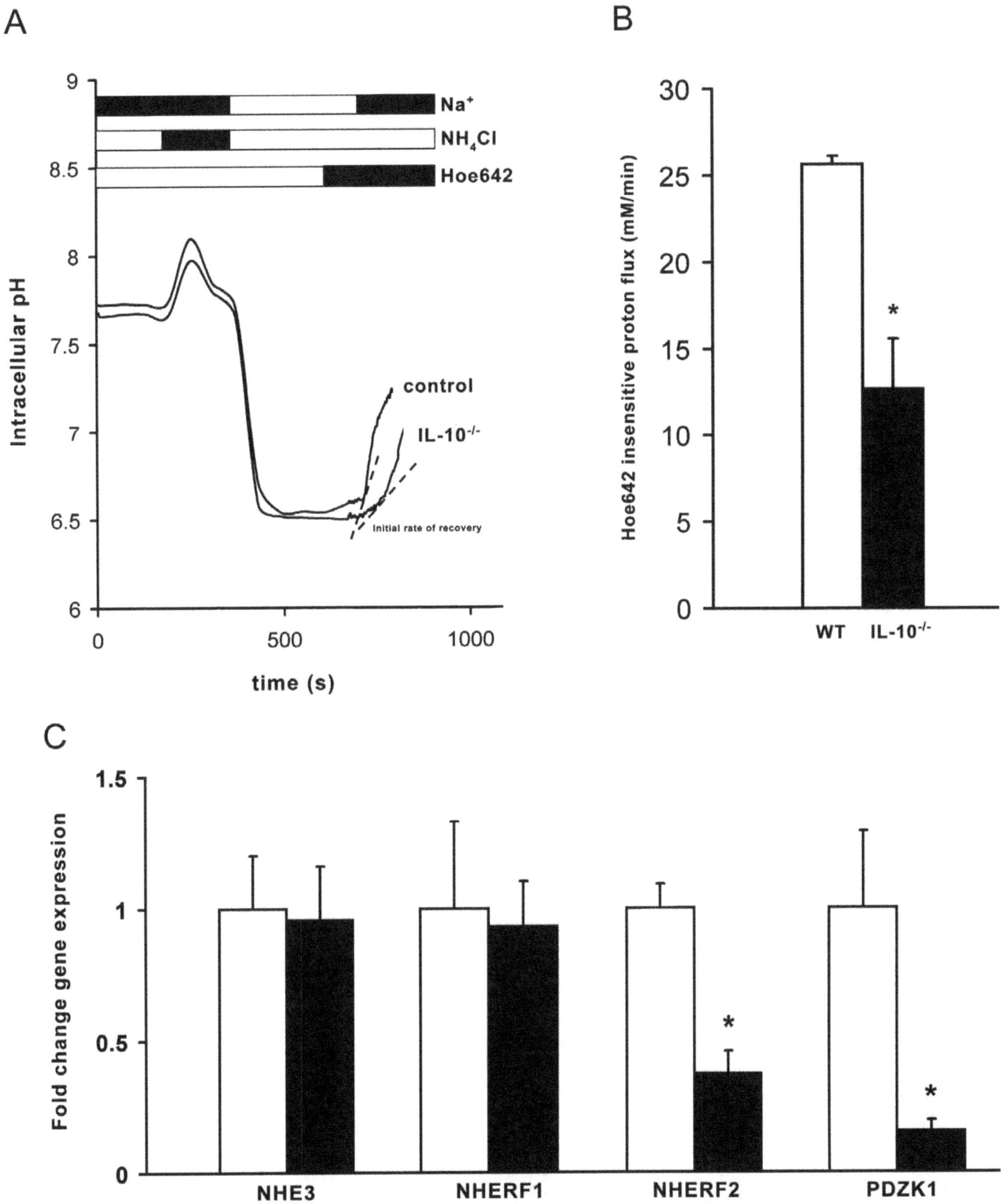

Figure 3. Fluorometric assessment of NHE3 activation by acid in colonic enterocytes in IL-10$^{-/-}$ mice. (A) Exemplary pH curve. (B) Reduced NHE3 activity as measured by acid-activated Hoe642-insensitive proton flux in colonic enterocytes in IL-10$^{-/-}$ mice (black columns) compared to healthy WT mice (open columns). n = 3 pairs of mice; * $p<0.05$ versus control. (C) Unaltered NHE3 gene expression but downregulation of the PDZ-adaptor proteins NHERF2 and PDZK1 in IL-10$^{-/-}$ mice. The expression of NHERF1 was not affected. Results are expressed as a comparison of fold change in expression of NHE3, NHERF1, NHERF2 and PDZK1 in the inflamed and noninflamed colon (from 5–6 experiments in each group). mRNA was quantified in relation to ß-actin. *$p<0.05$ versus control.

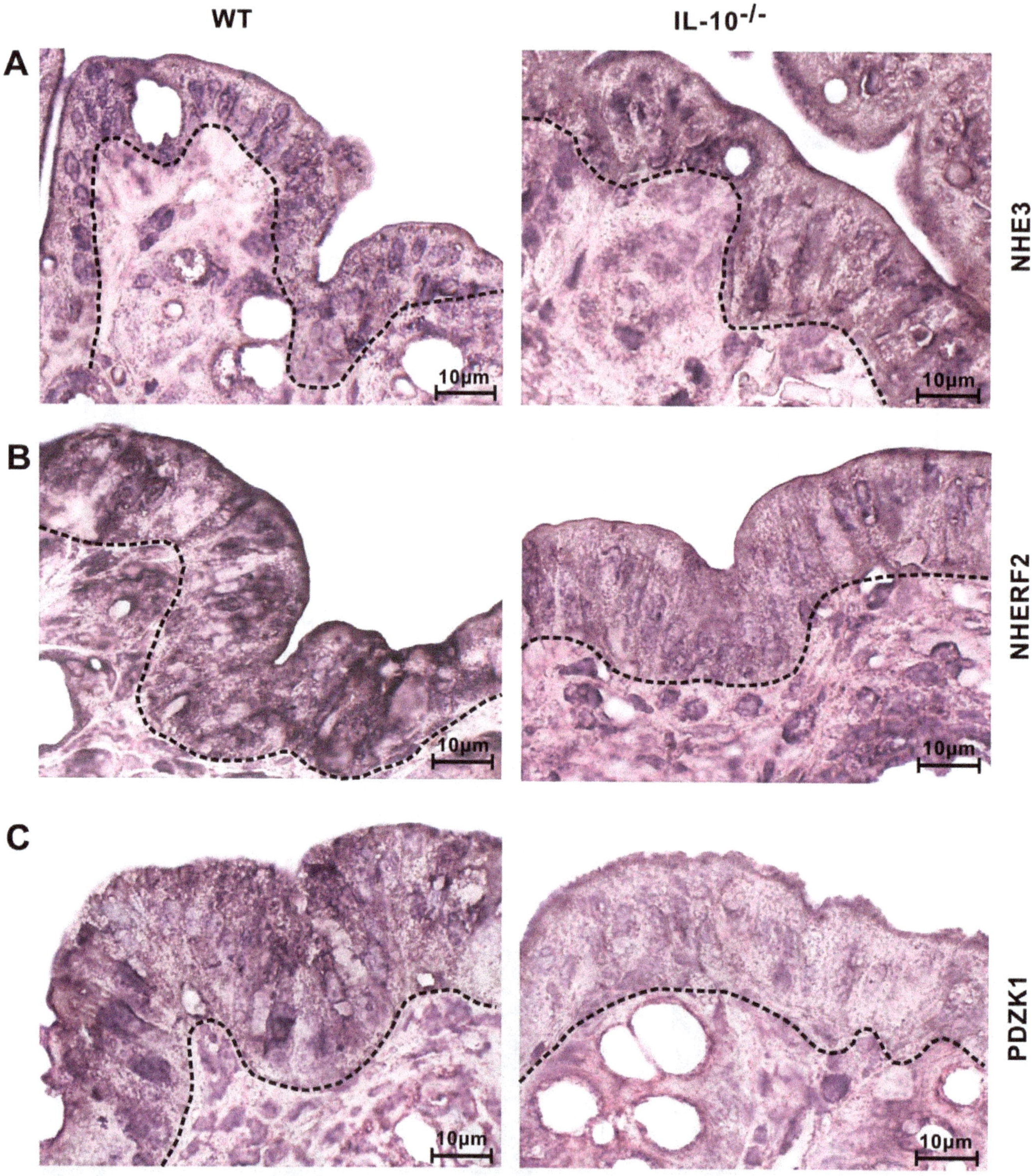

Figure 4. Gene expression by *in situ* RT-PCR of NHE3, NHERF2, and PDZK1 in the colonic mucosa. (A) Unaltered NHE3 expression levels in enterocytes of the epithelial layer of WT and IL-$10^{-/-}$ mice. (B) mRNA expression of NHERF2 and (C) PDZK1 in the epithelial enterocytes were markedly decreased in IL-$10^{-/-}$ mice. The dashed line separates the epithelial layer from the connective tissue of the lamina propria of the mucosa. Representative images of two independent experiments.

the gene and protein levels were significantly decreased. In addition to using *in situ* RT-PCR and immunofluorescence to demonstrate downregulation of these two PDZ-adaptor proteins, we also quantified for the first time NHE3, NHERF2, and PDZK1 protein expression in enterocytes using computer-assisted densitometry. These are the first data which document a NHERF

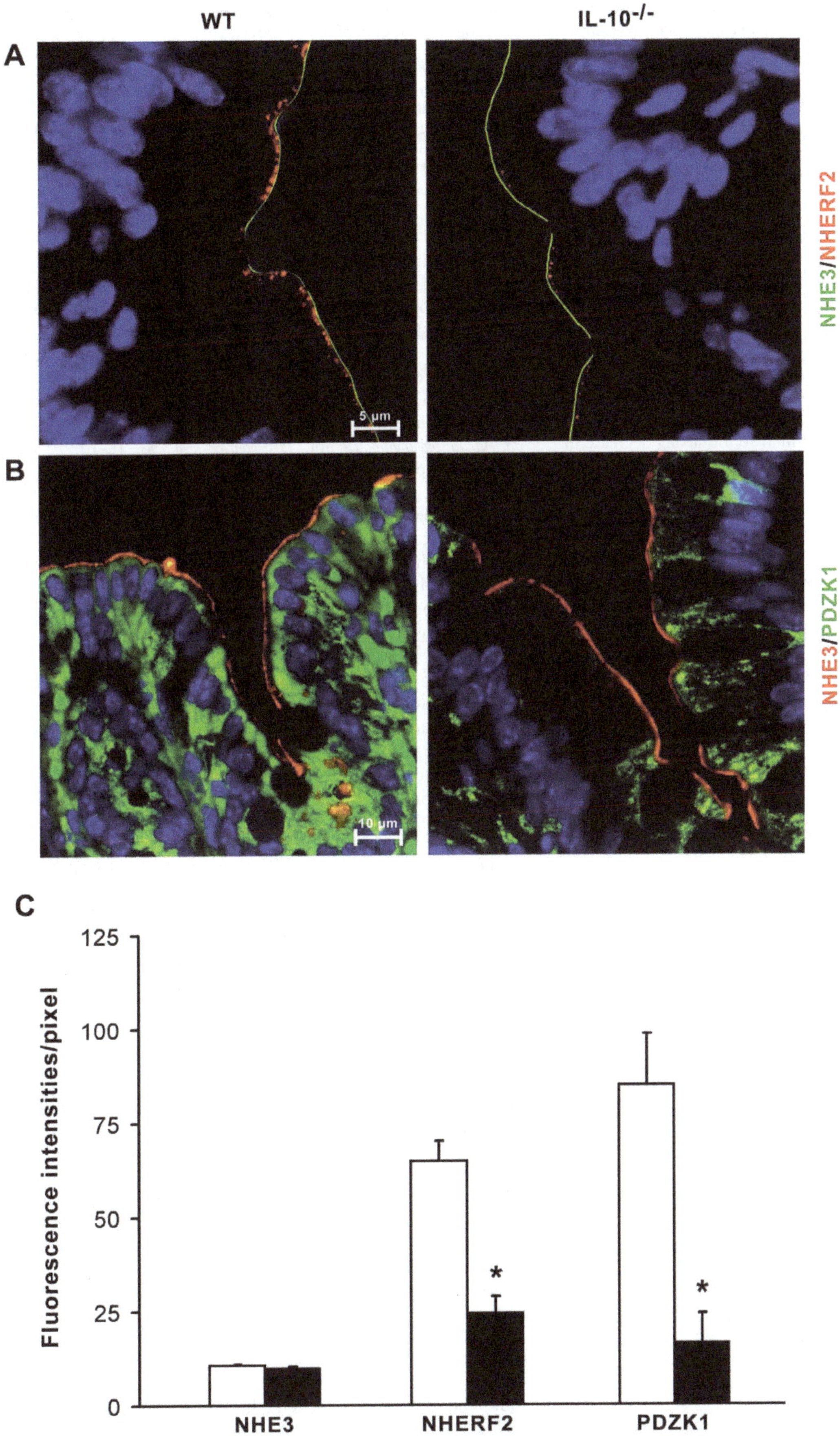

WT
IL-10-/-
A
NHE3/NHERF2
5 µm
B
NHE3/PDZK1
10 µm
C
Fluorescence intensities/pixel
125
100
75
50
25
0
*
*
NHE3
NHERF2
PDZK1

Figure 5. Double immunofluorescence staining and densitometric quantification of NHE3, NHERF2, and PDZK1 in enterocytes of the inflamed colon. (A) and (B) NHE3 protein expression was clearly restricted to the apical region of the enterocytes in colonic mucosa of diseased IL-10$^{-/-}$ mice and WT mice in comparable intensities. (A) NHERF2 protein expression (red) was restricted to the apical region of the enterocytes in a dotted-like fashion in association with the NHE3 staining (green). The number of red dots was markedly reduced in diseased IL-10$^{-/-}$ mice. (B) The PDZK1 immunostaining (green) was localized in the whole cytoplasm of the enterocytes under healthy and diseased conditions while the intensity of PDZK1 was markedly reduced in IL-10$^{-/-}$ mice. NHE3 staining (red) was not reduced in IL-10$^{-/-}$ mice. Nuclei of the cells were stained with DAPI (blue). A and B show representative images of three independent experiments. (C) Densitometric quantification of the NHE3, NHERF2, and PDZK1 protein expression in enterocytes of WT and IL-10$^{-/-}$ mice. Densities are expressed in mean fluorescence intensities per pixel as means ± SEM. n = 4 animals; in each animal, 9–23 enterocytes in the same cell section plane were analyzed. *p<0.01 versus control.

protein expression with cellular localization in the murine colonic epithelium.

How may the downregulation of these NHERF adaptors be related to the observed NHE3 dysfunction? NHERF2 deficiency in murine colon has been reported to selectively disturb certain regulatory features of NHE3, such as Ca^{2+}-dependent NHE3 transport inhibition, without a change in acid-activated NHE3 transport [19]. In contrast, PDZK1 deficiency results in a strong decrease in acid-activated NHE3 activity in murine colonic surface cells [18]. The latter defect is very similar to the strong decrease in acid-activated NHE3 activity observed in the surface colonocytes of the IL-10–deficient chronically inflamed colon in this study, as well as the decreased acid-activated NHE3 activity observed in surface colonocytes of moderately inflamed mucosa from ulcerative colitis patients [33,40]. We therefore assume that the very strong PDZK1 downregulation observed in IL-10$^{-/-}$ colonocytes is a likely contributory factor to NHE3 dysfunction. This assumption will have to be confirmed in future experimentation.

We also compared the results obtained in the spontaneous IL-10$^{-/-}$ mouse model with the situation in the DSS mouse, a chemically-induced IBD model. The histopathological scores were in the same range and the mucosal layer was preserved. The changes in the mRNA expression profile in the DSS mouse colon with significant increases of the proinflammatory cytokines IL-1β and TNF-α as well as a significantly decreased PDZK1 gene expression in spite of unchanged expression levels of NHE3 and NHERF1 were comparable to those in the IL-10$^{-/-}$ mouse colon. The only significant difference between the two animal models was the lack of a reduction of NHERF2 gene expression in the DSS mouse colon. Severe colonic NHE3 dysfunction in DSS colitis has previously been described by our group [41]. Thus, NHE3 dysfunction despite normal NHE3 gene expression, but strongly reduced PDZK1 expression, is seen in both mouse models of chronic colonic inflammation. Data obtained in control experiments from IL-10$^{-/-}$ mice kept under SPF conditions with non-inflamed colonic mucosa confirmed that there is no PDZK1 downregulation without inflammation.

Taken together, the present data support the idea of an interference of proinflammatory cytokines with NHE3 transport function despite unaltered NHE3 expression and membrane localization in the IL-10$^{-/-}$ mouse model. Similar findings were obtained in the chronic DSS colitis mouse model. Downregulation of the PDZ-adaptor protein PDZK1 of the NHERF family was observed in both models as well. We therefore propose that NHE3 functional dysregulation may, at least in part, be related to NHE3 protein network disruption. Inflammation-induced PDZK1 downregulation may therefore be a contributory factor in the pathogenesis of inflammatory diarrhea in IBD.

Materials and Methods

IL-10–deficient Mouse Model

IL-10–deficient (*Il10^{tm1Cgn}*, *Il10$^{-/-}$*) and wild-type (WT) mice on a C57BL/6J background were produced and maintained in a room with a controlled environment (21±2°C, 55±5% relative humidity, 12 hours light/dark cycle). Mice were housed separated by sex in cages with a 360-cm^2 floor area at a maximum of four animals on bedding of non-sterilized, dust-free softwood fibers. A pelleted diet (Altromin® 1314, Lage, Germany) containing 22.5% protein, 5.0% fat, and 4.5% fiber and tap water treated with UV light were provided *ad libitum*. Routine microbiological monitoring according to FELASA recommendations [42] did not reveal any evidence of infection with common murine pathogens except for *Pasteurella pneumotropica* and *Helicobacter hepaticus*. IL-10$^{-/-}$ mice developed a disease that became apparent by weight loss and pasty stool at the age of 3–4 months. Mice were used at 8±1 months of age with a significant body weight reduction (24.1 g versus 28.4 g in WT mice, p<0.01). Additional IL-10–deficient mice were bred and maintained under strict specific pathogen-free (SPF) barrier conditions (IL-10$^{-/-}$ SPF) as described previously [43]. IL-10$^{-/-}$ SPF mice showed no clinical signs of inflammation with a body weight not significantly different to WT mice (27.5 g versus 28.4 g).

DSS Mouse Model

12- to 14-weeks old male C57BL/6J mice (body weight: 21–22 g) were treated with 3% of dextran sodium sulfate (DSS; MW: 36,000–50,000 Da, MP Biomedicals, Eschwege, Germany) dissolved in autoclaved drinking water and subsequently sterilized by filtration. Drinking water was replaced by the DSS solution for five days followed by a 10-day recovery period. This treatment schedule was repeated for another three cycles. Body weight was monitored daily. Colitis manifested with typical clinical symptoms such as weight loss, diarrhea and rectal bleeding. Treatment caused a body weight loss of 2–3 g, which was normalized again towards the end of the treatment free intervals. Animal experiments were approved by the Local Institutional Animal Care and Research Advisory Committee at the Hannover Medical School and authorized by the local government for the regulation of animal welfare (Niedersächsisches Landesamt für Verbraucherschutz und Lebensmittelsicherheit).

RNA Isolation, cDNA Preparation, and Real-time PCR

Segments of proximal colonic mucosa were dissected free of seromuscular layers. Total RNA was obtained using the NucleoSpin RNA/Protein kit (Machery & Nagel, Germany). RNA was reverse transcribed into complementary DNA using an oligo-dT18TNV primer (Fermentas, St. Leon-Rot, Germany) and the Revert-Aid™ H-Minus M-MuLV reverse transcriptase (Fermentas, St. Leon-Rot, Germany). Quantitative real-time reverse transcription polymerase chain reaction (*q*RT-PCR) was performed with the QuantiTect SYBR Green™ technology (QIAGEN, Hilden, Germany) using the DNA Engine Opticon™ Sequence Detection System (Biozym Diagnostik, Hessisch-Oldendorf, Germany). ß-actin was used for normalization. Table S3 shows the *q*RT-PCR primers used in this study.

Fluorometric Analyses

Preparation of colonic crypts and pH measurements were performed as previously described [18,19]. In brief, for the pH_i measurements colonic crypts where loaded with BCECF and mounted onto a heated stage of an inverted microscope (Zeiss Axiovert 200, Carl Zeiss AG, Jena, Germany). Crypts were acidified using an ammonium prepulse (40 mM NH_4Cl isotonically replacing NaCl), then perfused with a Na^+-free buffer (TMA^+ isotonically replacing Na^+), until pH_i reached its lowest value plateau. Subsequently, 50 µM Hoe 642 was added to the Na^+-free buffer. After 2–3 min, the buffer was switched to Na^+-containing buffer, supplemented with 50 µM HOE642 and forskolin, if appropriate. Cells were exposed to alternating 440 and 495 nm light from a monochromator (Visichrome, Visitron Systems, Puchheim, Germany) with a 515-nm DCXR dichroic mirror and a 535-nm barrier filter (Chroma Technology, Rockingham, VT, USA) in the emission pathway and images digitalized. Calibration of the 440/495 ratio was performed as described [44]. Regions of interest (ROIs) were selected in the apical and basal part of the crypts. NHE3 activity was measured by calculating the initial rate of pH_i recovery (dpH/dt) from acidosis after re-administration of Na^+ (Figure 3B). For the fluorometric measurements, Hoe642 was kindly provided by Sanofi-Aventis (Frankfurt, Germany). Nigericin and 2′,7′-bis-(2-carboxyethyl)-5-(and-6)-carboxyfluorescein (BCECF) were purchased from Molecular Probes (Leiden, Netherlands).

Morphology

H&E staining was used for general assessment of intestinal inflammation. Histopathological scores were performed as previously described [20] to grade the degree of colonic inflammation from grade 0 to 4 with grade 0: no changes from normal tissue (no signs of inflammation); grade 1: very low level of leukocyte infiltration; grade 2: low level of leukocyte infiltration; grade 3: high level of leukocyte infiltration involving the submucosa and thickening of the colon wall; grade 4: transmural leukocyte infiltration, loss of goblet cells, thickening of the colonic wall.

For immunohistochemistry, tissue specimens of mouse colon were rinsed with ice-cold phosphate-buffered saline (PBS) and fixed in 4% paraformaldehyde in 0.15 M PBS, pH 7.3. Fixed tissue was embedded in paraffin. Mouse colon sections from the experimental groups were immunostained by a fluorescence method as previously described [45]. For the double fluorescence immunostaining, we used the following primary antibodies: CD3-T-cells (hamster anti-mouse, MCA1413 Serotec, Düsseldorf, Germany), CD68-macrophages (MCA1947 rat anti-mouse, Serotec, Düsseldorf, Germany), IL-1β, TNF-α (rabbit polyclonal, R&D Systems, Wiesbaden-Nordenstadt, Germany), NHE3 (rabbit polyclonal, Alpha Diagnostics, San Antonio, TX, USA), PDZK1 (M-16, sc-27289, goat polyclonal anti-mouse, Santa Cruz Biotechnology, Santa Cruz, CA, USA) and NHERF1 (rabbit polyclonal, Ab5199) and NHERF2 (rabbit polyclonal, Ab2170) (kindly provided by Prof. Chris Yun, Emory University, Atlanta, GA, USA). The primary antibodies were detected using species-specific secondary antibodies conjugated to the green fluorescent Cy2 and the red fluorescent dye Cy3 (MoBiTec, Göttingen, Germany), and by a counterstaining with 4′,6-diamidino-2-phenylindole (DAPI) in the mounting medium (Vectashield Mounting Medium with DAPI, Vector Laboratories, Burlingame, CA, USA).

Densitometric Measurements

In order to verify possible changes in the densities of NHE3, NHERF2 and PDZK1 protein expression in the enterocytes of the colonic mucosa was densitometrically quantified. A computer-assisted method (cell P software, Olympus) using fluorescence illumination (filters for carbocyanine dyes Cy2 and Cy3) was employed using the BX61 upright microscope (Olympus Optical, Hamburg, Germany). After separation for each channel the mean fluorescence intensities per pixel of the protein expression ranged between 8 and 85 for all epithelial cells (n = 4 in each group) after subtraction of background staining. The protein expression data were expressed from 9–23 epithelial cells in each group in comparable cell areas with a sectioned nucleus.

In situ RT-PCR

Sections from the colonic mucosa of IL-$10^{-/-}$ and WT mice were fixed on the same 3-Chamber SuperFrost Plus™ slides and subjected to *in situ* reverse transcription polymerase chain reaction (*in situ* RT-PCR) gene expression analysis using a two-step protocol with reverse transcription and PCR amplification on a specific thermal cycler (PTC-200 Twin Tower DNA Engine, MJ Research, Waltham, MA, USA) as described in detail before [22]. Table S4 lists the primer sequences.

Statistical Analysis

Analyses of the *q*RT-PCR data and of the standard curve for the genes were performed using the Opticon Monitor v. 1.07 (MJ Research, Inc., Waltham, MA, USA). Statistical analyses were performed using the Prism analysis program (Graphpad, San Diego, CA, USA). Data were tested for significance using the unpaired Student's *t*-test with $p<0.05$ as the limit of significance. All data are expressed as means ± SEM (standard error of the means).

Supporting Information

Table S1 Gene expression profile of the proinflammatory cytokines IL-1β, TNF-α, IFN-γ, iNOS, the cell death marker procaspase 3 and NHE3 and the PDZ-adaptor proteins NHERF1, NHERF2 and PDZK1 in the colonic mucosa of WT and IL-$10^{-/-}$ SPF mice.

Table S2 Gene expression profile of the proinflammatory cytokines IL-1β, TNF-α, IFN-γ and iNOS and the cell death marker procaspase 3 and the transporter and adaptor proteins NHE3, PDZK1, NHERF1 and NHERF2 in the colonic mucosa of control and DSS treated mice.

Table S3 *q*RT-PCR primer sequences.

Table S4 *In situ* RT-PCR primer sequences.

Acknowledgments

We gratefully acknowledge the technical assistance of Janina Bonhagen and Dagmar Lischke. The work was performed in part towards the fulfillment of the HBRS StrucMed thesis for the doctorate in medicine of Maria Lünnemann. We thank Brigitte Riederer for helpful discussions.

Author Contributions

Conceived and designed the experiments: HL US AJ. Performed the experiments: HL ML AJ. Analyzed the data: HL US AJ. Contributed reagents/materials/analysis tools: AB US MPM AJ. Wrote the paper: HL AJ. Assisted in writing: AB ML US MPM.

References

1. Podolsky DK (2002) Inflammatory bowel disease. N Engl J Med 347: 417–429.
2. Field M (2003) Intestinal ion transport and the pathophysiology of diarrhea. J Clin Invest 111: 931–943.
3. Rogler G, Andus T (1998) Cytokines in inflammatory bowel disease. World J Surg 22: 382–389.
4. Sanchez-Munoz F, Dominguez-Lopez A, Yamamoto-Furusho JK (2008) Role of cytokines in inflammatory bowel disease. World J Gastroenterol 14: 4280–4288.
5. Neurath MF, Fuss I, Pasparakis M, Alexopoulou L, Haralambous S, et al. (1997) Predominant pathogenic role of tumor necrosis factor in experimental colitis in mice. Eur J Immunol 27: 1743–1750.
6. Kollias G, Douni E, Kassiotis G, Kontoyiannis D (1999) The function of tumour necrosis factor and receptors in models of multi-organ inflammation, rheumatoid arthritis, multiple sclerosis and inflammatory bowel disease. Ann Rheum Dis 58 Suppl 1: I32–39.
7. Reimund JM, Wittersheim C, Dumont S, Muller CD, Baumann R, et al. (1996) Mucosal inflammatory cytokine production by intestinal biopsies in patients with ulcerative colitis and Crohn's disease. J Clin Immunol 16: 144–150.
8. Hanauer SB, Feagan BG, Lichtenstein GR, Mayer LF, Schreiber S, et al. (2002) Maintenance infliximab for Crohn's disease: the ACCENT I randomised trial. Lancet 359: 1541–1549.
9. Rutgeerts P, Sandborn WJ, Feagan BG, Reinisch W, Olson A, et al. (2005) Infliximab for induction and maintenance therapy for ulcerative colitis. N Engl J Med 353: 2462–2476.
10. Seidler U, Lenzen H, Cinar A, Tessema T, Bleich A, et al. (2006) Molecular mechanisms of disturbed electrolyte transport in intestinal inflammation. Ann N Y Acad Sci 1072: 262–275.
11. Schultheis PJ, Clarke LL, Meneton P, Miller ML, Soleimani M, et al. (1998) Renal and intestinal absorptive defects in mice lacking the NHE3 Na^+/H^+ exchanger. Nat Genet 19: 282–285.
12. Zachos NC, Tse M, Donowitz M (2005) Molecular physiology of intestinal Na^+/H^+ exchange. Annu Rev Physiol 67: 411–443.
13. Donowitz M, Li X (2007) Regulatory binding partners and complexes of NHE3. Physiol Rev 87: 825–872.
14. Lamprecht G, Seidler U (2006) The emerging role of PDZ adapter proteins for regulation of intestinal ion transport. Am J Physiol Gastrointest Liver Physiol 291: G766–777.
15. Seidler U, Singh A, Chen M, Cinar A, Bachmann O, et al. (2009) Knockout mouse models for intestinal electrolyte transporters and regulatory PDZ adaptors: new insights into cystic fibrosis, secretory diarrhoea and fructose-induced hypertension. Exp Physiol 94: 175–179.
16. Shenolikar S, Voltz JW, Cunningham R, Weinman EJ (2004) Regulation of ion transport by the NHERF family of PDZ proteins. Physiology (Bethesda) 19: 362–369.
17. Kühn R, Löhler J, Rennick D, Rajewsky K, Müller W (1993) Interleukin-10-deficient mice develop chronic enterocolitis. Cell 75: 263–274.
18. Cinar A, Chen M, Riederer B, Bachmann O, Wiemann M, et al. (2007) NHE3 inhibition by cAMP and $Ca2^+$ is abolished in PDZ-domain protein PDZK1-deficient murine enterocytes. J Physiol. 2007/03/31 ed. pp. 1235–1246.
19. Broere N, Chen M, Cinar A, Singh AK, Hillesheim J, et al. (2009) Defective jejunal and colonic salt absorption and altered Na(+)/H (+) exchanger 3 (NHE3) activity in NHE regulatory factor 1 (NHERF1) adaptor protein-deficient mice. Pflugers Arch 457: 1079–1091.
20. Berg DJ, Davidson N, Kühn R, Müller W, Menon S, et al. (1996) Enterocolitis and colon cancer in interleukin-10-deficient mice are associated with aberrant cytokine production and CD4(+) TH1-like responses. J Clin Invest 98: 1010–1020.
21. Rennick DM, Fort MM, Davidson NJ (1997) Studies with IL-$10^{-/-}$ mice: an overview. J Leukoc Biol 61: 389–396.
22. Jörns A, Günther A, Hedrich HJ, Wedekind D, Tiedge M, et al. (2005) Immune cell infiltration, cytokine expression, and beta-cell apoptosis during the development of type 1 diabetes in the spontaneously diabetic LEW.1AR1/Ztm-*iddm* rat. Diabetes 54: 2041–2052.
23. Bell EB, Westermann J (2008) CD4 memory T cells on trial: immunological memory without a memory T cell. Trends Immunol 29: 405–411.
24. Uno S, Imagawa A, Okita K, Sayama K, Moriwaki M, et al. (2007) Macrophages and dendritic cells infiltrating islets with or without beta cells produce tumour necrosis factor-alpha in patients with recent-onset type 1 diabetes. Diabetologia 50: 596–601.
25. Davidson NJ, Hudak SA, Lesley RE, Menon S, Leach MW, et al. (1998) IL-12, but not IFN-gamma, plays a major role in sustaining the chronic phase of colitis in IL-10-deficient mice. J Immunol 161: 3143–3149.
26. Dinarello CA (2009) Immunological and inflammatory functions of the interleukin-1 family. Annu Rev Immunol 27: 519–550.
27. Kolios G, Valatas V, Ward SG (2004) Nitric oxide in inflammatory bowel disease: a universal messenger in an unsolved puzzle. Immunology 113: 427–437.
28. Gratz R, Becker S, Sokolowski N, Schumann M, Bass D, et al. (2002) Murine monoclonal anti-TNF antibody administration has a beneficial effect on inflammatory bowel disease that develops in IL-10 knockout mice. Dig Dis Sci 47: 1723–1727.
29. Lohi H, Makela S, Pulkkinen K, Hoglund P, Karjalainen-Lindsberg ML, et al. (2002) Upregulation of CFTR expression but not SLC26A3 and SLC9A3 in ulcerative colitis. Am J Physiol Gastrointest Liver Physiol 283: G567–575.
30. Yang H, Jiang W, Furth EE, Wen X, Katz JP, et al. (1998) Intestinal inflammation reduces expression of DRA, a transporter responsible for congenital chloride diarrhea. Am J Physiol 275: G1445–1453.
31. Siddique I, Hasan F, Khan I (2009) Suppression of Na^+/H^+ exchanger isoform-3 in human inflammatory bowel disease: lack of reversal by 5′-aminosalicylate treatment. Scand J Gastroenterol 44: 56–64.
32. Sullivan S, Alex P, Dassopoulos T, Zachos NC, Iacobuzio-Donahue C, et al. (2009) Downregulation of sodium transporters and NHERF proteins in IBD patients and mouse colitis models: potential contributors to IBD-associated diarrhea. Inflamm Bowel Dis 15: 261–274.
33. Yeruva S, Farkas K, Hubricht J, Rode K, Riederer B, et al. (2009) Preserved Na(+)/H(+) exchanger isoform 3 expression and localization, but decreased NHE3 function indicate regulatory sodium transport defect in ulcerative colitis. Inflamm Bowel Dis 16: 1149–1161.
34. Heller F, Florian P, Bojarski C, Richter J, Christ M, et al. (2005) Interleukin-13 is the key effector Th2 cytokine in ulcerative colitis that affects epithelial tight junctions, apoptosis, and cell restitution. Gastroenterology 129: 550–564.
35. Mankertz J, Schulzke JD (2007) Altered permeability in inflammatory bowel disease: pathophysiology and clinical implications. Curr Opin Gastroenterol 23: 379–383.
36. Gawenis LR, Stien X, Shull GE, Schultheis PJ, Woo AL, et al. (2002) Intestinal NaCl transport in NHE2 and NHE3 knockout mice. Am J Physiol Gastrointest Liver Physiol 282: G776–784.
37. Murtazina R, Kovbasnjuk O, Zachos NC, Li X, Chen Y, et al. (2007) Tissue-specific regulation of sodium/proton exchanger isoform 3 activity in Na(+)/H(+) exchanger regulatory factor 1 (NHERF1) null mice. cAMP inhibition is differentially dependent on NHERF1 and exchange protein directly activated by cAMP in ileum versus proximal tubule. J Biol Chem 282: 25141–25151.
38. Lin S, Yeruva S, He P, Singh AK, Zhang H, et al. (2010) Lysophosphatidic acid stimulates the intestinal brush border Na(+)/H(+) exchanger 3 and fluid absorption via LPA(5) and NHERF2. Gastroenterology 138: 649–658.
39. Hillesheim J, Riederer B, Tuo B, Chen M, Manns M, et al. (2007) Down regulation of small intestinal ion transport in PDZK1- (CAP70/NHERF3) deficient mice. Pflugers Arch 454: 575–586.
40. Farkas K, Yeruva S, Rakonczay Z Jr, Ludolph L, Molnar T, et al. (2011) New therapeutic targets in ulcerative colitis: the importance of ion transporters in the human colon. Inflamm Bowel Dis 17: 884–898.
41. Ukena SN, Singh A, Dringenberg U, Engelhardt R, Seidler U, et al. (2007) Probiotic Escherichia coli Nissle 1917 inhibits leaky gut by enhancing mucosal integrity. PLoS One 2: e1308.
42. Nicklas W, Baneux P, Boot R, Decelle T, Deeny AA, et al. (2002) Recommendations for the health monitoring of rodent and rabbit colonies in breeding and experimental units. Lab Anim 36: 20–42.
43. de Buhr MF, Mahler M, Geffers R, Hansen W, Westendorf AM, et al. (2006) Cd14, Gbp1, and Pla2g2a: three major candidate genes for experimental IBD identified by combining QTL and microarray analyses. Physiol Genomics 25: 426–434.
44. Bachmann O, Rossmann H, Berger UV, Colledge WH, Ratcliff R, et al. (2003) cAMP-mediated regulation of murine intestinal/pancreatic $Na^+/HCO3$-cotransporter subtype pNBC1. Am J Physiol Gastrointest Liver Physiol 284: G37–45.
45. Arndt T, Wedekind D, Weiss H, Tiedge M, Lenzen S, et al. (2009) Prevention of spontaneous immune-mediated diabetes development in the LEW.1AR1-*iddm* rat by selective CD8+ T cell transfer is associated with a cytokine shift in the pancreas-draining lymph nodes. Diabetologia 52: 1381–1390.

IL-17A Signaling in Colonic Epithelial Cells Inhibits Pro-Inflammatory Cytokine Production by Enhancing the Activity of ERK and PI3K

Xiaoqin Guo[1,2], Xingwei Jiang[1], Yan Xiao[3], Tingting Zhou[1], Yueling Guo[4], Renxi Wang[1], Zhi Zhao[1], He Xiao[1], Chunmei Hou[1], Lingyun Ma[3], Yanhua Lin[1], Xiaoling Lang[1], Jiannan Feng[1], Guojiang Chen[1]*, Beifen Shen[1], Gencheng Han[1]*, Yan Li[1]

1 Department of Molecular Immunology, Beijing Institute of Basic Medical Sciences, Beijing, China, **2** Department of Immunology, Logistics College of Chinese People's Armed Police Forces, Tianjin, China, **3** Department of Respiratory Medicine, First Affiliated Hospital of the Chinese PLA General Hospital, Beijing, China, **4** Department of Medical Engineering, Military General Hospital of Beijing PLA, Beijing, China

Abstract

Our previous data suggested that IL-17A contributes to the inhibition of Th1 cell function in the gut. However, the underlying mechanisms remain unclear. Here we demonstrate that IL-17A signaling in colonic epithelial cells (CECs) increases TNF-α-induced PI3K-AKT and ERK phosphorylation and inhibits TNF-α induced expression of IL-12P35 and of a Th1 cell chemokine, CXCL11 at mRNA level. In a co-culture system using HT-29 cells and PBMCs, IL-17A inhibited TNF-âinduced IL-12P35 expression by HT-29 cells and led to decreased expression of IFN-γ and T-bet by PBMCs. Finally, adoptive transfer of CECs from mice with Crohn's Disease (CD) led to an enhanced Th1 cell response and exacerbated colitis in CD mouse recipients. The pathogenic effect of CECs derived from CD mice was reversed by co-administration of recombinant IL-17A. Our data demonstrate a new IL-17A-mediated regulatory mechanism in CD. A better understanding of this pathway might shed new light on the pathogenesis of CD.

Editor: Emiko Mizoguchi, Massachusetts General Hospital, United States of America

Funding: This work was supported by a National "973" Fund (grant number 2013CB530506), and the National Natural Sciences Foundation of China (grants 81072475, 81172800, and 31100961). The funders had no role in study design, data collection and analysis, decision to publish, or preparation of the manuscript.

Competing Interests: The authors have declared that no competing interests exist.

* E-mail: genchenghan@163.com (GH); guogangch@yahoo.com. (GC)

These authors contributed equally to this work.

Introduction

Crohn's disease (CD) and ulcerative colitis (UC) are two forms of inflammatory bowel disease (IBD) in man. The etiology of IBD remains unclear, but evidence indicates that it results from an interaction between genetic and environmental factors, which eventually lead to an excessive and poorly controlled mucosal inflammatory response directed against components of the normal microflora and mucosal constituents of the gut [1–2]. Studies over the last 2–3 decades have shown that different T cell differentiation patterns determine disease progression [3–4]. For example, it is known that CD is linked to a predominantly T helper cell (Th1) immune response (e.g., secretion of IFN-γ, TNF-α, and IL-12). Accordingly, therapeutic strategies targeting these cytokines have been widely investigated. Antibody against TNF-α attenuates colitis in IBD patients, but more than one third of IBD patients do not respond to anti-TNF-α therapy [5-6]. These observations suggest the need to identify novel targets for therapeutic intervention in IBD.

In addition to the classical Th1/Th2 pathways, a new pathway, the Th17 pathway, has been discovered as a result of the identification of a novel CD4 T cell subset, the Th17 cell [7]. It is now known that IL-17A has pro-inflammatory effects on a wide range of cellular targets, such as epithelium, endothelium, and monocytes/macrophages [8–10], and plays pathogenic roles in some organ-specific autoimmune diseases, such as rheumatoid arthritis (RA) and multiple sclerosis, as well as IBD [11]. Because of this, the therapeutic effects of an IL-17 neutralizing antibody, secukinumab (AIN457T), in RA are now being evaluated in phase II clinical trials [12]. As regards IBD, IL-17A is produced in the healthy gut, but high IL-17A mRNA expression is seen in inflamed colonic mucosa [13-14], suggesting a pathogenic role of IL-17A in the progression of IBD. Accordingly, IL-17A has been examined as a target for reducing autoimmune damage in IBD [15]. Unfortunately, clinical trials targeting IL-17A in IBD failed to show an effect, indicating that further studies are needed on its role in IBD.

It is now known that there is a complex and active interplay between IL-17A and colonic epithelial cells (CECs) during the progression of IBD. After stimulation by IL-17A, CECs release a wide range of pro-inflammatory cytokines and chemokines, e.g., CXCL8 for neutrophil chemotaxis and CCL20 to attract Th17 cells, further amplifying the gut inflammation [16]. On the other hand, IL-17A also has protective effects on the gut epithelial barrier, e.g., by upregulating the expression of antimicrobial peptides [17]. Recent data have also shown that IL-17A, by directly binding to its receptor (IL-17R) expressed on Th1 cells, inhibits Th1 cell-mediated colonic inflammation [18].Together, these data suggest that IL-17A plays both a pro-inflammatory and an anti-inflammatory role in IBD, which might explain the failure of the clinical trial targeting IL-17A. To explore more effective intervention strategies, the mechanisms by which IL-17A mediates its pathogenic or protective effects, especially the latter, need to be investigated.

In most target cells, IL-17A signaling activates the MAPK and NF-κB pathways through IL-17RA and increases the expression of inflammatory cytokines [16]. Act1 has been identified as an essential adaptor molecule in IL-17 signaling [19]. In addition, the results of a microarray screen suggested the involvement of the CCAAT/enhancer binding protein transcription factors C/EBPβ and C/EBPδ in the IL-17A-induced signaling cascade [20], while another report showed that the PI3K pathway is involved in IL-17A signaling, mainly in an Act1-independent manner [21], but the underlying mechanisms remain largely unclear. Further investigation of the signaling mechanisms of IL-17A will shed light on its biological functions and help in understanding and treating inflammatory diseases.

Our previous data suggested that IL-17A signaling inhibited the function of Th1 cell in IBD [22]. However, the underlying mechanisms remain largely unclear. Although some data suggest that IL-17A suppresses the development of colonic inflammation by directly inhibiting the differentiation of Th1 cells [18], we argue that other mechanisms may exist, since IL-17A binds to multiple target cells and stimulates complex intracellular cascades. In this study, CECs were used as the target for IL-17A and we demonstrated, for the first time, that IL-17A signaling in CECs can also trigger anti-inflammatory mechanisms by activating the PI3K-AKT and ERK-CEBP/β pathways in an Act1-dependent manner, finally leading to inhibition of TNF-α-induced expression of IL-12P35 and of a Th1 cell chemokine, CXCL11, and of Th1 cell function. This is the first report demonstrating the involvement of the Act1-PI3K-AKT pathway in the IL-17A-triggered signaling cascade. Further investigation of this pathway should shed new light on therapeutic strategies against many IL-17A–related clinical diseases

Materials and Methods

Cell culture and gene expression

HT-29 human colorectal cancer cells (ATCC) were cultured in McCoy's 5A medium (ATCC) supplemented with 10% fetal bovine serum (FBS), penicillin (10 U/ml), and streptomycin (10 μg/ml) (all from Sigma-Aldrich). For tests, they were plated in 12-well plates at a density of 3×10^5 cells per well in McCoy's 5A medium containing 10% FBS and antibiotics. Before cytokine treatment, the cells were incubated overnight in McCoy's 5A medium containing 0.5% FBS and antibiotics, then were incubated for 6 h with different dose of TNF-α (R & D Systems) and/or of IL-17 (eBiosciences, San Diego, CA). Here 0.5 ng/ml of TNF-α (suboptimal dose from which we can see the effects of IL-17A) and/or 50 ng/ml of IL-17 were used for in vitro cell stimulation. The cells were then harvested and RNA prepared using Trizol reagent (Invitrogen). RNA samples (2 μg) were then reverse-transcribed with Moloney murine leukemia virus reverse transcriptase (New England Biolabs) and real-time PCR performed using SYBR Green (TOYOBO) and a standard curve for quantization, as described previously [23].

The relative expression of cytokine mRNAs was evaluated by real-time PCR. The real-time PCR reaction mixture consisted of 10 μl of 2×SYBR green Master Mix, 0.5 μl of 10 pM primers, and 2 μl of cDNA in a total volume of 20 μl. The thermal cycling conditions were an initial denaturation step at 95°C for 3 min; 40 cycles at 95°C for 10 s, annealing at 60°C for 15 s, and extension at 72°C for 10 s; and 71 cycles at 60°C for 30s. The sequences of the primers used, produced by Assays-by-Design Service for Gene Expression Assays (Biomics Biotechnologies Co. Ltd., China), are listed in Table 1. At the end of the PCR cycles, the specificity of the amplification products was checked by dissociation curve analysis. mRNA levels in each sample were determined using the gene-specific threshold cycle (Ct) for each sample (ΔCt) corrected by subtracting the Ct for the GAPDH housekeeping gene. Untreated controls were used as the reference samples and the ΔCt for all experimental samples was subtracted from the ΔCt for the control samples (ΔΔCt). The magnitude of the change in levels of the test gene mRNA was expressed as 2-ΔΔCt. Each measurement was performed in duplicate.

Western blots

Western blotting was performed to evaluate levels of ERK, AKT, phospho-ERK, phospho-AKT, phospho-C/EBPβ, PI3K p110γ, Act1, and GAPDH. Briefly, 30 ug of protein was electrophoretically separated on a 12% sodium dodecyl sulfate-polyacrylamide gel and transferred to a polyvinylidene difluoride membrane, which was then blocked by incubation for 1 h at room temperature in 5% fat-free dry milk in Tris-buffered saline containing 0.1% Tween 20 (TBST). The blots were then incubated overnight at 4°C with rabbit antibodies against human ERK (1:1000), AKT (1:1000), phospho-ERK (1:1000), phospho-AKT (1:1000), phospho-C/EBP(1:1000), or PI3K p110γ(1:1000) (Cell Signaling Technology, USA), rat antibodies against human Act1 (eBiosciences, San Diego, CA), or mouse antibodies against GAPDH (1:5000) (Tianjin Sungene Biotech Co. Ltd) diluted in TBST containing 5% BSA, washed for 25 min with TBST, and incubated for 1 h at room temperature with alkaline phosphatase-conjugated anti-rabbit, anti-mouse, or anti-rat IgG antibodies (KPL, Gaithersburg, MD, USA) (1:2000 in TBST containing 5% BSA).

Act1 gene knockdown in the HT-29 cell line

To directly examine whether Act1 was involved in the IL-17 signaling pathway, Act1 gene expression in HT-29 cells was

Table 1. Sequences of the primers used for real-time PCR.

	Forward primer	Reverse primer
hCXCL11	GAGGACGCTGTCTTTG	GATTTGGGATTTAGGC
hIL-12P35	ACCACTCCCAAAACCTGC	CCAGGCAACTCCCATTAG
hAct1	AACAAGGAAGCATGAATTTCAGA	ATTCTTGGGCCAGCTGTAGA
hPI3K-CG	CTGGAAAGAAGACAAGCCCA	TTAACTGGGGCATTCCTGTC
hIFN-γ	ACTGACTTGAATGTCCAACGCA	ATCTGACTCCTTTTTCGCTTCC
hT-bet	CCACCTGTTGTGGTCCAAGT	AACATCCAGTAGTGGCTGGTG
hCCL20	CTGGCTGCTTTGATGTCAGT	CGTGTGAAGCCCACAATAAA
hGAPDH	AACGGATTTGGTCGTATTG	GGAAGATGGTGATGGGATT
mIFN-γ	AAGCGTCATTGAATCACACCTG	TGACCTCAAACTTGGCAATACTC
mIL-12a	CGCAGCACTTCAGAATCACA	TCTCCCACAGGAGGTTTCTG
mCXCL11	AAGGTCACAGCCATAGCCCT	CATTTTGACGGCTTTCATC
mCCL20	CCAAGTCTTCTCAGCGCCAT	GAATCTTCCGGCTGTAGGAGAAG
mGAPDH	TCTTGGGCTACACTGAGGAC	CATACCAGGAAATGAGCTTGA

h indicates human and m mouse.

blocked using short-hair RNA (shRNA). Three non-overlapping shRNA duplexes (Biomics Biotechnologies Co. Ltd, China) were individually tested for maximal knockdown of gene expression. The duplex sequences were CCATAGACACGGGATATGA (shRNA1), CCCTGAAACTTGCAAATC A (shRNA2), CTGCAATTGACATATTTGA (shRNA3), and TTCTCCGAACGTGTCACGT. (negative control (NC)). These sequences were inserted into the pRNAT-U6.1/Neo vector, then the purified recombinant vectors were transfected into HT-29 cells using Lipofectamine 2000^{TM} (Invitrogen) according to the manufacturer's protocol. The shRNA duplex giving maximal knockdown was identified and HT-29 cell clones stably express Act1 shRNA selected using G418 (Gibco) and analyzed for Act1 expression by Western blotting and RT–PCR.

Co-culture of peripheral blood mononuclear cells and HT-29 colonic epithelial cells

HT-29 cells were plated in 24-well plates at a density of 1.5×10^5 cells/well in McCoy's 5A medium containing 10% FBS and antibiotics and incubated for 24 h, then were treated with IL-17 (50 ng/ml; eBiosciences) and/or TNF- α(0.5 ng/ml; eBiosciences) for 24 h. Human peripheral blood mononuclear cells (PBMCs) were isolated by density gradient centrifugation and added to the culture in a ratio of 1 HT-29 cells to 10 PBMCs. The co-cultures were then stimulated for 24 h by a combination of monoclonal antibodies (mAbs) against CD3 (3 μg/ml) and CD28 (3 μg/ml) (eBiosciences) with or without IL-12 (12.5 ng/ml; eBiosciences), then non-adherent PBMCs and adherent HT-29 cells were harvested separately for analysis. The human PBMC used in this study have been described in our previous publication [22], and the study protocol was approved by the Ethics Committee of the General Hospital of the Air Force of the PLA, Beijing, China.

Induction of colitis in mice

Balb/C mice were originally obtained from the Jackson Laboratory, and bred in our facilities under specific pathogen-free conditions. The care, use, and treatment of mice in this study were in strict compliance with the guidelines for the care and use of laboratory animals of the Institute of Basic Medical Sciences, Beijing. The protocol was approved by the Committee on the Ethics of Animal Experiments of the Beijing Institute of Basic Medical Sciences (Permit Number: AMMS2012-0136). All surgery was performed under sodium pentobarbital anesthesia, and all efforts were made to minimize suffering. To induce colitis, 6- 8-week-old male mice were intrarectally injected with 0.2 mg of the hapten reagent 2, 4, 6-trinitrobenzene sulfonic acid (TNBS) (Sigma) in 50% ethanol as previously described [24–25]. In control experiments, mice received 50% ethanol alone. The total injection volume was 100 μl in both groups.

Anti-IL-17A antibody injection

To test the effect of anti-IL-17A antibody on TNBS--induced colitis, mice were injected intraperitoneally with 100 μg of anti-IL-17 mAb or the same amount of same isotype IgG (Tianjin Sungene Biotech Co. Ltd) on days 1, 3, 5, and 7, and the mice were weighed daily and checked for tissue injury.

Cell isolation and adoptive transfer

The isolation procedure for the mouse colonic epithelial cells (CEC) and colonic lymphocytes in this study has been described previously [26]. In brief, the muscle layer of the mouse colon was removed with forceps and the whole colon opened longitudinally and cut into sections approximately 0.5 cm long, which were then placed in a 150 ml conical flask containing 20 ml of 15 mM HEPES, 5 mM EDTA, 10% FBS, and 100 μg/ml of gentamycin and incubated at 37°C with shaking for 30 min. The sample was then filtered at room temperature through a 200 mesh filter, then the filtrates from three collections were combined and centrifuged at 850 g for 10 min at 37°C and the pellets (CECs) resuspended in phosphate-buffered saline (PBS). For the collection of lymphocytes from colonic lamina propria, colon tissue removed of CECs was further incubated with collagenase D (Roche) (0.6 mg/ml) in 20 ml RPMI-1640 medium at 37°C for about 3 hours. Finally, samples were filtered at room temperature through a 200 mesh filter, then the filtrates from three collections were combined and centrifuged at 850 g for 10 min at 37°C and the pellets (lymphocytes) resuspended in phosphate-buffered saline (PBS). For transfer assay, CECs (1×10^6 cells/mouse) from TNBS-induced colitis or control mice isolated on day 8 of TNBS treatment were injected into the peritoneum of previously untreated mice on day 1 of TNBS induction of colitis and again on day 4, then the mice were sacrificed on day 8. To test the in vivo effect of IL-17A on the activity of transferred CECs from these TNBS-induced colitis mice were injected intraperitoneally with mouse recombinant IL-17 (eBiosciences, San Diego, CA) at a dose of 500 ng/mouse on days 1,3,5 and 7 of induction of TNBS-colitis.

Flow cytometry

For staining for IL-17RA, CECs were collected from TNBS-induced colitis mice or control mice, and then were stained with phycoerythrin (PE)-conjugated anti-mouse IL-17RA antibodies (Biolegends). For staining IFN-r within $CD4^{+}T$ cells and IL-12 within monocytes/macrophage, cells were stimulated for 4 h with 50 ng/ml of phorbol 12-myristate 13-acetate, 1 μg/ml of ionomycin, and 1 μg/ml of brefeldin A (Sigma, St Louis, MO), then were washed and stained with fluorescein isothiocyanate (FITC)-conjugated anti-human CD4, anti-mouse CD4, anti-human CD14 or anti-mouse CD11b, then fixed for overnight with Fix/Perm buffer, washed with permeabilization buffer, stained for 30 min at 4°C with PE-conjugated anti-human IFN-γ, anti-mouse IFN-γ, anti-human IL-12P70 and anti-mouse IL-P70 antibodies(all from eBioscience) and analyzed on a FACSca-libur flow cytometer.

Histopathological analysis

For histopathological analysis, a specimen from the middle part of the colon was fixed in 10% phosphate-buffered formalin, embedded in paraffin, and sectioned and the sections stained with hematoxylin-eosin (H&E).

Mouse whole colon cultures

Colon tissue (200–300 mg) was washed in cold PBS containing penicillin and streptomycin and cut into small pieces (0.5×0.5 cm), which were cultured (three pieces per mouse) in 24-well flat bottom culture plates in serum-free RPMI 1640 medium (Gibco) at 37°C for 24 h. The culture supernatants were then centrifuged at 9000 g at 4°C for 5 min and stored at –80°C until use.

ELISA

The concentration of IFN-γ and IL-12P70 in mouse serum was measured using a sandwich ELISA according to the manufacturer's protocol (eBiosciences, San Diego, CA).

Statistical analysis

All data are presented as the mean±SD. Statistical analysis was performed using one way or two-way ANOVA. p values less than 0.05 were considered significant.

Results

IL-17A signaling in human HT-29 colonic epithelia cells inhibits TNF-α-induced expression of CXCL11 and IL-12P35 mRNA by enhancing phosphorylation of AKT, ERK, and CEBP/β

We previously found that levels of IL-17A mRNA and protein are increased and Th1 cell function decreased in patients with IBD [22]. In the present study, to test whether, and if so, how the increased IL-17A expression was responsible for inhibition of Th1 cell function in IBD, we used the human colonic epithelial cell line HT-29 cells, as we have found that the expression of IL-17A in and IL-17R on CEC cells is significantly increased in mice with TNBS-induced colitis, which is an animal model of Crohn's disease (CD). IL-17A alone had little effect on the activity of HT-29 cells, so we examined its synergistic effects with TNF-α. Treatment of HT-29 cells with IL-17A inhibited the TNF-α-induced increase in expression of mRNAs coding for CXCL11 (Fig. 1B) and IL-12P35 (Fig. 1C), two factors promoting Th1 cell function. We then examined how IL-17A signaling affected the TNF-α-induced activation of CECs. Our data showed that IL-17A signaling enhanced TNF-α induced phosphorylation of ERK (Fig. 1D), AKT (Fig. 1E), and CEBP/β (Fig. 1F). These data show that IL-17A signaling triggers intracellular cascades, which affect TNF-α-induced cytokine production.

To further characterize the intracellular cascades involved in IL-17A-induced negative regulation of TNFα-induced CXCL11 and IL-12P35 mRNA expression, specific inhibitors of ERK (U0126) or PI3K-AKT (wortmannin) were added for 30 minutes before and during cytokine treatment. As shown in Fig. 2, blockade of either ERK or PI3K blocked the inhibitory effect of IL-17A on TNF-α-induced CXCL11 or IL-12P35 mRNA expression. These data show that the ERK and PI3K-AKT pathways play essential roles in IL-17A-mediated negative regulation. We did not examine the effects of CEBP/β blockade on IL-17A mediated negative regulation, as no inhibitor is currently available.

Act1 is involved in the IL-17A-induced enhancement of the TNF-α-induced phosphorylation of ERK and AKT, and Act1 knockdown prevents IL-17A-induced inhibition of the TNF-α-induced increase in CXCL11 and IL-12P35 mRNA expression

Act1 (an activator of NF-κB) is an essential adaptor molecule in IL-17 signaling [19]. To examine whether Act1 was also involved in IL-17A-mediated negative regulation in CECs, Act1 stable knock down HT-29 cells were established. Silencing of Act1 led to decreased expression of Act1 at both the mRNA (Fig. 3A) and protein (Fig. 3B) level. In Act1 knockdown cells, IL-17A signaling failed to enhance TNF-induced phosphorylation of ERK (Fig. 3C) and AKT (Fig. 3D), showing that Act1 is involved in the IL-17A-induced phosphorylation of ERK and AKT. In contrast, Act1 knockdown did not significantly affect IL-17A-induced phosphorylation of CEBP/β (data not shown), suggesting that CEBP/β might be regulated by multiple signaling cascades. However, when HT-29 cells were incubated with the ERK inhibitor U026, IL-17A signaling failed to enhance the TNF-induced phosphorylation of CEBP/β(Fig. 3E), indicating that ERK is an upstream activator of CEBP/β.The band intensity analysis data clearly showed that Act1 is involved in the IL-17A-induced phosphorylation of ERK and AKT, and that ERK plays a role in IL-17A enhanced TNF-a induced phosphorylation of CEBP/β (Fig. 3F). Finally, the effects of Act1 knockdown on IL-17A-mediated negative regulation were examined and the data showed that Act1 knockdown blocked IL-17A-induced inhibition of TNFα-induced increase in CXCL11 (Fig. 3G) and IL-12P35 (Fig.3H) mRNA expression. These data show that Act1 is involved in IL-17A-induced enhancement of TNF-α-induced phosphorylation of ERK and PI3K-AKT and for IL-17A-mediated negative regulation.

Act1 knockdown decreases the expression of PI3K-cat-gamma and identifies a new pathway (IL-17A-Act1-PI3KIB-AKT) of IL-17A-mediated negative regulation in CECs

To investigate the mechanisms by which IL-17A induced negative regulation, microarray analysis was carried out. About 200 differentially expressed genes were present in the knockdown line compared to controls. Of these, expression of chemokines, such as CXCL1 and CXCL2, and cytokines, such as TNF-α, was found to be decreased by more than two-fold in Act1 knockdown HT-29 cells compared to control cells (Fig. 4A); these genes covered a wide range of cellular functions, such as macrophage recruitment. However, we were intrigued by the unexpected finding that PI3K-cat gamma (one subunit of PI3K- IB) expression was more than two-fold lower in Act1 knockdown HT-29 cells and this was confirmed by real-time PCR (Fig. 4B) and Western blotting (Fig. 4C). Notably, we found that IL-17A signaling in the absence of TNF-α increased PI3K-CG expression in control HT-29 cells, but not in Act1 knockdown cells. These data suggest that IL-17A signaling might induce phosphorylation of AKT by increasing PI3K-CG expression, a process dependent on Act1.

IL-17A negatively regulates Th1 cell activity in a human CEC and PBMC co-culture system

The above data demonstrated that IL-17A signaling inhibits TNF-α-induced mRNA expression of CXCL11 and IL-12P35. To further explore the possible effects of IL-17A signaling, we used an HT-29 cell and human PBMC co-culture system with or without addition of IL-17A. Firstly, human PBMCs were stimulated with anti-human CD3 and CD28 antibodies in the absence or presence of IL-17A and/or TNF-α. We found that recombinant IL-17A did not significantly affect the expression of IL-12P35 mRNA induced by TNF-α (data not shown). Secondly, HT-29 cells were incubated in the presence of IL-17A and/or TNF-α for 24 h, then human PBMCs were added and stimulated with anti-human CD3 and CD28 antibodies for another 24 h, then the non-adherent human PBMCs and adherent HT-29 cells were collected separately and analyzed for gene expression. Our data showed that TNF-α-induced IL-12P35 expression in the isolated adherent HT-29 cells was inhibited by IL-17A (Fig. 5A). And that expression of T-bet, a Th1 cell transcriptional factor, in the non-adherent PBMCs was significantly downregulated in the IL-17A/TNF-α-treated group compared to the TNF-α-treated group, a phenomenon can be reversed by adding recombinant IL-12 p70(Fig. 5B). Flow cytometry analysis examining the IFN-γ expression within CD4+ T cells showed the same tendency as that of T-bet (Fig. 5C). These data indicated that IL-17A signaling on HT-29 cells inhibited TNF-α induced Th1 cells function in the co-culture system, in which IL-12 plays an important role. It is known that bioactive form of IL-12 is IL-12 p70 (hetero dimer with p40 and p35). As there is no detectable IL-12P70 secretion in the supernatant and

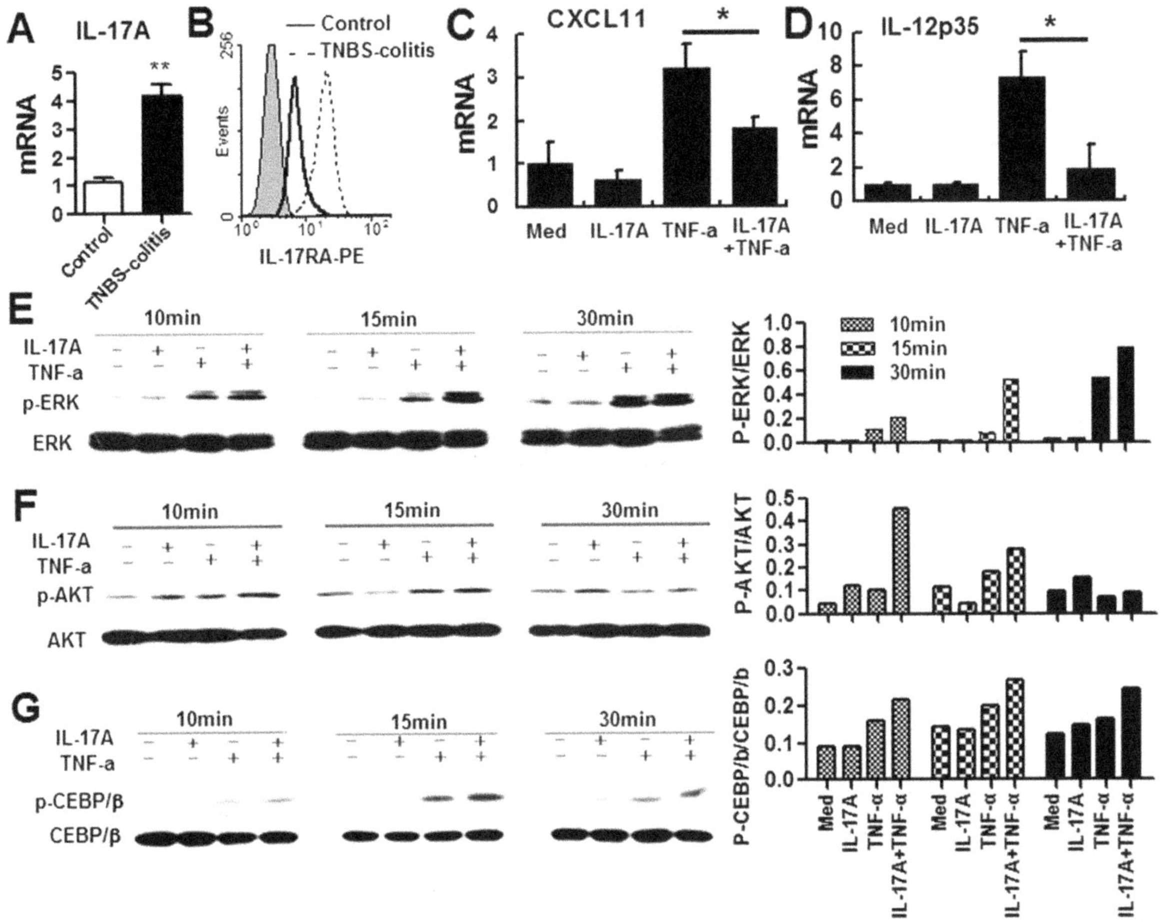

Figure 1. Effects of IL-17A signaling on TNF-α-induced HT-29 cell activation and the intracellular mechanisms. (A&B) CECs were collected from mice as described in the material and methods, and then expressions of IL-17A in and IL-17RA on CECs were examined using real time-PCR(A) or Flow cytometry analysis(B). (C and D) HT-29 cells were stimulated with recombinant IL-17A and/or TNF-a for 6h, then CXCL11 (C) and IL-12P35 (D) mRNA levels were examined by real-time PCR. (E-G) HT-29 cells were treated as above, but for 10 to 30 min, then were examined for the phosphorylation of ERK (E), PI3K-AKT (G), or CEBP/β (G). Band intensity data were shown as well. The results shown are representative of those obtained in three independent experiments.

there is no detectable IL-12p35 protein expression within adherent HT-29 cells, the possible source of IL-12 protein were then investigated. Our data showed that IL-17A inhibited TNF-α induced IL-12 protein expression (p70) by CD14+monocytes in the co-culture system (Fig. 5D). These in vitro data again indicated that IL-17A signaling on HT-29 cells may indirectly affect Th1 cell activity by altering the IL-12 expression by monocytes. However, the underlying mechanisms by which IL-17A negatively regulates Th1 cell activity in a human CEC and PBMC co-culture system remain to be investigated.

IL-17A blockade in vivo leads to exacerbated TNBS colitis and enhanced Th1 related gene/protein expression

To further examine the axis by which IL-17 mediates negative regulation through CEC cells, in vivo IL-17A neutralization was performed by injection of anti-IL-17A antibody on days 1, 3, 5, and 7 during induction of TNBS-induced colitis and the effects on the activity of CECs examined. Physical and histopathological examination of colon tissue revealed marked tissue injury and infiltration of inflammatory cells in TNBS colitis mice receiving anti-IL-17A antibody (Fig. 6A). IL-17A neutralization enhanced the mRNA expression of CXCL11, IL-12P35, and IFN-γ in splenocytes CECs (data not shown), indicating that neutralization of IL-17A in CD can systemically affect the activity of Th1 cells. It is worthy to note that IL-17A neutralization also enhanced the mRNA expression of CXCL11, IL-12P35, and IFN-γ in CECs (Fig. 6B), showing that CECs are important target for IL-17A mediated regulatory effects.

Adoptive transfer of CECs derived from TNBS-induced mice exacerbates colitis in mice, which can be inhibited by co-transfer of IL-17

Finally, CECs isolated from mice on day 8 of TNBS-induced colitis were transferred alone or together with recombinant IL-17A into previously untreated mice on days 1 and 4 of induction of TNBS-induced colitis to examine 1) possible roles of CECs in the pathogenesis of CD and 2) whether IL-17A can trigger anti-inflammatory mechanisms in CECs, thus blocking their pathogenic roles in vivo. Adoptively transferred CECs from TNBS-induced colitis mice exacerbated tissue damage (Fig. 7A) and led to increased mRNA expression of CXCL11, IL-12P35, and IFN-γmRNA by CECs of the recipient mice of TNBS colitis mice (Fig. 7B). In addition, transfer of CECs from colitogenic mice into mice without TNBS treatment is associated with an increase of Th1-

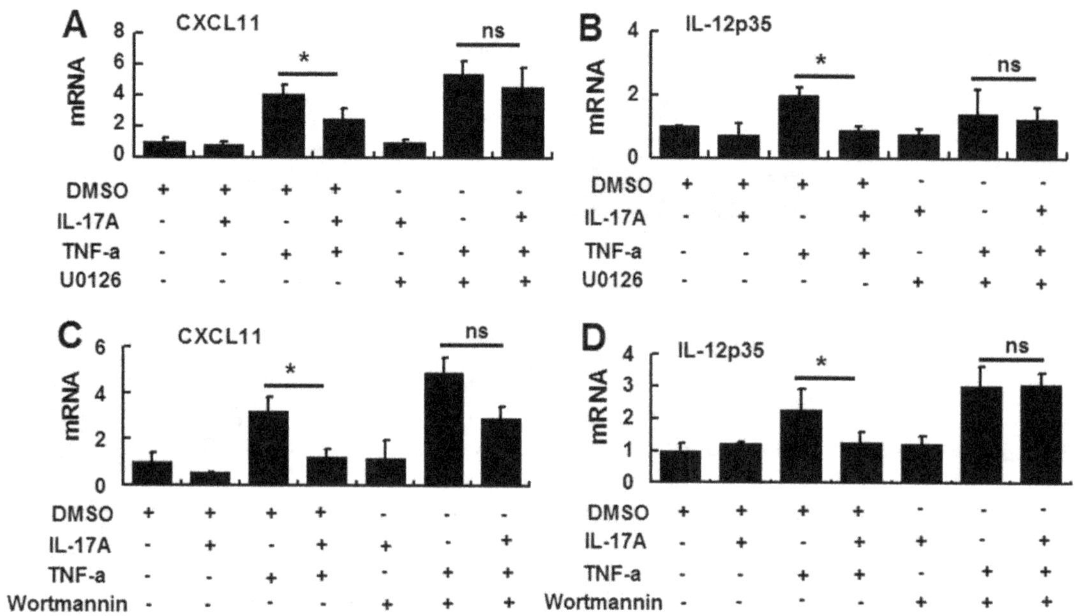

Figure 2. Effects of an ERK or PI3K inhibitor on IL-17A signaling-mediated negative regulation in HT-29 cells. HT-29 cells were incubated with or without an inhibitor specific for ERK(U0126) or PI3K(wortmannin) or DMSO (vehicle control) for 30 min, then IL-17A and/or TNF-α was added and the cells incubated for 6 h in the continued presence of the inhibitor. The cells were then examined for CXCL11 and IL-12P35 expression by real-time PCR. The results shown are representative of those obtained in three independent experiments. The bars are the SD.

related cytokines in comparison to mice transferred with CECs from non colitogenic mice (data not shown here). These data showed that CECs from colitogenic mice may affect the Th1 cell activity in vivo after injection. Interestingly, our data clearly showed that administration of IL-17A attenuated the ability of CECs from TNBS-induced colitis mice to induce colitis when transferred into recipients and decreased the expression of CXCL11, IL-12P35, and IFN-γ (Fig. 7B). To further investigate whether and how co administration of IL-17A with CECs affect Th1 cell activity in vivo, we firstly cultured colon tissues and found that colon tissues from TNBS-CECs injected mice produced more IL-12 and IFN-γ than those from Con-CECs injected controls, while co-administration of IL-17A with TNBS-CECs leads to decreased IL-12 and IFN-γ production (data not shown). Secondly, we isolated lamina propria cells and examined the expression of IL-12P70 by CD11b+F4/80+macrophage and of IFN-γ expression by $CD4^{+}T$ cells. Our data showed that transfer of CECs alone increased IL-12p70 expression by CD11b+F4/80+ macrophage from lamina propria cells. However, co administration of IL-17A with CECs reversed CECs transfer increased IL-12p70 expression by macrophage (Fig.7C). Co-administration of IL-17A lead to decreased IFN-γ expression within $CD4^{+}T$ cells (Fig.7D).These data suggested that TNBS-CECs injection with or without IL-17A affected local Th1 response, in which IL-12 might play an important role. Finally, we also examined how IL-17A signaling on CECs, following CECs and IL-17A i.p.injection, affect local Th1 response.

Discussion

IL-17A plays both pathogenic and protective roles in the progress of IBDs, but the mechanisms by which it mediates its protective effects remain largely unclear [27–29]. Here, we demonstrated that IL-17A signaling enhances the TNF-α-induced phosphorylation of the Act1-PI3K (IB)-AKT and Act1-ERK-CEBP/β pathways in CECs, finally inhibiting TNF-α-induced CXCL11 and IL-12P35 mRNA expression. Studies using our in vitro co-culture system and CEC adoptive transfer clearly demonstrated that IL-17A can act on CECs and trigger anti-inflammatory mechanisms against Th1 cells, thus contributing to colonic homeostasis.

Here CECs were selected as the target for IL-17A, as we previously found that, in mice with TNBS-induced colitis, expression of IL-17A in and IL-17RA on CECs was significantly increased (Fig.1A). Although the mechanisms for up-regulating IL-17A and IL-17R expression on CECs following CD remain to be determined, these data indicates that IL-17A/IL-17R pathway might be involved in the physiopathology of IBD. In addition, many reports suggest that, in inflammatory situations, CECs may also act as antigen-presenting cells in the local colonic immune response [30-31]. Here, we used a human CEC cell line, HT-29 cell, to investigate the mechanisms by which IL-17A mediated an anti-inflammatory response in CECs. This is the first report showing that IL-17A signaling inhibits the TNF-α-induced increase in IL-12P35 mRNA expression by CECs. Here CXCL11 is selected as it is reported that CXCL11 showed potent activity on activated T cells through selective high affinity binding to CXCR3 which is especially expressed on Th1 cells but not on Th2 cells [32-33]. And as an IFN-γ inducible chemokine, the effects of CXCL11 on Th1 cells can be amplified by IFN-γ, a Th1-related cytokine, as a positive feedback [33].

The biologic activity of IL-17A is dependent on a complex composed of IL-17RA and IL-17RC [34]. Here we did not investigate the roles of IL-17A receptor in IL-17A mediated anti-inflammatory effects. In fact, although there are many different reports demonstrating the oppose function of IL-17A [18,27-29,35], the roles of IL-17A receptor in IL-17A mediated pro-inflammatory and anti-inflammatory effects remain largely unclear.

We then focus on the intracellular mechanisms by which IL-17A signaling inhibits the TNF-a induced expression of IL-12 and

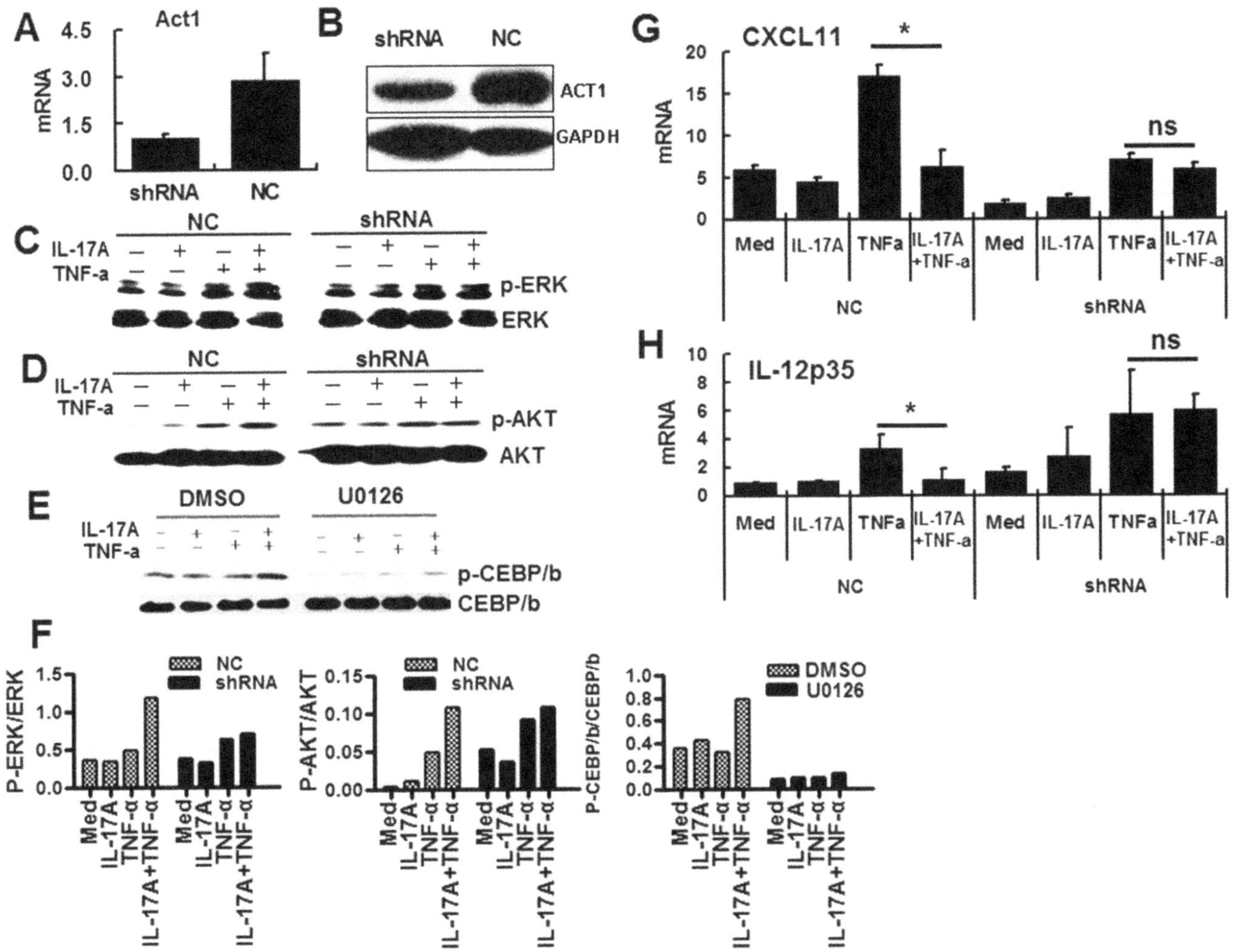

Figure 3. Roles of Act1 in IL-17A-mediated negative regulation in HT-29 cells. (A and B) An Act1 stable knockdown HT-29 cell line was established as described in the Materials and Methods and silencing of Act1 confirmed by real-time PCR (A) and Western blotting (B). (C and D) Act1 knock down or control HT-29 cells were treated with IL-17A and/or TNF-α for 15 min, then cells were examined for phosphorylation of ERK (C) or PI3K-AKT (D) by Western blotting. (E) HT-29 cells were treated with IL-17A and/or TNF-α for 15 min in the presence or absence of the ERK inhibitor, U026, then were lysed and examined for the phosphorylation of CEBP/β. The band intensity data for above western blot assay were shown in F. (G and H) Act1 knock down or control HT-29 cells were treated with IL-17A and/or TNF-α for 6 h, then were examined for levels of mRNAs for CXCL11 (G) or IL-12P35 (H) by real-time PCR. The results shown are representative of those obtained in three independent experiments. The bars are the SD.

CXCL11 by HT-29 cells. We first examined whether NF-κB pathway was involved in IL-17A mediated anti-inflammatory effects in CECs. However, our data showed that IL-17A signaling does not significantly affect the activity of NF-κB, nor it affects TNF-α induced activation of NF-κB (data not shown). So we then focus our manuscript on the MAPK/PI3K pathways. Although it has been reported that the P38 pathway is involved in the IL-17A-mediated pro-inflammatory response [16], we here demonstrated that P38 pathway were not involved in the IL-17A mediated anti-inflammatory response (CXCL11 and IL-12P35 inhibition) (data not shown). However, IL-17A signaling significantly enhanced TNF-α- induced phosphorylation of ERK in HT-29 cells (Fig. 1). In addition, we also demonstrated the involvement of PI3K-AKT pathway in IL-17A-mediated negative regulation (Fig.2).

Act1 (transcription factor NF-κ B activator 1) is an important adaptor protein in IL-17 receptor (IL-17R) signaling and IL-17A-dependent immune responses [36]. The facts that Act1 expression is increased in colon epithelial cells in mice with IBD and Act1-deficient mice show a delayed onset and much lower severity of DSS-induced colitis [19] suggest that Act1 is involved in the regulation of IBD, but whether or how it is involved in IL-17A-mediated negative regulation remained to be investigated. Our data showing that Act1 knockdown decreased IL-17A-induced enhancement of TNF-α-induced ERK and AKT phosphorylation and blocked IL-17A-mediated negative regulation demonstrate that Act1 plays an essential role in transducing the negative signal of IL-17A in CECs.

Previous report showed that PI3K pathway is involved in IL-17A signaling mainly in an Act1-independent manner [21]. However, here we found that Act1 knock down significantly lead to decreased expression of PI3K- cat gamma 1B (PI3K- 1B) in response to IL-17A stimulation (Fig.4). These data partially explains how Act1 knock down leads to decreased phosphorylation of AKT, and indicates that PI3K pathway might be involved in IL-17A signaling pathway in a manner partially dependent on Act1.

However, it was still not known how the enhanced phosphorylation of ERK and PI3K-AKT led to inhibition of CXCL11 and

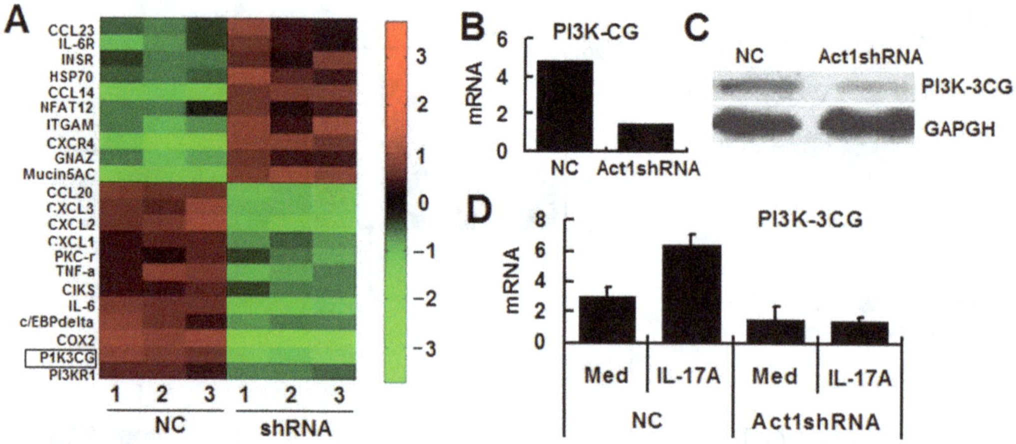

Figure 4. Microarray assay identifies involvement of an Act1--PI3K IB subunit (PI3K-cat gamma) pathway in IL-17A-mediated signaling cascades. (A) Gene chip assay identifies multiple genes differentially expressed in Act1 knock down and control HT-29 cells. (B and C) Act1 knock down decreases PI3K-cat gamma expression as shown by real-time PCR (B) and Western blotting (C). (D) Act1 knock down and control HT-29 cells were treated with recombinant IL-17A for 6 h, then PI3K-cat gamma expression was examined by real-time PCR. The results shown are representative of those obtained in three independent experiments. The bars are the SD.

IL-12P35 mRNA expression. To examine this, the transcriptional factors controlling CXCL11 and IL-12P35 mRNA expression were investigated, among which we focus on the function of C/EBPβ. Data suggest that C/EBPβ can bind to the region bp - 444 and - 392 of the IL-12P35 promoter and negatively regulate LPS-induced expression of the IL-12 subunit P35 [37]and that phosphorylation of C/EBPβ decreases its ability to bind to DNA [38]. As shown in Fig. 1, IL-17A signaling enhanced the TNF-α-induced phosphorylation of C/EBPβ, a process inhibited by blockade of the ERK pathway (Fig. 3), suggesting that ERK activation is the upstream signaling cascade accounting for the phosphorylation of C/EBPβ. Our above data showed that Act1 knockdown decreased IL-17A-induced enhancement of TNF-a-induced ERK phosphorylation (Fig.3). In such a scenario, IL-17A signaling activates Act1 and this enhances the TNF-α-induced phosphorylation of ERK, finally leading to phosphorylation of C/EBPβ, while decreases its ability to bind to the CXCL11 and IL-

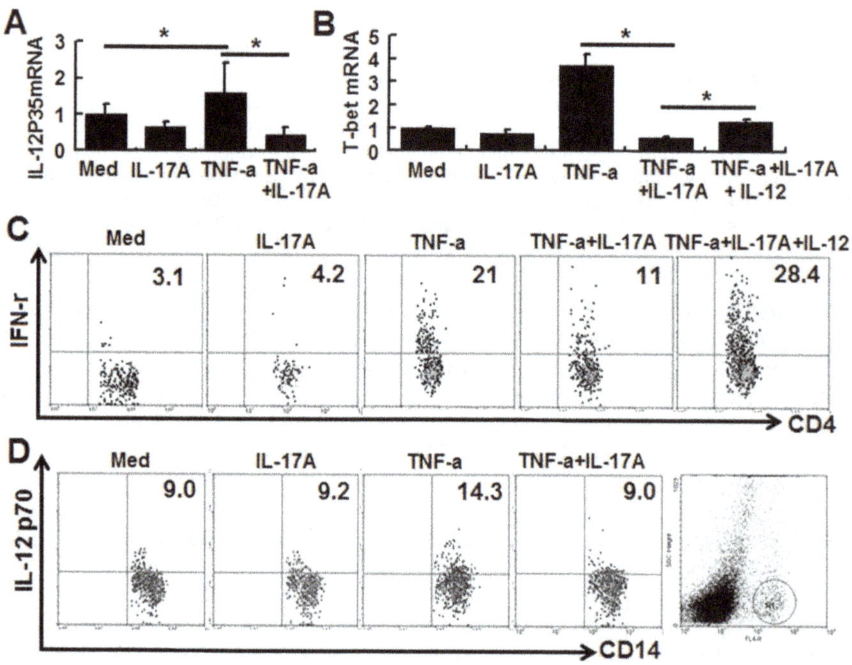

Figure 5. IL-17A signaling mediates negative regulation in a PBMC/HT-29 cell co-culture system. HT-29 cells were cultured in the presence of IL-17A and/or TNF-αfor 24 h, then human PBMCs were added and stimulated with anti-human CD3 and CD28 antibodies with or without recombinant IL-12 for another 24 h. Adherent HT-29 cells were analyzed for IL-12P35 mRNA (A) and non-adherent PBMCs were analyzed for T-bet (B) expression by real-time PCR. IFN-γ expressions within $CD4^{+}$T cells (C) and IL-12P70 expressions within CD14+monocytes (D) were examined by flow cytometry analysis. The results shown are representative of those obtained in three independent experiments. The bars are the SD.

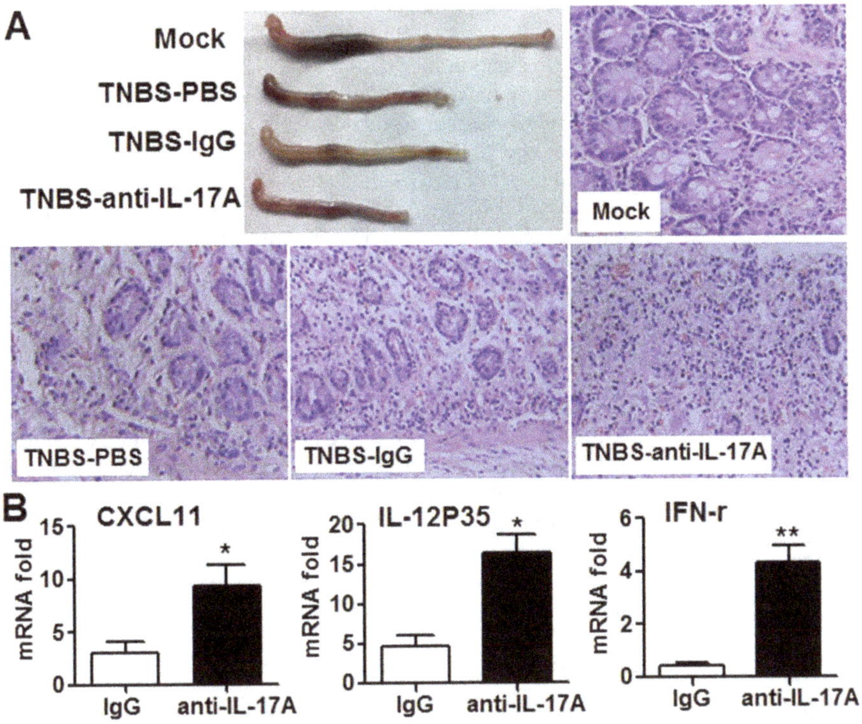

Figure 6. IL-17A blockade in vivo leads to exacerbated TNBS colitis and enhanced Th1 activity. (A-C) The TNBS-colitis model was established in C57BL/6 mice as described in the Materials and Methods and 100 ug of IL-17A neutralizing antibody or control IgG was injected i.p on days 1, 3, 5, and 7 (day 1 is the first day TNBS was administered in the drinking water). Mice were sacrificed on day 8 and examined for tissue damage (A) and CECs (B) isolated from the treated mice were analyzed for CXCL11, IL-12P35, and IFN-γ expression by real-time PCR. The results shown are representative of those obtained in three independent experiments using 8 mice per group. The bars are the SD.

12P35 promoters, leading to decreased CXCL11 and IL-12P35 mRNA expression.

We then further investigated how the enhanced PI3K-AKT phosphorylation contributes to IL-17A mediated negative regulation. One study in HT-29 cells has suggested that inhibition of

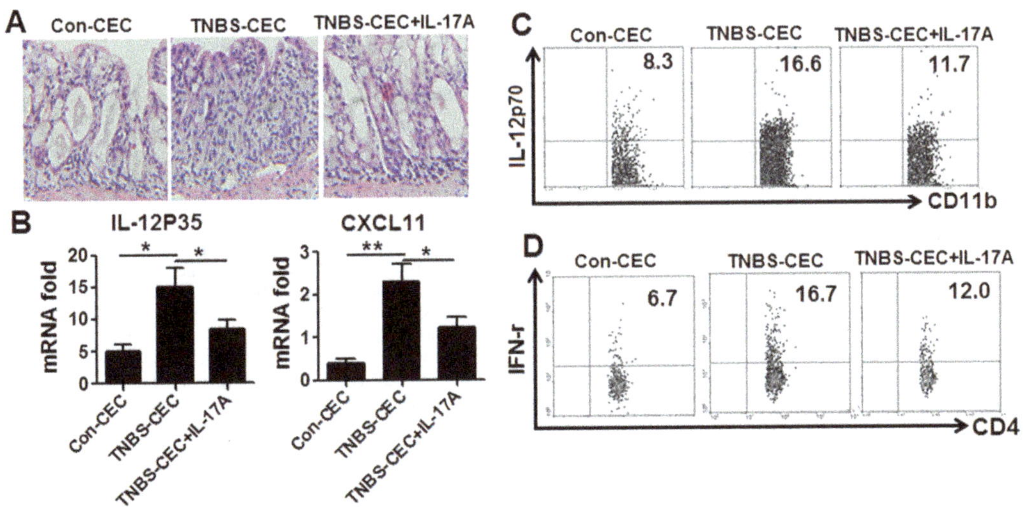

Figure 7. Adoptive transfer of CECs from TNBS-induced mice exacerbates colitis in mice, which can be inhibited by co-transfer of IL-17. CECs were collected from untreated mice (control CECs) or from mice with TNBS-induced colitis on day 8 of colitis induction (TNBS-CEC) and adoptively transferred into TNBS-induced mice (i.p, 1×10^6/mice) on days 1 and day 4 (TNBS treatment was started on day 1). On day 8, the mice were sacrificed and colon tissue collected for H&E staining (A), CECs were tested for IL-12P35 and CXCL11 mRNA levels by real-time PCR (B). Lymphocytes from colonic lamina propria cells were collected and expressions of IL-12P70 were examined within $CD11b^+$ macrophage (C), expressions of IFN-γ were examined within $CD4^+$T cells (D). The results shown are representative of those obtained in three independent experiments, each using 6 mice per group. The bars are the SD.

PI3-K results in induction of NF-κB binding activity [39]. Consistent with this, a mutation that inactivates PI3Kγ enzymatic activity ('kinase-dead') leads to less severe colitis in mice, which produce significantly more pro-inflammatory Th1 cytokines, such as IL-12, TNF-α, and IFN-γ. This suggests a role for PI3Kγ in the negative regulation of these cytokines [40]. In our study, IL-17A signaling alone did not markedly affect TNF-α-induced NF- κB phosphorylation, but wortmannin, a PI3K inhibitor enhanced this process (data not shown), suggesting that IL-17A may inhibit TNF-α-induced NF-γ B phosphorylation by increasing the phosphorylation of PI3K-AKT, although the underlying mechanism remains to be determined.

Whether and how IL-17A-mediated negative regulation affected the local immune response was then investigated. Our co-culture system clearly showed that IL-17A signaling in CECs inhibited the TNF-α-induced increase in IL-12P35 mRNA expression by adherent HT-29 cells, which led to inhibited Th1 cell function, suggesting that IL-17A signaling in CECs can affect the activity of Th cells (Fig.5B&C). Interestingly, our data showed that IL-17A signaling enhanced TNF-a induced IL-12p35 mRNA expression but not protein expression, while IL-17A signaling enhanced TNF-a induced IL-12p70 protein expression by monocytes in the co-culture system, indicating that IL-17A signaling on CECs may affect Th1 cell activity indirectly. A previous report which showed that IL-12 expressing epithelia cells (at mRNA level) promotes the Th1 cell response support our findings [41]. However, the underlying mechanisms by which IL-17A negatively regulates Th1 cell activity in a human CEC and PBMC co-culture system remain to be investigated. In addition, we blocked IL-17A in mice with TNBS- induced colitis in vivo and found that this enhanced CXCL11 and IL-12P35 mRNA expression by CECs. This is the first report demonstrating a negative regulation mechanism of IL-17A on CEC in vivo.

The above data indicate that CECs act as important mediators in the pathogenesis or regulation of IBD, which are consistent with previous reports [42–43]. To further demonstrate that CECs were a critical target of IL-17A-mediated negative regulation in vivo, we transferred CECs or co-transferred CECs and IL-17A into TNBS colitis mice. As shown in Fig. 7, transfer of CECs from TNBS colitis mice exacerbated colitis and increased the activity of Th1 cells in recipient mice, while co-transfer of these cells and IL-17A inhibited colitis by inhibiting Th1 cell function in recipient mice further demonstrating that CECs are critical target cells in IL-17A-mediated negative regulation.

In summary, we have demonstrated a regulatory mechanism of IL-17A in the progression of CD. By activating the Act1-ERK-CEBP/β and Act1-PI3K-AKT pathways in CECs, IL-17A signaling negatively regulates TNF-α-induced mRNA expression of CXCL11 and IL-12P35. Our in vivo assay also demonstrated the existence of an IL-17A-CEC- Th1 inhibition axis in IBD. Further investigation of this pathway will shed new light on the pathogenesis and regulation of IBD.

Author Contributions

Conceived and designed the experiments: GH Y. Li GC BS. Performed the experiments: XG XJ YX Y. Lin. Analyzed the data: JF XL TZ. Contributed reagents/materials/analysis tools: LM CH HX ZZ. Wrote the paper: GH. Obtained the permission for use of clinical samples: YG. Discussed the manuscript: RW.

References

1. Strober W, Fuss I, Mannon P (2007) The fundamental basis of inflammatory bowel disease. J Clin Invest 117: 514–521.
2. Kaser A, Zeissig S, Blumberg RS (2010) Inflammatory bowel disease. Annu. Rev. Immunol 28: 573–621.
3. Romagnani S (1999) Th1/Th2 cells Inflamm Bowel Dis 5(4):285–294.
4. Funakoshi K, Sugimura K, Sasakawa T, Bannai H, Anezaki K, et al (1995) Study of cytokines in ulcerative colitis. J Gastroenterol. 30 Suppl 8:61–63.
5. Schreiber S, Rutgeerts P, Fedorak RN, Khaliq-Kareemi M, Kamm MA, et al (2005) A randomized, placebo-controlled trial of certolizumab pegol (CDP870) for treatment of Crohn's disease. Gastroenterology 3: 807–818.
6. Rahimi R, Nikfar S, Abdollahi M (2007) Do anti-tumor necrosis factors induce response and remission in patients with acute refractory Crohn's disease? A systematic meta-analysis of controlled clinical trials. Biomed. Pharmacother. 1: 75–80.
7. Park H, Li Z, Yang XO, Chang SH, Nurieva R, et al (2005) A distinct lineage of CD4 T cells regulates tissue inflammation by producing interleukin 17. Nat Immunol 6: 1133–1141.
8. Jovanovic DV, Di Battista JA, Martel-Pelletier J, Jolicoeur FC, He Y, et al (1998) IL-17 stimulates the production and expression of proinflammatory cytokines, IL-1beta and TNF-alpha, by human macrophages. J. Immunol. 160: 3513–3521.
9. Fossiez F, Djossou O, Chomarat P, Flores-Romo L, Ait-Yahia S, et al (1996) T cell interleukin-17 induces stromal cells to produce proinflammatory and hematopoietic cytokines. J. Exp. Med. 183:2593–2603.
10. Awane M, Andres PG, Li DJ, Reinecker HC (1999) NF-kappa B-inducing kinase is a common mediator of IL-17-, TNF-alpha-, and IL-1 beta-induced chemokine promoter activation in intestinal epithelial cells. J. Immunol. 162: 5337–5344.
11. Onishi RM, Gaffen SL (2010) Interleukin-17 and its target genes: mechanisms of interleukin-17 function in disease. Immunology 129: 311–321.
12. Hueber W, Pate DD, Dryja T, Wright AM, Koroleva I, et al (2010) Effects of AIN457, a fully human antibody to interleukin-17A, on psoriasis, rheumatoid arthritis, and uveitis. Sci. Transl. Med. 2: 52ra72.
13. Fujino S, Andoh A, Bamba S, Ogawa A, Hata K, et al (2003) Increased expression of interleukin 17 in inflammatory bowel disease. Gut 52:65–70.
14. Rovedatti L, Kudo T, Biancheri P, Sarra M, Knowles CH, et al (2009) Differential regulation of interleukin 17 and interferon gamma production in inflammatory bowel disease. Gut 58:1629–1636.
15. Hueber W, Sands BE, Lewitzky S, Vandemeulebroecke M, Reinisch W, et al (2012) Secukinumab, a human anti-IL-17A monoclonal antibody, for moderate to severe Crohn's disease: unexpected results of a randomised, double-blind placebo-controlled trial. Gut. 61(12):1693–1700.
16. Lee JW, Wang P, Kattah MG, Youssef S, Steinman L, et al (2008) Differential regulation of chemokines by IL-17 in colonic epithelial cells. J. Immunol. 181: 6536–6545.
17. Liang SC, Tan XY, Luxenberg DP, Karim R, Dunussi-Joannopoulos K, et al (2006) Interleukin (IL)-22 and IL-17 are coexpressed by Th17 cells and cooperatively enhance expression of antimicrobial peptides. J. Exp. Med. 203: 2271–2279.
18. O'Connor W, Kamanaka M, Booth CJ, Town T, Nakae S, et al (2009) A protective function for interleukin 17A in T cell-mediated intestinal inflammation. Nat. Immunol. 10: 603–609.
19. Qian Y, Liu C, Hartupee J, Altuntas CZ, Gulen MF et al (2007) The adaptor Act1 is required for interleukin 17-dependent signaling associated with autoimmune and inflammatory disease. Nat. Immunol. 8: 247–256.
20. Ruddy MJ, Wong GC, Liu XK, Yamamoto H, Kasayama S, et al (2004) Functional cooperation between interleukin-17 and tumor necrosis factor-α is mediated by CCAAT/enhancer binding protein family members. J. Biol.Chem. 279: 2559–2567.
21. Huang F, Kao CY, Wachi S, Thai P, Ryu J, et al (2007) Requirement for both JAK-mediated PI3K signaling and ACT1/TRAF6/TAK1-dependent NF-kappaB activation by IL-17A in enhancing cytokine expression in human airway epithelial cells. J. Immunol. 179: 6504–6513.
22. Shi F, Guo X, Jiang X, Chen G, Zhou P, et al (2012) Dysregulated Tim-3 expression and its correlation with imbalanced CD4 helper T cell function in ulcerative colitis. Clinical. Immunology. 145: 230–240.
23. Lytle C, Tod TJ, Vo KT, Lee JW, Atkinson RW, et al (2005) The peroxisome proliferator-activated receptor γ ligand rosiglitazone delays the onset of inflammatory bowel disease in mice with interleukin 10 deficiency. Inflamm. Bowel. Dis. 11: 231–243.
24. Neurath MF, Fuss I, Kelsall BL, StiJber ER, Strober W (1995) Antibodies to IL-12 abrogate established experimental colitis in mice.J. Exp. Med. 182:1281–1290.
25. Li X, Chen G, Li Y, Wang R, Wang L, et al (2010) Involvement of T Cell Ig Mucin-3 (Tim-3) in the Negative Regulation of Inflammatory bowel diseases. Clin Immunol. 134:169–177;
26. Lefrançois L, Lycke N (2001) Isolation of mouse small intestinal, intraepithelial lymphocytes, Peyer's Patch, and lamina propria cells. Curr. Protoc. Immunol.3.19.1-3.19.16.
27. Ito R, Kita M, Shin-Ya M, Kishida T, Urano A, et al (2008) Involvement of IL-17A in the pathogenesis of DSS-induced colitis in mice. Biochem. Biophys. Res. Commun. 377: 12–16.

28. Ogawa A, Andoh A, Araki Y, Bamba T, Fujiyama Y (2004) Neutralization of interleukin-17 aggravates dextran sulfate sodium-induced colitis in mice. Clin. Immunol. 110: 55–62.
29. Yang XO, Chang SH, Park H, Nurieva R, Shah B, et al (2008) Regulation of inflammatory responses by IL-17F. J. Exp. Med. 205: 1063–1075.
30. Pallone F, Fais S, Capobianchi MR (1988) HLA-D region antigens on isolated human colonic epithelial cells: enhanced expression in inflammatory bowel disease and in vitro induction by different stimuli. Clin. Exp. Immunol. 74: 75–79.
31. Hansen JJ, Holt L, Sartor RB (2009) Gene expression patterns in experimental colitis in IL-10 deficient mice. Inflamm. Bowel. Dis. 15: 890–899.
32. Bonnechi RG, Bianchi PP, Bordignon DD (1998) Differential expression of chemokine receptors and chemotactic responsiveness of type 1 T helper cells (Th1s) and Th2s, J. Exp. Med, 187(1): 129–134.
33. Cole KE, Strick CA, Paradis TJ, Ogborne KT, Loetscher M, et al (1998) Interferon-inducible T cell alpha chemoattractant (I-TAC): a novel non-ELR CXC chemokine with potent activity on activated T cells through selective high affinity binding to CXCR3, J. Exp. Med, 187(12): 2009–2021.
34. Toy D, Kugler D, Wolfson M, Vanden Bos T, Gurgel J, et al (2006) Cutting edge: interleukin 17 signals through a heteromeric receptor complex. J Immunol. 177(1):36–39
35. Yamada S, Naito Y, Takagi T, Mizushima K, Hirai Y, et al (2011) Reduced small-intestinal injury induced by indomethacin in interleukin-17A-deficient mice. J Gastroenterol Hepatol.; 26(2):398–404.
36. Gaffen SL (2009) Structure and signalling in the IL-17 receptor family. Nat. Rev. Immunol. 9: 556–576.
37. Kollet J, Witek C, Gentry JD, Liu X, Schwartzbach SD, et al (2001) Deletional analysis of the murine IL-12 p35 promoter comparing IFN- g and lipopolysaccharide stimulation. J. Immunol. 167: 5653–5663.
38. Shen F, Li N, Gade P, Kalvakolanu DV, Weibley T, et al (2009) IL-17 receptor signaling inhibits C/EBPbeta by sequential phosphorylation of the regulatory 2 domain. Sci. Signal. 2 :ra8.
39. Wang Q, Kim S, Wang X, Evers BM (2000) Activation of NF-κB binding in HT-29 colon cancer cells by inhibition of phosphatidylinositol 3-kinase. Biochem. Biophys. Res. Commun. 273:853–858.
40. van Dop WA, Marengo S, te Velde AA, Ciraolo E, Franco I, et al (2010) The absence of functional PI3Kγ prevents leukocyte recruitment and ameliorates TNBS-induced colitis in mice. Immunol. Lett. 131: 33–39.
41. Ueno N, Fujiya M, Segawa S, Nata T, Moriichi K, et al (2011) Heat-killed Body of Lactobacillus brevis SBC8803 Ameliorates Intestinal Injury in a Murine Model of Colitis by Enhancing the Intestinal Barrier Function. Inflamm Bowel Dis 17: 2235–2250
42. Pallone F, Fais S, Capobianchi MR (1988) HLA-D region antigens on isolated human colonic epithelial cells: enhanced expression in inflammatory bowel disease and in vitro induction by different stimuli, Clin Exp Immunol, 74(1):75–79.
43. Brandtzaeg P, Halstensen TS, Huitfeldt HS, Krajci P, Kvale D, et al (1992) Epithelial expression of HLA, secretory component (poly-Ig receptor), and adhesion molecules in the human alimentary tract. Ann N Y Acad Sci. 664:157–179.

Intestinal Colonization by *Candida albicans* Alters Inflammatory Responses in Bruton's Tyrosine Kinase-Deficient Mice

Karin Strijbis[1*¤], Ömer H. Yilmaz[1], Stephanie K. Dougan[1], Alexandre Esteban[1], Andrea Gröne[2], Carol A. Kumamoto[3], Hidde L. Ploegh[1]

1 Whitehead Institute for Biomedical Research, Cambridge, Massachusetts, United States of America, 2 Department of Pathobiology, Faculty of Veterinary Medicine, Utrecht University, Utrecht, The Netherlands, 3 Department of Molecular Biology and Microbiology, School of Medicine, Tufts University, Boston, Massachusetts, United States of America

Abstract

The commensal yeast *Candida albicans* is part of the human intestinal microflora and is considered a "pathobiont", a resident microbe with pathogenic potential yet harmless under normal conditions. The aim of this study was to investigate the effect of *C. albicans* on inflammation of the intestinal tract and the role of Bruton's tyrosine kinase (Btk). Btk is an enzyme that modulates downstream signaling of multiple receptors involved in innate and adaptive immunity, including the major anti-fungal receptor Dectin-1. Colitis was induced in wild type and Btk-/- mice by treatment with dextran sodium sulfate (DSS) and the gastrointestinal tract of selected treatment groups were then colonized with *C. albicans*. Colonization by *C. albicans* neither dampened nor exacerbated inflammation in wild type mice, but colon length and spleen weight were improved in Btk-deficient mice colonized with *C. albicans*. Neutrophil infiltration was comparable between wild type and Btk-/- mice, but the knockout mice displayed severely reduced numbers of macrophages in the colon during both DSS and DSS/*Candida* treatment. Smaller numbers and reduced responsiveness of Btk-/- macrophages might partially explain the improved colon length of Btk-/- mice as a result of *Candida* colonization. Surprisingly, DSS/*Candida*-treated Btk-/- animals had higher levels of certain pro-inflammatory cytokines and levels of the anti-inflammatory cytokine TGF-β were reduced compared to wild type. A clustering and correlation analysis showed that for wild type animals, spleen TGF-β and colon IL-10 and for Btk-/- spleen and colon levels of IL-17A best correlated with the inflammatory parameters. We conclude that in Btk-/- immunocompromised animals, colonization of the gastrointestinal tract by the commensal yeast *C. albicans* alters inflammatory symptoms associated with colitis.

Editor: David R. Andes, University of Wisconsin Medical School, United States of America

Funding: The authors have no support or funding to report.

Competing Interests: The authors have declared that no competing interests exist.

* Email: K.Strijbis@uu.nl

¤ Current address: Department of Infectious Diseases & Immunology, Utrecht University, Utrecht, The Netherlands.

Introduction

The intestinal microflora plays an important not only in establishing immune tolerance but also in the development of inflammatory bowel disease (IBD) and obesity. While studies of the microbiome have mostly focused on commensal bacteria, several species of fungi are also major constituents of the mammalian gastrointestinal system, with highest fungal concentrations in the colon [1,2]. It is estimated that fungi are detectable in all gastrointestinal segments of about 70% of healthy adults [3], with *Candida* spp. being predominant [4,5]. *Candida albicans* is a commensal fungus of the human gastro-intestinal tract, capable of causing life-threatening opportunistic fungal infections [6]. *C. albicans* is considered opportunistic pathogen or a "pathobiont", a resident microbe with pathogenic potential yet harmless under normal conditions. Gut-colonizing *Candida* can cause candidaemia [7,8], but mucosal damage and neutropenia are required for *Candida* dissemination from the colon [9]. An increase in fungal load and *Candida* species was observed in patients suffering from Crohn's disease [10].

The C-type lectin Dectin-1, which recognizes cell wall β1,3-glucan, is the major receptor involved in antifungal immune responses [11]. While essential during antifungal immune responses during systemic *C. albicans* infections in mice, lack of Dectin-1 does not affect gastrointestinal colonization by *C. albicans* [12]. Dectin-1 knockout mice are more sensitive to chemically-induced colitis, presumably due to diminished immune surveillance of endogenous fungal species [1]. The contribution of fungi to the development of IBD is further illustrated by human polymorphisms in Dectin-1 associated with ulcerative colitis (UC) and its signaling molecule CARD9. The latter has been associated with both UC and Crohn's disease [1,13,14]. Serum antibodies against yeast cell wall components (anti-glucan, anti-laminarin and anti-chitin antibodies) are predictive for Crohn's disease and ulcerative colitis [15].

We previously identified Bruton's tyrosine kinase (Btk) as a signaling molecule in the Dectin-1-mediated immune response to *C. albicans* [16], where it contributes to macrophage phagocytosis and cytokine production. Btk-/- mice are more susceptible to systemic *C. albicans* infections. Btk also modulates downstream signaling of other immune receptors, including the Fcγ receptor [17] and the B-cell receptor, leading to reduced B cell numbers and antibody secretion [18,19]. For this study, we investigated the role of Btk during gastrointestinal colonization with *C. albicans*. Our findings add to a growing body of work that indicates probiotic effects of commensal yeasts in the gastrointestinal tract.

Materials and Methods

Candida cultures

C. albicans strain SC5314 was cultured in standard YPD medium (2% bactopeptone, 1% yeast extract, 2% glucose and 80 μg/ml uridine) for 16 hours at 30°C in a shaker.

Mouse models of *Candida* colonization

Animals used in this study were housed at the Whitehead Institute for Biomedical Research or at Tufts University, which are both certified by the United States Office of Laboratory Animal Welfare (OLAW) under the guidance of the Public Health Service (PHS) Policy on Humane Care and Use of Laboratory Animals. All experiments were done in compliance with regulatory guidelines defined by the Tufts University IACUC committee and Whitehead Institute IACUC committee and in accordance with procedures approved by the Massachusetts Institute of Technology Committee on Animal Care (Ploegh lab, CAC# 1011-123-14). Btk-/- animals were a kind gift from Whasif Khan [18]. For the Dectin-1 staining experiments, antibiotic-treated mice were colonized with *C. albicans* as described previously [20]. In short, 5–7 week-old BALB/c mice were treated with antibiotics (tetracycline, 1 mg/ml; streptomycin, 2 mg/ml; gentamicin, 0.1 mg/ml) in the drinking water and fed the purified diet AIN-93G containing glucose [21]. This diet was used because numerous yeast-form particles are found in the cecum contents of mice fed yeast extract-containing chow. Mice were inoculated with 0.1 ml *C. albicans* strain CKY101 and sacrificed at 4 and 18 days post-inoculation to obtain cecal contents for microscopy analysis [22]. Cecum contents was enriched for microbial cells by purification on Percoll gradients and stained with the Dectin1-CRD-Alexa^{647} probe [16]. For the DSS experiments, age-matched C57BL/6 mice were used as wild type control animals. To minimize differences in microbiota composition, all mice were bred and maintained in the same room at the Whitehead Animal Facility. All mice were 4 months old at the onset of experiments. Both males and females were used and genders were matched between wild type and Btk-/- groups. Chemically-induced colitis and *Candida* colonization experiments were performed as previously described [23,24]. In short, colitis was experimentally induced by administration of 5% Dextran sodium sulfate (DSS) in the drinking water from day 1. On day 3, mice were inoculated with *C. albicans* strain SC5314 by oral gavage with 1×10^7 colony forming units (CFU) in a final volume of 200 μl PBS. Mice were weighed and monitored daily and the experiment was terminated when animals had lost >20% of initial body weight. DSS was continuously administered until sacrifice. Colon and cecum were harvested for determination of colon length, cytokine levels and histology and cecum content for enumeration of fungal burdens. Spleens were harvested to determine weight and cytokine levels. To determine fungal burden, cecum contents were homogenized and plated on YPD plates with antibiotics.

Histology

For histology, tissues were fixed in 10% formalin in PBS, embedded in paraffin, sectioned and stained with Hematoxylin and Eosin (H&E) or Gomori Methenamine Silver (GMS). Immunohistochemistry was performed with antibodies directed against Myeloperoxidase (MPO) to detect neutrophils or CD68 to detect macrophages. For MPO staining, antigen retrieval was performed in Biocare's Pressure Cookers using EDTA, pH 8 solution, a polyclonal rabbit anti-human myeloperoxidase primary antibody (Dako) was diluted to 1:3500 and a Dako's Rabbit Envision detection kit was used. For CD68 staining antigen retrieval was performed with Borg Decloaker RTU solution (Biocare Medical) in a pressurized Decloaking Chamber (Biocare Medical) for 3 min. As a primary antibody rat monoclonal anti-CD68 [FA-11] antibody (Abcam) was diluted to 1:500 followed by biotin-conjugated secondary donkey anti-rat antibodies (Jackson ImmunoResearch). The Vectastain Elite ABC immunoperoxidase detection kit (Vector Labs PK-6101) followed by Dako Liquid DAB1 Substrate (Dako) was used for visualization. For quantification of neutrophil and macrophage numbers, 5×100 grids were counted at a 40x magnification for 3 individual animals.

Cytokine measurements

Colons and spleen were homogenized in 1 ml PBS followed by cytokine analysis using a Th1/Th2/Th17 mouse cytometric bead array (BD Biosciences) and LSR Flow Cytometer (Whitehead Institute Flow Cytometry Core) according to the manufacturer's directions. Separate ELISA assays were performed for IL-1β (BD Biosciences) and TGF-β (Abcam) according to the manufacturer's instructions.

Statistical analysis

For regular statistical analysis between samples within groups a one-way ANOVA test was performed with Holm-Sidak correction for multiple comparisons using Prism 6 software. We applied this test to 7 comparisons for all our experiments (colon length, spleen weight and cytokine data). 7 comparisons were: 1) wild type control vs wild type DSS. 2) wild type control vs wild type DSS/*Candida*. 3) wild type DSS vs wild type DSS/*Candida*. 4) Btk-/- control vs Btk-/- DSS. 5) Btk-/- control vs Btk-/- DSS/*Candida*. 6) Btk-/- DSS vs Btk-/- DSS/*Candida*. 7) wild type DSS/*Candida* vs Btk-/- DSS/*Candida*.

A student t test was used for a comparison between two values using Prism 6 software. For the clustering analysis, uncentered correlation with average linkage was performed using the program Cluster 3.0 [25]. Clustered matrices were visualized with Java TreeView [26]. Linear regression analysis was performed using R software (http://www.r-project.org/) to identify potential correlations between cytokine levels and colon lengths or spleen weights.

Results

C. albicans adapts to the gastrointestinal tract by formation of hyphae and exposure of β1,3-glucan

We first studied the adaptation of *C. albicans* to the gastrointestinal tract and the exposure of the Dectin-1 ligand β1,3-glucan in the yeast cell wall. To allow for colonization of the gastrointestinal tract in the absence of inflammation, we chose the previously described mouse model of *C. albicans* inoculation by oral gavage after antibiotics treatment [20]. Four or 18 days post-inoculation, *C. albicans* was retrieved from the caecum and stained with a fluorescent soluble carbohydrate recognition domain of Dectin-1 (Dectin1-CRD-Alexa647) [16]. At the 4-day time point, yeast morphology presented as short hyphae emanating from the yeast particles. The yeast-form mother cell stained extensively with Dectin1-CRD-Alexa647, while the germ tube showed less staining (**Figure 1A**). At the 18-day time point, we observed long hyphae that showed extensive staining with the soluble receptor domain (**Figure 1B**). We conclude that after an initial phase of adaptation to the gastrointestinal tract, *C. albicans* filaments contain β1,3-glucan that is accessible to Dectin-1.

Gastrointestinal colonization by *C. albicans* has protective effects in Btk-/- animals

Next we investigated the impact of *C. albicans* colonization on inflammation of the gastrointestinal tract. We chose the dextran sodium sulfate (DSS) colitis mouse model in conjunction with *C. albicans* colonization by oral gavage [23,24]. Colitis was induced in wild type and Btk-/- animals by provision of DSS in the drinking water, followed by an oral inoculum of 1×10^7 colony forming units of *C. albicans* on day 3 (**Figure 2A**). The experiment included control, DSS only and DSS/*Candida* treatment groups of wild type and Btk-/- animals. Animals were sacrificed 8 days after initiation of the experiment. DSS-treated and DSS/*Candida*-treated wild type and Btk-/- animals lost weight at a similar rate (**Figure 2B**). For both wild type and Btk-/- animals, *Candida* hyphae were visible when colons were stained with fungi-specific Gomori Methenamine Silver (GMS) (**Figure 2C**). The hyphal morphology observed in these histology slides corroborates our results that *C. albicans* adapts to the gastrointestinal tract by hyphae formation (**Figure 1**). We next quantified *C. albicans* colonization of the wild type and Btk-/- DSS/*Candida* groups. The numbers of *Candida* colony-forming units (CFUs) from caecum samples were slightly higher in the DSS/*Candida*-treated Btk-/- animals compared to wild type (**Figure 2D**). Addition of DSS to the drinking water resulted in statistically significant shortening of the colon of wild type animals (**Figure 2E**). Wild type animals that received the DSS/*Candida* combination treatment also showed significantly reduced colon lengths compared to the wild type control group. There was no difference in colon length between the wild type DSS and DSS/*Candida*-treated groups, suggesting that *C. albicans* neither increased nor decreased inflammation. Colon shortening as a result of DSS-only treatment was also observed for the Btk-/- mice. However, the DSS/*Candida*-treated Btk-/- animals displayed significantly longer colons compared to DSS-treated Btk-/- mice ($p<0.05$) and compared to DSS/*Candida*-treated wild type animals ($p<0.005$) (**Figure 2E**). These results suggest that in the Btk-/- animals, colonization by *C. albicans* may dampen inflammation. As a proxy for systemic inflammation we measured spleen weight, as increased leukocyte numbers enlarge the spleen. Wild type animals showed a significant increase in spleen weight upon treatment with the DSS/*Candida* combination (**Figure 2F**). Btk-/- animals treated with DSS had significantly enlarged spleens and spleen weight was reduced in the DSS/*Candida*-treated group, although this difference did not reach statistical significance. DSS/*Candida*-treated Btk-/- animals showed reduced spleen weight compared to the wild type DSS/*Candida*-treated animals ($p<0.05$). *Candida* colonization thus affords a measure of protection against DSS-induced colitis in Btk-/- animals.

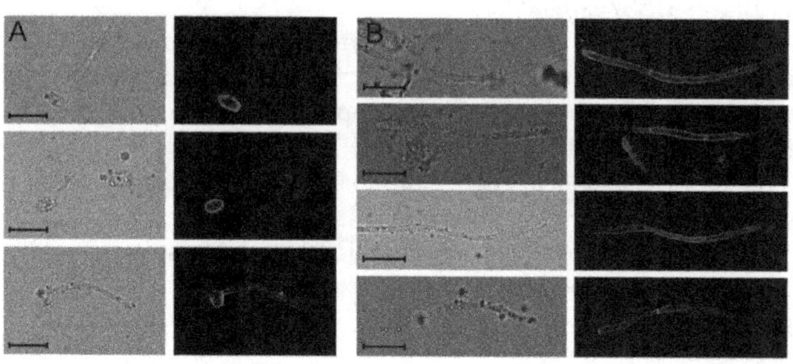

Figure 1. Morphology and β1,3-glucan exposure of *C. albicans* adapted to the gastrointestinal tract. A: *C. albicans* isolated from mouse cecum 4 days after inoculation and stained with Dectin1-CRD-Alexa^{647}. After 4 days of gastrointestinal adaptation, the majority of *C. albicans* display short (pseudo)hyphal morphology in which β1,3-glucan exposure is limimited. B: *C. albicans* isolated from cecum 18 days after inoculation and stained with Dectin1-CRD-Alexa^{647}. The majority of *C. albicans* display short (pseudo)hyphal morphology. After 18 days of gastrointestinal adaptation, the majority of *C. albicans* display long hyphal morphology with extensive β1,3-glucan exposure. Experiments were performed twice with two animals in each group, representative images are shown.

Colons of Btk-/- animals have reduced macrophage infiltrates

To further assess the severity of inflammation, we performed H&E staining of the distal colon of the wild type and Btk-/- control and treatment groups. Microscopy showed that all treatment groups suffered from severe cryptitis, crypt abscesses and (multi)focal ulcerations (**Figure 3A**). For a quantitative analysis, the H&E-stained colons were blindly graded for the presence of normal mucosa (1), cryptitis (2), crypt abscesses (3), focal ulcerations (4) and multifocal ulcerations (5). The colons of some Btk-/- animals of the DSS/*Candida* treatment groups showed improved histology, but the difference between groups did not reach statistical significance. To examine the composition of the colon inflammatory infiltrates we performed immunohistochemical analysis. Neutrophil invasion as measured by MPO staining was observed upon treatment with DSS and DSS/*Candida* in both wild type and Btk-/- colons and the number of neutrophilic infiltrates was comparable between groups (**Figure 3B**). A CD68 stain showed macrophage infiltrates in the wild type DSS and DSS/*Candida* condition, but a severely reduced number of macrophages in the colons of Btk-/- animals (**Figure 3C**).

Btk-/- animals show elevated pro-inflammatory cytokines and decreased TGF-β levels

We next investigated if colonization by *C. albicans* and the reduced macrophage numbers in the Btk-/- colons impact local cytokine levels in the colon and systemic cytokine levels in the spleen. Cytokine measurements were performed on lysates of the proximal colon (**Figure 4A**) and spleen (**Figure 4B**). Statistical differences between 7 selected groups were determined by one-way ANOVA test with Holm-Sidak's correction for multiple comparisons. In the colon of wild type animals, IL-10 levels were significantly lowered as a result of DSS or DSS/*Candida* treatment ($p<0.05$ and $p<0.005$, respectively) (**Figure 4A**). Colonic IL-6 was elevated in all wild type and Btk-/- treatment groups, but only the difference between Btk-/- control and DSS treatment was significant ($p<0.05$) (**Figure 4A**). In the spleens of Btk-/- mice, IL-17A levels were significantly decreased in both treatment conditions ($p<0.05$) (**Figure 4B**). This decrease is due mainly to the high levels of IL-17A in Btk-/- control spleens, suggesting elevated levels of this cytokine in the absence of any treatment or inflammation. Furthermore, IFN-γ levels in the spleen were significantly higher in DSS-treated wild type mice compared to the control group. Surprisingly, wild type spleen IL-1β levels were lowered in response to DSS/*Candida* treatment,

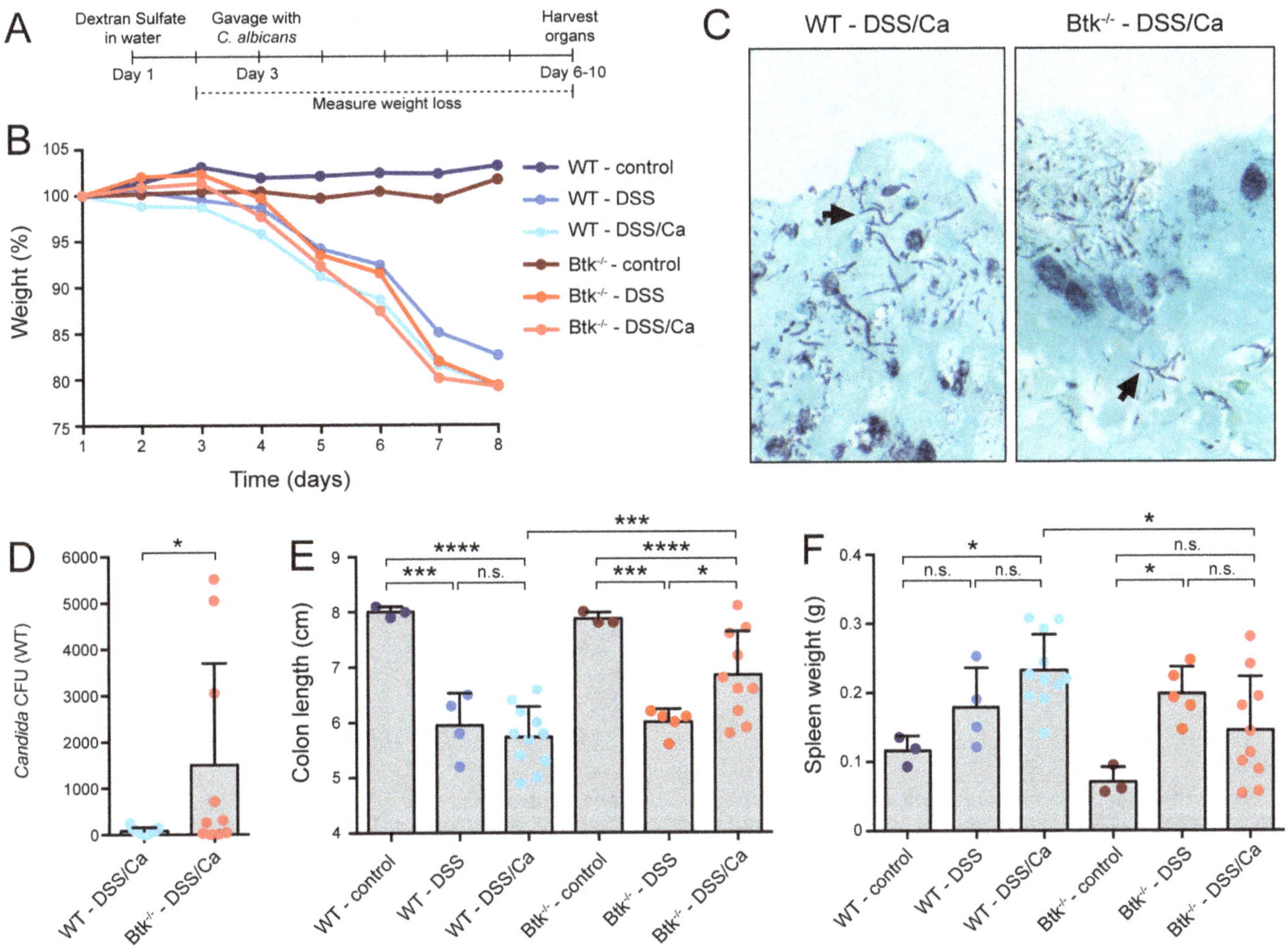

Figure 2. Colonization by *C. albicans* reduces DSS-induced inflammation in Btk-/- mice. A: Experimental design of DSS-induced colitis in combination with *C. albicans* colonization of the gastrointestinal tract. DSS was administered in the drinking water starting on day 1. On day 3, 1×10^7 CFU of *Candida albicans* was administered to the DSS/*Candida* treatment groups by oral gavage. Control groups included 3, DSS groups 5 and DSS/*Candida* groups included 10-11 animals. Animals were sacrificed on day 8 when the first animals reached 80% of initial body weight. B: Weight loss curve of the indicated groups of mice during DSS- or DSS/*Candida* treatment. C: Gomori Methenamine Silver (GMS) staining of wild type and Btk-/- colon after DSS/*Candida* treatment. Arrows indicate *Candida* hyphae. D: *C. albicans* colony forming units (CFUs) in cecum content in wild type and Btk-/- mice during DSS/*Candida* treatment. E: Spleen weights of all mice and treatment groups in DSS/*Candida* experiment. F: Colon lengths of all mice and treatment groups in DSS/*Candida* experiment. All graphs show individual data points, the means of the indicated groups and error bars depict standard deviations. *: $p<0.05$, **: $p<0.01$, ***: $p<0.005$, ****: $p<0.001$.

while Btk-/- animals showed a reverse trend. Of all cytokines analyzed, spleen TGF-β levels showed the most striking differences between treatment groups. TGF-β levels were similar in wild type and Btk-/- control groups and DSS/*Candida* treatment reduced TGF-β levels for both genotypes ($p<0.01$ and $p<0.001$, respectively). In Btk-/- animals, *C. albicans* colonization in combination with DSS treatment led to a significant decrease in TGF-β levels compared to DSS treatment alone ($p<0.01$). To investigate functional relationships between the investigated cytokines we performed clustering analysis of all cytokine measurements. The values of the wild type and Btk-/- control groups were averaged at 0 and other measurements were expressed as relative log values (**Figure 4C**). The first functional cluster of pro-inflammatory cytokines that emerged consisted of colon IL-1β, colon IL-17A, colon TNF, spleen IL-1β, colon IFN-γ, spleen IL-10 and spleen TNF. For this group of cytokines, a general upregulation was observed in the DSS and DSS/*Candida* conditions, which was more pronounced in the Btk-/- groups. A second cluster of pro-inflammatory cytokines consisted of colon IL-6, spleen IFN-γ and spleen IL-6 and was equally elevated in DSS and DSS/*Candida* groups of both wild type and Btk-/- animals. A third cluster of anti-inflammatory cytokines consisting of colon TGF-β, colon IL-10, spleen TGF-β and spleen IL-17A was downregulated in the DSS and DSS/*Candida* groups of both wild type and Btk-/- animals. In summary, Btk-/- treatment groups display a general increase in pro-inflammatory cytokine levels in colon and spleen and reduced levels of splenic TGF-β compared to wild type animals.

TGF-β, IL-10 and IL-17A are associated with inflammation

Because of the reduced inflammation seen in the Btk-/- animals, we were curious which of the cytokine profile best correlated with colon length or spleen weight in wild type and Btk-/- animals. We performed linear regression analysis and determined p and R^2 values of the correlation coefficients. For the wild type animals, TGF-β levels correlated with colon length and negatively

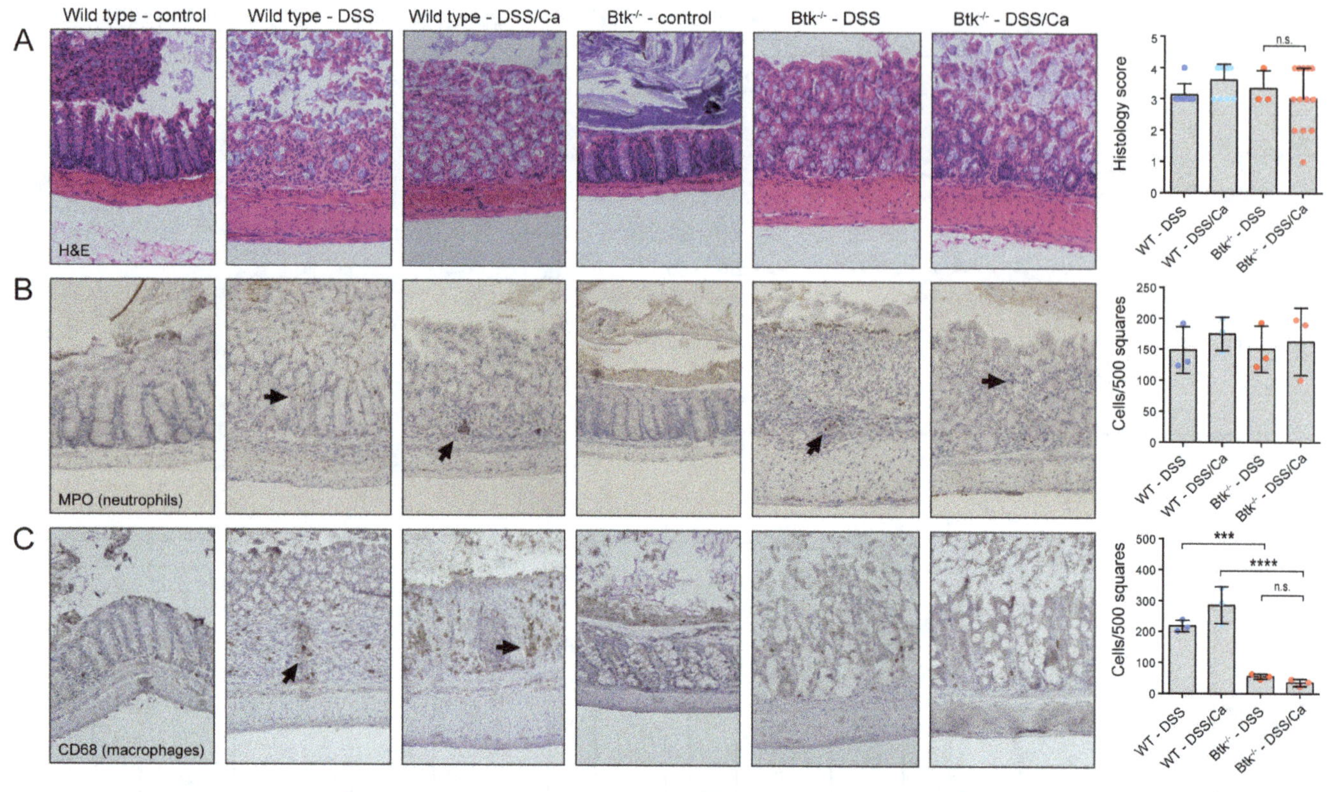

Figure 3. Btk-/- animals have reduced colonic macrophages, but not neutrophils. Mice were treated with DSS or the DSS/*Candida* combination as described in the legend of Figure 2. Sample size (number of animals): control groups (1), DSS groups (3), DSS/*Candida* groups (3). Animals were sacrificed on day 8 and the distal colons were fixed and prepared for histology. A: H&E staining of indicated mouse distal colon sections. Right: H&E stainings were blindly graded based on the following scheme: 1. Normal mucosa. 2. Cryptitis. 3. Crypt abscesses. 4. Focal ulcerations. 5. Multifocal ulcerations. B: Immunohistochemical staining using MPO antibody shows neutrophil infiltration in the indicated mouse distal colon sections. Right: Quantification of infiltrating neutrophils in DSS and DSS/*Candida* conditions. C: Immunohistochemical analysis with CD68 antibody showing macrophages in the indicated mouse distal colon sections. Right: Quantification of macrophages in DSS and DSS/*Candida* conditions. ***: $p<0.005$, ****: $p<0.001$. Representative pictures of each genotype and staining are shown.

correlated with spleen weight (**Figure 4D**). Colon IL-10 levels and colon length were also significantly correlated. In other words, lowering of the anti-inflammatory cytokines TGF-β and IL-10 best predicts inflammation in wild type animals. For the Btk knockout animals, spleen IL-17A correlated with colon length and negatively correlated with spleen weight, while colon IL-17A was negatively correlated with colon length (**Figure 4E**). We conclude that in Btk-/- animals, reduced inflammation is associated with high spleen IL-17A levels and decreased IL-17A in the colon.

Discussion

C. albicans is a commensal yeast that is part of the normal human microflora, although most studies have focused on the pathogenic properties of this opportunistic fungus. Here we show that colonization of the gastrointestinal tract by *C. albicans* alters inflammatory responses in a mouse model of colitis and improves some colitis parameters. Whereas wild type animals do not noticeably benefit (or suffer) from the presence of *C. albicans*, Btk-/- animals show a measure of protection as assessed by colon length and spleen weight (**Figure 2**). Macrophage, but not neutrophil, infiltration of the colon in response to DSS or DSS/*Candida* treatment is severely reduced in Btk-/- animals (**Figure 3**). We hypothesize that this reduction in combination with the lowered phagocytic capacity and reduced ROS production of Btk-/- macrophages causes the altered inflammatory responses of the Btk-/- animals during *C. albicans* colonization. In the colons and spleen of Btk-/- animals we find elevated levels of pro-inflammatory cytokines and reduced levels of anti-inflammatory cytokines during DSS or DSS/*Candida* treatment. For wild type animals, a reduction in colon IL-10 and spleen TGF-β is associated with increased inflammation. For Btk-/- animals, reduced inflammation is associated with elevated spleen IL-17A levels and reduced colon IL-17A levels (**Figure 4**).

We demonstrate that *Candida* adapts to the gastrointestinal tract by the formation of hyphae and exposure of the Dectin-1 ligand β1,3-glucan (**Figure 1A and B**). *C. albicans*, while in the gut, can therefore have potent immuno-stimulatory effects. Previous studies showed staining of fungal cells using a Dectin-1 CRD domain, but the identity and source of the stained cells was unknown [1]. In our experiments, mice were fed on feed devoid of yeast extract, thereby excluding an extraneous source of yeast-like particles. The combination of staining with the fluorescent Dectin-1 CRD domain allowed us to identify gut-adapted *C. albicans* in murine cecal contents. At 4 days post-inoculation, germ tubes produced by *C. albicans* cells colonizing the gastrointestinal tract stained poorly with Dectin-1, consistent with previous observations of differential exposure of β1,3-glucan in yeasts and hyphal elements grown in laboratory culture [27]. Later in the time course of colonization (day 18 post-inoculation), gene expression in colonizing cells changes [28] and we found numerous hyphal

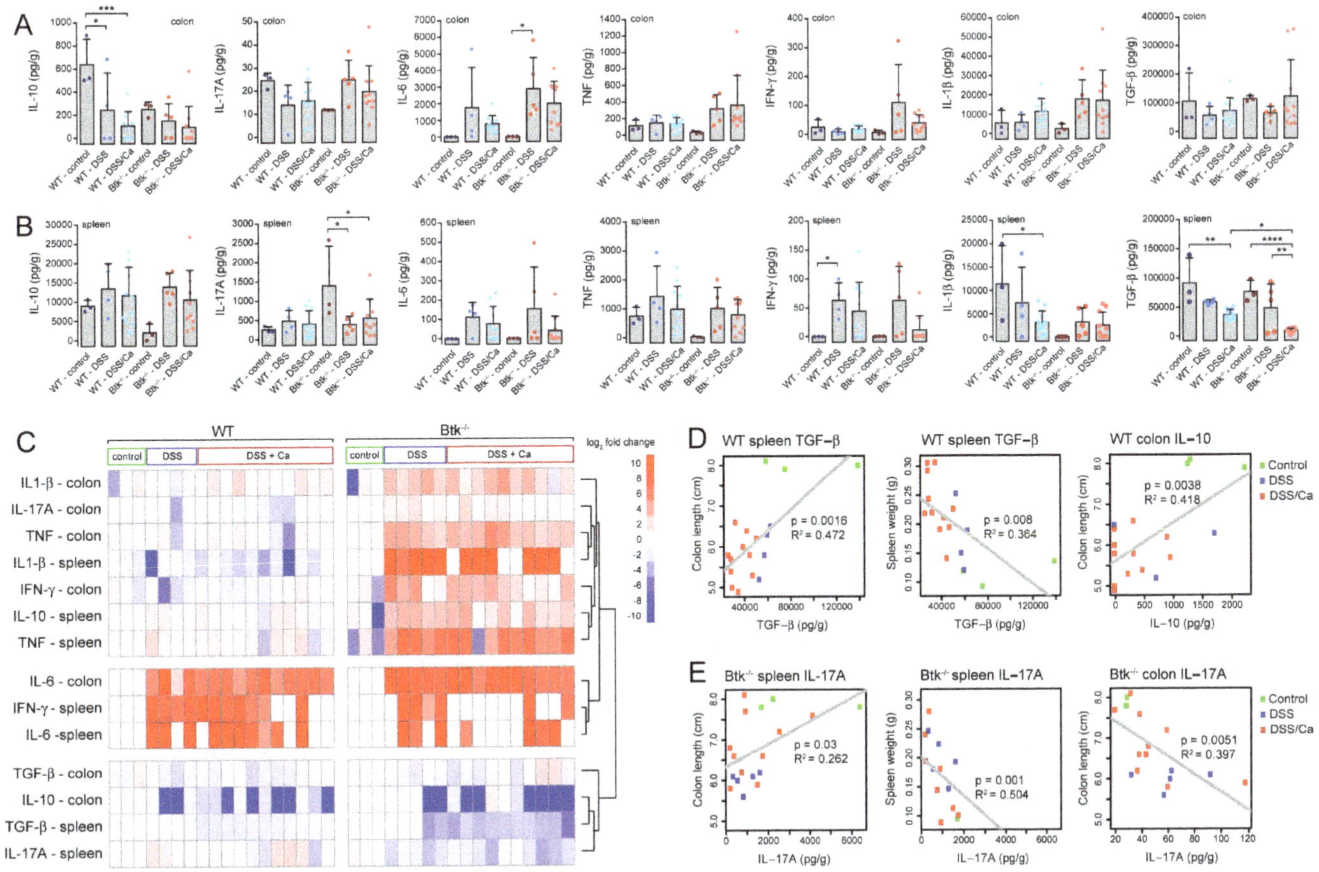

Figure 4. TGF-β, IL-10 and IL17A in colon and spleen are correlated with inflammatory parameters. Mice were treated with DSS or the DSS/*Candida* combination as described in the legend of Figure 2. Sample size (number of animals): control groups (3), DSS groups (5), DSS/*Candida* groups (10-11). Cytokine levels were determined in lysates of spleen and proximal colon. IL10, IL-17A, IL-6, TNF, IFN-γ, IL-1β and TGF-β cytokine levels in spleen lysates (A) and lysates of the proximal colon (B). Bars and error bars show the mean and standard deviation of the indicated groups and data points resembling individual mice are plotted. A one-way ANOVA test with Holm-Sidak correction for multiple comparisons was applied to determine statistical significance. *: $p<0.05$, **: $p<0.01$, ***: $p<0.005$, ****: $p<0.001$, C: Clustering analysis of all cytokine data. Each vertical column represents one animal and its respective cytokine values. The average value of the wild type and Btk-/- control groups was set at 0 and DSS and DSS/*Candida* data were expressed as relative log values. Color codes of relative log values ranging from -10 to 10 are indicated in the legend. D, E: Significantly correlated data after Pearson analysis of cytokine data versus colon length or spleen weight. For wild type animals, spleen TGF-β correlated with colon length and spleen weight and colon IL-10 correlated with colon length (D). For Btk-/- animals, spleen IL-17A correlated with both colon length and spleen weight, while colon IL-17A was correlated with colon length (E).

filaments that stained with Dectin-1. The observation of high β1,3-glucan exposure late during colonization replicates earlier findings of β1,3-glucan unmasking late during systemic infection [29]. Physiological changes that affect Dectin-1 binding occur as *C. albicans* adapts to growth in the gastrointestinal tract.

Conflicting data have been published on the importance of Dectin-1 during *Candida* colonization or the development of colitis. Dectin-1 knockout mice were found to be equally sensitive [30] or more susceptible to DSS-induced colitis [1]. The latter report points at the role of endogenous fungi of the gastrointestinal tract, therefore a different composition of the microbiome may explain the opposing results. However, in our hands the colon length of the DSS/*Candida*-treated Dectin1-/- animals was not significantly different from DSS/*Candida*-treated wild type animals (data not shown). In DSS-independent experiments, colonization of the gastrointestinal tract by *C. albicans* was not affected by the presence or absence of Dectin-1 [12]. Together, these results suggest that Dectin-1 plays a role in anti-fungal immunity only in conjunction with a diseased state of the colon. Besides Dectin-1, pattern recognition receptors like DC-SIGN, Mannose receptor and Mincle are known to be involved in cellular immune responses against *C. albicans*. Their roles during *C. albicans* colonization of the gastrointestinal tract remain to be investigated.

Which of the changes that result from the absence of Btk could explain the observed protective effect of the DSS/*Candida* treatment? Btk is an important component of B-cell receptor signaling and Btk-/- animals have reduced B cell numbers and impaired antibody secretion [18,19]. B cells are prominent immune cells in the small intestine's lamina propria where their ability to secrete IgA is crucial for normal intestinal gene expression [31]. Despite this, DSS induces colitis in B cell-deficient mice [32] without affecting composition of the gastrointestinal microbiome [31]. In addition to B cell defects, Btk deletion also leads to innate immune deficiencies. Btk-/- mice have reduced numbers of polymorphonuclear leukocyte (PMN) numbers and Btk-/- neutrophils are deficient in ROS and NO production [33–35]. Mangla *et al.* also reported reduced inflammatory responses of Btk-/- knockout mice in different infection models [33].

Our immunohistochemistry experiments show reduced numbers of macrophages in DSS- and DSS/*Candida*-treated Btk-/- colons while neutrophil numbers are comparable to wild type (**Figure 3**). Because infiltrating macrophages and neutrophils cause severe immunopathology during colitis, we hypothesize that their lower numbers and reduced reactivity contribute to the reduced inflammation in the Btk-/- DSS/*Candida* treatment group. We previously showed that Btk interacts with Dectin-1 and that Btk-/- macrophages have phagocytic defects [16], possibly leading to an increase in fungal load in Btk-/- animals (**Figure 2D**). In conjunction with the lower numbers of macrophage infiltrates in Btk-/- colons, these observations might explain the altered inflammatory response of Btk-/- animals in response to DSS treatment and *C. albicans* colonization.

Cytokine analysis of spleen samples showed a general pro-inflammatory response with upregulation of IL1-β, IL-17A (colon), TNF, IFN-γ, IL-10 (spleen) and IL-6) and down regulation of TGF-β, IL-10 (colon), IL17A (spleen) (**Figure 3A, B, C**). There was no clear-cut effect of *Candida* colonization on the cytokines measured. Clustering analysis showed that wild type and Btk-/- animals treated with DSS or DSS/*Candida* similarly induce expression of IFN-γ and IL-6, cytokines often associated with trauma induced by *C. albicans* infection/colonization (**Figure 3C**). However, Btk-/- animals treated with DSS or DSS/*Candida* showed a higher upregulation of IL1-β, IL-17A, TNF, IFN-γ and IL-10 compared to wild type treatment groups. Therefore we conclude that reduced inflammatory responses in Btk-/- animals during *Candida* colonization are associated with relatively high levels of pro-inflammatory cytokines. These observations support the hypothesis that reduced inflammatory responses in Btk-/- animals are due to less responsive innate immune cells.

Correlation analysis showed that inflammation in wild type mice is associated with decreased TGF-β and IL-10 levels (**Figure 4D**). TGF-β is an important anti-inflammatory cytokine that is involved in the induction of regulatory T cells and Th17 cells. Interestingly, it has been previously reported that TGF-β transgenic mice develop age-related autoimmune disease, characterized by T-cell activation and colitis [36–38]. The anti-inflammatory IL-10 is produced by monocytes and epithelial cells and plays an important role in immune regulation in relation to microbiota in the gastrointestinal tract [39]. Both TGF-β and IL-10 are important cytokines in maintenance of gut health, which fits with the negative correlation with DSS-induced inflammation in wild type animals. The cytokine that is most closely correlated with the inflammatory response of Btk-/- animals is IL-17A. Increased spleen IL-17A levels are associated with increased colon length and decreased spleen weight. On the contrary, low colon IL-17A levels are associated with increased colon length (**Figure 4E**). In other words, "healthy" Btk-/- animals have high spleen IL-17A levels and low colon IL-17A levels. When comparing IL-17A levels in control groups and DSS and DSS/*Candida* groups, Btk-/- animals show an opposite trend compared to wild type animals. In Btk-/- animals, colon IL-17A is upregulated during inflammation and in the spleen lower levels of IL-17A are observed (**Figure 4A, B**). IL-17A is a key cytokine in the Th17 anti-fungal immune response that can be produced by Th17 cells [40,41], but also to a minor extend by neutrophils [42] and innate lymphoid cells [43]. Th17 cytokines including IL-17A are generally linked to severity of colitis but also induce protective regulatory mechanisms in epithelial cells [44].

Considering it's central role in the development of colitis, altered regulation and secretion of IL-17A might contribute to the reduced inflammatory response in Btk-/- animals.

Favorable effects of *C. albicans* colonization of the gut were previously reported. β-glucan, a major *C. albicans* cell wall component and the ligand Dectin-1, was shown to have potent anti-inflammatory effects in a mouse colitis model [45]. In addition, in the recovery phase after antibiotics treatment, the presence of *C. albicans* promoted bacterial diversity in the mouse caecum, specifically enriching *Bacteroidetes* populations and reducing *Lactobacillus* species [46,47]. This link between *C. albicans* and Bacteroidetes is interesting, because *Bacteroides fragilis* was shown to induce Tregs and mucosal tolerance [48]. The pleiotropic effect of Btk deletion makes it difficult to pinpoint the mechanism of protection in the DSS/*Candida*-treated Btk-/- animals. Conditional knockout animals with Btk deletion in specific cell types might assist in future experiments. In addition, the available Btk inhibitors in combination with *Candida* colonization might replicate the protective phenotype and thus Btk could be a possible target for the treatment of inflammatory conditions such as ulcerative colitis and Crohn's disease.

Acknowledgments

We want to acknowledge George Bell of the Whitehead Bioinformatics and Research Computing (BARC) department for invaluable help with statistical analysis and John Jackson for his assistance with the mouse colony.

Author Contributions

Conceived and designed the experiments: KS CAK HLP. Performed the experiments: KS OHY SKD AE AG CAK. Analyzed the data: KS CAK HLP. Contributed reagents/materials/analysis tools: KS OHY. Wrote the paper: KS HLP.

References

1. Iliev ID, Funari VA, Taylor KD, Nguyen Q, Reyes CN, et al. (2012) Interactions between commensal fungi and the C-type lectin receptor Dectin-1 influence colitis. Science 336: 1314–1317.
2. Ghannoum MA, Jurevic RJ, Mukherjee PK, Cui F, Sikaroodi M, et al. (2010) Characterization of the oral fungal microbiome (mycobiome) in healthy individuals. PLoS Pathog 6: e1000713.
3. Schulze J, Sonnenborn U (2009) Yeasts in the gut: from commensals to infectious agents. Dtsch Arztebl Int 106: 837–842.
4. Ott SJ, Kuhbacher T, Musfeldt M, Rosenstiel P, Hellmig S, et al. (2008) Fungi and inflammatory bowel diseases: Alterations of composition and diversity. Scand J Gastroenterol 43: 831–841.
5. Hamad I, Sokhna C, Raoult D, Bittar F (2012) Molecular detection of eukaryotes in a single human stool sample from Senegal. PLoS One 7: e40888.
6. Gow NA, Hube B (2012) Importance of the Candida albicans cell wall during commensalism and infection. Curr Opin Microbiol 15: 406–412.
7. Miranda LN, van der Heijden IM, Costa SF, Sousa AP, Sienra RA, et al. (2009) Candida colonisation as a source for candidaemia. J Hosp Infect 72: 9–16.
8. Nucci M, Anaissie E (2001) Revisiting the source of candidemia: skin or gut? Clin Infect Dis 33: 1959–1967.
9. Koh AY, Kohler JR, Coggshall KT, Van Rooijen N, Pier GB (2008) Mucosal damage and neutropenia are required for Candida albicans dissemination. PLoS Pathog 4: e35.
10. Li Q, Wang C, Tang C, He Q, Li N, et al. (2013) Dysbiosis of Gut Fungal Microbiota is Associated With Mucosal Inflammation in Crohn's Disease. J Clin Gastroenterol.
11. Herre J, Marshall AS, Caron E, Edwards AD, Williams DL, et al. (2004) Dectin-1 uses novel mechanisms for yeast phagocytosis in macrophages. Blood 104: 4038–4045.
12. Vautier S, Drummond RA, Redelinghuys P, Murray GI, MacCallum DM, et al. (2012) Dectin-1 is not required for controlling Candida albicans colonization of the gastrointestinal tract. Infect Immun 80: 4216–4222.
13. Franke A, McGovern DP, Barrett JC, Wang K, Radford-Smith GL, et al. (2010) Genome-wide meta-analysis increases to 71 the number of confirmed Crohn's disease susceptibility loci. Nature genetics 42: 1118–1125.

14. McGovern DP, Gardet A, Torkvist L, Goyette P, Essers J, et al. (2010) Genome-wide association identifies multiple ulcerative colitis susceptibility loci. Nature genetics 42: 332–337.
15. Seow CH, Stempak JM, Xu W, Lan H, Griffiths AM, et al. (2009) Novel anti-glycan antibodies related to inflammatory bowel disease diagnosis and phenotype. The American journal of gastroenterology 104: 1426–1434.
16. Strijbis K, Tafesse FG, Fairn GD, Witte MD, Dougan SK, et al. (2013) Bruton's Tyrosine Kinase (BTK) and Vav1 contribute to Dectin1-dependent phagocytosis of Candida albicans in macrophages. PLoS Pathog 9: e1003446.
17. Jongstra-Bilen J, Puig Cano A, Hasija M, Xiao H, Smith CI, et al. (2008) Dual functions of Bruton's tyrosine kinase and Tec kinase during Fcgamma receptor-induced signaling and phagocytosis. J Immunol 181: 288–298.
18. Khan WN, Alt FW, Gerstein RM, Malynn BA, Larsson I, et al. (1995) Defective B cell development and function in Btk-deficient mice. Immunity 3: 283–299.
19. Kerner JD, Appleby MW, Mohr RN, Chien S, Rawlings DJ, et al. (1995) Impaired expansion of mouse B cell progenitors lacking Btk. Immunity 3: 301–312.
20. White SJ, Rosenbach A, Lephart P, Nguyen D, Benjamin A, et al. (2007) Self-regulation of Candida albicans population size during GI colonization. PLoS Pathog 3: e184.
21. Reeves PG, Nielsen FH, Fahey GC Jr. (1993) AIN-93 purified diets for laboratory rodents: final report of the American Institute of Nutrition ad hoc writing committee on the reformulation of the AIN-76A rodent diet. J Nutr 123: 1939–1951.
22. Brown DH Jr, Giusani AD, Chen X, Kumamoto CA (1999) Filamentous growth of Candida albicans in response to physical environmental cues and its regulation by the unique CZF1 gene. Mol Microbiol 34: 651–662.
23. Jawhara S, Thuru X, Standaert-Vitse A, Jouault T, Mordon S, et al. (2008) Colonization of mice by Candida albicans is promoted by chemically induced colitis and augments inflammatory responses through galectin-3. The Journal of infectious diseases 197: 972–980.
24. Jawhara S, Mogensen E, Maggiotto F, Fradin C, Sarazin A, et al. (2012) Murine model of dextran sulfate sodium-induced colitis reveals Candida glabrata virulence and contribution of beta-mannosyltransferases. J Biol Chem 287: 11313–11324.
25. de Hoon MJ, Imoto S, Nolan J, Miyano S (2004) Open source clustering software. Bioinformatics 20: 1453–1454.
26. Saldanha AJ (2004) Java Treeview—extensible visualization of microarray data. Bioinformatics 20: 3246–3248.
27. Gantner BN, Simmons RM, Underhill DM (2005) Dectin-1 mediates macrophage recognition of Candida albicans yeast but not filaments. EMBO J 24: 1277–1286.
28. Pierce JV, Kumamoto CA (2012) Variation in Candida albicans EFG1 expression enables host-dependent changes in colonizing fungal populations. MBio 3: e00117–00112.
29. Wheeler RT, Kombe D, Agarwala SD, Fink GR (2008) Dynamic, morphotype-specific Candida albicans beta-glucan exposure during infection and drug treatment. PLoS pathogens 4: e1000227.
30. Heinsbroek SE, Oei A, Roelofs JJ, Dhawan S, te Velde A, et al. (2012) Genetic deletion of dectin-1 does not affect the course of murine experimental colitis. BMC Gastroenterol 12: 33.
31. Shulzhenko N, Morgun A, Hsiao W, Battle M, Yao M, et al. (2011) Crosstalk between B lymphocytes, microbiota and the intestinal epithelium governs immunity versus metabolism in the gut. Nat Med 17: 1585–1593.
32. Dieleman LA, Ridwan BU, Tennyson GS, Beagley KW, Bucy RP, et al. (1994) Dextran sulfate sodium-induced colitis occurs in severe combined immunodeficient mice. Gastroenterology 107: 1643–1652.
33. Mangla A, Khare A, Vineeth V, Panday NN, Mukhopadhyay A, et al. (2004) Pleiotropic consequences of Bruton tyrosine kinase deficiency in myeloid lineages lead to poor inflammatory responses. Blood 104: 1191–1197.
34. Mukhopadhyay S, George A, Bal V, Ravindran B, Rath S (1999) Bruton's tyrosine kinase deficiency in macrophages inhibits nitric oxide generation leading to enhancement of IL-12 induction. J Immunol 163: 1786–1792.
35. Honda F, Kano H, Kanegane H, Nonoyama S, Kim ES, et al. (2012) The kinase Btk negatively regulates the production of reactive oxygen species and stimulation-induced apoptosis in human neutrophils. Nat Immunol 13: 369–378.
36. Li MO, Wan YY, Flavell RA (2007) T cell-produced transforming growth factor-beta1 controls T cell tolerance and regulates Th1- and Th17-cell differentiation. Immunity 26: 579–591.
37. Travis MA, Reizis B, Melton AC, Masteller E, Tang Q, et al. (2007) Loss of integrin alpha(v)beta8 on dendritic cells causes autoimmunity and colitis in mice. Nature 449: 361–365.
38. Gorelik L, Flavell RA (2000) Abrogation of TGFbeta signaling in T cells leads to spontaneous T cell differentiation and autoimmune disease. Immunity 12: 171–181.
39. Olszak T, Neves JF, Dowds CM, Baker K, Glickman J, et al. (2014) Protective mucosal immunity mediated by epithelial CD1d and IL-10. Nature.
40. Harrington LE, Hatton RD, Mangan PR, Turner H, Murphy TL, et al. (2005) Interleukin 17-producing CD4+ effector T cells develop via a lineage distinct from the T helper type 1 and 2 lineages. Nat Immunol 6: 1123–1132.
41. Park H, Li Z, Yang XO, Chang SH, Nurieva R, et al. (2005) A distinct lineage of CD4 T cells regulates tissue inflammation by producing interleukin 17. Nat Immunol 6: 1133–1141.
42. Katayama M, Ohmura K, Yukawa N, Terao C, Hashimoto M, et al. (2013) Neutrophils are essential as a source of IL-17 in the effector phase of arthritis. PLoS One 8: e62231.
43. Gladiator A, Wangler N, Trautwein-Weidner K, LeibundGut-Landmann S (2013) Cutting edge: IL-17-secreting innate lymphoid cells are essential for host defense against fungal infection. J Immunol 190: 521–525.
44. Monteleone I, Sarra M, Pallone F, Monteleone G (2012) Th17-related cytokines in inflammatory bowel diseases: friends or foes? Curr Mol Med 12: 592–597.
45. Jawhara S, Habib K, Maggiotto F, Pignede G, Vandekerckove P, et al. (2012) Modulation of intestinal inflammation by yeasts and cell wall extracts: strain dependence and unexpected anti-inflammatory role of glucan fractions. PLoS One 7: e40648.
46. Mason KL, Erb Downward JR, Mason KD, Falkowski NR, Eaton KA, et al. (2012) Candida albicans and bacterial microbiota interactions in the cecum during recolonization following broad-spectrum antibiotic therapy. Infect Immun 80: 3371–3380.
47. Erb Downward JR, Falkowski NR, Mason KL, Muraglia R, Huffnagle GB (2013) Modulation of post-antibiotic bacterial community reassembly and host response by Candida albicans. Sci Rep 3: 2191.
48. Round JL, Mazmanian SK (2010) Inducible Foxp3+ regulatory T-cell development by a commensal bacterium of the intestinal microbiota. Proc Natl Acad Sci U S A 107: 12204–12209.

19

Inflammation and MiR-21 Pathways Functionally Interact to Downregulate PDCD4 in Colorectal Cancer

Oliver Peacock, Andrew C. Lee, Fraser Cameron, Rebecca Tarbox, Natasha Vafadar-Isfahani, Cristina Tufarelli*, Jonathan N. Lund

Surgery Group, Division of Medical Sciences and Graduate Entry Medicine, School of Medicine, University of Nottingham, Royal Derby Hospital, Derby, United Kingdom

Abstract

Inflammation plays a direct role in colorectal cancer (CRC) progression; however the molecular mechanisms responsible for this effect are unclear. The inflammation induced cyclooxygenase 2 (COX-2) enzyme required for the production of Prostaglandin E2 (PGE_2), can promote colorectal cancer by decreasing expression of the tumour suppressor gene Programmed Cell Death 4 (PDCD4). As PDCD4 is also a direct target of the oncogene microRNA-21 (miR-21) we investigated the relationship between the COX-2 and miR-21 pathways in colorectal cancer progression. Gene expression profile in tumour and paired normal mucosa from 45 CRC patients demonstrated that up-regulation of COX-2 and miR-21 in tumour tissue correlates with worse Dukes' stage. In vitro studies in colonic adenocarcinoma cells revealed that treatment with the selective COX-2 inhibitor NS398 significantly decreased miR-21 levels ($p = 0.0067$) and increased PDCD4 protein levels ($p < 0.001$), whilst treatment with PGE_2 up-regulated miR-21 expression ($p = 0.019$) and down-regulated PDCD4 protein ($p < 0.05$). These findings indicate that miR-21 is a component of the COX-2 inflammation pathway and that this pathway promotes worsening of disease stage in colorectal cancer by inducing accumulation of PGE_2 and increasing expression of miR-21 with consequent downregulation of the tumour suppressor gene PDCD4.

Editor: Kalpana Ghoshal, The Ohio State University, United States of America

Funding: The work was supported by a donation from the Derby Colorectal Cancer Fund. The funders had no role in study design, data collection and analysis, decision to publish, or preparation of the manuscript.

Competing Interests: The authors have declared that no competing interests exist.

* Email: cristina.tufarelli@nottingham.ac.uk

Introduction

Colorectal cancer is the third most common cause of cancer related deaths worldwide [1]. Approximately half of all patients diagnosed with colorectal cancer ultimately die of the condition [2]. The five year survival rate has increased to approximately 50–55%, which is attributed mainly to an earlier diagnosis and better tailoring of treatments [3]. Death from colorectal cancer can be prevented by early stage disease detection, but unfortunately it is often detected at an advanced stage when prognosis is worse [4]. The prognosis in colorectal cancer patients is associated with disease stage at the time of diagnosis.

The exact "trigger" for the development of colorectal cancer is still unknown. In 1990, a series of morphological steps known as the normal mucosa-adenoma-adenocarcinoma sequence in colorectal cancer due to genetic alterations was proposed [5]. However, many genetic events lead to the development of sporadic colorectal cancer; no single event occurs in all cancers and therefore no single pattern is applicable to every tumour [6]. Therefore, understanding specific genetic events that occur in colorectal carcinogenesis may have significant implications for diagnosis, prognosis and potentially gene therapy in the future.

There has been a recent resurgence in interest into the causal link between inflammation and cancer. Epidemiological studies have shown that chronic inflammation predisposes individuals to various types of cancer [7]. It is estimated that 15% to 20% of all cancer deaths worldwide are linked with underlying chronic infections and inflammatory responses within such individuals [7]. There is evidence from animal studies and observations in humans that a daily aspirin might be effective in preventing several common cancers [8,9]. This has been confirmed recently in follow-up studies of patients recruited originally for randomised trials of daily aspirin versus control in the prevention of vascular events [10–12]. In these trials, allocation to aspirin resulted in a 40% reduction in cancer deaths from 5 years onwards [11] and a sustained reduction in cancer-related death at 20 year follow-up [10,12]. Observational studies have also shown that aspirin use is associated with reduced distant metastasis and recurrence in common adenocarcinomas [13–15], suggesting that inflammation could play a role in progression as well as in development of cancer.

One of the possible reasons for the observed chemo preventive effects of aspirin in colorectal cancer is its ability to reduce tumour development by inhibition of cyclooxygenase 2 (COX-2) [16]. There is increasing evidence linking the pro-inflammatory enzyme COX-2 with the development and progression of colorectal cancer. COX-2 is induced in colonic epithelium in active inflammatory bowel disease (IBD) [17] and its up-regulation results in elevated levels of prostaglandin (PG), in particular PGE_2 that is a downstream mediator of COX-2 and promotes many carcinogenic pathways including cellular proliferation, inhibition of apoptosis and angiogenesis [18]. This contributes to the chronic inflammatory process orchestrating a tumour-supporting micro-environment, further linking inflammation with carcinogenesis.

The mechanistic linkage between inflammation and cancer is still not completely clear. Increasing evidence suggests that micro-RNAs (miRNAs) are involved in the regulation of inflammatory processes and are dysregulated in inflammatory conditions [19], including ulcerative colitis [20]. Therefore miRNAs dysregulation represents a potential molecular mechanism for inflammatory pathways to mediate cancer development and progression [21]. In particular, expression levels of miR-21 are increased in active inflammation in ulcerative colitis, which may be associated with the increased risk of cancer development with this condition [22]. Up-regulation of miR-21 has also been reported in other inflamed states including allergic airway inflammation [23], inflammatory skin conditions [19] and *Helicobacter pylori* associated gastric cancer [24]. miR-21 has been recently demonstrated to be a genuine oncogene in pre-B-cell lymphoma [25] and found to be over-expressed in most tumour types [26]. miR-21 is a potent stimulator of tissue and vascular invasion in colorectal cancer and these effects appear in part mediated by its ability to prevent translation of one of the miR-21 target genes, Programmed Cell Death 4 (PDCD4) [27]. More recently, a study has also shown significant down-regulation of PDCD4 in active IBD compared with inactive IBD, which also correlated with up-regulation of miR-21 [28], further supporting the link between inflammation, miR-21 and carcinogenesis.

Our aim was to investigate whether a functional interaction exist between the COX-2 (pro-inflammatory enzyme with increased expression in CRC) and miR-21 (oncogenic miR overexpressed in CRC) pathways leading to downregulation of the tumour suppressor PDCD4 in colorectal cancer not associated with previous chronic inflammatory disease.

Materials and Methods

Human tissues

This study received ethical approval from the Derbyshire Research Ethics Committee for collection of colorectal cancer tissue and matched normal mucosa from patients who underwent surgical resection for colorectal cancer between August and December 2010 at the Royal Derby Hospital, Derby, UK.

All patients diagnosed with colorectal cancer were discussed at the Royal Derby Hospital colorectal Multidisciplinary Team Meeting after radiological staging, and those deemed suitable for resection with curative intent were eligible for inclusion. Written informed consent was taken and patients unable or not willing to provide informed consent were excluded from the study, as were those withdrawing consent at any stage.

Cell Culture

The HCA-7 cell line was obtained from the Health Protection Agency Culture Collection (HPACC, Porton Down, UK). Cells were cultured in Dulbecco's Modified Eagle Media (DMEM) (GIBCO, Paisley, UK) supplemented with 10% foetal bovine serum (Fisher Scientific, Loughborough, UK), 2mM L-Glutamine (Sigma-Aldrich, Poole, UK), penicillin (50 units/ml) and streptomycin (50 µg/ml) (Sigma-Aldrich). Cells were cultured in 75cm^3 vented flasks (TSZ Scientific, Framingham, MA, USA) in humidified incubators at 37°C with 5% CO_2 (Sanyo, Osaka, Japan).

Cell Line Transfections and treatments

Cells were seeded at 500,000 cells/well into a 6 well plate and incubated at 37°C with 5% CO_2 until they reached 70% confluence.

For miR-21 inhibition studies, cells were transfected with miR-21 inhibitor (100nM) or a negative scrambled control (100nM) (miRIDIAN, Dharmacon Lafayette, CO, USA), using Dharmafect 2 lipid transfection reagent (Dharmacon Lafayette, CO, USA) according to the manufacturer's instructions.

For COX-2 inhibition, cells were treated with serum free medium containing the control (0.1% DMSO) or 100 µM NS398 (selective COX-2 inhibitor, Cayman Chemical, Michigan, USA) for 72 hours. For Prostaglandin E_2 (PGE_2) treatment, cells were grown 24 hours with serum free medium containing DMSO vehicle alone or 1 µM PGE_2 so that the final concentration of DMSO in both conditions was the same (0.1%). For combined miR-21 inhibition and PGE_2 treatment, PGE_2 was added to the culture 48 hours after miR-21 inhibitor transfection and cells were cultured for a further 24 hours.

RNA analyses

Total RNA extraction was performed using TRI Reagent following the manufacturer's protocol (Sigma-Aldrich) and quantified using a Nanodrop spectrophotometer (Thermo Fisher Scientific, Wilmington, DE, USA).

For the miR-21 studies, a total of 6 ng of total RNA was used to reverse transcribe miR-21 and RNU44 control into cDNA following the TaqMan miRNA protocol (Applied Biosystems, Foster City, CA, USA), using hairpin primers directed to miR-21 and RNU44 as a control in a thermocycler (GeneAmp PCR System 9700, Applied Biosystems) for 30min at 16°C, 30 min at 42°C, 5min at 85°C. Real-time quantitative polymerase chain reaction was then performed using miRNAs specific TaqMan probe assays (miR-21, ID 000397; RNU44, ID 001094; Applied Biosystems) in a Chromo4 thermal cycler (Bio-Rad Laboratories LTD, Hemel Hempstead, UK). miR-21 expression levels were normalised to RNU44 and calculated using the $2^{-\Delta\Delta Ct}$ method [29] using commercially available normal colon RNA as a calibrator.

For *COX-2* and *PDCD4* analyses, 30ng of total RNA was converted to cDNA with random hexamers using the TaqMan high capacity cDNA reverse transcription protocol (Applied Biosystems, Foster City, CA, USA). Real time PCRs were performed according to the manufacturer instructions in a Chromo4 real time cycler (Bio-Rad Laboratories Ltd) using commercially available 20x TaqMan assays (Applied Biosystems) for *PDCD4* (Hs00377253_m1) and *COX-2* (PTGS2 - Hs00153133_m1), alongside the control genes *GAPDH* (Hs02258991_g1), *PGK1* (Hs00943178_g1) and *HPRT* (Hs01003267_m1). For the experiments in cell lines, quantification was performed in accordance to MIQE (Minimum Information for Publication of Quantitative Real-Time PCR Experiments) guidelines [30] relatively to the geometric mean of the reference genes *GAPDH*, *PGK1*, *HPRT* using the GenEX software (MultiD Analysis; Göteborg, Sweden). Due to limited sample's amounts, in human tissues expression was quantified relatively to *GAPDH* alone as described above for miR-21 analyses.

Protein analyses

Protein extractions and quantification were performed as previously described [31]. Western blotting was performed using the loading control anti-beta actin antibody (1:1000 dilution; Abcam, Cambridge, UK) in combination with anti-PDCD4 antibody (1:500 dilution; Sigma-Aldrich) or anti-COX-2 (1:1000

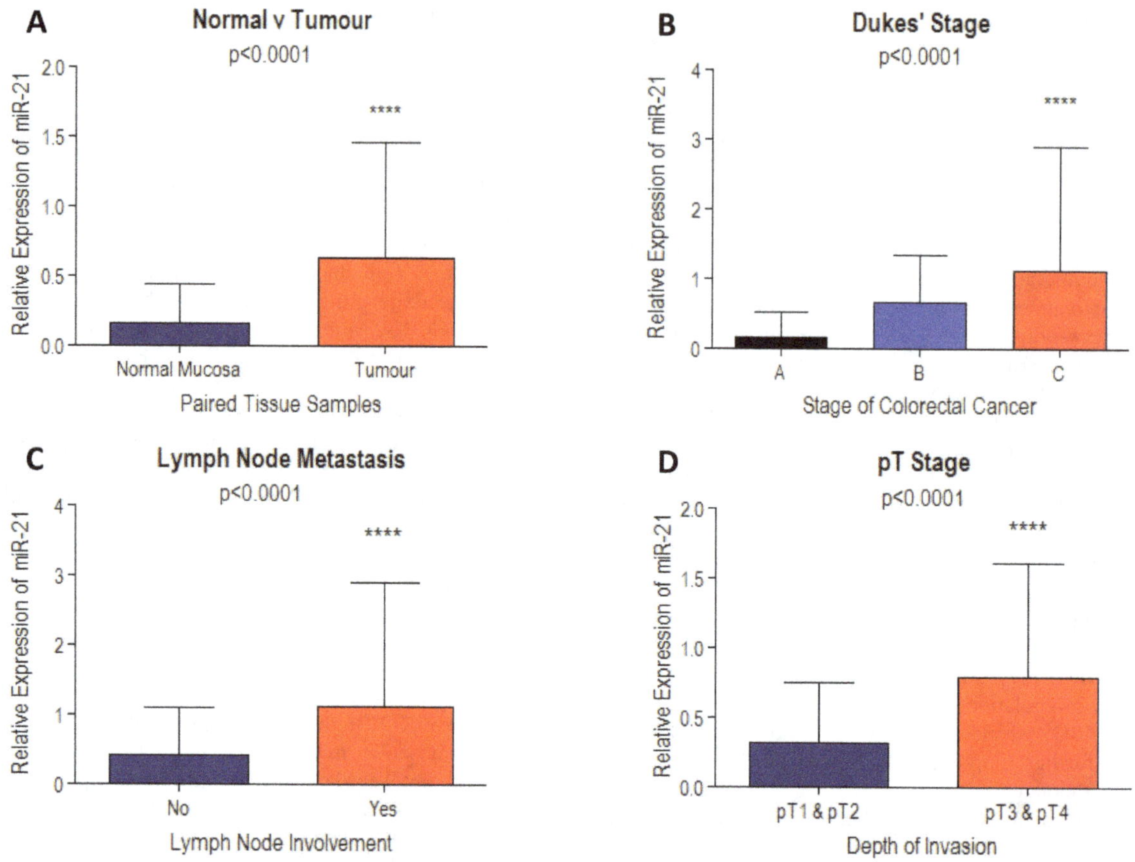

Figure 1. miR-21 expression in primary colorectal tissue samples, calculated relatively to that of the control miRNA RNU44, was studied in primary tumour and matched adjacent normal mucosa (n = 45; A); in Dukes' A (n = 9), B (n = 23) and C (n = 13) stages (B); in lymph node negative (No; n = 32) versus lymph node positive (Yes, n = 13) cases (C); and in tumours displaying lower (pT1 & pT2; n = 11) versus higher (pT3 & pT4; n = 34) depth of invasion (D). Column bar graphs indicate the median and whiskers demonstrate the IQR of miR-21 expression. Note that significant increase in miR-21 expression is observed in tumours, and this increases further with worsening stage, lymphnode involvement and depth of invasion. Statistical significance was calculated using the Wilcoxon signed-rank test in A, the Kruskall-Wallis test in B, and the Mann-Whitney U test in C and D.

dilution; Abcam). Anti-rabbit IgG antibody conjugated to alkaline phosphatase was used as secondary antibody (1:30,000 dilution; DAKO, Ely, UK) for detection of primary antibody binding. Immunocomplexes were visualised by enhanced chemiluminescence using the ECL kit (Bio-Rad) according to the manufacturer's protocol. The chemidoc system was used to capture images and Quantity One (Bio-Rad) software was used for quantification of bands' intensities.

Elisa Analysis

PGE_2 levels were measured in the media of HCA-7 treated and untreated cells using the PGE_2 elisa detection kit (Cayman Chemical, Ann Arbor, Michigan USA) according to the manufacturer's instructions. Plates were read with a plate photocytometer at 450 nm (Wallac 1420 Victor; Perkin-Elmer, Waltham, MA, USA).

Statistical Analysis

Statistical analysis was performed using GraphPad Prism Version 5.03 (GraphPad Software, La Jolla, CA, USA). The Kolmogorov-Smirnov test demonstrated all the tissue sample data to be non-parametric and all the cell line data to be parametric. Therefore patient's data is expressed as medians and range, whilst cell line data is expressed as mean and standard error of the mean. The Wilcoxon signed-rank test (paired data); the Mann-Whitney U test (unpaired) and the Kruskall-Wallis test were used for comparative analysis of patient's data. The paired t-test (paired data); the t-test (unpaired) and the ANOVA test were used for comparative analysis of cell line's data.

Statistical significance was determined at $p \leq 0.05$ for both patient's and cell line's data.

Results

Increase in miR-21 directly relates to increase in COX-2 mRNA levels in CRC patients

We performed our study on primary colorectal cancer tissue and paired normal mucosa collected between August and December 2010 from 45 elective patients with sporadic cases of CRC. A prospectively maintained database was populated with patient demographics, neoadjuvant therapies and tumour characteristics. The tumour histopathology was classified according to the national minimum data set for colorectal cancer designed by the Royal College of Pathologists, UK [32]. No patients were excluded or had withdrawn from the study and none had benign disease. The median age was 69 (range 51–88) years and the majority were male patients. Four patients with rectal cancer who received neo-adjuvant chemo-radiotherapy were also included based on previous studies demonstrating that expression of miR-21 is equivalent between radiated and non-radiated tissue [33]. All patients had a complete resection and histology confirmed all tumours were adenocarcinomas. (Table S1 and S2 in File S1)

Using by real time RT-PCR we studied expression of *COX-2* and miR-21 in tumour tissues as compared to normal mucosa in our cohort of CRC patients. Relative expression of miR-21 was significantly up-regulated in the CRC tissue compared with the matched normal mucosa ($p<0.0001$, Wilcoxon matched-pairs signed rank test; Fig. 1A). Moreover, expression levels of miR-21 were correlated with the commonly used clinical-pathological features for CRC (Table 1). Higher expression of miR-21 in tumour tissues significantly correlated with a worse Dukes' stage ($p<0.0001$, Kruskall-Wallis test; Fig. 1B), lymph node metastasis ($p<0.0001$, Mann-Whitney U test; Fig. 1C), and depth of tumour invasion (pT stage; $p<0.0001$, Mann-Whitney U test; Fig. 1D). These findings are in agreement with previous reports [34,35], and confirm that miR-21 is up-regulated in CRC with increasing expression levels correlating with increased severity of the disease.

Relative expression of *PDCD4* was significantly down-regulated in CRC tissues compared with matched normal mucosa ($p<0.0001$, Wilcoxon matched-pairs signed rank test; Fig. 2A). However, there was no correlation between *PDCD4* expression in tumour tissues and the Dukes' stage, with expression in Dukes'A stage being already significantly decreased as compared to normal tissue and no further decrease seen in more advanced stages (Fig. 2B). It is unlikely that the observed downregulation of *PDCD4* at the RNA level is caused by miR-21 given that this micro-RNA acts to prevent PDCD4 mRNA translation rather than induce its degradation or transcriptional repression [27]. Given that all the patients studied carried malignant tumours with an assigned Dukes' stage, the data suggest that during progression of malignancy increasing amounts of miR-21 lead to inhibition of translation of the already decreased levels of *PDCD4* mRNA. Ethics constraints prevented us from analysing PDCD4 protein levels in these patients to confirm this hypothesis and we recurred to *in vitro* studies to gain mechanistic insights (see next section).

Interestingly, relative expression of *COX-2* mRNA was significantly up-regulated in tumour tissues compared with their matched normal mucosa ($p<0.0001$, Wilcoxon matched-pairs signed rank test; Fig. 2C). Moreover, similarly to what was observed with miR-21, relative expression of *COX-2* mRNA in tumour tissues significantly correlated with a worse Dukes' stage ($p<0.0001$, Kruskall-Wallis test; Fig. 2D). Given that miR-21 and inflammation have both been shown to decrease PDCD4 protein levels [27,36], a possible interpretation of these findings is that increase in miR-21 and *COX-2* may be functionally related and that they could lead to downregulation of PDCD4 through a common pathway.

HCA-7 cells are a suitable system for analysing the relationship between miR-21 and COX-2 overexpression in CRC

To further investigate the potential of a functional relationship between COX-2 and miR-21 in the down-regulation of PDCD4 in CRC we recurred to an *in vitro* cell culture system. We chose the human colonic adenocarcinoma cell line HCA-7 isolated from a Dukes' B tumour [37] because it has high endogenous levels of COX-2 [38] and following treatment with the COX-2 inhibitor NS398 increases expression of *PDCD4* [39]. In order to determine whether HCA-7 cells are a good system in which to study the functional relationship between the miR-21 and COX-2 pathways, we first needed to determine whether miR-21 is expressed and is responsible for *PDCD4* downregulation in these cells. To achieve these we used RT-PCR to study the levels of miR-21 in untreated HCA-7 cells or in cells treated with 100nM of a miR-21 inhibitor or scramble control based on published work showing that this concentration is non-cytotoxic and effective in inhibitory studies [40].

We found that miR-21 is expressed at high levels in HCA-7 cells and these levels are not affected by treatment with scramble small RNAs but are significantly decreased ($p<0.0001$, unpaired t-test) following 72 hours treatment with a specific miR-21 small RNA inhibitor (Fig. 3A). No significant differences in PDCD4 mRNA

Table 1. Relative expression of miR-21 with common clinical-pathological features of colorectal cancer.

Variables	Patients	p-Value
Histological Type:		
Well Differentiated	4	
Moderate & Poorly Differentiated	41	p = 0.0002
Depth of Invasion:		
pT1 & pT2	11	p<0.0001
pT3 & pT4	34	
Dukes' Stage:		
A	9	
B	23	p<0.0001
C	13	
Lymph Node Metastasis:		
Positive	13	p<0.0001
Negative	32	
Vascular Invasion		
Positive	13	p = 0.01
Negative	32	

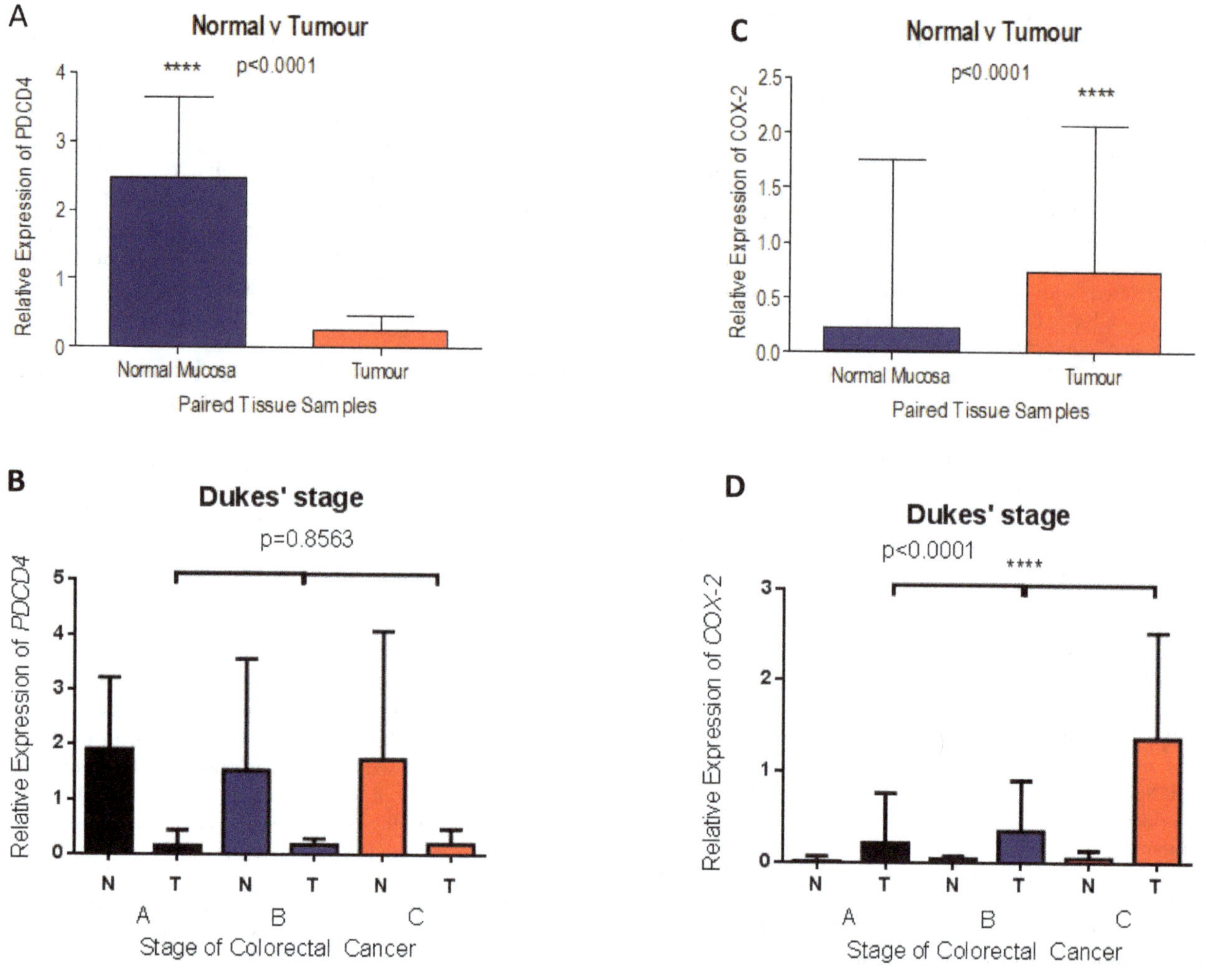

Figure 2. Expression of *PDCD4* and *COX-2* mRNA in primary colorectal tissue samples calculated relatively to that of the control gene *GAPDH*. Combined relative expression of PDCD4 and COX-2 was analysed in primary tumour versus matched adjacent normal mucosa (n = 45; A and C respectively), and in normal (N) and tumour (T) tissues from Dukes' A (n = 9), B (n = 23) and C (n = 13) stages (B and D respectively). The column bar graph indicates the median and the whiskers demonstrate the IQR of mRNA expression. Statistical significance was calculated using the Wilcoxon signed-rank test in A and C; the Kruskall-Wallis test in B and D. Note that *PDCD4* is downregulated in tumour versus normal, but no differences are seen in the remaining expression in tumours of different Dukes' stages. By contrast *COX-2* levels increase in tumour and with disease stage.

levels were observed by quantitative RT-PCR in any of the treatment conditions (Fig. 3B); by contrast, a significant increase ($p = 0.002$, unpaired t-test) in PDCD4 was observed at the protein level by western blot in the miR-21 inhibitor treated cells compared to untreated or scramble control treated cells. These findings are consistent with miR-21 acting to inhibit translation of PDCD4 mRNA rather than directing its degradation and confirm that miR-21 plays a role in PDCD4 downregulation in HCA-7 cells. Therefore both the COX-2 and miR-21 pathways contribute to downregulation of PDCD4 in HCA-7 cells, making them a suitable system in which to study whether a functional relationship exists between the two pathways.

Relation between miR-21 and COX-2 in the downregulation of PDCD4 in HCA-7 cells

To further investigate the functional interaction between the miR-21 and COX-2 pathways, we first analysed COX-2 mRNA and protein levels in HCA-7 cells after 72 hours treatment with the miR-21 inhibitor compared to scramble control and untreated cells. No difference in COX-2 expression was observed neither at the mRNA nor at the protein levels ($p = 0.62$ and $p = 0.83$ respectively, unpaired t test), showing that COX-2 is not a target of miR-21 (Fig. S1 in File S1).

We next treated HCA-7 cells with 100 μM NS398, a specific COX-2 inhibitor reported to be non-cytotoxic and effective at this concentration in cell culture [41], or with vehicle alone (0.1% DMSO). COX-2 plays a critical role during inflammation in the initial steps of the conversion of arachidonic acid to prostaglandins including prostaglandin E (PGE_2) and up-regulation of COX-2 in colorectal cancer has been shown to associate with marked increase in the production of PGE_2 [42]. Using Elisa to measure levels of PGE_2 we found a significant decrease ($p = 0.006$, unpaired t test) in the media of cells treated with NS398 compared to untreated cells or cells treated with vehicle alone, consistent with inhibition of COX-2 catalytic activity (Fig. S2 in File S1).

Having established effectiveness of the treatment we then measured the relative expression of miR-21 and we could detect a significant decrease in miR-21 following NS398 treatment for

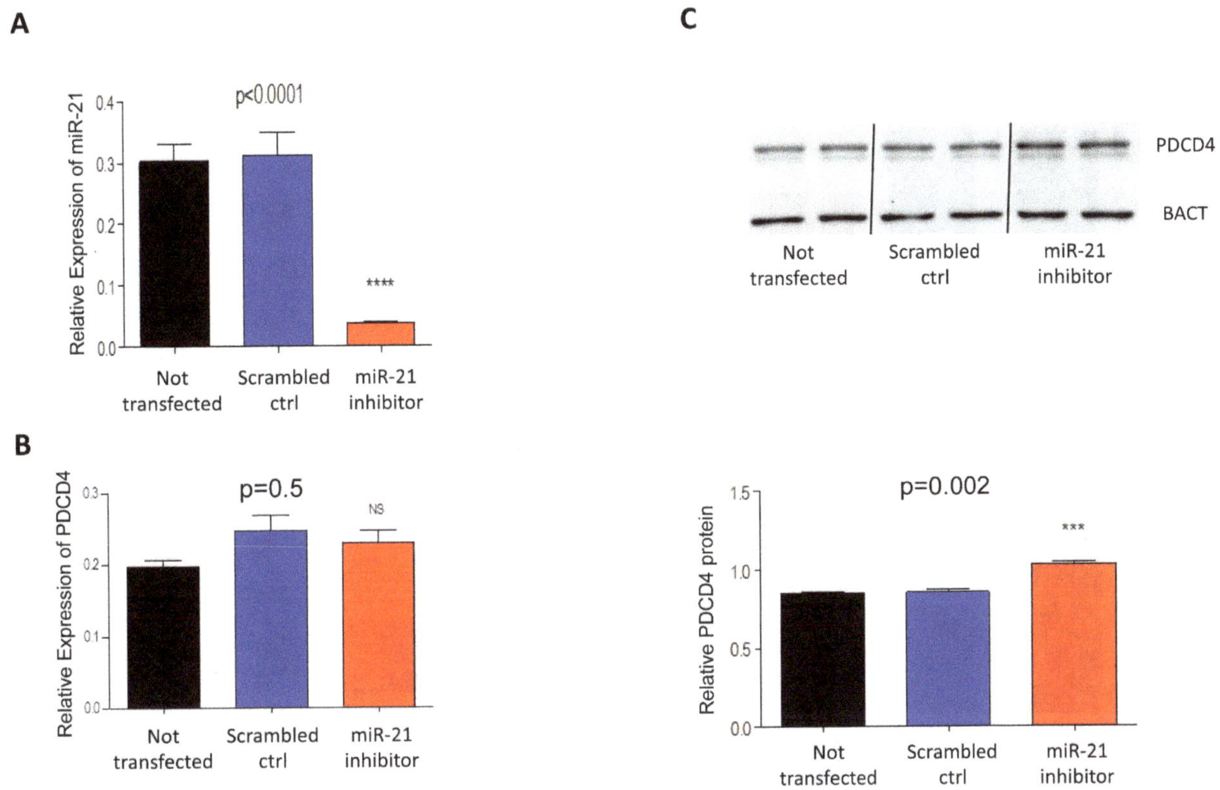

Figure 3. miR-21 and *PDCD4* expression in HCA-7 cells treated with miR-21 inhibitor. Following 72 hours from transfection significant decrease in miR-21 levels are seen only in cells transfected with miR-21 inhibitor (**A**). *PDCD4* mRNA levels were not affected by inhibition of miR-21 (**B**). Western blot analysis of PDCD4 (**C** top panel for a representative blot) reveals a significant increase in protein levels in cells transfected with the inhibitor as compared to untreated or scramble control treated cells, when quantified relatively to beta actin protein (BACT) as a loading control (**C** bottom panel). The column bar graph indicates the mean and the whiskers demonstrate the standard error of the mean (SEM). Statistical significance was calculated using the unpaired t-test. Experiments were repeated three times and analysed in duplicate. Untreated = cells culture in media; scramble = cells transfected with scramble RNA inhibitors; miR-21 inhibitor = cells treated with the miR-21 RNA inhibitor.

72 hours ($p<0.01$, unpaired t test; Fig. 4A). By contrast, treatment of HCA-7 cells with NS398 did not alter expression of PDCD4 mRNA ($p=0.74$, unpaired t test) (Fig. 4B), an observation that is in contrast to the previously reported 1.5 fold upregulation of PDCD4 mRNA following treatment of HCA-7 cells with NS398 [39]. The difference might be due to the methods used: the latter study analysed PDCD4 mRNA expression by northern blot and quantified it relatively to GAPDH, whilst in our study we have measured mRNA levels using quantitative RT-PCR and normalised the data using the geometric mean of three reference genes (GAPDH, PGK and HPRT) in accordance to the MIQE guidelines [30] (see methods). Our real time PCR data suggests that NS398 treatment leads to a decrease in GAPDH levels (Fig. S3 in File S1) and this change would result in an apparent increase in PDCD4 levels if GAPDH was used as the sole reference gene. Therefore we conclude that NS398 treatment does not alter PDCD4 transcription rate or mRNA stability; however, consistent with the observed decrease in miR-21, significant up-regulation in PDCD4 protein expression ($p<0.001$, unpaired t test) was observed in NS398 treated cells as compared to untreated or vehicle alone cells (Fig. 4C). These data indicate that down-regulation of PDCD4 by COX-2 is not a consequence of decreased PDCD4 mRNA synthesis or stability, but rather that COX-2 may act by promoting an increase in miR-21 which in turn inhibits translation of PDCD4 mRNA.

COX-2 activation of miR-21 in HCA-7 cells is mediated by PGE_2

Given the role of COX-2 in the production of prostaglandins, to investigate the mechanism underlying activation of miR-21 by COX-2 we treated HCA-7 cells with 1 μM PGE_2 for 24 hours as this concentration was shown to work effectively on these cells [38]. We found that miR-21 expression was significantly up-regulated ($p=0.019$, unpaired t test) in PGE_2 treated cells as compared to vehicle (0.1% DMSO) treated or untreated cells (Fig. 5A). No changes in PDCD4 mRNA levels were observed in PGE_2 treated cells (Fig. 5B); however a significant decrease ($p<0.05$, unpaired t test) in PDCD4 protein levels was observed which paralleled the increase in miR-21 (Fig. 5C). Combined treatment with PGE_2 and miR-21 inhibitor brought the levels of miR-21 down to levels comparable with those in untreated cells (Fig. S4 in File S1), and treatment with aspirin also led to a decrease in miR-21 levels (Fig. S5 in File S1). These data suggest that COX-2 driven downregulation of PDCD4 in this model system is mainly due to PGE_2 induced upregulation of miR-21.

Discussion

Dysregulation of miRNAs is a recognised step in the pathogenesis of many cancer types, including CRC. miR-21 is a miRNA frequently upregulated in CRC, whose increased expression levels are associated with poorer therapeutic outcomes in CRC [34]. We

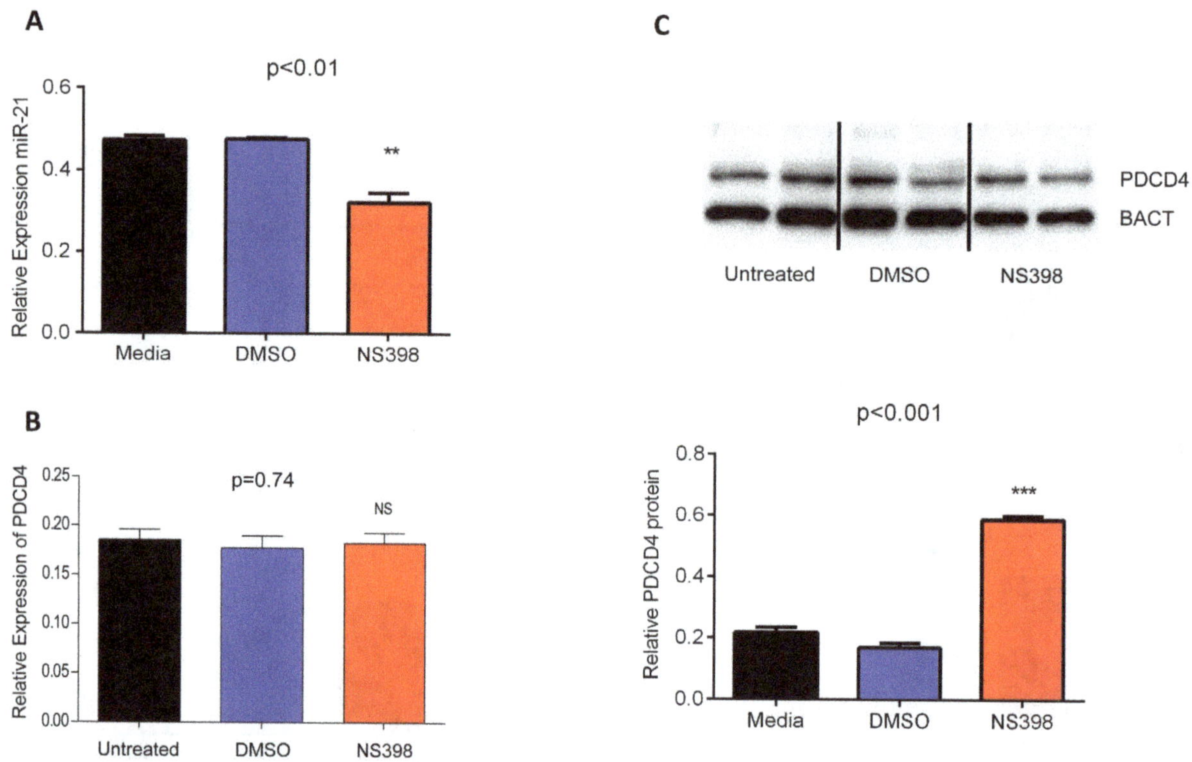

Figure 4. miR-21 and *PDCD4* expression in HCA-7 cells treated with the COX-2 inhibitor NS398. Following 72 hours treatment significant decrease in miR-21 levels is seen in NS398 treated cells (**A**). *PDCD4* mRNA levels are not affected by NS398 treatment (**B**). Western blot analysis of PDCD4 (**C** top panel for a representative blot) reveals a significant increase in protein levels in NS398 treated cells as compared to untreated or vehicle alone (DMSO) treated cells, when quantified relatively to beta actin protein (BACT) as a loading control (**C** bottom panel). The column bar graph indicates the mean and the whiskers demonstrate the standard error of the mean (SEM). Statistical significance was calculated using the unpaired t-test. Experiments were repeated three times and analysed in triplicate. Untreated = cells cultured in media; DMSO = cells cultured in media supplemented with 0.1% DMSO vehicle; NS398 = cells cultured in media supplemented with NS398 prepared in DMSO to a final concentration of 100 μM NS398 and 0.1% DMSO.

have confirmed that over-expression of miR-21 correlates significantly with worse pathological staging in our CRC patient's cohort (Fig. 1), comprised of patients who presented with tumours of an assigned Dukes' stage, suggesting an important role of miR-21 in cancer invasion and dissemination.

Few of the potential downstream targets regulated by miR-21 have been confirmed, and these include the programmed cell death 4 (PDCD4) tumour suppressor gene that inhibits neoplastic transformation [43]. Recent studies have shown a progressive reduction in PDCD4 expression from normal mucosa, to polyp, to colorectal tumour [33]. Interestingly a significant increase in miR-21 was seen in CRC compared to normal, but not between adenomatous polyps and normal, although a decrease in PDCD4 expression was evident at this transition [33]. In our cohort we observed a decrease in PDCD4 mRNA levels in the tumours relative to the normal tissues, but no changes as disease progressed by Dukes' stage (Fig. 2A). Taken together these observations suggest that at the transition from normal to hyperproliferation downregulation of PDCD4 might be due to regulation at the level of transcription and/or RNA and protein stability. However, in the transition to malignancy miR-21 mediated inhibition of translation of PDCD4 protein levels of the already decreased levels of *PDCD4* mRNA becomes predominant, thus promoting further progression of malignancy. Therefore determining the upstream factors that influence miR-21 expression is instrumental in establishing whether and how miR-21 contributes to malignancy progression and to provide potential therapeutic targets.

Given that in our cohort of CRC patients upregulation of miR-21 is positively related to that of COX-2 mRNA and with worse pathological staging (Fig. 1 and 2B), we hypothesised that miR-21 upregulation in CRC might be linked to an inflammatory response. Circumstantial evidence supporting this hypothesis includes the observations that inflammation can lead to down-regulation of PDCD4 in colorectal tissue [36] and that miR-21 upregulation in gastric cancer is due to PGE_2 induced activation of NF-kB [44]. Using an *in vitro* culture system we have shown that in HCA-7 cells PDCD4 downregulation is mediated by miR-21 at the post-transcriptional level as no change in PDCD4 mRNA levels were seen (Fig. 3). This confirms the work of a previous group who identified a conserved target site for miR-21 within the 3′-UTR of PDCD4 [27]. We found that whilst down-regulation of miR-21 by transfection of a miR-21 inhibitor had no effect on the expression of COX-2 (Fig. S1 in File S1), inhibition of COX-2 by the specific COX-2 inhibitor NS398 or use of the anti-inflammatory aspirin led to decrease in miR-21 levels (Fig. 3 and Fig. S5 in File S1). In NS398 treated cells, miR-21 downregulation correlates with an increase in PDCD4 protein without changes in PDCD4 mRNA levels (Fig. 4), further supporting a role of miR-21 in the downregulation of PDCD4. Previous studies have demonstrated that NS398 exerts several anti-carcinogenic effects in colon cancer by inducing apoptosis [45], whilst also inhibiting cell cycle progression [39], angiogenesis [46] and metastasis [47]. Our novel finding of a significant up-regulation in PDCD4 protein levels following NS398 treatment

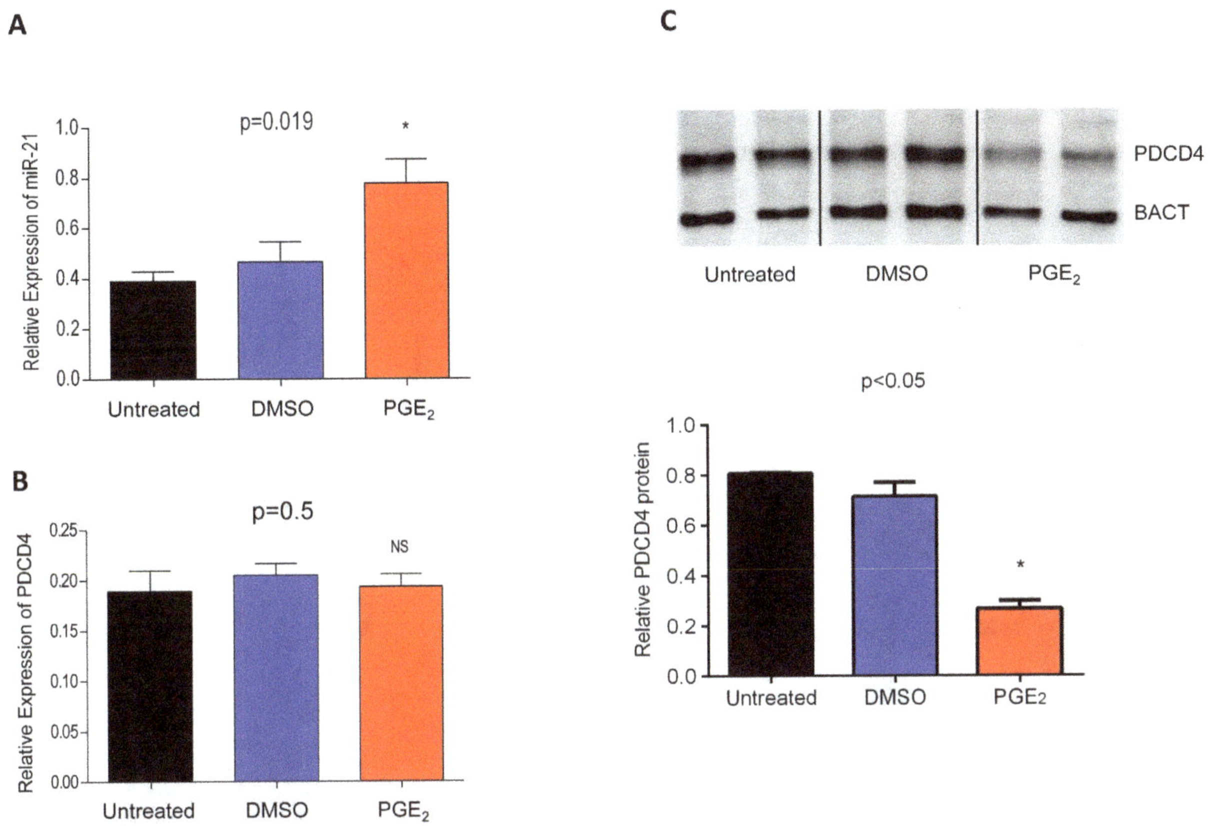

Figure 5. miR-21 and *PDCD4* expression in HCA-7 cells treated with PGE_2. After 24 hours treatment significant increase in miR-21 levels is seen in PGE_2 treated cells (**A**). *PDCD4* mRNA levels are not affected by PGE_2 treatment (**B**). Western blot analysis of PDCD4 (**C** top panel for a representative blot) reveals a significant decrease in protein levels in PGE_2 treated cells as compared to untreated or vehicle alone (DMSO) treated cells, when quantified relatively to beta actin protein (BACT) as a loading control (**C** bottom panel). The column bar graph indicates the mean and the whiskers demonstrate the standard error of the mean (SEM). Statistical significance was calculated using the unpaired t-test. Experiments were repeated three times and analysed in duplicate. Untreated = cells cultured in media; DMSO = cells cultured in media supplemented with 0.1% DMSO vehicle; PGE_2 = cells cultured in media supplemented with PGE_2 prepared in DMSO to a final concentration of 1 μM PGE_2 and 0.1% DMSO.

suggests that the chemo preventive effects of NS398 may in part be attributed to its action on PDCD4. Moreover, the relationship between COX-2 and miR-21 is unidirectional, whereby increase in COX-2 activity drives overexpression of miR-21; therefore miR-21 is a component of the COX-2 pathway, downstream of COX-2. Indeed we found that miR-21 upregulation is a consequence of COX-2 mediated PGE_2 production as treatment of cells with PGE_2 led to increase in miR-21 and decrease in PDCD4 protein, which was reversed by combining PGE_2 and miR-21 inhibitor treatments (Fig. 5 and Fig. S2 in File S1). These findings are in agreement with work by other groups indicating that COX-2 inhibitors induce apoptosis and inhibit angiogenesis *in vitro*, [48,49] whilst also attenuating invasion, angiogenesis and metastasis *in vivo* [50,51].

Our study provides mechanistic insights into the link between inflammation, miR-21 and PDCD4 expression and colorectal cancer progression. Based on our findings it is feasible to propose a model of one of the ways in which persistent inflammation at a site of invasive early stage colorectal tumour can induce progression to more malignant states (Fig. 6). According to our model, continued inflammation at the tumour site leads to progressive increase in COX-2 expression and consequent PGE_2 accumulation which can be blocked by the use of NS398 COX-2 inhibitor (Fig. 6, left side). PGE_2 induces increase in miR-21 expression causing further downregulation of PDCD4 protein levels (and potentially other miR-21 targets) thus facilitating further progression of the tumour to more malignant stages and these effects can be reversed using miR-21 inhibitors (Fig. 6, right side). Interestingly, it has just been reported that the 15-hydroxyprostaglandin dehydrogenase (15-PGDH) mRNA which codes for a key enzyme required for PGE_2 degradation, is a direct target of miR-21 in cholangiocarcinoma cells [52]. Although the presence of this miR-21 mediated effect remains to be proven in CRC, the observation suggests that a reinforcing positive feedback may exists whereby increase in miR-21 induced by PGE_2 favours further accumulation of PGE_2 by preventing its degradation.

Conclusions

In conclusion, we have highlighted the potential benefits of analysing COX-2 and miR-21 expression levels for tumour staging and of correlating these levels to therapeutic response or disease outcome. Moreover, this study has contributed to an improved understanding of the role of miR-21, PDCD4 and COX-2 in colorectal cancer progression. We have demonstrated a functional link between COX-2, miR-21 and PDCD4, which provides further understanding into the beneficial effects of COX-2 inhibitors in colorectal cancer control. Further investigation of the pathway linking inflammation to miR-21 will reveal key intermediate players and their potential to be targeted therapeutically, with the final goal to determine the feasibility of combining

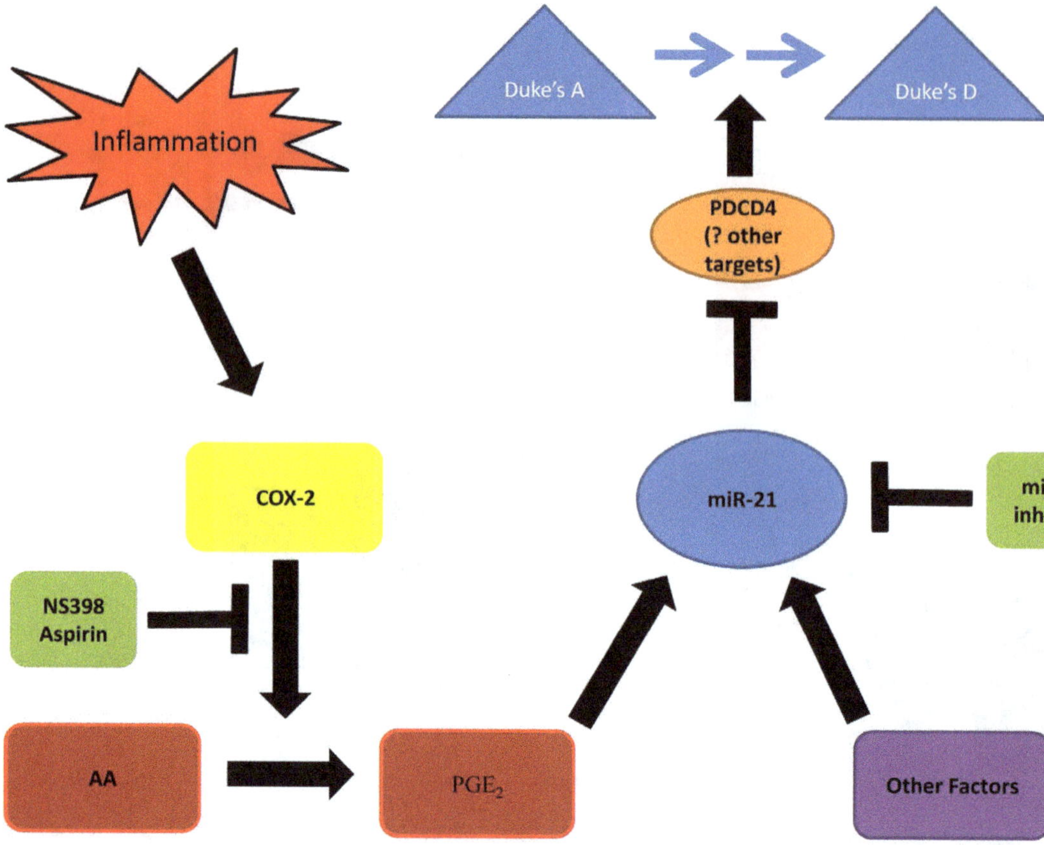

Figure 6. Proposed model of how the inflammation pathway can promote colorectal cancer progression by linking inflammation to downregulation of PDCD4 via miR-21 induction mediated by COX-2 driven accumulation of PGE_2. Persistent inflammation at the tumour site drives increase in COX-2 expression leading to accumulation of PGE_2. This in turn leads to the increase in expression of miR-21 and subsequent downregulation of PDCD4 protein levels facilitating progressive increase to more invasive and metastatic forms of colorectal cancer (from Dukes' A to B, C and D). Our experiments indicate that this pathway can be blocked by COX-2 inhibitors (NS398 and Aspirin) by preventing accumulation of PGE_2 as well as by miR-21 inhibitors. ↑ Activation, ⊤ Inhibition. See text for further details.

the use of anti-inflammatory drugs, with miR-21 inhibitors and strategies targeting intermediate components in the treatment of CRC. These findings therefore provide a basis for identification of potential therapeutic targets in the future management of colorectal cancer.

Supporting Information

File S1 Table of Contents: Method S1. Aspirin treatment of HCA-7 cells (page 1). **Figure S1.** *COX-2* mRNA expression in HCA-7 cells treated with miR-21 inhibitor (page 2). **Figure S2.** PGE2 levels in the media of cells treated with the COX-2 inhibitor NS398 (page 3). **Figure S3.** Expression of *GAPDH* in cells treated with NS398 (page 4). **Figure S4.** miR-21 expression in cells treated with PGE2 and miR-21 inhibitor (page 5). **Figure S5.** miR-21 expression in cells treated with Aspirin (page 6). **Table S1.** Demographics for the cohort of colorectal cancer patients (page 7). **Table S2.** Clinical-pathological staging (page 8).

Acknowledgments

We are grateful to Dr Raheela Khan for support and constructive discussions throughout the course of the project.

Author Contributions

Conceived and designed the experiments: OP CT JNL. Performed the experiments: OP ACL FC RT NV-I CT. Analyzed the data: OP ACL NV-I CT. Contributed reagents/materials/analysis tools: OP CT JNL. Wrote the paper: OP CT JNL. Study supervision: CT JNL.

References

1. Jemal A, Bray F, Center MM, Ferlay J, Ward E, et al. (2011) Global cancer statistics. CA Cancer J Clin 61: 69–90.
2. Figueredo A, Coombes ME, Mukherjee S (2008) Adjuvant therapy for completely resected stage II colon cancer. Cochrane Database Syst Rev: CD005390.
3. UK CR (2011) Bowel Cancer Survival Statistics.
4. Walsh JM, Terdiman JP (2003) Colorectal cancer screening: scientific review. JAMA 289: 1288–1296.
5. Fearon ER, Vogelstein B (1990) A genetic model for colorectal tumorigenesis. Cell 61: 759–767.
6. Smith G, Carey FA, Beattie J, Wilkie MJ, Lightfoot TJ, et al. (2002) Mutations in APC, Kirsten-ras, and p53–alternative genetic pathways to colorectal cancer. Proc Natl Acad Sci U S A 99: 9433–9438.
7. Pisani P, Parkin DM, Munoz N, Ferlay J (1997) Cancer and infection: estimates of the attributable fraction in 1990. Cancer Epidemiol Biomarkers Prev 6: 387–400.
8. Elwood PC, Gallagher AM, Duthie GG, Mur LA, Morgan G (2009) Aspirin, salicylates, and cancer. Lancet 373: 1301–1309.
9. Flossmann E, Rothwell PM (2007) Effect of aspirin on long-term risk of colorectal cancer: consistent evidence from randomised and observational studies. Lancet 369: 1603–1613.

10. Rothwell PM, Wilson M, Elwin CE, Norrving B, Algra A, et al. (2010) Long-term effect of aspirin on colorectal cancer incidence and mortality: 20-year follow-up of five randomised trials. Lancet 376: 1741–1750.
11. Rothwell PM, Price JF, Fowkes FG, Zanchetti A, Roncaglioni MC, et al. (2012) Short-term effects of daily aspirin on cancer incidence, mortality, and non-vascular death: analysis of the time course of risks and benefits in 51 randomised controlled trials. Lancet 379: 1602–1612.
12. Rothwell PM, Fowkes FG, Belch JF, Ogawa H, Warlow CP, et al. (2011) Effect of daily aspirin on long-term risk of death due to cancer: analysis of individual patient data from randomised trials. Lancet 377: 31–41.
13. Chan AT, Ogino S, Fuchs CS (2009) Aspirin use and survival after diagnosis of colorectal cancer. JAMA 302: 649–658.
14. Holmes MD, Chen WY, Li L, Hertzmark E, Spiegelman D, et al. (2010) Aspirin intake and survival after breast cancer. J Clin Oncol 28: 1467–1472.
15. Leitzmann MF, Stampfer MJ, Ma J, Chan JM, Colditz GA, et al. (2002) Aspirin use in relation to risk of prostate cancer. Cancer Epidemiol Biomarkers Prev 11: 1108–1111.
16. Chan AT, Ogino S, Fuchs CS (2007) Aspirin and the risk of colorectal cancer in relation to the expression of COX-2. N Engl J Med 356: 2131–2142.
17. Singer, II, Kawka DW, Schloemann S, Tessner T, Riehl T, et al. (1998) Cyclooxygenase 2 is induced in colonic epithelial cells in inflammatory bowel disease. Gastroenterology 115: 297–306.
18. Greenhough A, Smartt HJ, Moore AE, Roberts HR, Williams AC, et al. (2009) The COX-2/PGE2 pathway: key roles in the hallmarks of cancer and adaptation to the tumour microenvironment. Carcinogenesis 30: 377–386.
19. Sonkoly E, Stahle M, Pivarcsi A (2008) MicroRNAs: novel regulators in skin inflammation. Clin Exp Dermatol 33: 312–315.
20. Wu F, Zikusoka M, Trindade A, Dassopoulos T, Harris ML, et al. (2008) MicroRNAs are differentially expressed in ulcerative colitis and alter expression of macrophage inflammatory peptide-2 alpha. Gastroenterology 135: 1624-1635 e1624.
21. Schetter AJ, Heegaard NH, Harris CC (2010) Inflammation and cancer: interweaving microRNA, free radical, cytokine and p53 pathways. Carcinogenesis 31: 37–49.
22. Lin CJ, Gong HY, Tseng HC, Wang WL, Wu JL (2008) miR-122 targets an anti-apoptotic gene, Bcl-w, in human hepatocellular carcinoma cell lines. Biochem Biophys Res Commun 375: 315–320.
23. Lu TX, Munitz A, Rothenberg ME (2009) MicroRNA-21 is up-regulated in allergic airway inflammation and regulates IL-12p35 expression. J Immunol 182: 4994–5002.
24. Zhang Z, Li Z, Gao C, Chen P, Chen J, et al. (2008) miR-21 plays a pivotal role in gastric cancer pathogenesis and progression. Lab Invest 88: 1358–1366.
25. Medina PP, Nolde M, Slack FJ (2010) OncomiR addiction in an in vivo model of microRNA-21-induced pre-B-cell lymphoma. Nature 467: 86–90.
26. Volinia S, Calin GA, Liu CG, Ambs S, Cimmino A, et al. (2006) A microRNA expression signature of human solid tumors defines cancer gene targets. Proc Natl Acad Sci U S A 103: 2257–2261.
27. Asangani IA, Rasheed SA, Nikolova DA, Leupold JH, Colburn NH, et al. (2008) MicroRNA-21 (miR-21) post-transcriptionally downregulates tumor suppressor Pdcd4 and stimulates invasion, intravasation and metastasis in colorectal cancer. Oncogene 27: 2128–2136.
28. Ludwig K, Fassan M, Mescoli C, Pizzi M, Balistreri M, et al. (2013) PDCD4/miR-21 dysregulation in inflammatory bowel disease-associated carcinogenesis. Virchows Arch 462: 57–63.
29. Pfaffl MW (2001) A new mathematical model for relative quantification in real-time RT-PCR. Nucleic Acids Res 29: e45.
30. Bustin SA, Benes V, Garson JA, Hellemans J, Huggett J, et al. (2009) The MIQE guidelines: minimum information for publication of quantitative real-time PCR experiments. Clin Chem 55: 611–622.
31. Bhatti I, Lee A, James V, Hall RI, Lund JN, et al. (2011) Knockdown of microRNA-21 inhibits proliferation and increases cell death by targeting programmed cell death 4 (PDCD4) in pancreatic ductal adenocarcinoma. J Gastrointest Surg 15: 199–208.
32. The Royal College of Pathologists U (2007) Dataset for colorectal cancer (2nd edition).
33. Chang KH, Miller N, Kheirelseid EA, Ingoldsby H, Hennessy E, et al. (2011) MicroRNA-21 and PDCD4 expression in colorectal cancer. Eur J Surg Oncol.
34. Schetter AJ, Leung SY, Sohn JJ, Zanetti KA, Bowman ED, et al. (2008) MicroRNA expression profiles associated with prognosis and therapeutic outcome in colon adenocarcinoma. JAMA 299: 425–436.
35. Slaby O, Svoboda M, Fabian P, Smerdova T, Knoflickova D, et al. (2007) Altered expression of miR-21, miR-31, miR-143 and miR-145 is related to clinicopathologic features of colorectal cancer. Oncology 72: 397–402.
36. Schmid T, Bajer MM, Blees JS, Eifler LK, Milke L, et al. (2011) Inflammation-induced loss of Pdcd4 is mediated by phosphorylation-dependent degradation. Carcinogenesis 32: 1427–1433.
37. Kirkland SC (1985) Dome formation by a human colonic adenocarcinoma cell line (HCA-7). Cancer Res 45: 3790–3795.
38. O'Callaghan G, Kelly J, Shanahan F, Houston A (2008) Prostaglandin E2 stimulates Fas ligand expression via the EP1 receptor in colon cancer cells. Br J Cancer 99: 502–512.
39. Zhang Z, DuBois RN (2001) Detection of differentially expressed genes in human colon carcinoma cells treated with a selective COX-2 inhibitor. Oncogene 20: 4450–4456.
40. Wang P, Zou F, Zhang X, Li H, Dulak A, et al. (2009) microRNA-21 negatively regulates Cdc25A and cell cycle progression in colon cancer cells. Cancer Res 69: 8157–8165.
41. Foreman JE, Sorg JM, McGinnis KS, Rigas B, Williams JL, et al. (2009) Regulation of peroxisome proliferator-activated receptor-beta/delta by the APC/beta-CATENIN pathway and nonsteroidal antiinflammatory drugs. Mol Carcinog 48: 942–952.
42. Kutchera W, Jones DA, Matsunami N, Groden J, McIntyre TM, et al. (1996) Prostaglandin H synthase 2 is expressed abnormally in human colon cancer: evidence for a transcriptional effect. Proc Natl Acad Sci U S A 93: 4816–4820.
43. Cmarik JL, Min H, Hegamyer G, Zhan S, Kulesz-Martin M, et al. (1999) Differentially expressed protein Pdcd4 inhibits tumor promoter-induced neoplastic transformation. Proc Natl Acad Sci U S A 96: 14037–14042.
44. Shin VY, Jin H, Ng EK, Cheng AS, Chong WW, et al. (2011) NF-{kappa}B targets miR-16 and miR-21 in gastric cancer: involvement of prostaglandin E receptors. Carcinogenesis 32: 240–245.
45. Li M, Wu X, Xu XC (2001) Induction of apoptosis in colon cancer cells by cyclooxygenase-2 inhibitor NS398 through a cytochrome c-dependent pathway. Clin Cancer Res 7: 1010–1016.
46. Abdelrahim M, Safe S (2005) Cyclooxygenase-2 inhibitors decrease vascular endothelial growth factor expression in colon cancer cells by enhanced degradation of Sp1 and Sp4 proteins. Mol Pharmacol 68: 317–329.
47. Yao M, Lam EC, Kelly CR, Zhou W, Wolfe MM (2004) Cyclooxygenase-2 selective inhibition with NS-398 suppresses proliferation and invasiveness and delays liver metastasis in colorectal cancer. Br J Cancer 90: 712–719.
48. Nagatsuka I, Yamada N, Shimizu S, Ohira M, Nishino H, et al. (2002) Inhibitory effect of a selective cyclooxygenase-2 inhibitor on liver metastasis of colon cancer. Int J Cancer 100: 515–519.
49. Sheng H, Shao J, Kirkland SC, Isakson P, Coffey RJ, et al. (1997) Inhibition of human colon cancer cell growth by selective inhibition of cyclooxygenase-2. J Clin Invest 99: 2254–2259.
50. Leahy KM, Ornberg RL, Wang Y, Zweifel BS, Koki AT, et al. (2002) Cyclooxygenase-2 inhibition by celecoxib reduces proliferation and induces apoptosis in angiogenic endothelial cells in vivo. Cancer Res 62: 625–631.
51. Masferrer JL, Leahy KM, Koki AT, Zweifel BS, Settle SL, et al. (2000) Antiangiogenic and antitumor activities of cyclooxygenase-2 inhibitors. Cancer Res 60: 1306–1311.
52. Lu L, Byrnes K, Han C, Wang Y, Wu T (2014) MiR-21 Targets 15-PGDH and Promotes Cholangiocarcinoma Growth. Mol Cancer Res.

Permissions

All chapters in this book were first published in PLOS ONE, by The Public Library of Science; hereby published with permission under the Creative Commons Attribution License or equivalent. Every chapter published in this book has been scrutinized by our experts. Their significance has been extensively debated. The topics covered herein carry significant findings which will fuel the growth of the discipline. They may even be implemented as practical applications or may be referred to as a beginning point for another development.

The contributors of this book come from diverse backgrounds, making this book a truly international effort. This book will bring forth new frontiers with its revolutionizing research information and detailed analysis of the nascent developments around the world.

We would like to thank all the contributing authors for lending their expertise to make the book truly unique. They have played a crucial role in the development of this book. Without their invaluable contributions this book wouldn't have been possible. They have made vital efforts to compile up to date information on the varied aspects of this subject to make this book a valuable addition to the collection of many professionals and students.

This book was conceptualized with the vision of imparting up-to-date information and advanced data in this field. To ensure the same, a matchless editorial board was set up. Every individual on the board went through rigorous rounds of assessment to prove their worth. After which they invested a large part of their time researching and compiling the most relevant data for our readers.

The editorial board has been involved in producing this book since its inception. They have spent rigorous hours researching and exploring the diverse topics which have resulted in the successful publishing of this book. They have passed on their knowledge of decades through this book. To expedite this challenging task, the publisher supported the team at every step. A small team of assistant editors was also appointed to further simplify the editing procedure and attain best results for the readers.

Apart from the editorial board, the designing team has also invested a significant amount of their time in understanding the subject and creating the most relevant covers. They scrutinized every image to scout for the most suitable representation of the subject and create an appropriate cover for the book.

The publishing team has been an ardent support to the editorial, designing and production team. Their endless efforts to recruit the best for this project, has resulted in the accomplishment of this book. They are a veteran in the field of academics and their pool of knowledge is as vast as their experience in printing. Their expertise and guidance has proved useful at every step. Their uncompromising quality standards have made this book an exceptional effort. Their encouragement from time to time has been an inspiration for everyone.

The publisher and the editorial board hope that this book will prove to be a valuable piece of knowledge for researchers, students, practitioners and scholars across the globe.

List of Contributors

Jutta Schröder-Braunstein, Judith Gras, Sonja Schwarz, Guido Wabnitz, Antje Heidtmann, Yvonne Samstag, Thomas Giese and Stefan Meuer
Institute of Immunology, University Hospital Heidelberg, Heidelberg, Germany

Benedikt Brors
Division of Theoretical Bioinformatics, German Cancer Research Center (DKFZ), Heidelberg, Germany

Felix Lasitschka
Institute of Pathology, University Hospital Heidelberg, Heidelberg, Germany

Serin Schiessling
Institute of Immunology, University Hospital Heidelberg, Heidelberg, Germany
Department of Surgery, University Hospital Heidelberg, Heidelberg, Germany

Christine Leowardi, Mohammed Al-Saeedi and Alexis Ulrich
Department of Surgery, University Hospital Heidelberg, Heidelberg, Germany

Timea Szikszai
Institute of Immunology, University Hospital Heidelberg, Heidelberg, Germany
Department of Anesthesiology, University Hospital Heidelberg, Heidelberg, Germany

Antonia Engelke
Department of Surgery, Salem Hospital, Heidelberg, Germany

Johannes Winter
Department of Surgery, St. Vincentius Hospital, Speyer, Germany

Young-Seon Lee
Institute of Immunology, University Hospital Heidelberg, Heidelberg, Germany
Department of Gastroenterology, Hepatology, and Endocrinology, Hannover Medical School,Hannover, Germany

Yosuke Nishitani
Team of Health Bioscience, Organization of Advanced Science and Technology, Kobe University, Kobe, Japan

Ling Zhang, Kazuki Kanazawa, Takashi Hashimoto and Masashi Mizuno
Department of Agrobioscience, Graduate School of Agricultural Science, Kobe University, Kobe, Japan

Takeshi Azuma
Gastroenterology Division, Department of Internal Medicine, Graduate School of Medicine, Kobe University, Kobe, Japan

Masaru Yoshida
Gastroenterology Division, Department of Internal Medicine, Graduate School of Medicine, Kobe University, Kobe, Japan
The Integrated Center for Mass Spectrometry, Graduate School of Medicine, Kobe University, Kobe, Japan

Jutta M. Nagel, Brenda M. Geiger, Apostolos K. A. Karagiannis, Beatriz Gras-Miralles, David Horst, Robert M. Najarian, Dimitrios C. Ziogas, XinHua Chen and Efi Kokkotou
Division of Gastroenterology, Beth Israel Deaconess Medical Center, Harvard Medical School, Boston, Massachusetts, United States of America

Patricia M. Cano, Julie Seeboth, Isabelle P. Oswald and Laurence Guzylack-Piriou
INRA, UMR1331, Toxalim, Research Centre in Food Toxicology, Toulouse, France
Universitéde Toulouse, INPT, UMR1331, Toxalim, Toulouse, France

François Meurens
INRA, UMR1282 Infectiologie et Santé Publique, Nouzilly, France
Vaccine and Infectious Disease Organization, University of Saskatchewan, Saskatoon, Saskatchewan, Canada

Juliette Cognie
INRA, Physiologie de la Reproduction et des Comportements, Nouzilly, France

Roberta Abrami
INRA, UMR1331, Toxalim, Research Centre in Food Toxicology, Toulouse, France
Universitéde Toulouse, INPT, UMR1331, Toxalim, Toulouse, France
Universidade Estadual de Londrina, Lab Patologia Animal, Londrina, Brazil

Ute Hoffmann, Matthias Pink, Uta Lauer, Caroline Winsauer, Andrei Kruglov, Kerstin Schlawe, Claudia Leichsenring and Alf Hamann
Deutsches Rheumaforschungszentrum, Berlin, Germany

Markus M. Heimesaat and Oliver Liesenfeld
Institut für Mikrobiologie und Hygiene, Campus Benjamin Franklin, Universitätsmedizin Charité, Berlin, Germany

Uta Syrbe
Deutsches Rheumaforschungszentrum, Berlin, Germany
Klinik für Gastroenterologie, Infektiologie und Rheumatologie, Campus Benjamin Franklin, Universitätsmedizin Charité , Berlin, Germany

David Q. Shih, Robert Barrett, Nicole Yeager, Piangwarin Phaosawasdi, Brian Ko, Michelle H. Wong, Kathrin S. Michelsen, Gislaine Martins and Stephan R. Targan
Inflammatory Bowel and Immunobiology Research Institute, Cedars-Sinai Medical Center, Los Angeles, California, United States of America

Xiaolan Zhang
Inflammatory Bowel and Immunobiology Research Institute, Cedars-Sinai Medical Center, Los Angeles, California, United States of America
Department of Gastroenterology, The Second Hospital of Hebei Medical University, Shijianzuang, China

Hon Wai Koon, Yahui Song and Charalabos Pothoulakis
Division of Digestive Diseases, Inflammatory Bowel Disease Center, David Geffen School of Medicine, University of California Los Angeles, Los Angeles, California, United States of America

Emeran A. Mayer
Gail and Gerald Oppenheimer Family Center for Neurobiology of Stress, University of California Los Angeles, Los Angeles, California, United States of America
Pain and Interoception Imaging Network (PAIN), University of California Los Angeles, Los Angeles, California, United States of America
Department of Medicine, University of California Los Angeles, Los Angeles, California, United States of America
Department of Psychiatry, University of California Los Angeles, Los Angeles, California, United States of America
Brain Research Institute, University of California Los Angeles, Los Angeles, California, United States of America
Division of Digestive Diseases, University of California Los Angeles, Los Angeles, California, United States of America
Ahmanson Lovelace Brain Mapping Center, David Geffen School of Medicine, University of California, Los Angeles, California

Kirsten Tillisch Arpana Gupta and Cody Ashe-Mcnalley
Gail and Gerald Oppenheimer Family Center for Neurobiology of Stress, University of California Los Angeles, Los Angeles, California, United States of America
Pain and Interoception Imaging Network (PAIN), University of California Los Angeles, Los Angeles, California, United States of America
Department of Medicine, University of California Los Angeles, Los Angeles, California, United States of America

Suzanne R. Smith, Jean Stains and Nuwanthi Heendeniya
Gail and Gerald Oppenheimer Family Center for Neurobiology of Stress, University of California Los Angeles, Los Angeles, California, United States of America
Department of Medicine, University of California Los Angeles, Los Angeles, California, United States of America

Jui-Yang Hong
Gail and Gerald Oppenheimer Family Center for Neurobiology of Stress, University of California Los Angeles, Los Angeles, California, United States of America
Department of Medicine, University of California Los Angeles, Los Angeles, California, United States of America
Division of Digestive Diseases, University of California Los Angeles, Los Angeles, California, United States of America
Department of Bioengineering, University of California Los Angeles, Los Angeles, California, United States of America

Ivo Dinov
University of Michigan School of Nursing, Ann Arbor, Michigan, United States of America

Zhiguo Jiang
Department of Biomedical Engineering, New Jersey Institute of Technology, Newark, New Jersey, United States of America
Human Performance and Engineering Laboratory, Kessler Foundation Research Center, West Orange, New Jersey, United States of America

Yonggang Shi
Laboratory of Neuro-Imaging, University of Southern California, Los Angeles, California United States of America

Jeremy S. Schaefer, Dina Montufar-Solis, Niyati Nakra, Nadarajah Vigneswaran and John R. Klein
Department of Diagnostic and Biomedical Sciences, University of Texas Health Science Center School of Dentistry, Houston, Texas, United States of America

Shinta Mizuno, Nobuhiro Nakamoto, Tomohisa Sujino, Toshiro Sato, Katsuyoshi Matsuoka, Tadakazu Hisamatsu, Hirotoshi Ebinuma, Toshifumi Hibi and Takanori Kanai
Division of Gastroenterology and Hepatology, Department of Internal Medicine, Keio University School of Medicine, Tokyo, Japan

Yohei Mikami
Division of Gastroenterology and Hepatology, Department of Internal Medicine, Keio University School of Medicine, Tokyo, Japan
Department of Microbiology and Immunology, Keio University School of Medicine, Tokyo, Japan

Akihiko Yoshimura
Department of Microbiology and Immunology, Keio University School of Medicine, Tokyo, Japan

Atsushi Hayashi
Division of Gastroenterology and Hepatology, Department of Internal Medicine, Keio University School of Medicine, Tokyo, Japan
Research Laboratory, Miyarisan Pharmaceutical, Tokyo, Japan

Nobuhiko Kamada
Department of Pathology and Comprehensive Cancer Center, University of Michigan Medical School, Ann Arbor, Michigan, United States of America

Tonny Lagerweij and Lex Nagelkerken
Department of Metabolic Health Research, TNO, Leiden, The Netherlands

Rob Mariman
Department of Metabolic Health Research, TNO, Leiden, The Netherlands
Department of Immunohematology and Bloodtransfusion, Leiden University Medical Centrum, Leiden,The Netherlands

Bas Kremer
Department of Metabolic Health Research, TNO, Leiden, The Netherlands
Department of Microbiology and Systems Biology, TNO, Zeist, The Netherlands

Marjan van Erk
Department of Microbiology and Systems Biology, TNO, Zeist, The Netherlands

Stefan Bereswill, Melba Muñoz, André Fischer, Rita Plickert, Lea-Maxie Haag, Bettina Otto, Ulf B. Göbel and Markus M. Heimesaat
Institut für Mikrobiologie und Hygiene, Charité – Universitätsmedizin Berlin, Berlin, Germany

Anja A. Kühl and Christoph Loddenkemper
Institut für Pathologie, Charité- Universitätsmedizin Berlin, Berlin, Germany

Elisabetta Cavalcanti and Francesco Addabbo
Laboratory of Experimental Immunopathology, IRCCS "de Bellis," Castellana Grotte (BA), Italy

Elisa Vadrucci
Laboratory of Experimental Immunopathology, IRCCS "de Bellis," Castellana Grotte (BA), Italy
Laboratory of Mucosal Immunology, Mario Negri South, Santa Maria Imbaro (CH), Italy

Francesca Romana Delvecchio
Laboratory of Mucosal Immunology, Mario Negri South, Santa Maria Imbaro (CH), Italy
Laboratory of Translational Medicine, ARCHES, Castellana Grotte (BA), Italy,

Marcello Chieppa
Laboratory of Experimental Immunopathology, IRCCS "de Bellis," Castellana Grotte (BA), Italy
Laboratory of Mucosal Immunology, Mario Negri South, Santa Maria Imbaro (CH), Italy
Laboratory of Translational Medicine, ARCHES, Castellana Grotte (BA), Italy

Simona Bettini
Department of Engineering for Innovation, University of Salento, Lecce, Italy

Rachel Liou and Alex Yee-Chen Huang
Department of Pediatrics, Case Western Reserve University School of Medicine, Cleveland, Ohio, United States of America

Vladia Monsurrò
Department of Pathology and Diagnostic, University of Verona Medical School, Verona, Italy

Theresa Torres Pizarro
Department of Pathology, Case Western Reserve University School of Medicine, Cleveland, Ohio, United States of America

Angelo Santino
Institute of Science of Food Production, CNR, Lecce, Italy

Fu-Min Xue, Hui-Jie Hao, Zhao-Yang Shi, Chuan Zhou and Baisui Feng
Department of Gastroenterology, The First Affiliated Hospital of Zhengzhou University, Zhengzhou, China

Huan-Ping Zhang and Ping-Chang Yang
Department of Pathology & Molecular Medicine, McMaster University, Hamilton, Ontario, Canada

Efrat Harel, Abraham Rubinstein, Elena Khazanov, Mirela Nadler Milbauer and Boaz Tirosh
Institute for Drug Research, The Hebrew University of Jerusalem, Jerusalem, Israel

Aviram Nissan
Department of Surgery, Hadassah Hebrew University Medical Center, Mount Scopus, Jerusalem, Israel

Yechezkel Barenholz
The Laboratory of Membrane and Liposome Research, The Hebrew University of Jerusalem, Jerusalem, Israel

Elisabeth Wende, Robert Laudeley and Andreas Klos
Institute for Medical Microbiology and Hospital Epidemiology, Hannover Medical School, Hannover, Germany

André Bleich, Eva Bleich and Silke Glage
Institute for Laboratory Animal Science, Hannover Medical School, Hannover, Germany

Rick A. Wetsel
Brown Foundation Institute of Molecular Medicine, University of Texas, Health Science Center, Houston, Texas, United States of America

Henrike Lenzen, Maria Lünnemann, Michael P Manns and Ursula Seidler
Department of Gastroenterology, Hepatology and Endocrinology, Hannover Medical School, Hannover, Germany

Andre Bleich
Institute of Laboratory Animal Science, Hannover Medical School, Hannover, Germany

Anne Jörns
Institute of Clinical Biochemistry, Hannover Medical School, Hannover, Germany
Center of Anatomy, Hannover Medical School, Hannover, Germany

Xingwei Jiang, Tingting Zhou, Renxi Wang, Zhi Zhao,He Xiao, Chunmei Hou, Yanhua Lin, Xiaoling Lang, Jiannan Feng, Guojiang Chen, Beifen Shen, Gencheng Han and Yan Li
Department of Molecular Immunology, Beijing Institute of Basic Medical Sciences, Beijing, China

Xiaoqin Guo
Department of Molecular Immunology, Beijing Institute of Basic Medical Sciences, Beijing, China
Department of Immunology, Logistics College of Chinese People's Armed Police Forces, Tianjin, China

Yan Xiao and Lingyun Ma
Department of Respiratory Medicine, First Affiliated Hospital of the Chinese PLA General Hospital, Beijing, China

Yueling Guo
Department of Medical Engineering, Military General Hospital of Beijing PLA, Beijing, China

Karin Strijbis, Ömer H. Yilmaz, Stephanie K. Dougan, Alexandre Esteban and Hidde L. Ploegh
Whitehead Institute for Biomedical Research, Cambridge, Massachusetts, United States of America

Andrea Gröne
Department of Pathobiology, Faculty of Veterinary Medicine, Utrecht University, Utrecht, The Netherlands

Carol A. Kumamoto
Department of Molecular Biology and Microbiology, School of Medicine, Tufts University, Boston, Massachusetts, United States of America

Oliver Peacock, Andrew C. Lee, Fraser Cameron, Rebecca Tarbox, Natasha Vafadar-Isfahani, Cristina Tufarelli and Jonathan N. Lund
Surgery Group, Division of Medical Sciences and Graduate Entry Medicine, School of Medicine, University of Nottingham, Royal Derby Hospital, Derby, United Kingdom

Index

www.ingramcontent.com/pod-product-compliance
Lightning Source LLC
LaVergne TN
LVHW060604210926
848485LV00005B/1367